THE TEXTBOOK OF
Spinal Surgery

EDITORS IN CHIEF
Keith H. Bridwell, M.D.
Ronald L. DeWald, M.D.

ASSOCIATE EDITORS
John P. Lubicky, M.D.

David L. Spencer, M.D.

Kim W. Hammerberg, M.D.

Daniel R. Benson, M.D.

Michael G. Neuwirth, M.D.

ADMINISTRATIVE ASSISTANT TO
DR. BRIDWELL

Theresa M. Iffrig

60 CONTRIBUTORS

THE TEXTBOOK OF
Spinal Surgery
Volume One

J. B. LIPPINCOTT COMPANY
PHILADELPHIA   *New York   London   Hagerstown*

Acquisitions Editor: Darlene Barela Cooke
Developmental Editor: Delois Patterson
Project Editor: Tom Gibbons
Indexer: Katherine Pitcoff
Designer: Holly Reid McLaughlin
Design Coordinator: Doug Smock
Production Manager: Helen Ewan
Production Coordinator: Antoinette Bauer
Compositor: Circle Graphics
Printer/Binder: Arcata Graphics/Halliday

Library of Congress Cataloging-in-Publication Data
The textbook of spinal surgery/editors in chief, Keith H.
Bridwell, Ronald L. DeWald; associate editors, John P.
Lubicky . . . [et al.]; 60 contributors
     p.   cm.
Includes bibliographical references and index.
ISBN 0-397-51098-5 (set).—ISBN 0-397-51236-8 (v. 1).
—ISBN 0-397-51237-6 (v. 2)
    1. Spine—Surgery. 2. Spine—Diseases. I. Brid-
well, Keith H. II. DeWald, Ronald L., 1934–
    [DNLM: 1. Spinal Diseases—surgery. 2. Spine—
surgery. WE 725
T355]
RD533.T46   1991
617.3′75059—dc20
DNLM/DLC
for Library of Congress   91–6883
                                    CIP

6   5   4   3   2   1

The authors and publisher have exerted every effort to ensure that drug selection and dosage set forth in this text are in
accord with current recommendations and practice at the
time of publication. However, in view of ongoing research,
changes in government regulations, and the constant flow of
information relating to drug therapy and drug reactions, the
reader is urged to check the package insert for each drug for
any change in indications and dosage and for added warnings
and precautions. This is particularly important when the
recommended agent is a new or infrequently employed
drug.

To the patients who will benefit from our evolving understanding of surgical indications, techniques, and complications

Contributors

Max Aebi, MD
Associate Professor, Department of Orthopaedic Surgery,
University of Berne, Inselspital, Berne, Switzerland

Brent T. Allen, MD
Assistant Professor, General and Vascular Surgery,
Washington University School of Medicine; Attending
Surgeon, Barnes Hospital, St. Louis, Missouri

Paul L. Asdourian, MD
Chief, Section of Orthopaedic Spinal Surgery; Medical
Director, William H.M. Finney Spine Center; Clinical
Instructor in Orthopaedic Surgery, Johns Hopkins
University School of Medicine, Baltimore, Maryland

Richard B. Ashman, PhD
Director of Research, Texas Scottish Rite Hospital; Assistant
Professor of Orthopaedics, Orthopedic Surgery, University
of Texas Southwestern Medical School, Dallas, Texas

Daniel R. Benson, MD
Professor of Orthopaedic Surgery, Chief of Spine Surgery,
University of California, Davis, Sacramento, California

Heinrich Boehm, MD
Orthopaedic Surgeon, Oberarzt Department
Orthopaedics–Traumatology I, Rehabilitationskrankenhaus,
Karlsbad–Langensteinbach, Germany

Keith H. Bridwell, MD
Associate Professor of Orthopaedic Surgery, Washington
University School of Medicine; Director of Orthopedic
Spinal Surgery, Childrens, Barnes, and Shriners Hospitals,
St. Louis, Missouri

Courtney W. Brown, MD
Assistant Clinical Professor, Department of Orthopaedics,
University of Colorado, Denver, Colorado

Daniel Chopin, MD
Director of Spine Center, Institut Calot, Berck Plage,
France

Jozef Colemont, MD
Gemeinschaftspraxis, City Point, Orthopaedic,
Arthroscopic, General, and Cosmetic Surgery, Bochum,
Germany

Ronald L. DeWald, MD
Professor of Orthopaedic Surgery, Rush Medical College;
Director, Section of Spinal Surgery, Rush-Presbyterian–St.
Luke's Medical Center, Chicago, Illinois

David H. Donaldson, MD
Clinical Assistant Professor, University of Colorado; Spine
Consultant, Craig Rehab Hospital; Staff Physician,
St. Anthony Hospital; Physician, Children's Hospital,
Lakewood, Colorado

Jean Dubousset, MD
Hopital Saint-Vincent dePaul, Paris, France

Charles C. Edwards, MD
Professor of Orthopedic Surgery, University of Maryland, Baltimore, Maryland

Jean-Pierre C. Farcy, MD
Associate Clinical Professor of Orthopaedics, Columbia University College of Physicians and Surgeons; Associate Attending Orthopaedic Surgeon, Columbia–Presbyterian Medical Center, New York, New York

William Tallman Felmly, MD
Chief Resident and Assistant Instructor, Department of Orthopaedics, State University of New York, Health Science Center at Brooklyn, Brooklyn, New York

Lee T. Ford, MD
Professor Emeritus, Division of Orthopaedic Surgery, Washington University School of Medicine, St. Louis, Missouri

Robert W. Gaines, Jr., MD, FACS
Professor of Orthopaedic Surgery, University of Missouri School of Medicine, Columbia, Missouri

Johannes P. Giehl, MD
Orthopaedic Surgeon, Chief of Spine Surgery, Orthopaedic Department, University of Tubingen, Tubingen, Germany

Thomas R. Haher, MD
Associate Professor, Orthopaedic Surgery, State University of New York, Health Science Center at Brooklyn; Adjunct Professor of Civil Engineering, The Cooper Union School of Engineering, New York, New York

Kim W. Hammerberg, MD
Assistant Professor of Orthopaedic Surgery, Department of Orthopaedic Surgery, Rush Medical College; Attending Staff, Rush-Presbyterian–St. Luke's Medical Center; Attending Staff, Shriners Hospital for Crippled Children, Chicago, Illinois

Jurgen Harms, MD
Orthopaedic Surgeon, Medical Director, Department Orthopaedics–Traumatology I, Rehabilitationskrankenhaus, Karlsbad–Langensteinbach, Germany

Hans-Joachim Hehne, MD
Professor of Orthopaedics, Department of Surgery, Section of Orthopaedics, University of Freiburg, Freiburg, Germany

John A. Herring, MD
Chief of Staff, Texas Scottish Rite Hospital for Crippled Children; Professor of Orthopedic Surgery, University of Texas Southwestern Medical Center, Dallas, Texas

Charles E. Johnston II, MD
Staff Orthopedist, Texas Scottish Rite Hospital; Assistant Professor, Orthopedic Surgery, University of Texas Southwestern Medical School, Dallas, Texas

Kiyoshi Kaneda, MD, PhD
Professor and Chairman, Department of Orthopedic Surgery, Hokkaido University School of Medicine, Sapporo, Japan

Bruce A. Kaufman, MD
Department of Pediatric Neurosurgery, St. Louis Children's Hospital; Assistant Professor, Department of Neurosurgery, Washington University School of Medicine, St. Louis, Missouri

Shinya Kawai, MD
Chairman, Department of Orthopaedic Surgery, University of Yamaguchi School of Medicine, Yamaguchi Prefecture, Japan

John P. Kostuik, MD, FRCSC
Professor of Orthopaedics, University of Toronto; Director, Spinal Unit, Toronto Hospital; Director, Biomechanics Laboratory, Toronto Hospital, Toronto, Ontario, Canada

Keith R. Kuhlengel, MD
Assistant Professor of Neurosurgery and of Anatomy/Neuroscience, Milton S. Hershey Medical Center, The Pennsylvania State University, Hershey, Pennsylvania

Henry La Rocca, MD
Clinical Professor of Orthopaedic Surgery, Tulane University School of Medicine, New Orleans, Louisiana; Editor-in-Chief, *Spine*

John P. Lubicky, MD
Chief of Staff, Shriners Hospital for Crippled Children, Chicago Unit; Associate Professor of Orthopaedic Surgery, Rush Medical Center; Lecturer in Orthopaedic Surgery, Loyola University, Strich School of Medicine, Chicago, Illinois

Richard W. Maack, MD
Graduate Fellow with the American Academy of Facial, Plastic, and Reconstructive Surgery, American Academy of Otolaryngology–Head and Neck Surgery, Cincinnati, Ohio

Christian Mazel, MD
Chef de Clinique, Faculté de Medicine, Pitié-Saltpetriere, Paris, France

Daniel J. McGuire, MD
Orthopaedic Spine Surgeon, Des Moines Orthopaedic Surgeons, Des Moines, Iowa

Paul R. Meyer, Jr., MD
Professor of Orthopaedic Surgery, Northwestern University Medical School; Director, Spine Injury Center, Northwestern University, Chicago, Illinois

H. Dennis Mollman, MD, PhD
Shriner's Hospital–St. Louis; St. Luke's Hospital; Missouri Baptist Hospital; Chesterfield, Missouri

Michael R. Moore, MD
Colorado Spine Center, P.C., Aurora, Colorado

Christian Morin, MD
Head of Pediatric Orthopaedics Department, Institut Calot, Berck-sur-Mer, France

Ronald Moskovich, MD, MA, FRCS
Assistant Professor of Orthopaedic Surgery, New York University; Chief, Cervical Spine Surgery, Hospital for Joint Diseases Orthopaedic Institute, New York, New York

Michael G. Neuwirth, MD
Chief, Spine Services, Hospital for Joint Diseases Orthopedic Institute; Assistant Clinical Professor of Orthopedics, Mt. Sinai Medical School, New York, New York

W. Kirt Nichols, MD
Professor of Surgery, University of Missouri, Columbia, Missouri

Carl Helge Nielsen, MD
Assistant Professor of Anesthesiology, Washington University School of Medicine, Barnes Hospital, St. Louis, Missouri

Michael O'Brien, MD
Chief Resident and Assistant Instructor, Department of Orthopaedics, State University of New York, Health Science Center at Brooklyn, Brooklyn, New York

James W. Ogilvie, MD
Associate Professor, Department of Orthopedic Surgery, University of Minnesota; Director, Twin Cities Scoliosis Center–Spine Center, Minneapolis, Minnesota

Jeffrey H. Owen, PhD
Division of Orthopedic Surgery, Department of Surgery, Washington University School of Medicine, St. Louis, Missouri

Tae Sung Park, MD
Department of Neurology and Neurological Surgery, Washington University School of Medicine, St. Louis, Missouri

Mary Faut Rodts, RN, MS, ONC
Assistant Professor, Rush College of Nursing, Rush University, Chicago, Illinois

Raymond Roy-Camille, MD
Professeur de Chirurgie Orthopedique et Traumatologique a la Faculté, Pitié–Salpetriere a Paris; Chef du Service de Chirurgie Orthopedique, l'Hopital de la Pitie, Paris, France

Perry L. Schoenecker, MD
Associate Professor of Orthopedic Surgery, Washington University School of Medicine; Chief of Staff, St. Louis Shriners Hospital for Crippled Children, St. Louis, Missouri

James E. Shook, MD
Assistant Professor of Orthopedic Surgery and Pediatrics, Loma Linda University Medical Center, Loma Linda, California

J. Gershon Spector, MD
Professor of Otolaryngology–Head and Neck Surgery,
Washington University School of Medicine, St. Louis,
Missouri

David L. Spencer, MD
Associate Professor of Orthopaedic Surgery, University of
Illinois at Chicago; Attending Orthopaedic Surgeon,
Lutheran General Hospital, Park Ridge, Illinois

Dieter Stoltze, MD
Head Senior Surgeon, Rehabilitationskrankenhaus,
Karlsbad–Langensteinbach, Germany

Rudolph F. Taddonio, MD
Acting Vice Chairman, Department of Orthopaedic
Surgery; Clinical Associate Professor of Orthopaedic
Surgery; Director, Section of Scoliosis Surgery;
Orthopaedic Director, Section of Spinal Surgery,
Westchester County Medical Center, New York Medical
College, Hawthorne, New York

Ensor E. Transfeldt, MD, BCh, FRCS
Department of Orthopaedic Surgery, University of
Minnesota Hospital; Twin Cities Scoliosis Spine Center;
Abbott Northwestern Hospital, Minneapolis, Minnesota

Dennis G. Vollmer, MD
Department of Neurological Surgery, Washington
University School of Medicine, Barnes Hospital; Jewish
Hospital of St. Louis, St. Louis Children's Hospital,
St. Louis, Missouri

Mark Weidenbaum, MD
Assistant Professor of Orthopaedic Surgery, College of
Physicians and Surgeons, Columbia University, New York,
New York

John R. Whiffen, MD
Clinical Assistant Professor of Orthopaedic Surgery,
University of Wisconsin Medical School; Madison
Orthopaedic Associates, Madison, Wisconsin

Klaus Zielke, MD
Orthopaedic Surgeon, Former Director of German Center
for Spinal Surgery and German Scoliosis Center (retired),
Bad Wildungen, Germany

Preface

— ■ ■ ■ —

Until this publication, no single text has addressed all aspects of the surgical treatment of the spine. By "all aspects," we mean the pediatric and the adult spine, deformity and degenerative spinal disease, and all segments of the spine from the occiput to the sacrum. Moreover, the treatment options in spinal disease have evolved very quickly. Many surgical procedures are dramatically different today from only five years ago. Accordingly, in this book we endeavor to provide a comprehensive, up-to-date analysis and description of the surgical treatment of spine disease.

In an effort to be comprehensive, this text addresses (1) the cervical, thoracic, and lumbar spine; (2) both degenerative disease and deformities of the spine; and (3) spinal disease in all age groups. Our analysis includes (1) indications for surgery; (2) preoperative radiographic, social, and clinical evaluations; (3) associated conditions and concerns; (4) surgical techniques;

and (5) postoperative rehabilitation and recovery. We also discuss controversies and complications in connection with each surgical technique. Although nonsurgical measures are mentioned, the emphasis is on those spinal problems that require surgical treatment.

Each chapter includes an extensive review of the literature and current techniques and philosophies. We are fortunate to have an outstanding group of spine specialists from North America, Europe, and Asia contributing to this text. These authors describe the treatment methods they prefer and why, attempt to put current controversies in perspective, and provide a detailed description of the surgical procedures.

This book is intended to be of value to medical students, orthopedic and neurosurgery residents, and practicing orthopedic surgeons and neurosurgeons. It should also be useful to those specializing in spinal surgery.

Acknowledgments

This textbook is the product of the dedicated efforts of a great number of persons, all of whom we sincerely thank. We especially wish to acknowledge the contributing authors, without whom a work of this magnitude clearly is not possible. We thank them for allocating some of their very scarce time to this project. Not only do we appreciate their participation but also their adherence as a group to the time parameters set for this publication. Much thanks also goes to both the staff and the families of the contributors for the additional services and support required of them as a result of this textbook. Our special thanks also are extended to the associate editors and their wives (Karen Benson, Lucy Hammerberg, Vicky Lubicky, Linda Neuwirth, and Katie Spencer), whose support and assistance were essential and very much appreciated.

We also would like to express our gratitude to the following people: Terri Iffrig, for her tireless good cheer and her excellent organizational and technical skills as Administrative Assistant for this text; Christy Baldus, for her continuous good humor, competence, and energy as the "spine nurse" at Washington University; and our wives (Mala Bridwell and Mary DeWald), for their patience, love, and support. We would also like to thank the Lippincott staff, in particular Darlene Cooke, for their professional guidance through the publication process and their general enthusiasm for and assistance on this project: the photographers and illustrators, in particular Vicki Friedman and Ed Linn at Washington University, for their contributions to this text; and LaVinia Crabb, for her usual calm transcription of versions of several chapters.

Last, but not least, Dr. Bridwell extends his special thanks to Dr. DeWald not only for his invaluable services as coeditor of this textbook but also for the high standards and goals he instilled in him and in many of the contributors during their spine training.

Keith H. Bridwell, M.D.
Ronald L. DeWald, M.D.

Introduction

In 1961, Dr. Paul Harrington came to Chicago at the request of Dr. Claude Lambert to demonstrate his technique of internal instrumentation of the spine. It was October, and I was in my second year of residency training at the University of Illinois.

I observed as Dr. Harrington operated a 13-year-old boy afflicted with poliomyelitis. The spinal deformity and pelvic obliquity were partially corrected and stabilized in 4½ hours. What previously had taken months of plaster casts, traction, staged operations, and severe morbidity for both patient and surgeon had been changed dramatically and forever. It was evident that I was witness to the birth of the modern age of spine surgery.

Change is slowly accepted in surgery. Why change a technique when the old method still works? Similarly, spinal instrumentation was slowly accepted by surgeons treating spinal deformity. With the founding of the Scoliosis Research Society in 1966, however, spinal surgery clearly had entered its formative years.

Spinal surgery is currently growing and evolving so quickly that before a surgeon can learn a new technique, it may be considered obsolete or ineffective. The principles of spinal surgery remain the same, although the "semantics" may change. Our understanding of the anatomy and biomechanics of spinal deformity continues to improve. Spinal surgeons are quickly adopting the vocabulary of the engineer. Stress, strain, and column dynamics are now part of our daily discussions. Fixation, strength, and rigid are key engineering words, and stress shielding is beginning to enter our thinking. Can fixation of the spine be too rigid? The biology of fusion healing is not passé nor should it be forgotten; however, at present biology seems to be upstaged by the shine of spinal instrumentation.

The importance of sagittal plane balance, formerly underappreciated, now plays a central role in our appraisal of spinal deformity. We realize that a single instrumentation system cannot be universal. Each vertebra has its own unique spatial orientation in the spinal column. The surgical alteration of the position of one vertebra will, of necessity, affect the motion segments above and below it.

Spinal surgery has made tremendous advances in the last thirty years. In 1973, I started a Fellowship in Spinal Surgery, which continues to this date. The Fellowship was conceived because I felt there was not sufficient time in a residency training program to allow a young surgeon to become proficient in all the facets of spinal surgery. I had hoped to help create a new discipline—spine surgery—that would combine all of our knowledge of the spine, both orthopedic and neurosurgical. Fortunately, our neurosurgical colleagues have given their full support to the Fellowship, and some neurosurgical residents have applied for it. Nevertheless, the concept of spine surgery as a distinct discipline has not been fully achieved.

The Textbook of Spinal Surgery attempts to be as

comprehensive as possible. However, time is always a factor. If we try to encompass all, a section already written may become obsolete during the final preparation and publication.

I am proud that Dr. Keith Bridwell had the idea for this textbook and is the primary force in its completion. Dr. Bridwell and the associate editors are all experienced spine surgeons whom I have watched grow and mature. I hope that I have played some small part in the development of their careers.

Through the years it has been apparent that spinal surgery knows no national boundary. We are happy to include our international authors in this textbook and express our gratitude for their participation.

This textbook attempts to provide various strategies for the treatment of most spinal disorders with specific reference to the risks and benefits of specific surgical options. As well, it provides the personal treatment philosophies of many of the contributing authors. This book is not intended to define clinical policy but to share our accumulated experience in spine surgery. Future editions, naturally, will reflect the inevitable changes occurring in this field.

My personal thanks to all of our contributing authors.

Ronald L. DeWald, M.D.

Contents

■ ■ ■

VOLUME TWO
PART **V** DEGENERATIVE CONDITIONS   635

PART VI TRAUMA 855

PART **VII** TUMORS

CHAPTER

Index

THE TEXTBOOK OF
Spinal Surgery
Volume One

PART
I

GENERAL CONSIDERATIONS

CHAPTER

1

■ ■ ■

Nursing Care for the Spinal Surgery Patient

Mary Faut Rodts

■

Nursing care for the spinal surgery patient has changed dramatically during the last 10 years, requiring increased nursing expertise and clinical competence.[2, 5, 9, 17, 18] Although hemilaminectomies and percutaneous disc excisions have simplified or minimized the nursing care for patients undergoing routine disc surgical procedures, improved surgical techniques, instrumentation, and anesthesia are making surgery available for higher-risk patients with significant deformities and greater needs for specialized care.[7]

Appropriate nursing plans are based on six factors: (1) diagnosis, (2) age, (3) preoperative medical and social status, (4) surgical procedure, (5) physician orders, and (6) intraoperative complications. Understanding the impact each factor has on nursing decisions is imperative.[19] This reservoir of data allows the nurse to develop a comprehensive plan for hospitalization and home care (Table 1-1).

Spinal surgical procedures are recommended for treating significant deformity, fracture, osteomyelitis, tumor, or degenerative disease. After identifying the pathologic process, it is necessary to decide whether the spinal condition is stable or unstable. The classifications describing the stability of the spinal column after spinal fractures can be used as a guide in cases of spinal tumors or infections with bone destruction.[4, 8] Stability in spinal deformity is not as easily classified; one patient may have a kyphotic condition that is stable, as in Scheuermann's disease, and another may be at significant risk for neurologic deficit caused by instability or compromise, as in select congenital kyphosis or kyphosis from a tumor. The surgeon's determination of stability or instability provides the basis for developing the nursing care plan.

NURSING CONSIDERATIONS

Physiologic Balance

The patient's postoperative physiologic balance is influenced by his or her preoperative medical status. Understanding the patient's starting point helps the nurse set postoperative parameters and expectations. Ideally, the patient is evaluated by both the medical and nursing staff before surgery. A simple activity, such as sitting up in bed, becomes exceedingly difficult for the patient who has been in bed for several weeks before spinal stabilization. Preoperative status is especially

(text continues on page 8)

3

TABLE 1-1. Standardized Care Plan: Posterior Spinal Fusion with Instrumentation*

Patient Problems	Desired Patient Outcomes	Target Dates	Nursing Orders	Time
Preoperative Issues				
I. Anxiety resulting from hospitalization and scheduled surgery	Minimal anxiety as evidenced by verbalization of feelings about hospitalization and impending surgery and understanding preop teaching	24 h before surgery	a. Orient patient/significant other(s) and introduce primary nurse. b. Introduce to other scoliosis patients in same age group on floor. c. Encourage verbalization about surgery and impending body changes with staff and selected postop patients. d. Explain preop tests and routines to patient and significant other(s). e. Implement preop teaching. Include significant others. f. Assess patient's understanding of preop teaching.	Upon arrival/within 24 h Within 24 h Within 24 h On admission and prn On admission × 1 p teaching and prn
Postoperative Issues				
II. Hypovolemia resulting from blood loss	Maintains fluid volume as evidenced by maintenance of baseline vital signs, and Hgb > 10 and Hct > 30%, absence of bright red drainage on dressing, and hemovac drainage < 100 ml/ 4 h	24–48 h postop	a. Check vital signs—notify MD if not within prescribed parameters. b. Check hemovac drainage—notify MD if parameters exceeded. c. Keep patient in supine position. d. Check sheets for drainage. e. Observe dressing, mark drainage. f. Check bloodwork results.	q 15 min until stable, then q 2 h and prn Upon return from recovery room, then q 4 h × 2, then q shift First 8 h postop Upon return from recovery room, and q 2 h first 8 h q 2–4 h after first 8 h postop q shift × 3 days and prn
III. Neurologic impairment resulting from surgical procedure	Maintains preop movement and sensation of lower extremities and sphincter tones	72 h postop	a. Assess movement and sensation of lower extremities. b. Assess anal sphincter control. c. Assess urinary sphincter control when Foley catheter is removed.	q 2 h × 8, then q shift and prn q shift q shift
IV. Renal insufficiency resulting from hypotensive anesthesia	Maintains adequate renal function as evidenced by urine output > 150 ml/8 h, urine specific gravity of 1.010–1.030, absence of facial edema	72 h postop	a. Monitor urine otuput with specific gravity. b. Record accurate intake and output. c. Check for facial edema.	q 4 h × 24 h, then q shift q shift q 4 h
V. Pulmonary complications resulting from anesthesia,	Maintains ventilation and perfusion of lungs as	While on bedrest (3–4 days postop)	a. Assess respiratory status: auscultate lungs, check oral temperature; notify MD if > 101.5° F.	q shift q 2 h while in intensive care,

(continued)

TABLE 1-1 (continued)

Patient Problems	Desired Patient Outcomes	Target Dates	Nursing Orders	Time
Postoperative Issues (continued)				
narcotics, immobility, surgical correction of spine with subsequent alteration of thoracic cavity	evidenced by oral temperature < 100° F, respiratory rate 12–28/min, lungs clear on auscultation, breath sounds equal to or improved from preop		b. Provide respiratory care: cough, deep breathe, and use breathing exerciser; IPPB c. Turn patient: regular or logroll, maintain shoulder and hip alignment, use drawsheet d. Ensure adequate hydration (2000–3000 ml/24 h)	then q 4 h and prn q 2 h and prn qid × 24 h, then tid, per MD order After first 8 h postop, q 2–4 h prn q shift, per MD order
VI. Pain resulting from surgical trauma	Verbalizes or demonstrates decreasing level of pain	5–6 days postop	a. Assess pain level b. Provide comfort measures: back rub, positioning, and conducive environment c. Offer or medic\..te for pain. d. Evaluate effectiveness of pain medication.	Continuously prn prn per MD order With each administration
VII. Dislocation of hooks and rod(s) resulting from improper alignment or movement of back	Maintains location of hooks and rod(s) as evidenced by spinal x-ray film	5–7 days postop	a. Instruct patient on importance of maintaining body alignment and not lifting shoulders. b. Assess for sudden onset of sharp pain between shoulders; notify MD if present. c. Promote calmness through emotional support. d. Medicate to assist relaxation. e. Administer antiemetics for nausea. f. Brace patient at shoulders if vomiting occurs. g. Two nurses use drawsheet when sliding patient up or down in bed. h. Use fracture bedpan. i. Assist turning patient for spinal x-ray examination.	Initially and prn prn Continuously prn per MD order prn per MD order prn Continuously prn Per MD order
VIII. Infection resulting from interruption of skin integrity or invasive catheters	Absence of infection as evidenced by oral temperature < 100° F, incision or IV site(s), hemovac sites free of erythema, edema, tenderness, purulent drainage, clear yellow urine	5–6 days postop	a. Check oral temperature—notify MD if > 101.5° F. b. Assess back incision after initial dressing. c. Check hemovac sites and IV sites for signs and symptoms of infection. d. Administer antibiotics. e. Cleanse incision with alcohol. f. Prevent urinary tract infection: Foley catheter care while in place (see Policy and Procedure), pericare, and ensure adequate hydration (2000–3000 ml/24 h)	q 2 h while in intensive care, then q 4 h and prn q 4 h × 24 h, then q shift q 4 h and prn Per MD order q 4 h q shift With q void q shift, per MD order

(continued)

TABLE 1-1 (continued)

Patient Problems	Desired Patient Outcomes	Target Dates	Nursing Orders	Time
Postoperative Issues (continued)				
			g. Assess for signs and symptoms of urinary tract infection: check urine characteristics, instruct patient to report symptoms of UTI, and send urine for C & S and check for results	q 4 h × 24 h, then q shift upon removal of Foley; 24 h after Foley is removed, per MD order
IX. Thrombophlebitis resulting from venous stasis	Maintains adequate venous return from lower extremities, as evidenced by nontender lower extremities, even skin temperature, or negative Homans' sign	While on bedrest (3–5 days postop)	a. Inspect lower extremities for signs and symptoms of phlebitis. b. Encourage active range of motion. c. Perform passive range of motion. d. Reapply TED stockings. e. Administer anticoagulant therapy.	q shift q 4 h q 4 h q shift and prn Per MD order
X. Decreased peristalsis resulting from surgical procedure, anesthesia, or immobility	Demonstrates return of peristaltic activity as evidenced by flat abdomen on inspection, presence of bowel sounds on auscultation, absence of nausea, passage of flatus and/or stool	5–6 days postop	a. Assess gastrointestinal status. b. Administer antiemetics. c. Administer stool softeners/laxatives.	q shift prn per MD order prn per MD order
XI. Skin breakdown resulting from immobility	Maintains skin integrity	While on bedrest (3–5 days postop)	a. Assess for signs of skin breakdown. b. Massage bony prominences and pressure areas. c. Logroll (see problem V, Nursing Order c.) d. Maintain hydration (2000–3000 ml/24 h).	q shift q turn and prn p first 8 h postop, q 2–4 h prn q shift
XII. Decreased muscle tone resulting from immobility	Exhibits optimal muscle tone as evidenced by preop muscular strength and function	While on bedrest (3–5 days postop)	a. Encourage active range of motion of extremities. b. Perform passive range of motion of extremities.	q 4 h q 4 h
XIII. Dependency resulting from difficulty in performing activities of daily living	Demonstrates increased participation in activities of daily living	7 days postop	a. Assess patients feelings about level of dependency. b. Encourage and assist with increased participation in activities of daily living.	q shift prn

(continued)

6

TABLE 1-1 (continued)

Patient Problems	Desired Patient Outcomes	Target Dates	Nursing Orders	Time
Postoperative Issues (continued)				
XIV. Altered body image resulting from deformity of spine and surgical procedure	Verbalizes adaptation to body image	Entire stay	a. Encourage verbalization of changes in body image with staff and other scoliosis patients on unit.	q shift and prn
			b. Promote positive body image by supporting patient's positive attitudes about self or assisting with measures to improve physical appearance (i.e., washing hair, shaving, and grooming)	prn
Casting or Bracing				
I. Anxiety resulting from casting or bracing	Describes casting procedure or verbalizes feeling	24 h before casting	a. Discuss with patient and significant other(s) casting procedure and appearance of cast.	2–3 days before casting
			b. Encourage questions and verbalization of feelings.	Initially and prn
II. Compromised respiratory status resulting from confinement in body cast or brace	Maintains adequate ventilation as evidenced by respiratory rate of 16–18/min, absence of shortness of breath and dyspnea	24 h or until abdominal window trimmed	a. Assess respiratory status.	Upon return from casting, q 1 h × 2, then q 4 h, and prn
			b. Promote calmness through emotional support.	prn
			c. Instruct patient to report shortness of breath immediately, if indicated; notify MD to trim abdominal window.	Upon return to floor
III. Improper body alignment resulting from cast or brace breakdown	Maintains corrected body alignment	24–48 h or until cast dry	a. Instruct patient to keep cast uncovered.	Continuously
			b. Reposition patient on sides, back, and abdomen.	q 2 h and prn
			c. Check cast for areas that may need reinforcing (especially the shoulders).	q shift
IV. Skin irritation resulting from rough or tight edges of body cast/brace	Maintains skin integrity	Until discharge	a. Inspect skin around edges of cast for signs of irritation.	q 4 h
			b. Pad areas causing irritation until trimmed.	prn
			c. Petal edges and sew stockinette over cast.	When cast dry
V. Difficulting ambulating resulting from altered body image, prolonged immobility, or weight of body cast/brace	Verbalizes or demonstrates adaptation to ambulation as evidenced by maintenance of baseline vital signs, absence of vertigo, or minimal assistance when ambulating	24–48 h after casting	a. Elevate head of bed, then dangle.	× 2, 2–4 h after casting, as tolerated
			b. Encourage and assist with weight bearing and ambulation after dangling.	qid, as tolerated
			c. Check vital signs with initial ambulation.	× 1 and prn
			d. Provide positive reinforcement for progress in ambulation.	q ambulation

(continued)

TABLE 1-1 (continued)

Patient Problems	Desired Patient Outcomes	Target Dates	Nursing Orders	Time
Postoperative Issues (continued)				
Casting or Bracing				
VI. Anxiety about impending discharge resulting from lack of knowledge of home care	Verbalizes understanding of cast/brace care and activity restrictions	24 h before discharge	a. Discuss with patient/significant other(s): cast/brace care, need to maintain restrictions imposed during hospitalization (until first MD visit), patient's concern about sexual activities.	Begin 2 days prior to discharge
			b. Encourage questions and verbalization of feelings.	Initially and prn

* These model criteria are guidelines for nursing care and do not constitute standards of care governing the nurse's or hospital's obligation to the patient.

important for the nurses who provide the initial evaluation and care after surgery. Same-day admission policies abrogate assessment the night before surgery, denying useful information about the patient to the surgeon and the postoperative nursing staff.[10] Alternative arrangements, such as prehospital consultations with the surgeon and nursing staff, must be made in order to acquire this indispensable data.

Preoperative assessment consists of a thorough history, including the reason for admission and surgery, past medical history, past surgical history, family and social history, current medication requirements, and previous positive or negative experiences during hospitalization.

Baseline vital signs should be recorded. The patient should have certain laboratory tests and procedures done before surgery, including anterior-posterior and lateral chest x-ray films; an electrocardiogram; a complete and differential blood count, sedimentation rate, complete blood chemistry panel, and coagulation profile, and a urinalysis. Pulmonary function testing and arterial blood gas determinations are necessary for patients with impaired respiratory function. Thoracic scoliosis greater than 65° by Cobb measurement, emphysema, polio, muscular dystrophy, and myotonia are just a few of the disorders that can impair pulmonary function, increasing the likelihood of ventilatory assistance in the postoperative period. If the need for ventilatory assistance is suspected, a preoperative discussion with the patient and family is warranted to reduce anxiety after surgery.

Blood loss during spinal surgery is expected and unavoidable. Every effort is made to reduce the amount of blood loss during the surgical procedure through positioning of the patient, hypotensive anesthesia (see Chapter 2), meticulous use of cautery, and precise surgical technique. Posterior surgery usually demands that the patient be placed in the prone position, which produces pressure on the abdominal vascular structures and causes increased bleeding into the back wound. To minimize blood loss, Wilson or Relton-Hall frames are used to allow the patient's abdomen to be free (Fig. 1-1A,B). Blood loss is monitored closely by the surgical team, and blood is replaced as needed. Additional blood loss into the wound is expected in the early postoperative period. Accurate accounting of blood loss through drainage systems is necessary to predict the appropriate replacement amount.

Because of concerns about communicable diseases like hepatitis C and HIV, autologous blood donation provides an alternative to traditional blood bank transfusions.[3] Certain parameters allow safe blood donation: hematocrit above 34; weight above 100 pounds for a full unit, above 80 pounds for a partial unit; being at 10 years of age, with no upper age limit if there is no history of hypertension or hypotension or cardiac arrhythmias.

The number of units of blood requested is determined by the surgeon after reviewing the surgical procedure that is recommended and the patient's preoperative hemoglobin level. A one-level posterior spinal fusion may only require 1 unit of blood, but a two-

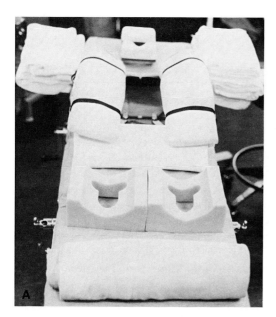

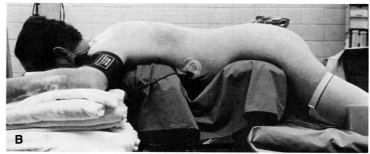

FIG. 1–1. **A.** The Wilson frame appropriately placed on the operating table with padding for arms and knees and a roll to support the ankles. **B.** A patient placed on a Relton-Hall frame, demonstrating the padding for extremities, the head support, and no pressure on the abdomen.

staged anterior and posterior spinal fusion with instrumentation may require 10 units.

A thorough explanation of the need for blood replacement, the probability of blood transfusions, and the phlebotomy procedure decreases fears about blood transfusion and encourages the patient to participate in an autologous blood program for elective spinal surgery.

Specific instructions about the dietary intake of iron and an iron supplement should be given before blood donation. The nurse should encourage a diet emphasizing green leafy vegetables, liver, and red meat. If the patient's diet is questionable, a consultation with a nutritionist may be in order.

Neurologic Assessment

One of the most important roles for the surgical nurse is monitoring and evaluating the neurologic status of the spinal surgery patient. Ideally, the preoperative assessment should be performed by the same nurse that will care for the patient during the postoperative period so that the nurse can identify deficits.[16] In most institutions this is not possible. Instead, the initial assessment is recorded on a neurologic nursing assessment form, which is compared with follow-up assessments. The neurologic examination should assess muscle strength, reflexes, and sensation. Perfecting the neurologic examination comes with practice. Memorizing the correct terms used for the examination is critical (Table 1-2).

TABLE 1-2. Grading Muscle Strength and Reflexes

Grades			Description
Reflex Grading			
4+			Extremely brisk; hyperactive
3+			Brisker than normal
2+			Average; normal
1+			Diminished
0			No response
Muscle Grading			
5	N	Normal	Full range of motion against gravity with extreme resistance
4	G	Good	Full range of motion against gravity with some resistance
3	F	Fair	Full range of motion against gravity; no resistance
2	P	Poor	Full range of motion with gravity eliminated
1	T	Trace	Slight contraction visible
0	0	Zero	No contraction

The first neurologic assessment after surgery should include the upper and lower extremities, regardless of what levels of the spine have been operated, to detect postsurgical deficits and deficits incurred from positioning during the procedure. If the results are normal, the nurse performs another examination based on the location of the surgical procedure: upper and lower extremities for a cervical spine procedure or lower extremities for a routine procedure for a thoracic scoliosis.

Rectal tone and bladder function are important indicators of neurologic competence. Bowel and bladder problems are often noticed before any other manifestation of neurologic deficit. Changes in bladder habits may be caused by bed rest, the use of a catheter, or narcotics. Changes should be evaluated to rule out neurologic compromise. Incontinence of stool or urine is assumed to be due to a neurologic cause until it is ruled out by a rectal examination. Rectal tone is defined as the ability to voluntarily tighten the anal sphincter muscles around the examiner's gloved index finger. Normal rectal tone can be observed during the routine administration of suppositories. If abnormal rectal tone is noticed, it should be reported immediately.

Accurate, concise communication of the neurologic examination is necessary to identify an evolving problem. A phrase such as "the patient seems to be a little weaker" is not as informative as stating that "the patient's left dorsiflexors are now Grade 3, which has decreased from Grade 5 in the past 3 hours; the patient is cooperative; pain is not a problem at the moment; and the patient understands my commands."

The neurologic examination should be performed every 2 hours for the first 24 hours; every 4 hours for the next 48 hours; and then once during every shift until discharge. The onset of neurologic deterioration has been documented 72 hours after a surgical procedure in patients that had been thought to be neurologically stable.[11, 13] Subjective complaints from the patient, such as the feeling of sleepiness or heaviness in the extremities or complaints of extreme pain, numbness, tingling, or the inability to move an extremity, are cause for immediate attention. Any of these complaints demand an immediate neurologic assessment. If no deficit is found, comfort measures should be taken, and the assessment should be repeated in 30 minutes. If the patient persists with the same complaints despite a normal assessment, the attending surgeon should be notified. Astute nursing evaluation can identify early neurologic change and prevent permanent neurologic deficits.

Respiratory Assessment

Prolonged anesthesia with subsequent atelectasis, changes in chest cage geometry, or iatrogenic hemothorax or pneumothorax can cause respiratory compromise after spinal surgery. Assessment of lung status should be performed during every shift for the first 72 hours and continued longer if indicated (e.g., shortness of breath, chest pain, declining hemoglobin, elevated temperature).

Pain after spinal surgery often prevents the patient from voluntarily coughing and deep breathing. Atelectasis and pneumonia are complications that occur if vigorous and consistent chest physical therapy is not instituted. The nurse should assist with frequent pulmonary hygiene sessions by offering pain medicine before the exercise, providing comfort measures by splinting the chest or abdominal wounds, and explaining why pulmonary secretions build up and become a problem. The patient who understands the necessity of pulmonary hygiene will cooperate much more actively.

Hemothorax or pneumothorax may exist even when the surgical approach has been posterior. During the posterior surgical procedure, the chest cavity may be entered intentionally, as in rib resections or the placement of intrathoracic and extrapleural instrumentation, or inadvertently when costotransversotomies are performed to decrease rib prominence. This must be considered for any patient who has pulmonary symptoms.

Abdominal Assessment

Postoperative ileus may occur because of significant correction of a scoliosis or kyphosis, manipulation of bowel during anterior surgery, general anesthesia, or the prolonged use of narcotic analgesics. An abdominal assessment should be performed before the initiation of a diet. The patient should not be vomiting and have bowel sounds. Once bowel patency has been confirmed, ice chips may be given to the patient. If this is tolerated, the patient may progress to having a clear liquid diet. This intake routine should be observed for 24 hours before advancing the diet.

Superior mesenteric artery syndrome (cast syndrome) has been seen in patients undergoing spinal surgery. The bowel obstruction occurs where the superior mesenteric artery crosses over the third portion of the duodenum. In most patients, this problem will resolve if a normal diet is slowly resumed. In general, the patients who develop problems will be thin with a significant correction of deformity. This type of patient warrants extra attention and dietary limitations until bowel patency has been confirmed. Physical examination reveals hyperactive, high-pitched bowel sounds. The symptoms are nausea and emesis. After superior mesenteric artery syndrome has been identified, treatment is complete restriction of oral intake, gastric decompression by use of a nasogastric tube and intermittent low suction, adequate intravenous nutrition, and sedation to allow the tight structures to adjust to the new position. In most cases, this treatment will be sufficient, but if the course is prolonged, hyperalimentation may be necessary.

Pain Management

Pain management is a problem for the spinal surgery patient. The use of narcotics to adequately relieve preoperative pain often increases the requirement for narcotics in the immediate postoperative period. After reviewing the patient's prior analgesia schedule, an appropriate pain management regime can be developed. The patient often is asked before surgery to decrease the use of narcotics to facilitate postoperative pain management.

Intramuscular or intravenous narcotics (e.g., morphine sulfate or meperidine hydrochloride) are necessary for the first 48 to 72 hours after spinal surgery. In our experience, the use of patient-controlled analgesia using morphine provides the most consistent and adequate pain relief. The average 150-lb (56-kg) patient is begun on a PCA routine consisting of 1 mg of morphine sulfate available every 6 minutes, with a maximum of 14 to 20 mg of morphine in a 4-hour period. If pain relief is not accomplished, these parameters can be adjusted, allowing 2 mg of morphine with a longer interval between doses.

Children, afraid of intramuscular injections, occasionally defer pain medication and subject themselves to significant discomfort. The astute nurse should encourage the use of pain medicine. Although the pediatric patient should be allowed to help make decisions

about his or her care, the nurse must assume control for the child who refuses pain medication. Adolescents who have been instructed on the use of patient-controlled analgesia have successfully used this mode of medication administration.[15]

By providing the patient control over his or her own analgesic administration, there is less fear about the intervals for pain medication and pain relief.[6, 12] Muscle relaxants (e.g., diazepam, cyclobenzaprine hydrochloride) provide additional comfort and should be used as adjunctive therapy, but not in place of narcotics. By providing a consistent medication routine, a rehabilitation program may be established earlier, and the patient will progress more quickly.

On approximately the third postoperative day, the use of intramuscular or intravenous narcotics may be changed to oral analgesics (e.g., acetaminophen and codeine or hydrocodone bitartrate), depending on the status of the abdomen. If the patient is tolerating fluids, oral medications may be instituted for the use of pain management, muscle relaxation, and stool softening. Additional medications, such as an iron supplement and vitamins, should be deferred until a less-restrictive diet is resumed.

At the time of discharge, oral narcotics will be necessary for an additional 2 to 4 weeks. During this period, the patient is encouraged to decrease the amount of medication by lengthening the interval between medications or by decreasing the dose of medication. The approach is based on the amount of activity performed each day, the time of day that is more of a problem, and how well the patient is sleeping. One person should be responsible for overseeing the pain medication schedule to assure continuity and to reinforce the goal of complete withdrawal from medications. In selected situations, medications may be necessary for longer periods and should be monitored by a physician with an understanding of chronic pain management.

Stabilization Procedures

Traction

Although used less frequently with deformity patients, the use of traction is necessary for patients with cervical instability caused by trauma, tumor, infections, or degenerative spinal disease. The purpose of halo or tong traction depends on the underlying diagnosis. For example, in deformity patients, the halo is applied to provide a stable point of traction from which to apply significant weight through the skull to the torso to correct the deformity. A halo is used because it provides several points of fixation into the skull, which are necessary if applying significant weight. In general, if applied gradually, one half of the body weight, but no more than 40 lb (15 kg), can be used to correct a deformity. Radiographs of the cervical spine are necessary to assure that overcorrection of the cervical spine is not occurring. Tong traction is not sufficient for this magnitude of weight.

Tong traction and halo traction are used for the treatment of the unstable cervical spine. If continued immobilization of the cervical spine is anticipated, the halo is often the better device to use. If surgery is required in the occipital area of the spine, a cervical halo facilitates the necessary exposure.

Any patient who is placed in halo or tong traction requires skilled nursing care and observation. Maintenance of traction and the airway, assessment of neurologic function, continuation of nutrition, preservation of muscle tone, and constant reassurance and emotional support are key nursing responsibilities.

The principles of skeletal traction for the spine must be understood to maintain the desired traction. As in traction for other orthopedic problems, the pull should be consistent, direct, and unencumbered. The initial weight applied is based on the diagnosis and the size of the patient. Initially, 10 to 15 lb (4–6 kg) is recommended, with increasing increments of 2 lb (0.75 kg) each day; depending on the patient's ability to tolerate the traction, the neurologic function, and whether correction or maintenance of alignment is being sought. It is the responsibility of the nurse to assess the traction, correcting problems such as fraying ropes, weights resting on the floor, incorrect patient positioning, or the knot against the pulley. It is also the nurse's responsibility to maintain the traction schedule as ordered. This becomes difficult when the patient is uncomfortable or noncompliant. Traction may need to be abandoned (only with a physician's order) if the patient is unable to tolerate the procedure.

Controversy exists about the best way to care for halo or tong pin sites. Most people agree that daily cleansing is necessary, but the exact procedure differs. The most important aspect of all pin care is that something is done consistently and completely on a daily basis. Pins should not be allowed to become encrusted with drainage or antibiotic ointment. The pins should

be cleansed with hydrogen peroxide every 8 hours after initial placement. If the surgeon prefers the application of antibiotic ointment around the pin site, this must be completely swabbed away at the next cleaning. If the pin sites become locally irritated, we recommend a more aggressive approach consisting of cleansing of the pin sites with hydrogen peroxide followed by sterile saline. Betadine wraps should be applied at each site and allowed to dry, thus debriding the area when it is removed. Prevention of pin-site infection with subsequent loosening can be avoided with good nursing care.

Protecting the patient's airway is mandatory. When completely recumbent in traction, the patient needs to be reassured that adequate ventilation is occurring. For patients who find it difficult to breathe while lying supine, discuss with the treating physician whether the patient is a candidate for a partial reversed Trendelenburg or side-lying position. In most cases, if the patient's spinal problem is stable, alteration of the position may be easily achieved, although the patient will never be totally comfortable in traction. Patients with unstable spinal problems require greater immobilization with less possibility for changes.

Neurologic assessment becomes especially critical for the patient in traction. Patients who are undergoing correction of deformity or realignment of a spinal fracture are at risk for developing a neurologic deficit. Neurologic assessment should be performed every 2 hours while traction is being increased, always including upper and lower extremities and cranial nerves. Asking the patient to wiggle his or her toes is not sufficient. A complete assessment should be performed, and the patient should be asked if he or she has noticed anything unusual.

An order from the surgeon about whether traction may be discontinued or decreased if neurologic deterioration occurs is helpful. Traction should never be removed without a physician's order, but if neurologic deterioration is noted in a patient undergoing corrective traction for deformity, traction is usually removed immediately to restore the former neurologic status. The surgeon should be notified as soon as possible.

Adequate nutrition is necessary for proper wound healing and to provide the necessary energy to begin a rehabilitation program. Constant attention is essential to maintain adequate nutrition for the patient who is recumbent in traction. Assessment of gastrointestinal status before instituting oral intake can identify potential problems with nausea and vomiting. Allowing the head of the bed to be raised, even a small amount, facilitates eating and decreases the anxiety associated with eating while lying flat. The patient should be attended during meals to simplify and encourage oral intake and to guard against aspiration. Oral intake should not be encouraged in patients who have an active problem with nausea or emesis; delay oral intake until the problem has subsided or been treated with antiemetics. A patient in traction who is actively vomiting should be given nothing by mouth, be placed in the side-lying position, and possibly have a nasogastric tube inserted to avoid aspiration.

Another important issue for the patient undergoing long-term traction is the preservation of as much stamina and muscle strength as possible. This is accomplished by early initiation of a physical therapy regime.

Patients undergoing halo or tong traction need constant emotional support by the nurse. The nurse's confidence, expertise, and knowledge of traction will allay the patient's fears about the situation. Frequent bedside visits by the primary nurse and other staff nurses will also show the patient that he or she is not isolated. All staff members should be aware that a patient in traction is on the nursing unit, and they should be readily available to assist the patient or family. Simple measures, such as positioning the patient to watch television or look out a window, never leaving the patient's room without providing the nurse call button, and frequent assistance to offer nutrition, are necessary. Although the patient should be encouraged to participate in some activities (e.g., hygiene), he or she has significant limitations and maximal nursing assistance is required.

Immobilization Devices

With the advent of newer internal fixation devices for the spine, the need for external immobilization in the postoperative period has decreased for patients undergoing deformity corrections or low back surgical procedures. In the past, plaster casts with the possible addition of a Minerva collar or thigh extension was almost always used. Today, a thoracolumbar sacral brace is often sufficient, depending on the location of the instrumentation (Fig. 1-2). A Milwaukee neck ring may be added for the patient whose instrumentation extends up to T1; a thigh extension may be added for a lumbosacral fusion. A light-weight plastic material is customized to fit the patient. This is less cumbersome

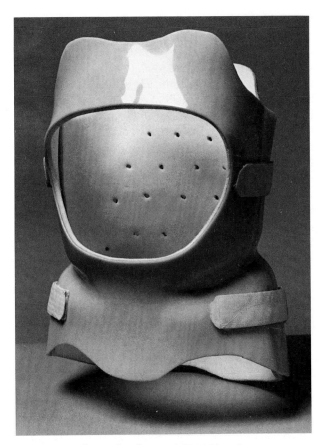

FIG. 1–2. Thoracolumbosacral (TLSO) orthosis.

than a traditional cast and facilitates hygiene. In most cases, daily showers are allowed after wound healing; in more restrictive circumstances, the brace may be removed from the supine patient for a bed bath. This determination is made by the surgeon based on the stability and location of the instrumentation.

In most cases, the unstable cervical spine still requires the use of a device such as a halo vest, Somi brace, or Philadelphia collar to augment the surgical stabilization. Depending on the stability of the spine, the brace or collar may be partially removed for hygiene. The anterior portion is removed first with the patient in the supine position to facilitate skin care. To avoid skin breakdown, the chin should be checked often. The skin should be assessed at least three times each day, allowing the brace to be off for 20 minutes each time. With the patient in the side-lying position, the posterior aspect of the brace should be removed daily to cleanse the skin.

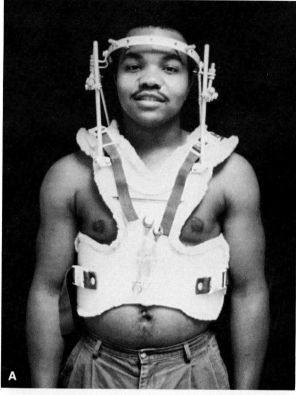

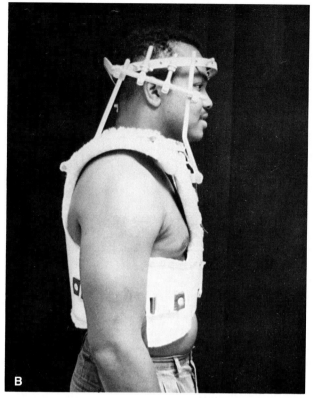

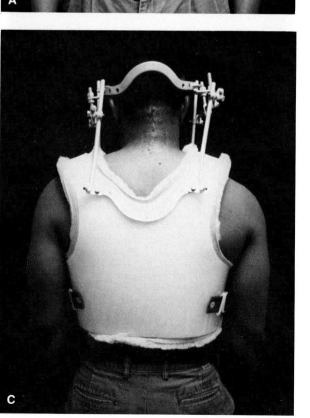

FIG. 1–3. **A.** Patient in a halo vest, anterior view. **B.** Lateral view. **C.** Posterior view. The posterior aspect of the halo ring allows access to the upper cervical spine.

Care of the patient in the halo vest is not as complex as one would anticipate after looking at the apparatus (Fig. 1-3). Halo pin care has already been discussed in this chapter. The same guidelines should be followed two times each day for long-term care. The skin under the vest needs cleaning daily. Use a thin, soft cloth that has been saturated in rubbing alcohol, with the excess expressed. Place it under the brace and gently rub the skin. Alcohol, rather than soap and water, is used to avoid a filmy build-up on the skin.

The patient in a halo vest should be instructed to notify his or her physician immediately if any motion occurs or if drainage appears around the pin sites. Headaches, temperature, dizziness, or blurry vision should be reported. Close observation of the patient in a halo vest is necessary to avoid problems with loosening of the pins or vest. Under no circumstances should the patient remove any portion of the vest. In the event of cardiopulmonary resuscitation, the anterior chest plate is fabricated to allow easy access to the chest. The necessary wrenches to remove the halo vest should be taped to the vest, and the patient should be instructed that these must be available at all times.

Stryker Frame

Most spinal surgery patients can be managed on a standard hospital bed because of the stability achieved through surgical instrumentation. However, the patient with an unstable spinal problem may require the use of a turning frame. The frame that is most commonly used is the Stryker frame (Fig. 1-4). The Stryker frame permits immobilization of the cervical and upper thoracic spine. Skin care is facilitated by the frame, which maintains traction and permits positioning of the supine or prone patient, allowing pressure to be relieved from bony prominences.

No frame can substitute for good nursing care, and problems can arise from the use of a turning frame. The patient must be turned every 4 hours or more frequently if the skin condition is in question.

When the patient is in the prone position, check the position of the arms to prevent hyperextension of the shoulders or pressure in the axilla. This avoids brachial plexus palsy. Correct placement of the anterior forehead strap aids in support of the head and comfort of the patient. In the supine position, the feet should be properly positioned to prevent contractures in those patients who are neurologically compromised. As is the case for using any device for patients with insensate

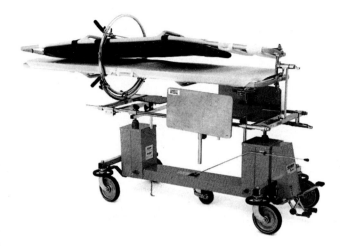

FIG. 1–4. The Stryker Wedge Turning Frame allows the patient to be turned from supine to prone without placing stress on the spine.

skin, observation is imperative to avoid skin breakdown.

Special patient supports, such as the Relton-Hall, Wilson, or Andrews frames, are used intraoperatively to stabilize the torso and protect from pressure on the abdomen and vena cava. This lack of pressure decreases intraoperative bleeding. Special attention is directed at correctly positioning the patient to avert pressure problems in the axillary area or over the breasts (Fig. 1-1A,B). The skin in these areas should be assessed immediately after the patient has been turned prone to identify pressure problems.

Neurologically Compromised Patients

Paraplegic or quadriplegic patients present with more complex medical and nursing problems. Observation for physiologic balance and prevention of complications like skin breakdown and contractures are important initial nursing goals. After these have been accomplished and the spine has been stabilized, the more sophisticated needs of the neurologically impaired patient can be addressed. These include bowel and bladder training, counselling, and rehabilitation. This subject is more fully covered in texts on spinal cord injury.[1, 14]

Rehabilitation

Goals of postoperative rehabilitation should be established before surgery if possible. Identifying the expected goals and the time required to meet them provides the patient a framework for his or her activities in the first few weeks after spinal surgery.

Before elective spinal surgery, the patient should be evaluated for his spinal condition and for his underlying strength and stamina, which will be important in the postoperative rehabilitation phase. Most children have an active lifestyle, but most adults will display significant strength and stamina problems. For decreased strength and stamina, the preoperative patient is placed on a conditioning program to increase endurance. Postoperative recovery occurs more rapidly in patients who have undergone such a program. The period during which patients donate autologous blood for elective procedures is a convenient time to institute an exercise program. Even those patients with significant pain and disability benefit from a modified aerobic program before surgery. The patient also develops a different philosophy about his own health during this period of time and eagerly looks forward to resuming exercise postoperatively.

For the first 48 hours, the patient is log rolled every 2 to 4 hours to alleviate discomfort and protect the skin. A draw sheet is placed from shoulder to pelvis to provide uniform support to the back as the patient is turned (Fig. 1-5). Limited exercise, begun within the first 48 hours after surgery, consists of simple arm and leg exercises. The progress of the exercise program depends on the diagnosis, surgical procedure, and the patient's tolerance.

The key to rehabilitation is a consistent program with small increments in activity. Physical therapy and nursing staff should work together in developing the rehabilitation program to assure patient follow-through. The daily plan of care for mobilization activities like sitting and walking is as important to the patient's progress as nutrition and wound care.

Ambulation after spinal surgery should proceed slowly. Assessment of the patient's hemoglobin can alert the nurse to potential problems with orthostatic hypotension such as lightheadedness and dizziness. Initially, the patient should be shown how to sit and stand. The patient should be taught to roll into the side lying position, and then with the use of his arms, push up from the lying to the sitting position (Fig. 1-6A–C).

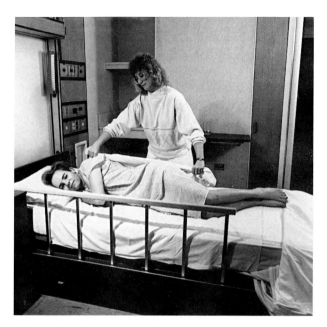

FIG. 1–5. Draw sheet, placed from shoulders to pelvis, provides uniform support for the back as the patient is turned from side to side.

The patient will require assistance at first because of discomfort. Although discouraged as a long-term solution, elevating the head of the bed will make the patient's first attempts easier. Before discharge, the patient should be ambulating with limited assistance, taking care of his or her hygiene activities, taking in an adequate diet, and ready to participate in a limited exercise routine, such as a walking program. Guidelines should be established for the continuation of an increasing activity program after discharge, with one person familiar with the patient overseeing and encouraging the progress of the home program.

Three weeks after discharge from the hospital, a more structured physical therapy program may be instituted. This depends on the patient's status when evaluated. Most children will be ready to return to a school program with no need for continued physical therapy, but adults require additional time to return to preoperative status. The number of surgical procedures directly correlates to the amount of time necessary to achieve full rehabilitation.[17] The patient who requires two or three surgical procedures will require 2 or 3 months before returning to a relatively active lifestyle.

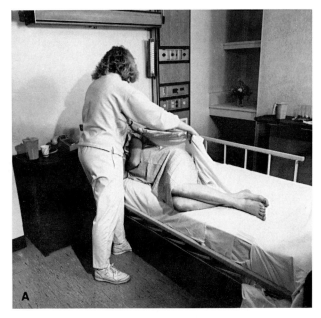

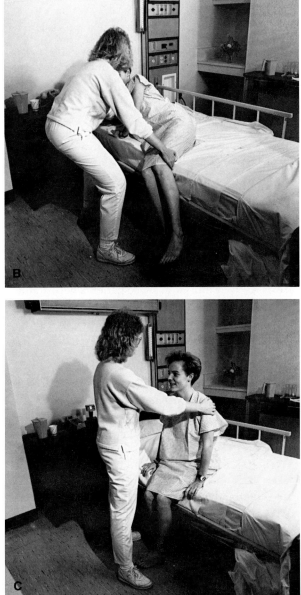

FIG. 1–6. Mobilization activities include sitting. **A.** Using an appropriately placed draw sheet, the patient is turned to the side-lying position. **B, C.** The patient pushes up with the arms as the legs swing over the side of the bed in one motion.

CONCLUSION

The nursing care of the spinal surgical patient should not be viewed as mundane, simple, or for the novice. Complex diagnoses and treatment of patients undergoing spinal surgery require the expertise of all members of the nursing team. The nurse plays an important role in the successful outcome for the patient and should be included in planning conferences or rounds to assure continuity of care. As more complex cases are accepted for surgery, the role of interested and competent nursing staff becomes even more critical—development and preservation of that interest is a formidable task and should be encouraged.

References

1. Bedrook GW: The Care and Management of Spinal Cord Injuries. New York, Springer-Verlag, 1981
2. Berke L, Weidenbaum M: Diastematomyelia and congenital scoliosis. Orthop Nurs 6:46, 1987
3. Brinkley LB: Predeposit autologous blood for elective orthopaedic surgery. Orthop Nurs 8:25, 1989
4. Denis F: The three column spine and its significance in the classification of acute thoracolumbar spinal injuries. Spine 8:817, 1983
5. Doheny MO, Sedlak CA: Body image considerations for the adult scoliosis patient having spinal fusion surgery. Orthop Nurs 6:18, 1987
6. Dunwoody CJ: Patient-controlled analgesia: rationale, attributes, and essential factors. Orthop Nurs 6:31, 1987
7. Gates SJ: Update: Nursing care following percutaneous posterolateral discectomy. Orthop Nurs 6:37, 1987
8. Haher T, Felmly W, Star M, et al: The contribution of the columns of the spine to rotational stability: A biomechanical model. Presented at the 23rd Annual Meeting of the Scoliosis Research Society Meeting, Baltimore, MD, September 30, 1988
9. Jacobs-Zacny JM: Nursing care of adolescents having posterior spinal fusion with Cotrel–Dubousset instrumentation. Orthop Nurs 7:17, 1988
10. Johnson K: Same day surgery: Ensuring pre-admission patient preparation. Nurs Econ 5:258, 1987
11. Johnston CE, et al: Delayed paraplegia complication sublaminar segmental spinal instrumentation. J Bone Joint Surg [Am] 68A:556, 1986
12. Kresl JS: Patient controlled analgesia. A new system for pain management. AORN J 48:481, 1988
13. Letts RM, Hollenberg C: Delayed paresis following spinal fusion with Harrington instrumentation. Clin Orthop 125:45, 1977
14. Meyer PR (ed): Surgery of Spine Trauma, pp 121–305. New York, Churchill Livingstone, 1989
15. Rauen KK, Ho M: Children's use of patient-controlled analgesia after spine surgery. Pediatr Nurs 13(5):589, 1989
16. Rodts MF: Musculoskeletal assessment. Nursing 83:65, 1983
17. Rodts MF: Surgical intervention for adult scoliosis. Orthop Nurs 6(6):11, 1987
18. Rodts MF: Cotrel–Dubousset instrumentation for scoliosis. In Nursing Yearbook 1988, pp 77–78. Springhouse, PA, Springhouse Corporation, 1988
19. Rush Presbyterian–St. Luke's Medical Center Standardized Nursing Care Plans, 1753 Congress Parkway, Chicago, IL 60612

CHAPTER 2

Anesthesia for Spinal Surgery

Carl Helge Nielsen

■

Rapid improvement and proliferation of fixation devices have promoted an increasing number of spinal column operations. It is now possible to correct pathologic conditions that in the past were considered beyond therapeutic reach. For anesthesiologists, this means a higher volume of anesthesia for spinal surgery and designing anesthesia plans for more patients with concomitant diseases.

Optimal management of anesthesia for spinal surgery is only possible after a thorough evaluation of the patient's status. The anesthesia care must be based on sound theoretical concepts, and the plan must be one the anesthesiologist can administer skillfully.

EVALUATION AND RISK ASSESSMENT

The preanesthetic evaluation of the patient for spinal surgery is not unique; it follows the general approach used before any patient is given an anesthetic. There are three goals for the evaluation. The first is to acknowledge the patient's physical status and the extent of concomitant illnesses. Second, therapies may be suggested or further consultations and laboratory studies may be requested before the operation. Third, an assessment of the goals and risks involved allows the physician to formulate an anesthesia management plan.

A basic preanesthesia evaluation is not elaborated here because it can be found in standard anesthesia textbooks, but a few pertinent details of the cardiac and pulmonary evaluation are discussed because they often predict the success of the procedure.

Cardiac Evaluation

Pediatric patients and young adults presenting for spinal operations have a low incidence of coronary artery disease. However, degeneration of cardiac muscle is a common problem in the late stage of patients with muscular dystrophy. This may cause mitral regurgitation due to papillary muscle dysfunction and decreased myocardial contractility.[42] The changes on the electrocardiograms (ECG) of many of these patients presumably reflect progressive myocardial necrosis.[38] The degree of cardiac dysfunction can be assessed with echocardiography or with radioisotope imaging.

Most adult cardiac disease is caused by coronary artery disease, and the patients usually have one of the many symptom complexes associated with ventricular dysfunction. The patient's history, ECG, and Goldman risk index may all be helpful in indicating conditions that can be corrected or optimized preoperatively, but they may not be accurate predictors.[9, 18] Dipyridamole-thallium cardiac imaging is currently enjoying a reputation as one of the best noninvasive tests for prediction of perioperative ischemic events.[12] However, it can be argued that exercise electrocardiography provides similar information at much lower cost.

Pulmonary Evaluation

The incidence of restrictive lung disease is higher than normal in patients presenting for spinal operations (e.g., the pediatric patient with muscular dystrophy or the adult with a thoracic scoliosis). The incidence of chronic obstructive pulmonary disease is significant among the geriatric patients presenting for spinal operations. Arterial blood gas analysis and spirometry are valuable for preoperative assessment and as a guide for postoperative management. Spirometry repeated after a dose of nebulized bronchodilator may indicate reversible obstructive pulmonary disease.[7] It is difficult to assign values that accurately indicate risk, and no study has successfully correlated data from any test or combination of tests with rates of morbidity or mortality. The preoperative vital capacity is clinically used as a predictor of postoperative pulmonary status. Patients with a vital capacity of less than 35% of predicted value are likely to need postoperative ventilatory support.

Preoperative management of patients who are at risk includes antibiotic treatment, bronchodilator therapy, and aggressive pulmonary hygiene, including cessation of smoking (Table 2-1). The optimal duration of this treatment has not been established, but it is considered cost-effective for 1 to 3 days before surgery.[7]

I do not recommend asking consultant internists to review all patients preoperatively. When consultants are requested to evaluate a patient, they should be asked to answer a specific question and to identify ways to reduce risk and manage the problem. The overall preoperative evaluation is the responsibility of the anesthesiologist.

ANESTHETIC PLAN

The goal of premedication is to have a mentally relaxed and comfortable patient arriving in the operating room. No single drug or dose will accomplish this

TABLE 2-1. Guidelines for Estimated Pulmonary Risk

Risk Factors	Moderate Risk	High Risk	Extreme Risk
FVC*	<50%	<35%	<35%
FEV$_1$	<50%	<25%	<25%
FEV$_1$/FVC	<50%	<35%	<35%
MMV	<50%	<50%	<50%
FEF$_{25-75\%}$	<50%	<30%	<30%
ABGs	Normal	Normal	Pa$_{O_2}$ < 50 mm Hg < Pa$_{CO_2}$

* Abbreviations: FVC, forced expiratory capacity; FEV$_1$, forced expiratory volume in first second; MMV, maximal mandatory ventilation; FEF$_{25-75\%}$, forced expiratory flow between 25% and 75% of FVC; ABGs, arterial blood gases; Pa$_{O_2}$, oxygen tension in arterial blood; Pa$_{CO_2}$, carbon dioxide tension in arterial blood. Pulmonary risk is expressed as a function of the ABG values and actual spirometry values in percent of predicted values.

satisfactorily. What and how much to use must be decided for each patient. The patient in pain preoperatively should be offered opioid analgesics, administered at a time when they can provide beneficial therapeutic effect during the transport to the operating area. If the patient is currently getting appropriate analgesics, it seems logical to continue these. Anxiolytic drugs (e.g., benzodiazepines) are used to reduce the patient's fear. Oral benzodiazepines (e.g., midazolam, diazepam, lorazepam) are effective for this purpose. By selecting the drug with the most favorable pharmacokinetics, the physician can tailor sedation, lasting from a few minutes to several hours.

The plasma half-lives for diazepam for geriatric patients may last up to four times longer than those for young adults. Difficulties with the selection of the correct drug and dosage of premedicants are a result of both pharmacokinetic and pharmacodynamic variability, and titration may be necessary, dictated by prescribing information and physical status.

Antisialagogues (i.e., saliva-reducing agents like atropine) are not prescribed as premedicants routinely. Their use cannot be justified with modern anesthetics.

Clonidine, a centrally acting antihypertensive drug, administered orally as a preoperative medication, reduces the increase in blood pressure and heart rate associated with intraoperative stimulation. This agent also prevents reflex sympathetic activation in response to vasodilators.[32] This yields more stable hemodynamics, avoiding nadirs and peaks in arterial blood pressure and in heart rate.[26]

A useful regimen for premedication of patients for spinal operations is a relatively large dose of oral diazepam (10–25 mg) with oral clonidine (5 μg/kg) 1 to 2 hours before arrival in the preoperative holding area.

Anesthetic management has several goals. The technique must provide intense analgesia with adequate sedation, amnesia, and muscular relaxation. It must allow control of blood pressure to minimize bleeding associated with hypertension. It must allow uncompromised monitoring of the somatosensory evoked potentials. It must allow a wake-up test during surgery, if desired, and permit awakening in the operating room after surgery to assess fully the patient's neurologic status.

The anesthesia literature describes many techniques that, with careful administration, can live up to these goals. A balanced technique with continuous infusion of opioid is currently favored. To this is added nitrous oxide, an inhalation agent in low concentration, or a continuous intravenous infusion of a sedative. Muscle relaxation is facilitated with intermittent boluses or continuous infusion of nondepolarizing muscle relaxants. Hypotension is produced by using vasodilating agents. No single drug and technique can satisfy all the goals.

The technique with ketamine is similar to opioid administration in many respects, but it does not depend on nitrous oxide or an inhalation anesthetic.[35, 36] Anesthesia is induced with diazepam (total dose of 0.3 mg/kg including the premedication), followed 1 to 2 minutes later with D-tubocurarine (0.5 mg/kg injected over 30–60 s) and with ketamine (100–200 mg given by bolus). All three drugs are administered intravenously. The anesthesia is maintained with a continuous infusion of ketamine, initially at 4 mg/kg/h. The rate is reduced during the procedure, usually to 0.5 mg/kg/h, during the final 30 minutes of the procedure.

MONITORING

Basic monitoring includes ECG, blood pressure, breath and heart sounds, temperature, and the use of pulse oximetry. Monitoring also includes checking direct arterial pressure by an indwelling catheter in a radial artery, neuromuscular blockade with a peripheral nerve stimulator, end-expiratory carbon dioxide concentration, and airway pressure. Somatosensory evoked potentials are also monitored. Blood gases are drawn as needed, which is usually only one time after anesthesia has been induced. I have not found the information provided by repeated blood gas analyses to be diagnostically valuable for the cardiovascularly stable patient if an inspired oxygen fraction of 0.25 to 0.30 yields pulse oximeter readings above 95% and stable end-expiratory carbon dioxide readings.

Venous access must be secured and catheters for monitoring central venous and pulmonary artery pressures must be inserted before starting the operation. Access is difficult after the patient is positioned for the operation. I have found monitoring of central venous and pulmonary artery pressures unnecessary unless dictated by concomitant disease.

Depth of anesthesia cannot be monitored accurately, a problem that is further complicated by the use of hypotensive techniques. It is not surprising that occasionally a patient may recall part of the intraoperative experience or that a patient is slow to wake up.

Meticulous attention must be paid to all details of fluid management during spinal operations, and third-space losses are often larger than blood loss. The operations are frequently long, and even small deviations may accumulate and cause disasters. Third spacing in a case with exposure of many segments of the posterior thoracic and lumbar spine or in a case with a transthoracic transdiaphragmatic approach may require infusion of crystalloids in the range of 12 to 15 ml/kg/h. Urine output is monitored with an indwelling catheter inserted in the urinary bladder at the time of anesthesia induction. Because deliberate hypotensive anesthesia decreases renal blood flow and glomerular filtration rate, the urine output does not accurately reflect the patient's level of hydration. Minimal or no urine output is common during deliberate hypotensive anesthesia. The urine flow should increase to a normal level immediately after the patient resumes spontaneous ventilation. Continuous low urine output in the recovery room is probably a sign of hypovolemia.

Somatosensory Evoked Potentials and Anesthesia

The success of somatosensory evoked potential monitoring depends on the expertise and cooperation of the anesthesiologist. This is particularly true for the potentials monitored over the sensory cortex. The potentials monitored at the subcortical level (e.g., over the cervical spinal cord) are more robust. Pharmacologic intervention and cardiovascular changes introduce variability in the somatosensory evoked potentials that may not be distinguished from the changes indicating spinal cord compromise. The major disadvantage of somatosensory evoked potential monitoring is that only sensory pathways are monitored. It is not surprising to find case reports of motor deficit after an operation in which evoked potentials remained normal throughout the procedure.

Accurate monitoring and interpretation require considerable experience by the anesthesiologist, and the monitoring also requires full attention. A full-time, well-trained technician is a necessity; even better is an electrophysiologist who simultaneously can interpret the results and discern artifacts.

The effect of anesthetics appear to be dose related, with increasing doses of anesthetic agents producing increasing degrees of alteration in the evoked response, until no response is measurable. A study conducted to determine the concentration of volatile anesthetics at which somatosensory evoked potential monitoring is still possible concluded that 0.5 MAC of halothane or up to 1.0 MAC of isoflurane or enflurane (each with 50% nitrous oxide) are compatible with wave generation adequate for spinal cord monitoring during scoliosis operations.[37] Unfortunately, a study like this does not address the clinical problem, because inhalation anesthetics in those concentrations are inadequate for this degree of surgery; 1 MAC is the minimal alveolar concentration at which 50% of patients do not move during skin incision and is not a reliable indicator for the quality of intraoperative anesthesia.

The significant increase in latency and decrease in amplitude seen at reportedly acceptable concentrations of inhalation agents make wave form recognition difficult and decrease the specificity and sensitivity of the monitoring.[37] The effects of enflurane, isoflurane, and nitrous oxide on cortical somatosensory evoked potentials during fentanyl anesthesia were compared.[28] Induction of anesthesia with fentanyl increased latency. The latency was further increased by isoflurane and enflurane. Neither fentanyl, enflurane, nor isoflurane changed the amplitude. Nitrous oxide decreased the amplitude. The study concluded that, for cases in which somatosensory evoked potentials are important, enflurane or isoflurane offer better conditions for monitoring than 50% nitrous oxide. In my judgment, inhalation anesthetics and nitrous oxide have no place in anesthesia for patients for whom monitoring of somatosensory evoked potentials is employed.

Another key to successful monitoring of somatosensory evoked potentials is the maintenance of a physiologically stable patient. Supervising the patient's temperature, oxygenation, hematocrit, glucose, and circulating blood volume is paramount in providing optimal neural survival and maintaining a stable monitoring environment. Conversely, insufficient oxygen delivery may cause deteriorating evoked potentials, which may be used as a warning of impending ischemia.[16, 17]

Motor pathway evoked potentials are being studied. The results may allow monitoring of the anterior part of the spinal cord.

Wake-Up Test

The wake-up test provides a reliable measure of gross motor function of the upper and lower extremities after spinal column operations.[44] Advantages of the wake-up test include no special equipment, low cost, and definite evidence of intact motor function while most electrophysiologic measurements reflect only sensory function. If compromise is discovered during the wake-up test, the surgeon can decrease the corrective force, and another wake-up test can be performed. Removal or modification of the spinal instrumentation within 3 hours after onset of a neurologic deficit decreases the risk of permanent neurologic sequelae.[10] The disadvantages are that the test can only be used intermittently and infrequently. The patient may wake up agitated, move too much, and disconnect life support devices, monitoring devices, or the spinal instrumentation. Spontaneous inspiration can produce air emboli. The wake-up test may be emotionally distressing to the patient, and the possibility of resulting psychological problems must be considered.

Inhalation anesthetics make timing of a wake-up test difficult. Opioid with nitrous oxide anesthesia is widely used to accomplish reliable tests. Substitution of nitrous oxide with oxygen usually yields a responsive patient within 5 minutes. Rehearsal of the wake-up test before the procedure greatly increases its speed and success, and it is an integral part of the preoperative visit and a necessity immediately before inducing anesthesia. I have found the wake-up test also works reliably with ketamine anesthesia.

INTUBATION

Fiberoptic Intubation

Fusion of cervical vertebral joints and fixed deformity of the head and neck can make endotracheal intubation extremely difficult. Patients presenting with fractures or dislocations of the neck may not tolerate the positioning necessary for direct laryngoscopy. Blind nasal intubation may be successful, but in difficult cases, the fiberoptic laryngoscope must be used. When difficulty is expected, adequate planning and preparation, including good anesthesia of the airway, are the keys to success. All the necessary equipment should be available before beginning the procedure. If the neck is unstable, greater support is necessary during the intubation. This can be provided by an assistant supporting the neck manually.

The use of local anesthesia for this procedure allows continuous monitoring of the patient's neurologic status. For intubation under local anesthesia, a suitable technique begins with 1% dyclonine applied to the nasal mucosa and 2% viscous lidocaine kept in the back of the mouth until it provides anesthesia for the back of the tongue and the oropharynx. Then 1 to 2 ml of 1% lidocaine is injected bilaterally superficial and deep to the thyrohyoid membrane, just inferior to the major cornu of the hyoid bone. This anesthetizes the two superior laryngeal nerves. Finally, 4 ml of 1% dyclonine is injected through the cricothyroid membrane in the midline. Guided by direct vision, the fiberoptic scope can be advanced either through the mouth or through the nose, after which the endotracheal tube is passed over the fiberoptic scope into the trachea. Visualization of the carina at the end of the tube assures that the tube is in an optimal position.

The fiberoptic scope is also helpful for assessing the correct placement of an endobronchial tube.

Double-Lumen Tubes

Procedures involving the anterior thoracic spine may be facilitated by endobronchial intubation and single-lung ventilation. The benefits appear obvious for the upper two thirds of the thoracic spine, but retraction of the lung may be sufficient for procedures below T8.[13]

Disposable tubes made of polyvinyl chloride have a blue endobronchial cuff that makes identification easy during bronchoscopy, a high-volume, low-pressure cuff that may reduce the risk for pressure-induced injury in the trachea, user-friendly packaging with a removable stylet and nonadhering suction catheters, and a clear plastic construction that permits observation of condensation from the exhaled water vapor. These features are not found in the traditional reusable endobronchial tubes.

The endobronchial tubes have left-sided and right-sided conformations for intubation of the left and right main bronchus, respectively. The left-sided endo-bronchial approach should always be used for spinal operations because the margin of safety during placement of this tube is twice that of the right-sided approach.[5] Once inserted, the position of the double-lumen tube must be confirmed. This can reliably and simply be done with auscultation of the lungs while first one and then the other tube is clamped during ventilation.[8] The current state of the art for verification of endobronchial tubes is fiberoptic bronchoscopy, but a size 37 French endobronchial tube requires a bronchoscope with an external diameter of 4.9 mm or less. Any flexion or extension of the patient's head will produce an inward or outward movement of the endobronchial tube, respectively, which may require repositioning of the tube.

Two-lung ventilation should be continued as long as possible, and the adequacy of gas exchange during one-lung ventilation should be documented with continuous monitoring of oxygen saturation with the pulse oximeter and, if needed, arterial blood gas analysis. Hypoxic pulmonary vasoconstriction improves the ventilation and perfusion matching during one-lung ventilation, but this benefit may unfortunately be eliminated by inhalation anesthetics and by the use of vasodilators added to induce deliberate hypotensive anesthesia.[11]

The use of ketamine does not interfere with hypoxic pulmonary vasoconstriction and the mixture of air and oxygen can be adjusted to the lowest possible inspired oxygen fraction producing satisfactory oxygen saturation. This technique has, in my experience, not necessitated the use of 100% inspired oxygen, positive end-expiratory pressure, nor continuous positive airway pressure with oxygen to the deflated lung to keep the oxygen saturation above 0.95.

POSITIONING FOR SPINAL SURGERY

Posterior spinal operations are performed with the patient in the prone position, and the lateral and supine positions are used for operations on the anterior spine. The prone position carries with it a degree of risk, which is only surpassed by the risk of anesthesia in the sitting position. The lateral position produces considerable alterations in cardiorespiratory physiology, which may be exacerbated by the nature of the surgery.[2]

Lateral stabilizers may be used to maintain the lateral position, but their use is frequently impossible because they interfere with the surgical field. Better results are possible with an evacuatable mattress. When air is sucked out, it becomes firmer and holds its shape until opened again. The evacuated mattress offers several advantages. First, the patient is securely supported in almost any position. Second, folding the bag under the dependent axilla relieves pressure on the adjacent deltoid muscle and pressure on the brachial plexus. Third, this mattress increases the surface area supporting the patient's weight, and the pressure on the skin is evenly and widely distributed. Fourth, the polystyrene granules in the bag have excellent insulating properties, and heat loss is minimized.

Proper support of the head is essential; rotation and angulation of the head must be minimized. No unnecessary pressure should affect the dependent ear. The upper arm must be positioned without any stretching of the brachial plexus. A Mayo stand covered with a pillow may be used for this purpose. Bony prominences on the dependent leg are supported with a pillow because the common peroneal nerve is at risk as it crosses the proximal fibula. Both legs are protected by pillows between them.

Arterial blood pressure monitoring is reliable from either of the two arms if correctly positioned. Similarly, intravenous infusion is obstructed only if the arm is incorrectly positioned.

The prone position can lead to external pressure on the abdomen, which increases the pressure on the vena cava. This leads to increased pressure in the epidural veins and promotes hemorrhage. Suitably placed pillows and foam pads beneath the chest and pelvis provide good support for short operations on superficial structures, but more complex operations carried out on the vertebral column demand a much more sophisticated approach. The main objective is to eliminate any mechanical pressure on the abdomen and the large blood vessels. This is achieved by raising the patient above the level of the operating table with a support mechanism exerting pressure only on the chest and pelvis. Another objective is to provide the optimal position for the operation. It is important to preserve lumbar lordosis (by extending the hips) for cases involving instrumentation and fusion. On the other hand, if the patient is having lumbar disc surgery, it is helpful to flex the hips in order to flex the lumbar spine and widen the interlaminar space to improve the surgical exposure.

The patient's head in the prone position must be kept as close to neutral as possible. A patient with a normal range of movement of the neck will tolerate a prolonged operation with the head turned either to the right or the left. The neck and head should usually be supported without flexion or extension on the same plane as the rest of the spine. Too much flexion may stretch the cervical cord. Too much extension in the patient with cervical spondylosis may compromise the blood supply to the spinal cord. These compromises may be significant enough to cause deterioration of the somatosensory evoked potentials.

Posterior operations on the cervical spine, as well as support of the patient's head with limited range of movement of the neck, require positioning of the head without any rotation of the neck. Foam pads have been developed for this purpose, but they provide limited access to the face, which makes frequent checking of the head position a difficult task. The "horseshoe" head rest allows easy access to the entire face and head, making it readily apparent when the patient is misplaced or displaced. The "horseshoe" head rest must be properly padded and be allowed to rest principally on the forehead. It is necessary to check the position frequently to assure that no pressure is applied to the orbits.

Careful positioning of the shoulders prevents damage to the joint capsule or the brachial plexus. Although it is preferable to replicate the normal prone sleeping position with the arms resting on the table at the side of the head, this is impossible without additional width of the operating table for all but the smallest patients. Extra width can be provided with arm boards positioned parallel to the table. The patient's arms should be positioned along the sides of the body for operations requiring access to the cervical spine.

Anesthesia is induced before the patient is positioned prone. This is conveniently done on a stretcher, which can be positioned along the operating table to allow the patient to be "rolled" over to the prone position. All arterial and venous access should be secured before positioning. A wake-up test is helpful after positioning patients with rheumatoid cervical spine deformities and C1–C2 instabilities to assure that no new neurologic deficit has occurred during the turning and repositioning of the head. This can be accomplished with an awake intubation and judicious administration of analgesics before the patient is "rolled" to the prone position.

The choice of frame or positioner for the prone position is most commonly made by the surgeon and is not discussed in this chapter about anesthetic implications.

CONTROLLED HYPOTENSION

Blood loss during spinal fusion and instrumentation may be considerable. A loss of up to 1.5 times the estimated blood volume has been reported.[1, 41] Several approaches have been made to reduce blood loss, including infiltration of the surgical field with epinephrine-containing solutions, the use of negative end-expiratory pressure, hemodilution, careful positioning, hypotensive anesthesia, and the use of desmopressin. The latter two approaches appear to be the most successful, but only the technique of deliberate hypotensive anesthesia has been used long enough to allow accurate assessment of its results. One physician advised a combination of surgical and anesthetic techniques, including the use of autotransfusion, to control blood loss during scoliosis surgery.[39]

Hypotensive anesthesia for spinal column operations has been shown to decrease blood loss, the need for transfusion, and the operating time.[23, 43] However, hypotension may decrease spinal cord blood flow and predispose the spinal cord to ischemic injury, particularly if corrective force is applied during the operation.[25] Deliberate hypotension is best induced by means familiar to the anesthesiologist. This frequently means a higher inspired concentration of an inhalation agent, which may be impossible to combine with monitoring of somatosensory evoked potentials and a timely wake-up test.

An opioid anesthetic with nitrous oxide or an intravenous sedative has become a popular technique because it allows both monitoring of the somatosensory evoked potentials and a wake-up test. Blood pressure can be reduced by using intravenous vasodilators and beta-blockers. The three most commonly used vasodilators are nitroprusside, nitroglycerin, and trimethaphan.

Sodium nitroprusside is a potent peripheral vasodilator that relaxes the smooth muscles in the walls of arterioles and venules. It has a fast onset, transient duration, and predictable effect. Sodium nitroprusside carries with it the risks of cyanide toxicity, tachyphylaxis, reflex tachycardia, abolition of cerebral autoregulation, hypoxic pulmonary vasoconstriction, and systemic rebound hypertension through direct activation of the renin-angiotensin system. Treatment with a beta-blocking agent or angiotensin-converting enzyme inhibitor reduces the dose requirement for nitroprusside and ameliorates its risks.[3, 46]

Nitroglycerin is slower in onset and less potent than nitroprusside. It relaxes arteriolar and venous smooth muscle directly, and it may favorably affect the endomyocardial blood flow. Nitroglycerin use avoids toxic side-effects, but it is frequently not potent enough to produce the desired level of hypotension, and a ceiling effect has been demonstrated.[47]

Trimethaphan has a ganglion-blocking action, and it may also be a vasodilator mediated by histamine release. It has a favorable hemodynamic and hormonal response.[22] The maximal dose is not limited by toxicity, but tachyphylaxis may occur.

All of these drugs have been used clinically with good results. However, no single drug is an ideal agent for induction of deliberate hypotension. In animals, differences have been noted in each drug's effects on spinal cord blood flow. Nitroprusside-induced hypotension in dogs to 50% of the baseline mean arterial blood pressure caused an initial decrease in spinal cord blood flow, but 30 minutes later it returned to baseline level.[20] In contrast, spinal cord blood flow during trimethaphan-induced hypotension decreased and paralleled the decrease in mean arterial blood pressure. No autoregulatory compensation was documented with trimethaphan.[21] How much data can be extrapolated from the canine spinal cord blood flow model to clinical cases is uncertain.[39] These two studies using dogs had significantly different baseline spinal cord blood flows, and the anesthesia included halothane for the nitroprusside study and an opioid nitrous oxide anesthetic for the trimethaphan study. Moreover, we do not know the minimal critical spinal cord blood flow. This controversy will continue because there are too many factors that vary from one study to another to allow for any rigid conclusions.[33]

Various other techniques may be combined with induced hypotension to control blood loss during scoliosis surgery. Hemodilution can be used routinely in elective surgical procedures.[14] Although hemodilution may decrease the need for transfusions, it does nothing to decrease the rate of blood loss. Without induced hypotension, rapid blood loss often obscures the surgical field and slows the surgery. Blood with a low hematocrit is as difficult to see through as blood with a high hematocrit. Autotransfusion of preoperatively collected autogenic blood and reinfusion of intraoperatively salvaged blood likewise should be encouraged, but neither technique decreases the bleeding into the surgical field.

Desmopressin is a synthetic analogue of the antidiuretic hormone vasopressin. It raises the circulating levels of factor VIII coagulant and von Willebrand factor and shortens prolonged bleeding times. There is evidence from controlled clinical trials that desmopressin can reduce surgical blood loss and transfusion requirements. The usual dose is 0.3 μg/kg administered over 15 to 30 minutes. Tachyphylaxis occurs in some patients. If hypotension and tachycardia occur, they can be abolished by slowing the rate of infusion.[29] The current role of desmopressin is unclear. Should it be used prophylactically or only therapeutically? Should concern about thrombosis preclude its widespread use?

A novel approach is to give the patients instructions on how to decrease bleeding during spinal operations. Patients are informed about the procedure and given statements about the importance of blood conservation. They are told to concentrate on moving their blood away from the operative field from the beginning until the end of the procedure, after which the blood must return normally. A study in which 30 of 90 patients were randomized to this technique reported a reduction in the estimated blood loss from a mean of 1090 ml to 650 ml.[4] This technique has been routinely used by my patients since it was published 3 years ago.

When trimethaphan is used for deliberate hypotension with the aim of achieving a mean arterial blood pressure of 60 mm Hg, the following technique may be used. The infusion of trimethaphan is started as early as possible to allow hypotension from the time of skin incision. The infusion rate is controlled with a volumetric pump. Tachyphylaxis and lack of sufficient effect are occasionally seen, and if the infusion for more than 5 minutes has exceeded a rate of 1 g/h, the patient is given intravenous hydralazine (5–10 mg intravenous bolus). A pulse rate above 100 beats each minute is treated with propranolol (1 mg by intravenous bolus). Patients with chronic obstructive lung disease who may not tolerate propranolol are given verapamil (1.25 mg by intravenous bolus).

REGIONAL ANESTHESIA FOR SPINAL OPERATIONS

Regional anesthesia for surgical treatment of spinal disease is unfortunately not considered very often. General anesthesia, with its myriad drugs and their effects and side-effects, can be substituted by spinal or epidural anesthesia. Strong emotions, uncertainty about legal implications, and ignorance among anes-

thesiologists and surgeons are just a few of the hurdles that must be overcome; it may seem infinitely easier to give a general anesthetic.

The anesthetic management for spinal operations must produce safety and comfort for the patient and facilitate the operation. It must provide intense analgesia with adequate sedation, amnesia, and muscular relaxation. It must allow controlled blood pressure to prevent bleeding associated with hypertension. Regional anesthesia can accomplish all these goals, but because adequate spinal and epidural anesthesia blocks transmission of nerve impulse in the spinal cord, it cannot allow monitoring of somatosensory evoked potentials or a wake-up test. It is therefore contraindicated when these types of monitoring are necessary.

Hypotensive anesthesia is superb with the regional technique. A spinal or epidural anesthetic gives sympathetic blockade and relaxes the splanchnic and lower extremity vessels, causing pooling of blood in these capacitance vessels, and the epidural veins collapse. Spontaneous ventilation, with its lower mean intrathoracic pressure than that for controlled artificial ventilation, produces a lower central venous pressure, which also reduces epidural venous pressure.

Regional anesthesia requires skill and experience. Unfortunately, the technique is rarely taught for spinal surgery. My experience with spinal and epidural anesthesia for a large number of laminotomies and laminectomies for resection of herniated discs has been quite good. Epidural anesthesia is administered with a single injection with placement of an 18-gauge Tuohy- or Crawford-tip needle. Injection of a total of 20 to 30 ml of 0.75% bupivacaine with 1:200,000 epinephrine provides 3 to 4 hours of anesthesia. Spinal anesthesia for similar procedures is best accomplished with a hypobaric technique and 6 to 10 mg of tetracaine in 5 to 10 ml of water with 200 μg of epinephrine; this provides 3 to 4 hours of anesthesia.

POSTOPERATIVE PAIN MANAGEMENT

Anesthetic management in the United States has traditionally been completed with the patient's discharge from the recovery room. However, the development of patient-controlled analgesia systems and epidural opioid analgesia has motivated many anesthesiologists to participate in postoperative pain management. Conventional administration of intramuscular analgesics is not obsolete, but it has often failed.[30, 45]

The patient-controlled analgesia technique does not differ in any essential way from conventional analgesic therapy, but the approach offers improvement in the method of administration. Although small doses of opioid with rapid onset can be given manually in response to the patient's request, delays often occur because the nurse may not be readily available and because it takes time to give the injection. Furthermore, the patient may not wish to inconvenience the personnel and may wait too long before calling for another dose. These problems are eliminated with patient-controlled analgesia.

Several systems are available, and they all work well. The choice of opioid is not important. Our postoperative patients have for the past 2 years used a disposable, mechanical, patient-controlled analgesia device that delivers 2 mg of morphine intravenously or subcutaneously every 6 minutes, as needed. Primed with meperidine, it can deliver 20 mg every 6 minutes, as needed. This is potentially a very large dose, but patients do not activate the system unless they have pain, and smaller doses may be inadequate. Most patients can be switched to oral analgesics on the third or fourth postoperative day.

Epidural opioid analgesia, the other major development in pain management in the past decade, can also successfully be used after spinal operations.[40] Controlled studies comparing the conventional techniques with patient-controlled analgesia and epidural analgesia are frequently biased. Perhaps conventional techniques would work much better if they were applied with the same amount of effort and enthusiasm.

Intrapleural analgesia is a new technique in which a small catheter is percutaneously inserted and placed between the parietal and visceral pleura. It is intermittently injected with local anesthesia. It is too early to judge if this technique is of value after an anterior spinal operation requiring a thoracotomy.

A continuous intercostal nerve block with intermittent injection of local anesthesia causes spread of the drug along the nerve next to the catheter and into the paravertebral space a couple of segments above and below. Thus, analgesia is unilateral, and a 30-ml injection covers approximately five ribs.[31] All patients who have had an operation on the spine with an anterior approach have received continuous intercostal nerve blocks for postoperative analgesia. The combination of patient-controlled analgesia given intravenously and 30 ml of 0.5% bupivacaine with 1:200,000 epinephrine injected every 12 hours in the continuous intercos-

tal catheter gives excellent analgesia, allowing deep breaths and strong coughs.

EPIDURAL STEROID INJECTION

Reports about the apparent success of epidural administration of steroid preparations first appeared about 30 years ago.[19, 24] The technique is widely used, and more than 100 reports have been published reporting success rates between 0 and 100%. Despite their widespread use, epidural steroids remain controversial.[6] There have been few studies constructed to meet the standards of a randomized, double-blind trial. The patients with the best results have certain characteristics: radicular pain, recent onset of pain, absence of opioid dependence, young or middle age, no previous spinal operation, and a lack of environmental reinforcers like pending disability compensation. This set of characteristics also describes the group of patients who have a good chance of spontaneous resolution of pain.

Epidural steroid injections have the potential for complications: headache secondary to dural puncture, water retention, skin lesions, Cushing's syndrome secondary to steroid use, and steroid-induced depression.

The rationale for epidural steroid injection has never been satisfactorily explained. The practice was introduced simultaneously with the technique of intra-articular steroid injection for rheumatoid diseases. However, the anti-inflammatory role for epidural steroid is presumptive, and the small amount of supporting evidence is circumstantial and inferential.[34] A single study reported intense inflammation occurring in the dural sac, adjacent nerve roots, and nerve root sleeves after small doses of autologous nucleolus pulposus material were injected into the epidural space.[27]

The injection of steroids into the epidural space should not be passively accepted simply because it has been used for a long time. I suggest that we adopt an attitude of cautious skepticism and thoroughly communicate this to patients before performing the procedure, ensuring that their consent is truly informed consent.

Epidural steroid injections should be administered only after the patient has been thoroughly evaluated by a surgeon or a neurologist. The patient with radicular pain to one of the lower extremities often receives the epidural steroid with a caudal approach to deliver the most drug around the sacral nerve roots. All other patients with back pain receive an epidural injection at or just below the area with the most pain. Methylprednisolone acetate (80 mg in 1 or 2 ml) is administered with a dose of local anesthesia. The local anesthetic gives mild, transient epidural anesthesia, which eliminates the pain and documents correct administration of the injection.

References

1. Abbott TR, Bentley G: Intraoperative awakening during scoliosis surgery. Anaesthesia 35:298, 1980
2. Anderton JM, Keen RI, Neave R: Positioning of the Surgical Patient: The Lateral Position, the Prone Position, pp 31–61. Scarborough, Ontario, Butterworth & Co., 1988
3. Bedford RF, Berry FA, Longnecker DE: Impact of propranolol hemodynamic response and blood cyanide levels during nitroprusside infusion: a prospective study in anesthetized. Anesth Analg 58:466, 1979
4. Bennett HL, Benson DR, Kuiken DA: Preoperative instructions for decreased bleeding during spine surgery. Anesthesiology 65:A245, 1986
5. Benumof JL, Partridge BL, Salvatricrra C, et al: Margin of safety in positioning modern double-lumen endotracheal tubes. Anesthesiology 67:729, 1987
6. Bogduk N: Back pain: Zygapophysial blocks and epidural steroids. In Cousins MJ, Bridenbaugh PO (eds): Neural Blockade in Clinical Anesthesia and Management of Pain, pp 935–954. Philadelphia, JB Lippincott, 1988
7. Boysen PG: Evaluation of pulmonary risk. In American Society of Anesthesiologists Refresher Course Lectures, vol 261, pp 1–5, 1988
8. Brodsky JB, Mark JBO: A simple technique for accurate placement of double-lumen endobronchial tubes. Anesth Rev 10:26, 1983
9. Carliner NH, Fisher ML, Plotnick GD, et al: Routine preoperative exercise testing in patients undergoing major noncardiac surgery. Am J Cardiol 56:51, 1985
10. Chamberlain ME, Bradshaw EG: The "wake-up test": A new approach using drug infusions. Anaesthesia 40:780, 1985
11. Domino KB, Borowec L, Alexander CM, et al: Influence of isoflurane on hypoxic pulmonary vasoconstriction in dogs. Anesthesiology 64:423, 1986
12. Eagle KA, Coby CM, Newell JB, et al: Combining clinical and thallium data optimizes preoperative assessment of cardiac risk before major vascular surgery. Ann Intern Med 110:859, 1989
13. Ebert J: Anterior spinal surgery—anesthetic reflection. In Wheler AS (ed): Anesthesia for New Surgical Procedures. Anesthesiology Clinics of North America, vol 7, pp 653–673. Philadelphia, WB Saunders, 1989
14. Fahmy NR: Hemodilution and hypotension. In Enderby GEH (ed): Hypotensive Anaesthesia. New York, Churchill Livingstone, 1985
15. Goldman L, Caldera DL, Nussbaum SR, et al: Multifactorial index of cardiac risk in noncardiac surgical procedures. N Engl J Med 297:845, 1977
16. Grandy BL, Nash CL, Brown RH: Arterial pressure manipulation alters spinal cord function during correction of scoliosis. Anesthesiology 54:249, 1981
17. Grundy BL: Intraoperative monitoring of sensory evoked potentials. Anesthesiology 58:72, 1983
18. Jeffrey CC, Kunsman J, Cullen DJ, Brewster DC: A prospective evaluation of cardiac risk index. Anesthesiology 58:462, 1983
19. Joebert HW Jr, Julio ST, Gardner WS: Painful radiculopathy treated with epidural injections of procaine and hydrocortisone acetate: Results in 113 patients. Anesth Analg Curr Res 40:130, 1961
20. Kling TF, Ferguson NV, Leach AB, et al: The influence of induced hypotension and spine distraction on canine spinal cord blood flow. Spine 10:878, 1985
21. Kling TF, Wilton N, Hensinger RN, et al: The influence of trimethaphan (Arfonad) induced hypotension with and without spine distraction on canine spinal cord blood flow. Spine 11:219, 1986
22. Knight PR, Lane GA, Hensinger RN, et al: Catecholamine and renin-angiotensin response during hypotensive anesthesia induced by nitroprusside or trimethaphan camsylate. Anesthesiology 59:248, 1983
23. Lam AM: Induced hypotension. Can Anaesth Soc J 31:S56, 1984
24. Lievre JA, Bloch-Michel H, Pean G, et al: L'hydrocortisone en injection locale. Rev Rheum 20:310, 1953
25. Lindop MJ: Complication and morbidity of controlled hypotension. Br J Anaesth 47:799, 1975
26. Longnecker DE: Alpine anesthesia: Can pretreatment with clonidine decrease the peaks and valleys? Anesthesiology 67:1, 1987
27. McCarron RF, Wimpce MW, Hudkins PG, et al: The inflammatory effect of nucleus pulposus. A possible element in the pathogenesis of low back pain. Spine 12:760, 1987
28. McPherson RW, Mahla M, Johnson R, et al: Effects of enflurane, isoflurane, and nitrous oxide on somatosensory evoked potentials during fentanyl anesthesia. Anesthesiology 62:626, 1985
29. Mannucci PM: Desmopressin: A nontransfusional form of treatment for congenital and acquired bleeding disorders. Blood 72:1449, 1988
30. Marks RM, Sachar EJ: Undertreatment of medical inpatients with narcotic analgesics. Ann Intern Med 78:173, 1973
31. Middaugh RE, Menk EJ, Reynolds WJ, et al: Epidural block using large volumes of local anesthetic solution for intercostal nerve block. Anesthesiology 63:214, 1985
32. Mitchell HC, Pettinger WA: The hypernoradrenergic state in vasodilator treated hypertensive patients: Effect of clonidine. J Cardiovasc Pharmacol 2:1, 1980
33. Murphy JM, Sage JI: Trimethaphan or nitroprusside in the setting of intracranial hypertension. Clin Neuropharmacol 11:436, 1988

34. Nachemson A: The natural course of low back pain. In White AA, Gordon SL (eds): Symposium on Idiopathic Low Back Pain, pp 46–51. St. Louis, CV Mosby, 1982

35. Nielsen CH: Anesthesia for orthopedic surgery in the geriatric patient. In Felts JA (ed): Anesthesia for the Geriatric Patient. Clin Anesthesiol 4(4):959, 1986

36. Nielsen CH: Hypotensive anesthesia during somatosensory evoked potentials. Surv Anesthesiol 34:51, 1990

37. Pathak KS, Ammadio BS, Kalamchi MD, et al: Effect of halothane, enflurane and isoflurane on somatosensory evoked potentials during nitrous oxide anesthesia. Anesthesiology 66:753, 1987

38. Perloff JK, de Leon AC, O'Doherty D: The cardiomyopathy of progressive muscular dystrophy. Circulation 33:625, 1966

39. Phillips WA, Hensinger RN: Control of blood loss during scoliosis surgery. Clin Orthop 229:88, 1988

40. Ray CD, Bagley R: Indwelling epidural morphine for control of post-lumbar spinal surgery pain. Neurosurgery 13:388, 1983

41. Relton JES, Conn AW: Anesthesia for the surgical correction of scoliosis by the Harrington method in children. Can Anaesth Soc J 10:604, 1963

42. Sanyal SK, Johnston WW, Dische MR, et al: Dystrophic degeneration of papillary muscle and ventricular myocardium. Circulation 62:430, 1980

43. Sivarajan M, Amory DW, Everett GB, et al: Blood pressure, not cardiac output, determines blood loss during induced hypotension. Anesth Analg 59:203, 1980

44. Vauzelle C, Stagnara P, Jouvinrouk P: Functional monitoring of spinal cord activity during spinal surgery. Clin Orthop 93:173, 1973

45. Weis OF, Sriwatanakul K, Alloza JL, et al: Attitudes of patients, housestaff, and nurses toward postoperative analgesic care. Anesth Analg 62:70, 1983

46. Woodside J, Garner L, Bedford RF, et al: Captopril reduces the dose requirements for sodium nitroprusside induced hypotension. Anesthesiology 60:413, 1984

47. Yaster M, Simmons RS, Tolo VT, et al: A comparison of nitroglycerin and nitroprusside for inducing hypotension in children: A double blind study. Anesthesiology 65:175, 1986

CHAPTER

3

Evoked Potential Monitoring During Spinal Surgery

Jeffrey H. Owen

■

Evoked potential monitoring during surgery for spinal deformity offers reliable and valid measures of spinal cord function. By monitoring, it is possible to determine the onset of spinal cord damage, the involvement of sensory or motor tracts, whether specific nerve roots are involved, and if the damage is structural or ischemic in origin.

This chapter reviews the theories and techniques of evoked potential monitoring and describes the status of these procedures. Although behavioral measures will always be the "gold standard" of clinical status, evoked potential monitoring can provide the surgeon with a valid measure of spinal cord function and avoid the difficulties associated with other intraoperative assessments of clinical status.

MIXED-NERVE SOMATOSENSORY EVOKED POTENTIALS

Anatomy and Physiology

To understand the use of somatosensory evoked potentials as a measure of spinal cord function during surgery, it is necessary to review the anatomy and physiology of the somatosensory system.

The somatosensory system is naturally stimulated by mechanical receptors in the skin, muscles, and joints. However, it is possible to elicit activity within this system by electrically stimulating a peripheral nerve (e.g., median or posterior tibial nerves). Elicited activity, regardless of the method of elicitation, is conveyed into the spinal cord by fibers by way of the dorsal roots (Fig. 3-1). The cell bodies for these fibers compose the dorsal root ganglia, and their central branches ascend the spinal cord. Although both the dorsomedial and the anterolateral tracts convey sensory-based information, it is generally assumed that electrically elicited activity is conveyed by the dorsomedial column (Fig.3-2).

The ascending fibers within the dorsomedial tracts remain ipsilateral to their side of entry.[32] The majority of these fibers are first-order neurons, and approximately 15% are second-order neurons.[32] The gracilius nucleus is the site of termination for fibers from the lower portion of the body (lumbar and sacral regions); the cuneatus nucleus is the termination point for fibers from the upper portion of the body (thoracic and cervical regions).

The fibers that leave the gracilius and cuneatus

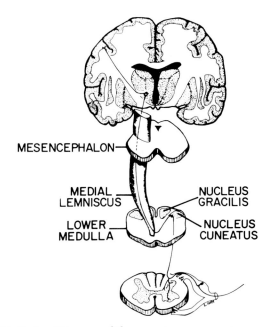

FIG. 3–1.   Diagram of the somatosensory system.

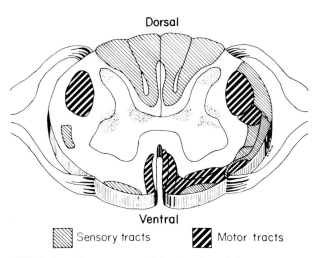

FIG. 3–2.   Cross-section of the spinal cord showing sensory and motor tracts.

nuclei decussate and form the contralateral medial lemniscus. The medial lemniscus ascends into the brain stem and terminates within the thalamus, which forms a second point of synapse. The third-order fibers that leave the thalamus eventually terminate within the sensory cortex in a somatotopic arrangement, with legs represented in areas closest to the midline and the trunk, arms, and hands represented more laterally (Fig. 3-3). This arrangement must be kept in mind when placing recording electrodes at their appropriate locations.

The activity within the somatosensory system originates from either axonal or dendritic sources. Axonal responses can be recorded peripherally from the stimulated nerve or over the central axis distal to the cortex. Dendritic activity is recorded over the somatosensory cortex. The functional characteristics of axonal and dendritic activity are significantly different and must be considered when eliciting and recording an evoked potential. Axonal responses are of short duration and morphologically succinct, but dendritic activity is relatively long and morphologically broad. Because of these differences, the frequency compositions of the two responses are different, and the parameters used to record them must be adjusted.

According to the Heisenberg Principle, the temporal duration of a signal influences its frequency compo-

sition.[16] In general, the shorter the duration of the signal, the greater its frequency composition. Because axonal activity has a shorter duration, it contains a much wider band of frequencies than dendritic activity. Therefore, when recording an axonal response, the filters used should be adjusted to pass a wide band of frequencies. Conversely, because dendritic activity is typically of a much longer duration than axonal activity, the width of the band-pass filters should be much

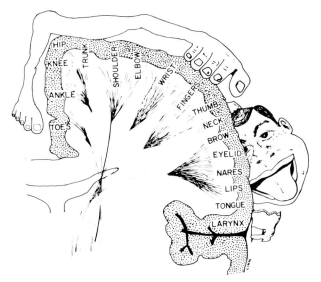

FIG. 3–3.   Topographic arrangement of body areas representative of the primary sensory and motor cortex.

narrower and centered over the lower frequencies. The lower frequencies are emphasized because most of the frequencies within this activity are between 1 and 200 Hz.[23]

Axonal and dendritic activity are differentially sensitive to the presentation rate of the eliciting stimulus. Axonal activity is more resistant to the fatigue and desynchronization associated with faster presentation rates than dendritic activity. Because dendritic activity is more susceptible to fatigue and desynchronization, the rate at which stimuli are presented must be "slowed down" to optimize the cortical response.

The anatomic sources of axonal and dendritic activity also display a differential sensitivity to anesthetic agents. In general, depression of axonal activity by anesthetics occurs infrequently, which supports the use of a noncortical recording site. However, dendritic activity is very susceptible to these agents. Of the various anesthetic agents available, high-dose inhalation agents, alone or in combination with more than 60% nitrous oxide, or bolus injections of narcotics demonstrate a significant influence on evoked potentials of dendritic origin (see Chapter 2).

Instrumentation Requirements

Instruments used to elicit and record the evoked potential consist of three major systems: stimulus control, recording, and storage (Fig. 3-4). Each system demonstrates certain characteristics that facilitate testing and that require adjusting when developing a monitoring program.

Stimulus Control System

The stimulus control system generates the signal delivered to the patient. All of the signal's characteristics are controlled by this system, including whether the signal is constant current or constant voltage, the intensity level of the signal, and the presentation rate of the signal.

When electricity is used to stimulate a nerve, it is the amount of current within the stimulus that determines the number of neural fibers stimulated. Because there is always a certain amount of impedance between the nerve and the contact points of the stimulator, there is a reduction in the signal's effective intensity level. A system that uses a constant current signal automatically adjusts voltage to overcome the resistance at the point of stimulation. The signal is subsequently indicated in amperage and remains constant regardless of changes in resistance.

An evoked potential system that uses a constant voltage signal applies a stimulus of a known voltage but adjusts current as a function of resistance. Because the intensity of the signal is indicated in volts, the amount of current contained within the signal is unknown.

In addition to the obvious advantage of knowing the amount of current being applied, responses elicited

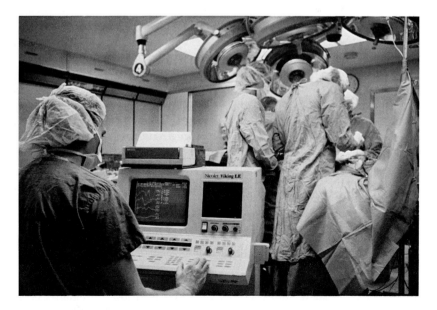

FIG. 3–4. Orientation of a commercially available signal-averaging system in the operating room.

with constant current stimuli demonstrate better interlaboratory agreement than responses elicited using constant voltage. If, for example, a patient is evaluated at two laboratories, it is much easier to replicate testing conditions if the amount of current used to stimulate the nerve is known.

A constant voltage system produces a recording that may be less contaminated by stimulus artifact when the distance between stimulating and recording electrodes is very small. This is advantageous for monitoring during the exploration of peripheral nerves (e.g., neuroma incontinuity). It is now possible to purchase a system in which both current and voltage types of stimuli are available. The systems my colleagues and I use (Nicolet) have this capability, allowing greater flexibility in monitoring a wider variety of cases.

The intensity level of the signal must be adjusted so that the maximal number of neurons are being stimulated, an intensity known as the point of saturation. To ensure that saturation is reached, the system must produce a signal of adequate intensity. If constant current is used, there should be at least 79 mA of available current. However, the probability of damaging the skin increases when higher-intensity stimuli are used.

The stimulus control unit must allow the examiner to control the duration of the stimulus. In most monitoring situations, a signal duration of 200 microseconds is adequate. However, a slightly longer duration may improve the reliability and morphology of a response, especially in cases of peripheral neuropathy. However, longer durations increase the effective intensity of the signal.

The rate at which stimuli are presented must also be adjustable. Two criteria determine presentation rate: how often data need to be interpreted and the operating characteristics of the nervous system. At certain times during spinal surgery (e.g., passing of sublaminar wires), data should be interpreted more frequently. One way of acquiring data more frequently is to present the signal at a slightly faster presentation rate. However, the operating characteristics of the nervous system are not uniform, and faster presentation rates degrade the amplitude and morphology of the dendritic-cortical response. We have found that a presentation rate of 4.1 to 4.8 each second allows frequent updating of data without unwanted degradation of response reliability or morphology.

The presentation rate must not be a multiple of the line current or other periodic signal. Every time a stimulus is presented, *all* of the electrical activity at the

recording electrodes is recorded and averaged. If some type of periodic, nonbiologic electrical activity is present, it will also be recorded and averaged with the stimulus-elicited activity. This may yield a sinusoidal artifact within the averaged response. To avoid this problem, the presentation rate is adjusted to include a decimal component (e.g., 4.1/s or 4.8/s).

Recording System

The recording system consists of a headbox, differential amplifiers, band-pass filters, and the signal-averaging computer. The headbox is the device that acts as the interface between the recording electrodes and differential amplifiers (Fig. 3-5). The headbox used in the operating room should have a cable that is at least 6 m long. This will ensure that the evoked potential equipment and personnel are not near the operative field. The headbox should also contain a "bovie-protector" circuit that will protect the system's computer during the use of electrocautery equipment. Consequently, headboxes designed for diagnostic purposes are not appropriate for intraoperative use.

The neurologic activity that is elicited by a stimulus is very small in amplitude, especially compared with ongoing electroencephalographic (EEG) and myogenic activity. To improve the ratio between the desired re-

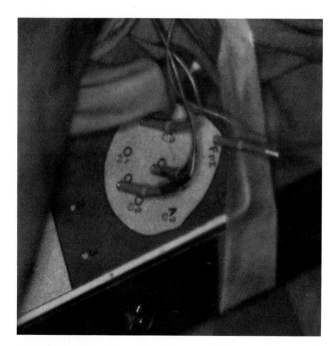

FIG. 3–5. Location of headbox used for interfacing with recording electrodes.

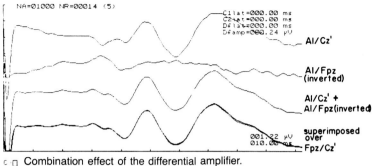

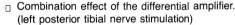

FIG. 3–6. Effect of differential recording amplifiers and montages on the evoked response. Combination effect of the differential amplifier. (left posterior tibial nerve stimulation)

sponse and the undesired noise, differential amplifiers, band-pass filters, and signal-averaging techniques are used.

Differential amplifiers require two inputs, one from the active electrode and the other from the reference electrode. Signals that are common at both electrode sites are cancelled, and uncommon signals are amplified and delivered to the band-pass filters (Fig. 3-6). Because differential amplifiers are used to improve the signal-to-noise ratio of a response, it is necessary to place the active electrode as close to the biologic origin of the signal as possible. Placement of the reference electrode in a "quiet" or biologically inactive location also improves the signal-to-noise ratio. The absolute impedance of the recording electrode must be as low as possible and the impedances between electrodes should be less than 2 kΩ.

The output from the differential amplifier is then filtered. Because various responses contain different frequencies, the acquisition filters require adjustment. We use a filter setting of 10 to 250 Hz for dendritic-cortical data and 10 to 2000 Hz or 10 to 3000 Hz for subcortical axonal data (Table 3-1).

After being filtered, the signal is delivered to a signal-averaging computer, which averages the repetitive samples of neurologic activity. Based on the principles of signal averaging, any activity that is time locked to the presentation of the signal is enhanced, and random activity is "averaged out." By averaging an adequate number of samples, it is possible to improve on the morphology and reliability of the response. In most cases, a reliable mixed-nerve somatosensory evoked potential can be achieved with as few as 300 samples of averaged data.

One subsystem of the signal-averaging computer governs the sensitivity used to record data. By using appropriate sensitivity, it is possible to improve the signal-to-noise ratio. However, if sensitivity is too

TABLE 3-1. Parameters for Recording a Four-Channel SEP to Posterior Tibial Nerve Stimulation*

Parameters	Chn. 1	Chn. 2	Chn. 3	Chn. 4
Sensitivity (μV)	50–100	50–100	50–100	50–100
Low linear filter	10	10	10	10
High linear filter	250	250	250	2000
Notch filter	Off	Off	Off	Off
Referential	Fpz	Fpz	Fpz	Fpz
Active	C3′	Cz′	C4′	Crv
Artifact reject.	On	On	On	On
Timebase (msec)	125			
Rate	4.8/sec	Swp: 300	Trigger: Int	
Duration	200 μsec			

*Recording included 1 cervical/peripheral channel and 3 cortical SEPs. A 65-msec timebase was used in recording the ulnar nerve responses.

great, a higher proportion of data is rejected and averaging takes longer. Conversely, if sensitivity is too low, noise is accepted by the computer with the signal, and the resultant average contains an unacceptable amount of noise. I recommend setting the sensitivity of the signal averager so that 10% of the elicited activity is rejected.

Storage System

After data have been collected and displayed on the screen, they are stored and printed. Large amounts of data can be stored on a floppy disk or a hard disk. Although there are advantages and disadvantages to both forms of storage, it is more important that the evoked potential system have a mass storage capability. We print all of the data acquired during surgery. This means that the data are recalled from storage, the pertinent points identified and labeled, and the data printed. Significant amounts of time can be saved if data are printed during surgery. Although printing all of the data produces a large printout, it provides ready access to all of the patient's records.

Elicitation and Recording

Electrodes

There are two types of electrodes that can be used to elicit and record data: cup and subdermal needles. Cup electrodes are made of silver or gold and are approximately 3 mm in diameter (Fig. 3-7). Gold is

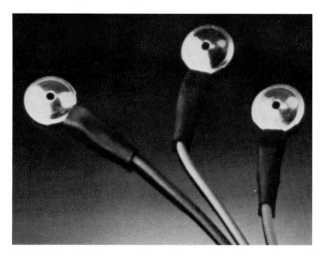

FIG. 3–7. Surface cup electrodes used to elicit and record evoked potentials.

preferred because it has a better frequency response and does not need chloride treatment.

If cup electrodes are used during surgery, collodion is used to attach them to the skin. Because collodion is flammable, the electrodes must be applied before the patient is taken into the operating room. After ascertaining the recording sites (Table 3-2), the skin is cleaned and the electrode held in place. A small (1 cm^2) gauze pad, impregnated with collodion, is applied over the electrode and allowed to dry. Drying time of the collodion can be decreased if an air compressor is used to blow air over the electrode. After the collodion dries, a blunt-tip hypodermic needle is inserted through the electrode, and the skin underneath the cup is slightly abraded. An electrolyte is then introduced under the cup. During the surgery, the impedance of cup electrodes should be periodically checked. If the electrolyte dries out, impedance will increase, causing an unacceptable interelectrode impedance in that channel and a noisier recording. To resolve this problem, the examiner refills the electrodes with electrolyte. After surgery, the electrodes are removed by dissolving the collodion with acetone.

Alternative to cup electrodes are sterile subdermal needle electrodes (Fig. 3-8). Subdermal needle electrodes are usually 26 gauge, 0.5 in (1.3 cm) long, and made from various types of metal (e.g., stainless steel, platinum-iridium). These electrodes are usually applied after the patient has been anesthetized. After cleaning the electrode site with alcohol, the electrode is inserted under the skin and taped in place. There is no need to use an electrolyte with subdermal needle electrodes.

We use subdermal needle electrodes for eliciting and recording all of our evoked potentials because they demonstrate the several advantages over cup electrodes. First, although absolute impedance of the needle electrode tends to be slightly higher, the interelectrode impedance is nearly identical. Second, the impedance of the needle electrode remains more stable throughout the surgery, especially because there is no electrolyte to dry out. Third, needle electrodes are much easier to place and do not require collodion or acetone.

There are several disadvantages associated with subdermal needle electrodes. First, the needle can break off in the skin. Second, it is possible to develop an infection at the electrode site. Third, needles pose a danger to the examiner, especially in the presence of

TABLE 3-2. **Primary and Secondary Recording Sites for SEPs Elicited by Stimulating Upper or Lower Limbs**

Sites	Surgical Level	
	Above C8	*Below C8*
Primary stimulation	Median nerve	Posterior tibial nerve
	Ulnar nerve	
Secondary stimulation	Posterior tibial nerve	Ulnar nerve
Recording	Fpz = C3'	Fpz = C3' (at 10%)
	Fpz = Cz'	Fpz = Cz'
	Fpz = C4'	Fpz = C4' (at 10%)
	Fpz = Crv	Fpz = Crv
	Erb's Point	Popliteal Fossa

contagious diseases. Fourth, high-intensity stimulation through a needle electrode could produce a small lesion at the stimulation site.

I do not recommend mixing cup and needle electrodes during a procedure. For example, recording electrodes should be all needles or all cups, but not some of each. Also, the same type of metal should be used (e.g., all silver electrodes).

Recording Sites

My procedure for recording a mixed nerve-somatosensory evoked potential requires four channels. However, I apply recording electrodes at a minimum of five sites: peripherally, over the fourth and fifth cervical vertebrae (Crv4 and Crv5), and at C3', Cz', and C4' (10–20 Recording Method; see Table 3-2 for specific recording sites).[18] Each recording site demonstrates

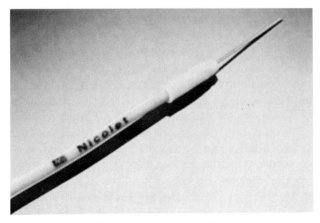

FIG. 3–8. Subdermal needle electrodes used to elicit and record evoked potentials during surgery.

certain strengths that make it an invaluable aid in collecting and interpreting data.

The peripheral channel provides the examiner with information about the appropriateness of the signal's intensity and about the encoding of the stimulus into the peripheral nervous system. There are several methods for determining the intensity of the eliciting stimulus. Some are based on motor threshold, sensory threshold, or some combination of these thresholds. My colleagues and I believe that stimulus intensity should be the minimal level adequate to saturate all of the peripheral nerve's fibers. This is determined by recording the peripheral response at various intensity levels. Start at a low intensity and increase it in 5-mA steps, until the amplitude of the peripheral response plateaus. This method determines the saturation level of the peripheral fibers and avoids unnecessarily high intensities that could damage the skin.

The peripheral recording channel also provides the examiner with information about the neurologic encoding of the stimulus. For example, if cortical and subcortical data are lost during surgery, the peripheral response allows the examiner to determine if instrumentation, stimulus encoding, or something else is the cause. In most cases, we only collect data from this channel immediately after incision or in the event of the loss of cortical and subcortical potentials. This is not an active recording site most of the time.

Our primary recording channels are over Crv4 and Crv5 and at C3', Cz', and C4'. All four channels are referenced to Fpz (International 10–20 Method).[18] These channels provide information about whether the nerve impulse, elicited peripherally, has successfully propagated through the site of surgery. The cervical channel is more resistant to the effects from anesthesia than the cortical channels. However, the cervical response can be slightly more difficult to record. If the proximal end of the incision extends into the high cervical region, it may not be possible to place a recording electrode cervically. An alternative is to use linked mastoid electrodes or a nasopharyngeal electrode. Figure 3-9 depicts an x-ray film of a nasopharyngeal lead in place. We have obtained reliable responses using this recording method.

There are several reasons for using an array of cortical channels. First, they provide redundant confirmation of arrival of the nerve impulses at the somatosensory cortex. Second, the intraoperative procedure requires monitoring of brachial plexus function to avoid a plexopathy caused by improper positioning of the patient's shoulders. This requires placing stimulating electrodes in all four extremities, regardless of level of surgery. Simultaneously recording from three cortical

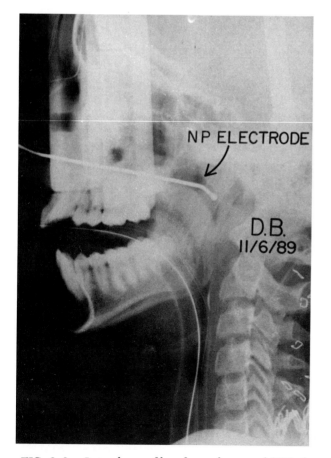

FIG. 3–9. Lateral x-ray film of nasopharyngeal (NP) electrode used during surgery.

sites avoids the need to switch recording channels as different sites are stimulated. Third, the Fpz-Cz' recording site does not always provide the largest response to lower-limb stimulation (Fig. 3-10).

Stimulation Sites

Our intraoperative monitoring method calls for stimulating the upper and lower limbs during *all* surgeries. This necessitates the labeling of stimulation sites as either primary or secondary, based on the level of surgery. If surgery is at or distal to Crv7, the posterior tibial nerve is designated as the primary site of stimulation. Although a secondary site would be the peroneal nerve, I have found that the response from the peroneal nerve is not as robust or reliable as that from the posterior tibial nerve.

During surgeries that are proximal to Crv7, the primary stimulation sites are the median and ulnar nerves. The ulnar nerve response provides more complete information on cervical spine function because it enters the spinal cord at a lower level than the median, but both nerves are continuously monitored during cervical spine surgery. I also stimulate the posterior tibial nerve to obtain additional information on spinal cord function.

During all surgeries, regardless of the level, I monitor brachial plexus function using the ulnar nerve response. The major source of brachial plexus dysfunction is improper positioning of the arms and shoulders on the operating table. I use the ulnar nerve, rather than the median, to monitor brachial plexus function

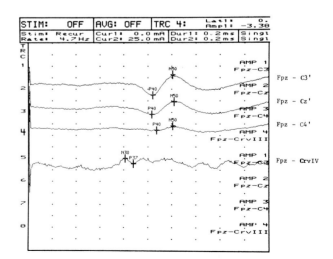

FIG. 3–10. Effect of recording montage on the cervical (Crv IV) and cortical somatosensory evoked potentials.

because it is more frequently involved in surgically induced plexopathies. Cortically recorded ulnar nerve responses are also helpful in ruling out the influence of presurgical variables (e.g., anesthetic effects) on data elicited by lower-limb stimulation. Only one nerve should be stimulated at a time. Bilateral, simultaneous stimulation reduces the sensitivity and specificity of the response to spinal cord damage.

A problem encountered during monitoring is the effect of peripheral neuropathies on the somatosensory evoked potential. Because the synchronicity of an evoked potential can be significantly influenced by this condition, it may be very difficult to record a reliable response. Although such a condition can make monitoring more difficult, it is still possible to obtain reliable data by modifying the elicitation and recording parameters: stimulating at sites more proximal than usual, such as the sciatic notch instead of the medial malleolus; using a slower presentation rate; increasing the duration and intensity of the stimulus; and collect-

ing smaller samples. It also helps to avoid fatiguing the response by alternating among the various stimulation sites.

Response Characteristics

Every response demonstrates certain characteristics that form the basis for interpretation. Figure 3-11 depicts a normal somatosensory evoked potential recorded during surgery after left and right posterior tibial nerve stimulation. Data were recorded between Crv4 and Crv5 and at C3', Cz', and C4'. Labeled on each of these traces are the latency and amplitude of the response, the two characteristics traditionally used for interpretation.

A reliable baseline response is essential for determining whether a response is abnormal. I recommend that the data recorded after skin incision be used as baseline, rather than using preoperative data. However, this is still in dispute. Keith, studying the effects

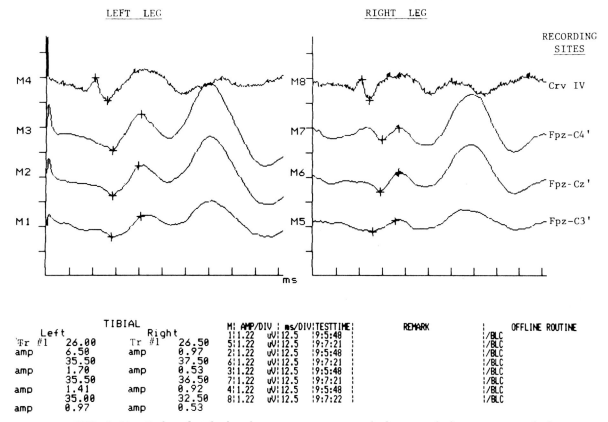

FIG. 3–11. Left and right baseline somatosensory evoked potentials from posterior tibial nerve stimulation, recorded during surgery.

of acquisition time on the response, found that the amplitude and latency of a response vary over time.[22] The greatest amount of variability occurred when preoperative data were compared with results obtained immediately after incision. He recommended that preoperative data be used to ascertain stimulation sites and to determine gross abnormalities in the response, but that postincisional data be used as baseline information during surgery.

To be considered a response, the data must meet four criteria. First, response morphology must be appropriate. Signals from a more central origin tend to be "slower" and last longer than peripheral signals (Fig. 3-11). For example, the P40 cortical response, after posterior tibial nerve stimulation, usually demonstrates a polyphasic, W-shaped pattern that is relatively long. Second, the within-leg test-retest latency of a suspected response must be reliable. The latency of a suspected response is reliable if the latencies of two responses are within 10% of each other. Third, the test-retest amplitude of a suspected response must demonstrate certain characteristics: the amplitude of the two trials from the same limb must be within 30% to 40% of each other, and the amplitudes of the responses from either limb must not differ by more than 50%. If the amplitude of the response from one limb is more than 50% smaller than the response from the other limb, the reduced data are considered to be abnormal.

As a fourth criterion, silent control periods are used to determine the existence or lack of a suspected response. In a silent control period, stimuli are presented at 0 mA and "data" recorded. The amplitude of a suspected response is then measured, and the cursor points are moved to the same latency points on the silent control data. To be considered a response, the amplitude of the suspected response must be at least twice that of the silent control. If amplitude of the suspected response is less than 50% of the silent control, then no response is present.

During surgery, I continuously monitor the spinal cord, especially during critical periods. Critical periods depend on the type of case, surgical approach, instrumentation used, and other factors, but they always include passing sublaminar wires, applying corrective force or derotation, and placement of a bone graft.

Interpretation

A review of the literature reveals a wide range of criteria being used to interpret data. In most methods,

amplitude of the response is considered to be a more valid indicator of the functional integrity of the nervous system than latency. Nuwer suggests warning the surgeon of a possible neurologic problem if response amplitude degrades by at least 50%.[34] Engler reported that amplitude degradation must be greater than 50% before warning the surgeon.[10] A more sensitive guideline has been recommended by Cohen and Huizenga.[5] They recommended warning the surgeon if the amplitude is reduced by only 20% and latency increases by 4%. However, these criteria may be too sensitive and may generate an unacceptable false-positive warning rate. Jones and colleagues investigated the criteria for pathologic changes in the somatosensory evoked potential during spinal cord monitoring.[19] The two response characteristics analyzed were amplitude and latency. Of these two characteristics, it was concluded that amplitude was more valid and sensitive than latency. They recommended that an amplitude reduction criteria of 60% of baseline values be used. They did not consider latency to be an adequately sensitive characteristic.

Lubicky and co-workers analyzed the normal within-subject variability of cortically recorded somatosensory evoked potentials, recorded from Fpz-Cz, during 291 consecutive spinal column surgeries.[26] Patients were classified according to diagnosis, neuromuscular status, age, and surgical procedure. Results indicated that normal variability of response latency and amplitude was associated with the type of pathology and the presence of neurologic disorders. For example, response variability, as indicated by the standard deviation, was least in patients with idiopathic scoliosis, but greatest in patients with cerebral palsy. The standard deviations of response amplitude were always greater than those of latency. Of the various components of the response, the P1-NI (P40) amplitude demonstrated greater variability than N1-P2 or P2-N2, but these differences were not statistically significant.

Described within the article was an interpretation method known as the Monitoring Quality Score (MQS).[26] The MQS is based on the repeatability of the response and its qualitative (morphology) and quantitative (latency and amplitude) characteristics. By using the MQS, the examiner is able to use more of the information contained within the response for interpretive decisions. Lubicky and colleagues concluded that cortically recorded somatosensory evoked potentials demonstrated too much variability to be considered a reliable method for routine use on all patients undergoing spinal surgery. They recommended that intraoperative monitoring is most appropriate for patients with high MQS ratings.

In a similar study, Abel and co-workers reported their experience using subcortical brainstem responses elicited by stimulating the posterior tibial nerve.[1] They reported similar difficulties in recording a cortical-somatosensory evoked potential in certain patient groups, especially those with cerebral palsy and neuromuscular diseases. However, instead of limiting the application of somatosensory evoked potential monitoring only to certain groups, they recommended that a subcortical brainstem response be used in conjunction with the cortical-somatosensory evoked potential. By using a subcortical brainstem response, a reliable and valid estimate of spinal cord function could be obtained from all groups of difficult-to-test patients.

Although I agree with Lubicky regarding the difficulty in obtaining a reliable cortical response in certain patient populations, I do not think that intraoperative monitoring should be limited to certain groups. Rather, our procedure makes use of multiple cortical recording sites and a subcortical brainstem site, similar to that of Abel's group and others.[1] It would seem appropriate to apply the MQS method of Lubicky to the cervical brainstem data described by Abel.[1, 26]

Based on published recommendations and personal experience, I have developed the following criteria for interpreting somatosensory evoked potentials:

1. Amplitude is the primary response characteristic used for interpreting data. If amplitude is reduced by 60% of baseline values, warn the surgeon of degraded data. If amplitude remains stable, without further degradation, no additional warnings are made.
2. If signals continue to demonstrate reductions in amplitude, inform the surgeon, and the appropriate intervention can be decided.
3. Inform the surgeon if absolute latency increases by more than 10%. However, latency is not considered a primary interpretative criterion.

In response to a warning, there are four possible intervention strategies available to the surgeon: no action can be taken; the surgeon can wait to determine if data will improve; a Stagnara wake-up test can be administered; or instrumentation can be immediately removed.

Taking no action implies that the surgeon has little confidence in the somatosensory evoked potential. Although early somatosensory evoked potential procedures demonstrated unacceptable false-positive and false-negative rates, current methods have reduced these rates significantly.

Waiting to see if data improve implies that the degradation was valid but due to a transient phenomenon. The primary, presurgical variables that can produce a significant but transient reduction of data are anesthesia, severe hypotension, and temperature. These influences can be easily ascertained through accurate record keeping and interpretation of the pattern of response degradation. To keep accurate records, graph cortical and cervical response amplitudes chronologically (Fig. 3-12). This is used to determine the onset of amplitude degradation and correlate it with possible surgical maneuvers.

The pattern of response degradation is used in determining whether the cause was surgical or presurgical. Table 3-3 lists the patterns that can occur and the

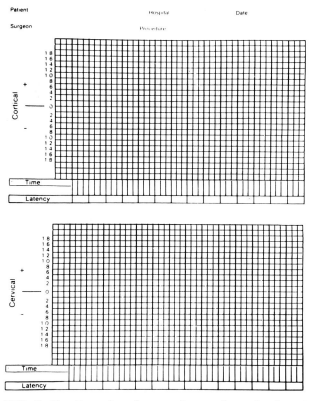

FIG. 3–12. Recording form used to track amplitudes of the cervical and Cz' cortical response.

TABLE 3-3. Possible Results from SEP Recordings
and Required Actions

Situation	Peripheral	Cervical	Cortical	Probable Source/Action
1	OK	OK	OK	No action required
2	OK	OK	NR*	Perisurgical/contact anesthesia
3	OK	NR	OK	Perisurgical/contact anesthesia
4	OK	NR	NR	Surgical/contact anesthesia and surgeon
5	NR	OK	OK	Instrumentation
6	NR	NR	NR	Instrumentation

*NR, no response.

steps the examiner should take in response to them. If data were lost due to anesthetic effects, only the cortical response(s) should be degraded, not the cervical. If this pattern occurs, the examiner needs to contact the anesthesiologist and not the surgeon. If severe hypotension occurs (usually a mean arterial pressure of 50 mm Hg), the cervical and cortical data are degraded or lost. However, levels of hypotension this severe may indicate a more serious condition. Although temperature affects the somatosensory evoked potential, it is easy to ascertain by checking the patient's temperature. As indicated by Table 3-3, most conditions that affect the somatosensory evoked potential are presurgical. By using the various patterns of responses, it is possible to determine that response degradation is due to surgical or presurgical variables. It is very important to ascertain the reason(s) for the degraded data before informing the surgeon.

If response degradation is due to a surgical event, the surgeon will typically administer a Stagnara wake-up test by reversing all anesthetic agents and muscle relaxants and waking the patient to a level of consciousness adequate to determine the motor status of upper and lower limbs. To conduct a successful wake-up test, it is necessary to keep the anesthesiologist informed of the possibility of conducting this test. It often requires 10 to 15 minutes to awaken the patient to a level of consciousness adequate to assess motor status. This test should be rehearsed with the patient before surgery.

Although the Stagnara wake-up test provides information about the patient's motor status, the test has weaknesses. It may require more than 15 minutes for the patient to achieve an adequate level of consciousness for determining motor status. If the cause for the

loss of evoked potentials is not removed as soon as possible, the probability of permanent neurologic deficit increases. In 1989, my colleagues and I reported the incidence of paraplegia in hogs based on the duration of lost evoked potentials.[38] We found that the longer the evoked potentials were absent, the greater the likelihood of paraplegia. Therefore, motor function and the need to remove spinal instrumentation should be determined as soon as possible.

The timing of the wake-up test is also important. In the same 1989 study, we found that it required approximately 20 minutes to lose the somatosensory evoked potentials after the onset of overcorrection and an additional 6 minutes for paraplegia to occur.[38] If the wake-up test is administered before the onset of the neurologic deficit, test results will be negative and instrumentation may not be removed, but the patient could still demonstrate a neurologic deficit after recovery from anesthesia.

The two benefits associated with the wake-up test are that its administration raises blood pressure and that it provides a behavioral indication of motor status. If the cause for the degraded somatosensory evoked potential is ischemia of the spinal cord, increasing blood pressure may re-establish spinal cord perfusion if done as soon as possible. In a second study, we demonstrated that if spinal cord perfusion was reduced by more than 65% for more than 6 minutes, all of the animals demonstrated a wake-up test positive for paraplegia. However, if blood flow was maintained above this value, there was a greater probability of a negative wake-up test.[38]

The final option available to the surgeon is releasing the corrective force produced by spinal instrumentation. This appears to be the quickest way to alleviate many of the deleterious forces acting on the spinal cord.

Brachial Plexus Monitoring

A problem associated with spinal surgical procedures is the possible compression of peripheral nerves caused by the patient's position on the operating table. Although compression of any nerve can occur, one of the most frequent sites is the brachial plexus.

Brachial plexus compression typically results from pressure exerted by the frame that the patient is lying on or from "rolls" placed under the shoulders. It appears that this type of compression or stretch occurs most frequently in patients who are very heavy or very thin.

The traditional method to avoid brachial plexus injuries is to position the upper arms so that there is a 90° flexion angle at the elbow and at the shoulder. Although this "90–90" approach usually is adequate, some patients still have nerve compression. Therefore, my colleagues and I prefer a "60–60" position.

We monitor brachial plexus function throughout surgery by stimulating the ulnar nerve and recording the response at C4. We use the ulnar nerve, rather than the median, because this nerve enters the spinal cord at a lower level and provides additional information about that structure. By monitoring the ulnar nerve, we are also able to ascertain if a degraded cortical-somatosensory evoked potential to posterior tibial nerve stimulation is the result of surgical or presurgical

variables. We typically stimulate the ulnar nerve at the ulnar groove to avoid the intravenous lines placed for anesthesia. We have had several cases in which the ulnar nerve response was degraded due to pressure on the brachial plexus. The effects were reversed by repositioning the patient's arm and shoulder (see Clinical Example 5).

Clinical Examples

Example 1. Normal Variability

Somatosensory evoked potentials demonstrate a certain amount of variability that is not attributable to any specific event and that is considered to be normal. Figure 3-13 demonstrates the normal variability of the somatosensory evoked potential recorded from Crv4 and from the Fpz-Cz' cortical site. Both responses demonstrate fluctuations in amplitude and latency that should be taken into consideration when developing criteria for interpreting test results.

Example 2. Anesthetic Effects

Somatosensory evoked potentials were recorded from Crv4 and from cortical sites at Fpz-C3', -Cz, and -C4' (Fig. 3-14). Data were recorded midway through surgery, after administering 0.75% of forane (Isoforane), and 30 minutes after the cessation of this anesthetic agent. Nitrous oxide levels remained constant at 40%. Cervical (Fpz-Crv 4) data remained well-formed and

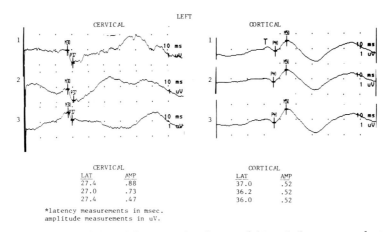

FIG. 3–13. Normal variability of the cervical and cortical (Fpz-Cz') responses during surgery.

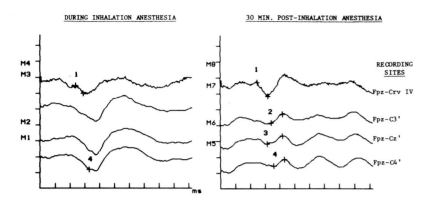

FIG. 3–14. Response to inhalation anesthesia (0.6% halothane) by cervical and cortical somatosensory evoked potentials.

morphologically robust compared with the cortical data. These results suggest that subcortical recording sites, proximal to the level of surgery, must be used in conjunction with cortical sites if the effects from anesthesia are to be discriminated from surgical variables.

Example 3. True-Positive Somatosensory Evoked Potential

Figure 3-15 depicts the test-retest reliability of the somatosensory evoked potential to stimulation of the right posterior tibial nerve after skin incision. Reliable data were obtained from the popliteal fossa (PF), Crv4, and Fpz-Cz'. Left leg data (not shown) were equivalent to right leg results.

Figure 3-16 depicts the right leg somatosensory evoked potentials, from the patient depicted in Figure 3-15, after overcorrection of the cauda equina while reducing a high grade spondylolisthesis. A reliable

response was still present at the popliteal fossa, but no reliable response was present at the cervical or cortical recording sites. The results from the left leg remained unchanged. Results from an initial intraoperative Stagnara wake-up test demonstrated no gross motor movement in the right leg, but grossly normal movement in the left. Instrumentation was removed, and a second wake-up test was initiated. Before conducting the second wake-up test, right leg somatosensory evoked potentials returned to baseline values. Results on the second wake-up test revealed normal motor function bilaterally. No further attempts to place instrumentation were made, and an in situ fusion was accepted.

Example 4. Lesioning of Dorsomedial Tract

Figures 3-17 and 3-18 depict the somatosensory evoked potentials recorded between T10 and T11 and cortically during a surgery to biopsy an intramedullary

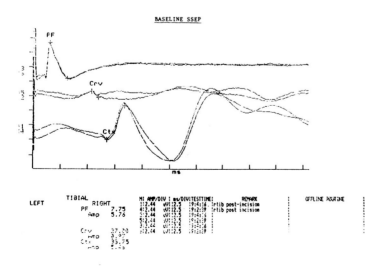

FIG. 3–15. Baseline somatosensory evoked potentials recorded during surgery after skin incision. Only data following right posterior tibial nerve stimulation are shown; left leg data were equivalent.

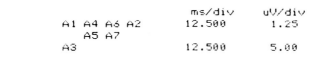

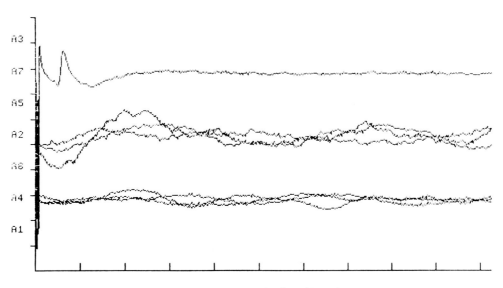

True Positive SSEP Indication

FIG. 3–16. Somatosensory evoked potentials (SEP) in response to right leg stimulation after too much distractive force was applied to the spinal cord. Left leg data were lost also.

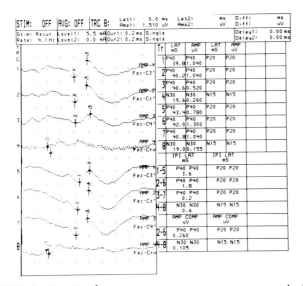

FIG. 3–17. Baseline intraoperative somatosensory evoked potentials in response to left and right leg stimulation, recorded at T10–T11 and cortically.

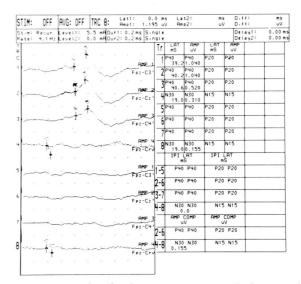

FIG. 3–18. Left and right somatosensory evoked potentials in response to lesioning right dorsal column. These data are from the same patient as in Figure 3-17.

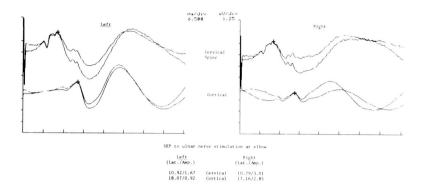

FIG. 3–19. Baseline intraoperative somatosensory evoked potentials (SEP) in response to ulnar nerve stimulation at the ulnar groove.

tumor at T2. Somatosensory evoked potentials were elicited by unilaterally stimulating the left and right posterior tibial nerve.

Baseline values (Fig. 3-17) depict reliable and well-formed data from all recording sites. Data remained stable until the surgeon attempted to biopsy the tumor. The right leg data demonstrated minor, nonsignificant fluctuations during manipulation of the spinal cord.

Figure 3-18 depicts the somatosensory evoked potentials elicited by left and right leg stimulation after removal of the biopsy material from the spinal cord. Right leg data were immediately lost from recording sites proximal to the biopsy site. The more distal thoracic site remained stable, as did the data from the left leg stimulation. After awakening from anesthesia, the patient demonstrated normal gross motor movements bilaterally. Sensory status was grossly normal in the left leg, but paresthesia was present in the right leg.

Example 5. Brachial Plexus Compression

A complication associated with positioning a patient on the operating table, especially when a four-post frame is used, is compression or stretch of the brachial plexus. Figures 3-19, 3-20, and 3-21 depict somatosensory evoked potentials elicited by right and left ulnar nerve stimulation at the elbow, recorded from the cervical vertebra and cortically. Because of our recording techniques, only cervical data were used to interpret the functional integrity of the brachial plexus.

Baseline values (Fig. 3-19) demonstrate reliable, well-formed, and robust proximal data. Midway through the surgery, data from right ulnar nerve stimulation demonstrated a significant degradation attributed to the position of that arm (Fig. 3-20). The right arm and shoulder were repositioned, and the ulnar nerve response for that arm returned almost to the baseline value (Fig. 3-21).

MOTOR EVOKED POTENTIALS

An important limitation of monitoring techniques using somatosensory evoked potentials is that the response only measures the integrity of the sensory system. Based on the anatomic proximity of the motor and sensory tracts, it was assumed that a surgical variable affecting motor tract function would also affect the sensory tracts and that damage to the motor tracts would degrade the somatosensory evoked potentials. However, a number of studies have reported false-negative results for paraplegia when using somatosensory evoked potentials as a measure of "total" spinal cord function.

In 1985, Ginsburg and co-workers reported a case

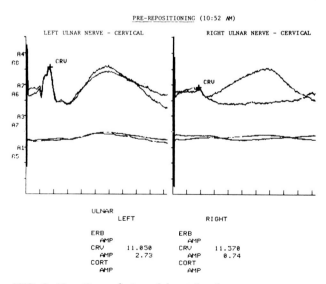

FIG. 3–20. Degradation of the right ulnar nerve response due to improper positioning of that arm. Left arm data show no significant change.

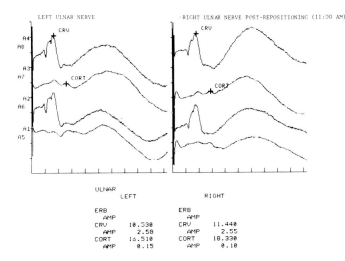

FIG. 3–21. Effects from repositioning of the right arm on the right ulnar somatosensory evoked potential.

study of a 12-year-old achondroplastic dwarf undergoing a two-stage procedure for progressive kyphosis.[11] Before surgery, the patient was neurologically normal. During the initial surgery, somatosensory evoked potentials remained stable, and the patient demonstrated no postoperative neurologic deficits. During the second surgery 3 weeks later, somatosensory evoked potentials remained stable, and data at closure were equivalent to baseline values. After awakening from anesthesia, the patient had severe motor deficits.

Dinner and colleagues reported on the correlation rates of somatosensory evoked potentials with postoperative clinical status.[7] Of the 220 cases monitored, there was a true-negative agreement in 209 (95%) of the patients. This means that there were no significant changes in the somatosensory evoked potentials or clinical status of the patients. In 3 (1.36%) of the remaining 11 cases, the somatosensory evoked potentials demonstrated a significant change during surgery, and the patients were found to have postoperative neurologic deficits. Two of these patients demonstrated paraparesis, and the third had a flaccid paraplegia. Four (1.82%) of the remaining 8 patients demonstrated a significant change in the somatosensory evoked potential, but no postoperative neurologic deficits. In the remaining 4 patients (1.82%), the somatosensory evoked potentials remained stable during surgery, but the patients demonstrated postoperative neurologic deficits. No delineation of the types of deficits was provided.

Although studies and case reports indicate that somatosensory evoked potentials do provide information about the functional integrity of the spinal cord, dam-

age to the motor tracts can occur without influencing the somatosensory evoked potentials. Motor evoked potentials must also be monitored to ensure the integrity of the spinal cord. Procedures that can elicit a motor evoked potential can be grossly divided into methods that use cortical or spinal cord stimulation.[25, 28, 31, 36]

Anatomy and Physiology

The motor cortex demonstrates an arrangement similar to that of the somatosensory system. The neural architecture of the lower extremities is arranged medially, and the array for the face, tongue, and related parts occurs more laterally. This arrangement is also maintained within the spinal cord tracts: lower extremity representation is medial and upper extremity organization is lateral.

The pathway that leads from the motor cortex to the spinal cord without interruption is the corticospinal tract. The other efferent pathways are interrupted in the basal ganglia and brain stem. Because the corticospinal tract proceeds through the section of the brainstem called the pyramids, this pathway is also known as the pyramidal tract. The remaining efferent pathways that do not pass through the pyramids are known as the extrapyramidal tracts.

The axons that leave the motor cortex first run through the internal capsule, between the thalamus and basal ganglia, and into the brainstem. Upon entering the brainstem, the majority of the fibers decussate and travel down the spinal cord in the posterolateral quadrant. The remaining fibers run uncrossed down the anterolateral sections of the spinal cord. Most of the fibers in the crossed and uncrossed tracts terminate within the spinal cord. Only a few of the crossed fibers synapse directly on a motoneuron.

After terminating within the spinal cord, the majority of the first-order neurons synapse on an interneuron. The interneuron subsequently synapses on the motoneuron located within the anterior horn of the spinal cord. Crossed efferent fibers synapse on interneurons located ipsilateral to the descending tract. The uncrossed fibers, however, can synapse with interneurons ipsilateral and contralateral to its side of descent.

The physiology of the motor systems reflects the rapid motor requirements of the peripheral musculature, which is afforded by anatomic efficiency. Consequently, it is possible to stimulate the motor system using typical stimulation rates without a significant degradation of the evoked potential. The rate used to elicit a motor evoked potential varies with the site of stimulation and the type of response recorded. For example, my colleagues and I have elicited a reliable neurogenic motor evoked potential using high rates, but our typical clinical rate is much less. When implementing a motor evoked potential procedure, it is necessary to use rates appropriate for that method.

Cortical Stimulation

One of the first reports of cortical stimulation was that of Penfield and Jasper.[41] In that report, direct stimulation of the cerebral cortex was performed to identify the motor cortex. More practical cortical stimulation techniques use transosseous rather than direct stimulation of the cerebral cortex.

Transosseous stimulation of the cerebral cortex uses stimulating electrodes placed on the surface of the skull. A stimulus of adequate intensity is administered, and an electromyographic response is recorded peripherally. Various arrays of stimulating electrodes have been reported in the literature. Merton and Morton reported using a bipolar stimulation method that used two leads placed on the scalp over the motor strip.[31] An alternative transosseous stimulation method reported by other research teams uses a singular anodal lead placed over the motor strip and a cathode "ring" electrode placed around the scalp.[15, 43, 44] According to Rossini, regardless of the location of the stimulating electrodes, anodal stimulation elicits motor evoked potentials at lower-intensity levels than cathode stimula-

tion.[44] Motor evoked potentials are elicited at lower-intensity levels using the unipolar method described by Rossini and colleagues than with the bipolar stimulation described by Merton and Morton.[31, 43]

Levy and co-workers reported several studies that used spinal cord and transosseous stimulation to elicit the motor evoked potential.[24, 25] Initial studies used direct stimulation of the spinal cord. This method was considered to be too invasive, motivating the development of a bipolar transosseous method. The transosseous method was administered to animals and humans undergoing various surgeries, and the results were found to be more consistent with the patient's motor status than somatosensory evoked potentials.

Although transosseous stimulation of the motor cortex elicits a motor evoked potential, there has been a general reluctance by the clinical community to accept this technique. Nuwer reported that this method of stimulation elicits contraction of large muscle groups, which reduces the sensitivity and specificity of the response.[34] Additionally, fears of triggering an epileptic seizure or kindling patterns exist. Levy and his colleagues monitored the EEG before and after stimulation and did not detect any changes in this activity. However, Nuwer recommends preoperative and postoperative monitoring of the EEG in patients administered this procedure. This type of stimulation should be avoided if the patient's EEG shows inherent abnormalities.

Because transosseous stimulation of the cortex also elicits activity in the brainstem, in the cerebellum, and antidromically in the sensory system, there is an antidromic sensory component to the recorded peripheral response.[2, 49] Another limitation is that it is very difficult to record a reliable lower limb response after electrical stimulation of the brain. Although a reliable upper limb response is easily elicited and recorded, lower limb data are much more difficult to elicit and record, limiting the application of the procedure to surgeries involving the cervical spine.

An alternative method for stimulating the cortex is to use magnetic rather than electrical stimulation.[4] Magnetic elicitation requires a wire coil to be placed in the proximity of the motor strip and electrical current delivered to the coil. The resultant magnetic field produces lines of flux that stimulate underlying tissue, causing excitation.

To determine the relationship between the electromyographic motor evoked potentials elicited by electrical and magnetic stimulation, Cracco and associates elicited upper limb electromyographic motor evoked potentials in two awake humans.[6] The responses elicited by the stimuli were similar in morphology and amplitude, but the magnetically elicited response was longer in duration. However, the electrically induced response was obtained at lower intensity levels than the magnetically elicited response. Patient discomfort, attributed to contraction of facial musculature, was less with the magnetic stimulus than with the electrical.

Investigation of magnetic elicitation techniques is accelerating, but this method is still considered to be investigative. There are several limitations associated with its intraoperative use. The most significant limitation is the influence of anesthesia on the response. In the awake individual, it is possible to record an electromyographic-motor evoked potential elicited by a magnetic pulse from the upper and lower limbs. However, after anesthesia, the response quickly fades, and it is very difficult to record a reliable response, especially from the lower limbs. Consequently, this method for eliciting motor evoked potentials is not yet considered to be clinically applicable.

Spinal Cord Stimulation

An alternative to cortical stimulation is stimulation of the spinal cord. Several methods have been reported in the literature. Levy and colleagues reported a method that used direct stimulation of the motor tract between the intermediolateral sulcus and the dentate ligament in cats and humans.[25] This method required exposure and direct stimulation of the spinal cord. This method is considered to be too invasive for practical use, especially during corrective spinal surgery for scoliosis.

A less invasive method for stimulating the spinal cord was reported by Machida and co-workers.[28] A pair of stimulating electrodes was placed within the epidural space, proximal to the level of surgery. Stimulating electrodes must be placed midline and on the posterior side of the spinal cord. Placed in this position, reliable electromyographic-motor evoked potentials can be simultaneously recorded from both lower extremities. In a later study, Machida reported on the relationship between electromyographic-motor evoked potentials elicited by stimulating the spinal cord and mixed-nerve somatosensory evoked potentials.[29] In every case of postoperative paraplegia, the electromyographic-motor evoked potentials demonstrated

significant degradation and eventual loss, but somatosensory evoked potentials were not lost.

Several limitations are associated with the use of epidural stimulating electrodes. First, placement of the stimulating electrodes requires that the epidural space of the spinal cord be accessible proximal to the site of surgery. To accomplish this, a laminectomy is made, and the electrodes are inserted into the epidural space. A second limitation is the orientation of the stimulating electrode to the spinal cord. In a 1988 study, Machida's group reported that orientation of the stimulating electrode to the spinal cord can influence test results.[30] If the electrodes were placed midline and on the posterior side of the spinal cord, reliable data could be simultaneously recorded from both lower limbs. However, as the location of the stimulating electrodes became more anterior, the electromyographic-motor evoked potential from the contralateral limb was lost. No reliable lower-limb response could be elicited from either leg if the stimulating electrodes were placed on the anterior side of the spinal cord.

Tamaki and colleagues described a method of stimulating the spinal cord using an epidural technique, but recording from the spinal cord. This spine-to-spine response is neurogenic in origin, polyphasic in morphology, but smaller, in amplitude than the myogenic-motor evoked potential.[50-52] According to Tamaki, the response is more sensitive than somatosensory evoked potentials to the patient's clinical motor status. The approach demonstrates several advantages over motor evoked potential procedures that record a myogenic response. Although an electromyographic-motor evoked potential is considered to be a true motor evoked potential, its clinical application is very difficult. During surgery, the total muscle relaxation by the patient that is advantageous to the surgeon makes it very difficult to record the myogenically based electromyographic-motor evoked potential. If muscle relaxant levels are titrated, a response can be recorded, but because the level of relaxation is not constant, the amplitude and morphology of the response varies. Consequently, these two characteristics cannot be used for interpretation. Responses can only be interpreted as "present" or "absent," which reduces the sensitivity of the response to changes in neurologic status. The method reported by Tamaki, however, records a response that is neurogenic in origin, which permits the use of muscle relaxants during the surgery and avoids the problems associated with monitoring a myogenic response.

Although recording a neurogenic response avoids the problems associated with a myogenic-motor evoked potential, it also demonstrates several limitations. Like the Machida method, epidural electrodes are used to elicit the response, and the limitations associated with the Machida method also affect the Tamaki method. Sabato and co-workers reported the influence of placement of the stimulating electrode on spinal cord integrity.[45] In their study, pairs of stimulating electrodes were placed within the epidural space and into the base of the spinous process. The latter case, known as translaminar stimulation, was described by my colleagues and me.[36] Sabato reported that histologic and neurologic changes occurred in the spinal cord of 50% of the rats in which epidural placement was used. None of the animals demonstrated any histologic, structural, or biochemical changes in their spinal cords when translaminar placement was used. Translaminar placement appears to be a safer way of stimulating the spinal cord than epidural placement of electrodes.

Orientation of the epidural stimulating electrodes to the spinal cord also influences test results.[30] Because spinal cord stimulation elicits activity within both lower limbs simultaneously, it is necessary to ensure that stimulating electrodes are placed at midline. If placement is off midline, data from the contralateral limb will be degraded. Although a stiffer electrode can reduce placement problems, it is possible to introduce it into the spinal cord during epidural placement.

A response recorded from the spinal cord after spinal cord stimulation contains orthodromic motor activity and antidromic sensory activity. This is a limitation of all motor evoked potential responses that record a neurogenic response. Consequently, it is difficult to discriminate between these two components if the distance between stimulating and recording electrodes is small. If the distance between stimulating and recording electrodes can be increased, it is possible to take advantage of the conduction velocity differences exhibited by the sensory and motor fibers. This can be accomplished by recording a spine-to-peripheral nerve response.

To determine the relative sensitivity of spine-to-spine and spine-to-peripheral nerve responses to spinal cord lesioning, both potentials were recorded in hogs before and after overdistraction of the spinal cord.[37] Results indicated that if the spine-to-spine response was used as the index of onset of overdistraction, 100% of the animals demonstrated nonreversible

paraplegia. If, however, the peripheral nerve response was used as the index, it was possible to reverse the deleterious effects in 100% of the cases. This suggests that spine-to-spine recordings are not as sensitive to the onset of overdistraction as a spine-to-peripheral nerve response.

In 1988, my colleagues and I reported the development of a procedure that stimulated the spinal cord with an electrical stimulus to elicit a motor evoked potential.[36] Rather than eliciting a myogenic-motor evoked potential, the method elicited a motor evoked potential that was neurogenic in origin. By using electrical stimulation of the spinal cord, we avoided the numerous problems associated with transosseous stimulation of the motor cortex using electrical or magnetic stimuli. By recording a neurogenic response, total muscle relaxation could be achieved during surgery, which facilitated the surgical technique and allowed us to use amplitude and morphology to interpret test results. Based on its neurogenic origins, the response was labeled the neurogenic-motor evoked potential.

To elicit the response, stimulating electrodes are placed into the spinous process at the proximal end of the incision. The response is recorded using bipolar electrodes placed over the sciatic nerve, at the sciatic notch, and at the popliteal fossa. More distal recording sites can also be used to record the response.

Elicitation and Recording

Electrodes

My colleagues and I have tried different brands of commercially available stimulating electrodes, and they each have limitations. For example, because the electrode is being inserted into bone, the needle portion must be very strong. Because of this and other limitations we have developed a 0.5-in (1.3-cm) needle electrode that is approximately 23 gauge and made of stainless steel (The Electrode Store, Yucca Valley, CA). We strongly recommend our JO-5 electrode for eliciting the neurogenic-motor evoked potentials.

Recording Sites

We use several sites to record the neurogenic-motor evoked potential during surgery, including the sciatic notch and popliteal fossa. Because both legs are considered to be "active," after spinal cord stimulation, it is necessary to use a bipolar recording montage. Figure 3-22 displays typical responses obtained at these two sites. Recording electrodes at the sciatic notch consist

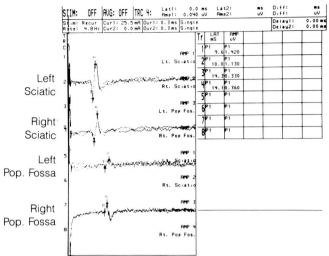

Left
Sciatic

Right
Sciatic

Left
Pop. Fossa

Right
Pop. Fossa

FIG. 3–22. Baseline intraoperative neurogenic motor evoked potentials recorded from the right and left legs at the sciatic notch and popliteal fossa.

of "monopolar" electromyographic electrodes. The entire electrode, except for 0.5 in (1.3 cm) at its distal end, is insulated (The Electrode Store, Yucca Valley, CA). The electrodes at the popliteal fossa are subcutaneous needle electrodes and are the same ones used to record the peripheral somatosensory evoked potential after posterior tibial nerve stimulation.

Table 3-4 displays the acquisition parameters we use to elicit and record the neurogenic-motor evoked potential. To keep acquisition parameters simple, we use the same presentation rate used with the somatosensory evoked potential. However, much faster presentation rates can be used to elicit the neurogenic-motor evoked potential without significant response degradation.[35] The major differences between the so-

matosensory evoked potential and neurogenic-motor evoked potential settings are the filter band widths used, time base, and sample size. We use filter settings typical of those used for the peripheral somatosensory evoked potential. The time base is much shorter than that used with the somatosensory evoked potentials because of the smaller distance between stimulating and recording electrodes. We used much smaller sample sizes because the neurogenic-motor evoked potential is much larger and easier to distinguish than the somatosensory evoked potential.

Stimulation Sites

To elicit the neurogenic-motor evoked potential, we place stimulating electrodes into the spinous processes

TABLE 3-4. Parameters for Recording Four-Channel NMEPs to Spinal Cord Stimulation*

Parameters	Chn. 1	Chn. 2	Chn. 3	Chn. 4
Sensitivity (μV)	10–25	10–25	10–25	10–25
Low linear filter	10	10	10	10
High linear filter	2000	2000	2000	2000
Notch filter	Off	Off	Off	Off
Referential	L-Sci 1	R-Sci 1	L-PF 1	R-PF 1
Active	L-Sci 2	R-Sci 2	L-PF 2	R-PF 2
Artifact reject.	On	On	On	On
Timebase (msec)	55	55	55	55
Rate	4.8/sec	Swp:100	Trg:Int	
Duration	200 μsec			

*Recording included 2 sciatic and 2 popliteal fossa NMEPs.

(Fig. 3-23). There are two possible placement sites: the base of the spinous process or in the process after its tip has been removed. Both stimulation sites yield reliable, well-formed responses. However, if the electrodes are placed in the base of the process, fluids in the surgical site can accumulate and shunt current away from the spinal cord. We prefer to place the electrodes into the cancellous bone of the spinous process. At either site, the stimulating electrodes must be within 1 cm of the cord, and we place the electrodes so that there is a minimum of 2.5 cm between them. This can be conveniently achieved by placing each electrode at a different spinal level. We do not recommend placing the electrodes into the interspinous ligament because they could inadvertently damage the spinal cord.

The surgeon places the anode electrode proximal to the cathode. Otherwise, greater intensity levels are needed to elicit the neurogenic-motor evoked potential. The eliciting stimulus should always be set at the lowest level required for a reliable response. This minimal effective level varies among patients. We routinely perform an intensity-output function determination for each patient to assess the appropriate presentation level.

Response Characteristics

Figure 3-22 depicts the normal neurogenic-motor evoked potential elicited during surgery and recorded at the sciatic notch and at the popliteal fossa. The response consists of a sharp, biphasic component at both sites. The response at the popliteal fossa also contains a smaller, polyphasic component that typically overlaps the larger, biphasic component.

Based on lesioning and collision studies, my colleagues and I have found that the large, biphasic component originates in motor neurons and that the smaller, polyphasic component is sensory.[39] This morphologic relationship is supported by the conduction velocities of the motor and sensory fibers making up the sciatic nerve. In general, the motor fibers demonstrate a faster conduction velocity than the sensory fibers. The sensory fibers can be divided into a greater number of small groups based on size and conduction velocity than the motor fibers. This breakdown according to velocity contributes to the polyphasic characteristics of the sensory component.

Interpretation

To interpret the neurogenic-motor evoked potential during surgery, we base our judgments primarily on the amplitude of the motor component and secondarily on its latency. Results from our animal studies indicated that amplitude demonstrates a greater sensitivity than latency to the functional integrity of the spinal cord motor tracts. Unlike the mixed-nerve somatosensory evoked potential, however, the continued presence of the neurogenic-motor evoked potential indicates that the motor tracts are still intact and that paraplegia has not occurred. We inform the surgeon of amplitude degradations of at least 60%, but this does

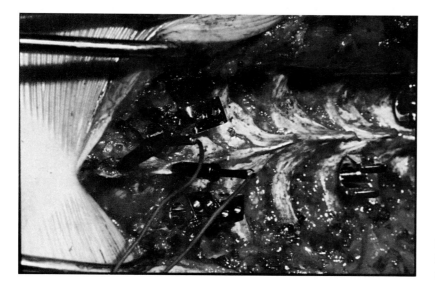

FIG. 3–23. Photograph of the stimulating electrode used to elicit the neurogenic motor evoked potential.

not warrant the administration of a wake-up test. However, if amplitude continues to degrade after this initial warning, some form of intervention is considered. The most typical form of intervention is the administration of the Stagnara wake-up test.

Research in Neurogenic-Motor Evoked Potentials

Since 1988, my colleagues and I have investigated the relationship between sensitivity and specificity of neurogenic-motor evoked potentials, somatosensory evoked potentials, and clinical status in animals.[36, 38, 39] To determine this relationship, we administered various maneuvers (e.g., overdistraction, compression, ischemia) to the spinal cord and recorded their effects on the evoked potentials and the animal's clinical status. Clinical status was based on results from the Stagnara wake-up test. Because the effects from overdistraction are directly applicable to spinal deformity surgery, the results from these studies are reported here. The two variables that we investigated were the level of overdistraction and duration of lost neurogenic-motor evoked potentials.

Level of Overdistraction

To determine the relationship between level of overdistraction and spinal cord function, we segregated 22 hogs into three groups based on their level of osteotomies: T5–T6 (n = 9), T12–L1 (n = 7), and L3–L4 (n = 6). In the hog, the spinal cord extends to S4. Before osteotomy, pairs of Kostuik screws were placed proximal and distal to the level of osteotomy. After osteotomy, Harrington rods were inserted into the screws and distractive force was applied. At the onset of overdistraction, as indicated by a reduction in neurogenic-motor evoked potentials, we determined spinal cord blood flow using hydrogen clearance methods. Neurogenic-motor evoked potentials were elicited by stimulating the spinal cord proximal to the level of overdistraction; somatosensory evoked potentials were elicited by stimulating the equivalent of the posterior tibial nerve. Evoked potentials were recorded from the high and low spine and from each sciatic nerve. Clinical status was determined by administering the Stagnara wake-up test.

Results indicated that the amount of distractive force that could be administered varied with the level of the spine. In the stiffer thoracic segments of the spine, only two to three ratchets of distraction could be

applied before neurogenic-motor evoked potentials were lost. In the more flexible lumbar spine, four to six ratchets could be applied before data were lost.

Results from the Stagnara wake-up test indicated that neurogenic-motor evoked potentials always correlated with clinical status but the somatosensory evoked potentials did not. Specifically, neurogenic-motor evoked potentials demonstrated no false-positive or false-negative responses; somatosensory evoked potentials demonstrated no false-positive responses but did have a 14% false-negative rate, confirming that the somatosensory evoked potentials could not guarantee that the animal's motor tracts were functionally intact.

The time-to-loss of the evoked potentials fell into two categories: fast and slow. In the fast-loss group, neurogenic-motor evoked potentials were lost within 2 minutes and were always associated with structural changes in the spinal cord. In the slow-loss group, neurogenic-motor evoked potentials required almost 24 minutes to be lost and were associated with a reduction of spinal cord perfusion but no structural changes. The fast-loss group occurred in the stiffer segments of the spine, and the slow-loss group occurred in the more flexible segments.

Duration of Lost Evoked Potentials

To determine the relationship between duration of lost evoked potentials and clinical status, we administered an osteotomy to 20 hogs at L3–L4. Distractive force was applied by using Kostuik screws and Harrington rods. Neurogenic-motor evoked potentials and somatosensory evoked potentials were elicited and recorded as described in the previous section.

Neurogenic-motor evoked potentials were lost about 2 minutes sooner than somatosensory evoked potentials. All animals demonstrated a slow rather than a fast loss of data. After data were lost, the percentage of positive results on the Stagnara wake-up test increased with the duration of lost neurogenic-motor evoked potentials. If neurogenic-motor evoked potentials were lost more than 6 minutes, 100% of the animals demonstrated a positive wake-up test (i.e., neurologic deficits); for 5 to 6 minutes, 75% demonstrated a positive wake-up test; and for 5 minutes, 25% demonstrated a positive wake-up test. If neurogenic-motor evoked potentials were lost less than 4 minutes, none of the animals demonstrated any gross neurologic problems on the wake-up test. These values indicate that the longer the neurogenic-motor evoked potentials are lost, the greater the likelihood of positive results on the

Stagnara wake-up test. However, total times (i.e., time to loss plus duration of lost data) are more important than the duration of lost data alone. This point is important because it helps define the relationship between efficacy of intervention and the elapsed time following the deleterious maneuver..

Clinical Examples

Figure 3-24 depicts the baseline neurogenic-motor evoked potential recorded from a patient undergoing surgery for a bilateral motor tract cordotomy for uncontrolled spasticity of the lower limbs. Baseline values were well-formed and reliable. Somatosensory evoked

potentials (not pictured) were well-formed and within normal limits bilaterally.

Figure 3-25 depicts the neurogenic-motor evoked potentials after lesioning of the primary motor tracts. Data were lost immediately, and the patient awoke with and maintained lower-limb flaccidity. Somatosensory evoked potentials to posterior tibial nerve stimulation remained unchanged.

DERMATOMAL EVOKED POTENTIALS

Although mixed-nerve somatosensory evoked potentials and motor evoked potentials can be used to moni-

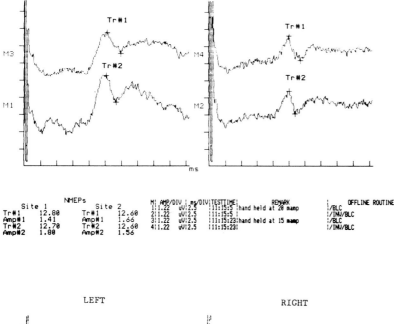

FIG. 3–24. Baseline intraoperative neurogenic motor evoked potentials (NMEPs).

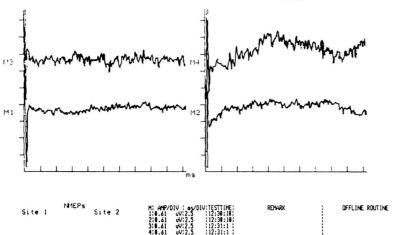

FIG. 3–25. Abnormal neurogenic motor evoked potentials (NMEPs) after bilateral rhizotomy of all the ventral roots innervating the lower limbs.

tor spinal cord function during surgery, neither of these procedures provides information about single nerve root function. The purpose of this section is to describe other electrophysiologic techniques used to monitor single nerve root function during surgery.

More than 200,000 patients undergo some type of surgery for herniated disks each year; 56% to 95% of the patients had relief from pain after surgery.[43, 51] To improve the surgical outcome of these cases, attempts were made to monitor single nerve root function using somatosensory evoked potentials. Because of multiple levels of innervation, the effects from degraded activity at one level is "masked" by normal activity at other levels. Consequently, mixed-nerve somatosensory evoked potentials demonstrate unacceptably low levels of sensitivity and specificity to single nerve root dysfunction.

To improve the sensitivity and specificity of detecting single nerve root dysfunction, two methods that elicit a dermatomal-somatosensory evoked potential have been developed: stimulating specific nerves (i.e., sural) or stimulating specific dermatomal fields.[8,27] Each method has advantages and disadvantages that must be taken into consideration when monitoring dermatomal-somatosensory evoked potentials.

Specific Nerve Stimulation

One of the first studies that attempted to ascertain single nerve root function was by Eisen and Elleker in 1980.[8] They stimulated peripheral nerves (i.e., ulnar, sural) in the upper and lower extremities and recorded the response peripherally and over the somatosensory cortex. The conduction velocities of the peripheral and cortical components were determined and interpreted as indicating the presence of a peripheral or intra-axial dysfunction. Data were recorded from 102 normal patients and 6 patients demonstrating various neurologic conditions, including lumbar radiculopathies (n = 2). Dermatomal-somatosensory evoked potentials from the 2 patients with lumbar radiculopathies correlated well with the physiologic and myelographic findings.

In a later study, Eisen and Horich recorded dermatomal-somatosensory evoked potentials from two groups of patients: Group 1 (n = 27) demonstrated various types of root lesions; Group 2 (n = 12) demonstrated plexopathies.[9] In addition to dermatomal-somatosensory evoked potentials, electromyographic responses, F-wave procedures, and myelograms were administered. Dermatomal-somatosensory evoked potentials agreed with clinical status in 70% and 75% of

the patients in these two groups, respectively. Compared with the other procedures administered, dermatomal-somatosensory evoked potentials correlated better with clinical status than F-waves, but slightly less than electromyographic responses or myelograms. False-positive results for all procedures were few, but normal dermatomal-somatosensory evoked potentials were recorded in 26% of patients for whom the responses should have been abnormal.

In a procedure similar to that reported by Eisen, Seyal and co-workers stimulated the saphenous, superficial peroneal, and sural nerves to obtain information about the L4, L5, and S1 nerve roots, respectively.[8, 9, 48] Responses were recorded at the root entry zone and over the somatosensory cortex. The rationalization for recording the response at the entry zone was the poor correlation between cortically recorded dermatomal-somatosensory evoked potentials and clinical status.[3] Results from 30 neurologically normal subjects indicated that the root potential was more reliable and less affected by the subject's state (e.g., sleep) than the cortical potential. Unfortunately, data on the correlation of the entry zone response with clinical status in patients demonstrating radiculopathies were not presented.

A limitation of stimulating the nerves cited in these studies is that no information is provided for the S2 to S4 segments. These nerve roots are directly involved with bowel and bladder control, and they must be monitored during surgeries that place them at risk (e.g., spondylolisthesis). In 1988, Neuwirth and colleagues used dermatomal-somatosensory evoked potentials from stimulation of the pudendal nerve to monitor the integrity of S2 to S4 segments during surgery in 16 patients.[33] This method, previously described by Haldeman and colleagues, consisted of stimulating the pudendal nerve with various electrode arrangements.[13, 14] In men, the response was elicited by placing ring electrodes at the base of the penis; in women, surface electrodes straddled the clitoris. In the Neuwirth study, responses were recorded over the somatosensory cortex, whereas in the Haldeman studies, responses were recorded over the spine and over the somatosensory cortex. Haldeman recommended using a spinal recording site because it allows the examiner to determine the time required by the nerve impulse to travel from the low spine to the somatosensory cortex. This measurement, known as the central conduction time, provides the examiner with information about the integrity of the peripheral and central segments of this neural pathway. Results indicated that a reliable response could be obtained from all recording sites using this stimulation technique, permitting the S2 to S4 segments to be monitored when necessary.

Methods that use specific nerve stimulation to elicit a dermatomal-somatosensory evoked potential demonstrate certain strengths and limitations that need to be considered when interpreting test results. By stimulating a peripheral nerve, such as the sural, the response is larger and more reliable than from stimulating a dermatomal field. Consequently, subject state (e.g., anesthetized) will demonstrate less influence on test results. A second advantage of stimulating a specific nerve is that peripheral (i.e., entry zone data) and cortical data can be recorded, allowing the examiner to determine the functional characteristics of the peripheral and central nervous systems. Typically, it is very difficult to record a reliable peripheral dermatomal-somatosensory evoked potential after stimulation of a dermatomal field.

Although dermatomal-somatosensory evoked potentials using specific nerves have certain advantages, there are also limitations associated with the procedure. First, by stimulating a specific nerve, no information about single nerve root function is obtained because the nerves enter the spinal cord at multiple levels. For example, superficial peroneal nerve stimulation elicits activity at L4, L5, and S1, and sural nerve stimulation evokes activity at S1 and S2. Multilevel activity reduces the sensitivity and specificity of the results to single nerve root involvement. Procedures that use this method of stimulation acknowledge this limitation, but proponents contend that the stimulated nerve consists of fibers predominately from one spinal level.[48] A second limitation is that this method of stimulation may activate the faster conducting group I muscle afferents rather than the slower conducting cutaneous afferents. This may explain the differences in the response latencies reported in several studies.[3, 8, 9, 48] A third limitation is that, during surgery for degenerative disc disease, it may not be possible to place a recording electrode at the root entry zone because of interference with the surgical field. This allows only the cortical response to be recorded and eliminates the use of a peripheral and central response for interpreting test results.

Dermatomal Field Stimulation

In an effort to improve the specificity of dermatomal-somatosensory evoked potentials to single nerve root

involvement and to avoid stimulation of multiple nerve roots, procedures that stimulate dermatomal fields have been developed.[17, 21, 26, 47] These methods consist of stimulating a dermatomal field at an intensity two to three times that of the sensory threshold and recording a cortical response. The exact site of stimulation is based on sites of commonality among dermatomal fields. For example, the common site for eliciting S1 activity is the dermatomal field located at the base and side of the fifth metatarsal (Fig. 3-26).

The correlation between clinical status and results from dermatomal field stimulation has been extensively studied. Scarff and co-workers reported the dermatomal-somatosensory evoked potential correlations for 38 patients who underwent myelography and surgery for herniated disks.[47] Dermatomal-somatosensory evoked potentials, elicited by stimulating the L5 and S1 dermatomal field, were recorded cortically. The evoked potentials correlated with the surgically confirmed level of specific nerve root involvement in 35 (92%) of these patients. Of the remaining patients, dermatomal-somatosensory evoked potentials were normal in two, and the third demonstrated an abnormal dermatomal-somatosensory evoked potential in the contralateral root only. Myelograms were normal or nondiagnostic in 5 of the 38 patients, and electromyographic responses were positive in fewer than 50% of the patients.

Katifi and Sedgwick reported the correlations among dermatomal-somatosensory evoked potentials, radiologic findings, and surgically confirmed results for 21 patients complaining of back pain and sciatica.[21] Dermatomal-somatosensory evoked potentials, elicited by stimulating the L5 and S1 dermatomes, were

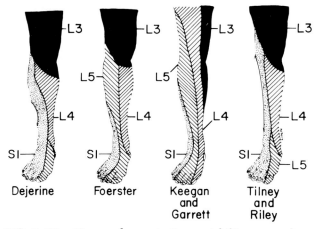

FIG. 3–26. Figures demonstrating variability among dermatomal fields.

recorded cortically. In 19 of the patients, dermatomal-somatosensory evoked potentials were abnormal. In 1 of the remaining cases, the evoked potentials were normal but the disc was surgically confirmed as abnormal. In the remaining case, no disc involvement was noted at the time of surgery, and it was concluded that preoperative radiologic results had been overinterpreted. Similar results have been reported by others.[46]

Green and colleagues investigated the correlation between dermatomal-somatosensory evoked potentials and radiculopathy in the cervical and lumbar regions of 129 patients.[12] The dermatomal fields attributed to Crv6, Crv7, Crv8, L5, and S1 were used to elicit the response, and the results were correlated with clinical symptoms. No surgical confirmation was obtained. Of the 129 patients administered dermatomal-somatosensory evoked potential procedures, 87 (67%) had a normal results, and 42 (33%) had abnormal results. For patients with abnormal responses, dermatomal-somatosensory evoked potentials correlated correctly for 38 (91%) with the side of involvement. In the remaining 4 patients, dermatomal-somatosensory evoked potentials were abnormal on the side opposite the complaint.

A comparison of the correlation of dermatomal-somatosensory evoked potentials and clinical status as a function of cervical or lumbar involvement revealed 51 (81%) of 63 patients with normal upper dermatomal-somatosensory evoked potentials and 12 (19%) with abnormal responses. In the abnormal cervical dermatomal-somatosensory evoked potential group, 11 (92%) responses correctly correlated with the side of the complaint, but 1 (8%) indicated the contralateral side.

In the lumbar group, 36 (55%) of 66 patients had normal dermatomal-somatosensory evoked potentials, and 30 (45%) had abnormal responses. In the abnormal group, results correctly correlated with the side of involvement in 27 (90%) of the patients, but they indicated the contralateral side in the remaining 3 (10%). Green concluded that dermatomal-somatosensory evoked potentials demonstrated a low sensitivity but a high specificity to cervical and lumbar radiculopathies.[12]

Herron investigated the sensitivity of dermatomal-somatosensory evoked potentials to the adequacy of lateral decompression in patients undergoing surgery for spinal stenosis.[17] Patients who had good, fair, or poor surgical relief demonstrated mean latency improvements of the dermatomal-somatosensory evoked potential of 9.9, 8.2, or 6.0 milliseconds, respectively. The differences in the amount of latency change were not statistically significant. The authors concluded that, although surgical success was influenced by many anatomic and psychosocial variables, adequate neural decompression was essential, and adequacy of decompression was best determined using dermatomal-somatosensory evoked potentials.

In a study similar to Herron's, my colleagues and I determined the percentage of nerve roots that demonstrated a significant improvement in dermatomal-somatosensory evoked potential after decompression.[17, 40] Data were elicited by stimulating either L3, L4, or L5 levels in 80 patients undergoing surgery for degenerative diseases of the spine. We found that the percentage of nerve roots demonstrating a significant improvement varied with the level of involvement, ranging from 75% to 91%.

To determine the variables influencing improvement, we compared results with the type of anesthesia used and the duration of pain experienced by each patient. If ketamine was used, reliable but not necessarily normal dermatomal-somatosensory evoked potentials could be obtained in 100% of the patients. However, if other anesthetic agents were used, reliable data could be obtained in only 69% of the patients.

Using only those patients for whom reliable data were recorded, we found that intraoperative improvement of the dermatomal-somatosensory evoked potential was correlated with duration of symptoms. For patients who had symptoms less than 1 year, 73% demonstrated an improved dermatomal-somatosensory evoked potential during surgery and relief of pain postoperatively; 18% demonstrated no significant change in dermatomal-somatosensory evoked potential, but relief of some pain postoperatively; and 9% demonstrated no change in dermatomal-somatosensory evoked potential or in pain relief postoperatively. For patients who had pain for more than 1 year before surgery, 40% demonstrated an improved dermatomal-somatosensory evoked potential during surgery and relief of pain postoperatively. The remaining 60% had no change in dermatomal-somatosensory evoked potentials, but they did have some improvement in pain postoperatively.

A possible explanation for these findings is based on the relationship between time to relief and time to electrophysiologic confirmation of the relief. As reported by Katifi and Sedgwick, pain relief is almost immediate after peripheral nerve decompression, but nerve conduction changes take time to resolve.[21] Electrophysiologic procedures measure a different aspect of nerve function resulting from compression, which does not necessarily reflect the pain experienced by the patient.

A second explanation of our findings is based on the duration of pain experienced by the patient before surgery. The correlation between experiencing symptoms less than a year and greater likelihood of intraoperative improvement of the dermatomal-somatosensory evoked potential suggests there may be a patient "profile" that should be monitored and that may indicate when adequate decompression has been achieved.

Although dermatomal-somatosensory evoked potentials elicited by dermatomal field stimulation avoid many of the problems associated with specific nerve stimulation, they also have limitations. First, a peripheral response is very difficult to record. Consequently, interpretations are based primarily on cortical data that can be influenced by anesthesia, subject state, or other factors. Second, several studies have reported on the lack of sensitivity and specificity of dermatomal-somatosensory evoked potentials to radiculopathy.[3, 42] Aminoff and co-workers reported 19 patients with surgically confirmed unilateral radiculopathy at L5 or S1.[3] Dermatomal-somatosensory evoked potentials correctly identified the level and side of involvement in 5 (26%) of these patients. In 1 patient, the dermatomal-somatosensory evoked potential was abnormal on the involved side, but at the wrong level. In 10 patients (53%), dermatomal-somatosensory evoked potentials indicated either the wrong side of involvement or were interpreted as being normal. In the remaining 3 patients (16%), dermatomal-somatosensory evoked potentials and radiologic studies were normal, but level and side of involvement were correctly identified with electromyographic recordings. It was concluded that more sensitive and specific information was currently available using other electrophysiologic tests.

Several studies have reported that dermatomal-somatosensory evoked potentials lack adequate sensitivity and specificity to the level and side of radicular pain. However, most studies indicate that this method demonstrates sensitivity and specificity comparable to radiologic and other electrophysiologic procedures. Dermatomal-somatosensory evoked potentials can be administered continuously during surgery, which can provide the surgeon with ongoing information about the adequacy of lateral decompression. Consequently, dermatomal-somatosensory evoked potentials provide the surgeon with information not available with other techniques.

Elicitation and Recording

To elicit the dermatomal-somatosensory evoked potential, my colleagues and I stimulate specific dermatomal fields and record the response cortically. Table 3-5 lists the elicitation and recording parameters we administer in this procedure. We do not typically record a peripheral or cervical response, and we stimulate only one dermatomal field at a time. However, Machida and co-workers have stimulated both dermatomal fields at a specific level simultaneously.[27] Dermatomal-somatosensory evoked potentials are recorded simultaneously from both hemispheres. Machida believes that bilateral, simultaneous stimulation improves the detection of slight asymmetry that could be missed by using sequential methods. However, no data comparing the relative sensitivity of these two methods of stimulation were presented.

Figure 3-27 depicts cortical-dermatomal-somatosensory evoked potentials recorded during surgery after stimulation of the L4, L5, and S1 dermatomal fields. The response demonstrates morphologic characteristics essentially identical to those of the cortical-somatosensory evoked potential after mixed-nerve stimulation. We use the first major, positive (downward) deflection as the absolute latency of the response. Peak-to-peak amplitude is measured from the initial positive deflection to the following negative

TABLE 3-5. Parameters for Recording a Three-Channel, Cortical DSEP After Stimulation of Lower-Limb Dermatomes*

Parameters	Chn. 1	Chn. 2	Chn. 3
Sensitivity (μV)	50–100	50–100	50–100
Low linear filter	10	10	10
High linear filter	250	250	250
Notch filter	Off	Off	Off
Referential	Fpz	Fpz	Fpz
Active	C3′	Cz′	C4′
Artifact reject.	On	On	On
Timebase (msec)	125	125	125
Rate	4.8/sec	Swp:300	Trg:Int
Duration	200 μsec		

* A 65-msec timebase is used to record upper-limb DSEPs.

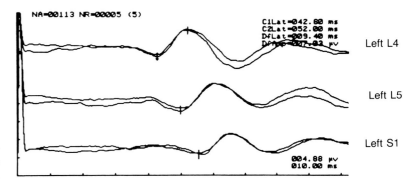

NA=00113 NR=00005 (5)

C1Lat=042.60 ms
C2Lat=052.00 ms
D#Lat=009.40 ms
DAmp=007.83 µV

Left L4

Left L5

Left S1

004.88 µV
010.00 ms

FIG. 3–27. Baseline intraoperative dermatomal somatosensory evoked potentials recorded cortically after stimulation of the L4, L5, and S1 dermatomal fields.

Normative dermatome data elicited in the OR during surgery.

wave. Two responses, recorded at each level, demonstrate reliability.

Interpretation

Interpretation of the dermatomal-somatosensory evoked potential follows the same guidelines for reliability as the mixed-nerve somatosensory evoked potential. However, unlike the mixed-nerve somatosensory evoked potential, latency is the primary characteristic of interpretation instead of amplitude. Because dermatomal-somatosensory evoked potentials demonstrate abnormalities before surgery, responses usually improve during surgery.

Because interpretation criteria influence the sensitivity and specificity of dermatomal-somatosensory evoked potentials, criteria must be carefully chosen. Typically, criteria are prioritized as follows:

1. A response is present and morphologically appropriate.
2. Within-limb latencies demonstrate a gradual prolongation in a proximal to distal direction. Usually, there is a difference of 3 milliseconds in the latency of the response as a function of level. Anything greater is considered abnormal.
3. Between-limb latencies of the response should be within 3 to 6 milliseconds of each other. Anything greater is considered abnormal.

Clinical Examples

Figures 3-28 through 3-32 demonstrate the relative sensitivity of mixed-nerve somatosensory evoked potentials and dermatomal-somatosensory evoked potentials to decompression of the right L4 nerve root. Base-

line mixed-nerve data (Fig. 3-28) were well-formed and reliable. There were no abnormalities in the response from either leg, nor were there any significant between-limb differences.

Baseline dermatomal-somatosensory evoked potentials to stimulation of the L4 dermatomal fields revealed a reliable L4 response on the left, but no response right (Fig. 3-29).

Baseline dermatomal-somatosensory evoked potentials to stimulation of the L5 dermatomal fields revealed reliable responses bilaterally. There were no significant differences in responses from either leg (Fig. 3-30).

After decompression of the right L4 nerve root, a reliable dermatomal-somatosensory evoked potential

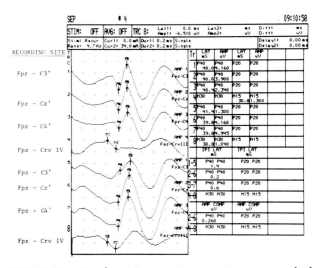

FIG. 3–28. Baseline intraoperative somatosensory evoked potentials in response to posterior tibial nerve stimulation after incision.

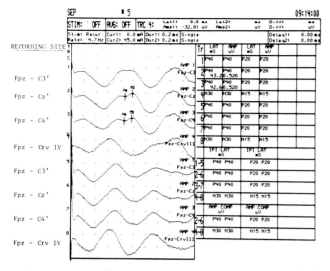

FIG. 3–29. Baseline intraoperative somatosensory evoked potentials in response to L4 stimulation, following incision. No reliable right L4 response is present.

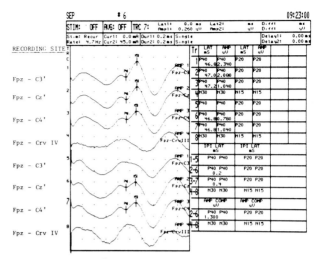

FIG. 3–30. Baseline intraoperative somatosensory evoked potentials in response to L5 stimulation after incision. The reliable response is bilateral.

from that field was recorded. The left L4 response remained unchanged.

The left and right L5 dermatomes remained unchanged after decompression.

RECOMMENDATIONS

Based on our clinical and research experience, my colleagues and I have developed the following guidelines for monitoring spinal cord and nerve root function during surgery.

Monitoring Mixed-Nerve Somatosensory Evoked Potentials

1. All four extremities are stimulated. The "primary" and "secondary" stimulation sites are determined by the level of surgery. To maintain adequate sensitivity and specificity, only one limb should be stimulated at a time. This method provides information about spinal cord function and detects the onset of effects from compression of the brachial plexus.

2. A minimum of five recording sites are required: a peripheral site, cervical site, and three cortical sites. Multiple recording sites allow the examiner to determine whether a degradation in the response is due to presurgical or surgical vari-

ables. Multiple cortical recording sites improve the chances of obtaining a reliable and morphologically robust response.

3. Acquisition parameters must consider the origin and functional characteristics of the recorded response. This requires that the evoked potential system demonstrate within-channel programmability.

4. Baseline values should be obtained after administration of anesthesia, positioning on the operating table, and incision. Data obtained preoperatively is helpful in determining the functional characteristics of the somatosensory system, but they should not be used as a baseline reference during surgery.

5. Mixed-nerve somatosensory evoked potentials should be monitored continuously and recorded at least every 10 minutes during noncritical portions of the procedure. Critical portions of surgery include times during which the spinal cord is at risk. Although these times vary, data should be monitored during periods of compression, application of distractive force, derotation, sublaminar wire passing, and placement of bone grafts. During critical periods, data should be recorded and stored continuously. We believe that data should be collected for at least 30 minutes after the last maneuver of the spinal column or cord.

6. Primary interpretation criteria should be based

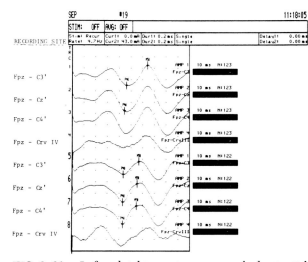

FIG. 3–31. Left and right somatosensory evoked potentials in response to L4 stimulation after decompression of the right L4 nerve root. A reliable L4 response is demonstrated.

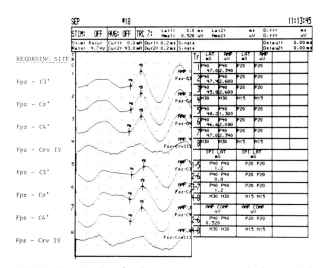

FIG. 3–32. Left and right somatosensory evoked potentials in response to L5 stimulation at closure.

on the amplitude of the response. Response latency should be monitored, and if significantly degraded, the surgeon should be informed of the changes. However, latency shifts are considered to be a secondary interpretation characteristic. Contingency plans based on the significant degradation of the response should be developed before surgery.

7. The surgeon and monitoring team must be aware of the limitations associated with monitoring spinal cord function using only mixed-nerve somatosensory evoked potentials, especially for determining motor tract functioning. Moreover, mixed-nerve somatosensory evoked potentials do not provide any information about the functional integrity of single nerve roots.

Monitoring Motor Evoked Potentials

1. The stimulation site for the motor evoked potential should be proximal to the level of surgery. The motor evoked potential method we use stimulates the spinal cord by placing stimulating electrodes into the spinous processes at the proximal end of the incision.

2. We believe that the recording sites for motor evoked potentials should be in the periphery, specifically over the sciatic nerve, at the sciatic notch, and at the popliteal fossa. A spinal re-

cording site may be used, but the response contains antidromic sensory activity that is difficult to discriminate and may reduce the sensitivity and specificity of the response to motor tract functioning.

3. The motor evoked potential recorded can be either myogenic or neurogenic in origin. Although a myogenic response appears to have a solely motor origin, it demonstrates several limitations that reduce its clinical feasibility. A neurogenic response contains some antidromic sensory activity, but this activity can be discriminated from motor activity if a distant, peripheral recording site is used. A neurogenic response avoids the limitations associated with a myogenic response.

4. Motor evoked potentials should be recorded as often as possible. However, because of the relative strengths and weaknesses of somatosensory evoked potentials and motor evoked potentials, we alternately record these two potentials. During critical periods of surgery, when the spinal cord is at most risk, we try to record the motor evoked potentials more frequently than the somatosensory evoked potentials.

5. Our primary criterion for interpretation criteria is amplitude; latency is a secondary consideration.

6. The major limitation of all motor evoked potential procedures is that they do not provide infor-

mation about the functional integrity of sensory system nor about cortical function. Therefore, the examiner should alternately collect somatosensory evoked potential and motor evoked potential data throughout the surgery.

Monitoring Dermatomal-Somatosensory Evoked Potentials

1. To monitor individual nerve root function, we recommend that dermatomal fields be stimulated to elicit the dermatomal-somatosensory evoked potential.
2. Because of their small size and lack of synchronicity, dermatomal-somatosensory evoked potentials should be recorded using the same cortical montages used for mixed-nerve somatosensory evoked potentials.
3. Baseline values, on which intraoperative decisions are based, should be collected after incision.
4. Data should be collected during surgical periods that place individual nerve roots at risk.
5. Interpretation criteria should take into consideration the latency and amplitude characteristics of the response.
6. There are several limitations associated with dermatomal-somatosensory evoked potentials, including lack of information about total spinal cord function, adverse effects from certain anesthetics, and variability in the representation of peripheral dermatomal fields.

SUMMARY

Evoked potential monitoring during surgeries for spinal deformities provides continuous information about the functional integrity of the spinal cord. Traditionally, mixed-nerve somatosensory evoked potentials have been used to monitor spinal cord function, but continued experience indicates that this response lacks the sensitivity to provide information regarding motor tract functioning.

The development of procedures that elicit a motor evoked potential allows the examiner to obtain information about motor tract functioning. However, motor evoked potential procedures do not provide any information about the sensory tracts or the functional integrity of the sensory cortex. Consequently, we recommend that motor evoked potential and mixed-nerve somatosensory evoked potentials be used to monitor total spinal cord function during surgeries that place that structure at risk.

To obtain information on single nerve root function, it is necessary to stimulate dermatomal fields and record the response cortically. Mixed-nerve somatosensory evoked potentials do not provide this information. However, during surgeries that are intended to decompress nerve roots, it is still necessary to monitor spinal cord function using mixed-nerve somatosensory evoked potentials.

An adequately trained examiner can provide the surgeon with reliable information about total spinal cord or nerve root function by using appropriate methods, which can reduce the postoperative neurologic deficits associated with maneuvers of the spinal cord.

References

1. Abel MF, Mubavak SJ, Wenser OR, et al: Brainstem evoked potentials for scoliosis surgery: A reliable method allowing use of halogenated anesthetic agents. J Pediatr Orthop 10:208, 1990
2. Adamson J, Zappulla RA, Ryder J, Malis LI: The effect of selective spinal cord lesions on the rat spinal motor evoked potential (MEP). Poster presentation at the Meeting of the American Academy of Neurosurgery, Toronto, Canada 1988
3. Aminoff MJ, Goodin DS, Barbaco NM, et al: Dermatomal somatosensory evoked potentials in unilateral lumbosacral radiculopathy. Ann Neurol 17:171, 1985
4. Barker AT, Freeston IL, Jalinous R, et al: Magnetic stimulation of the human brain. J Physiol 9P:369, 1985
5. Cohen BA, Huizenga BA: Dermatomal monitoring for surgical correction of spondylolisthesis. A case report. Spine 13:1125, 1988
6. Cracco RQ, Amassian VE, Maccabee PJ, Cracco JB: Comparison of human transcallosal responses evoked by magnetic coil and electrical stimulation. Electroencephalogr Clin Neurophysiol 74:417, 1989
7. Dinner DS, Luders H, Lesser RP, et al: Intraoperative spinal somatosensory evoked potential monitoring. J Neurosurg 65:807, 1986
8. Eisen A, Elleker G: Sensory nerve stimulation and evoked cerebral potentials. Neurology 30:1097, 1980
9. Eisen A, Horich M: The electrodiagnostic evaluation of spinal root lesions. Spine 8:98, 1983
10. Engler G: Personal communication, 1989
11. Ginsburg HH, Shetter AG, Raudzens PA: Postoperative paraplegia with preserved intraoperative somatosensory evoked potentials. J Neurosurg 63:296, 1985
12. Green J, Hamm A, Benfante P, Green S: Clinical effec-

tiveness of dermatomal evoked cerebrally recorded somatosensory responses. Clin EEG 19:14, 1988

13. Haldeman S, Bradley WE, Bhatia NN, Johnson BK: Pudendal evoked responses. Arch Neurol 39:285,1982
14. Haldeman S, Bradley WE, Bhatia WN, Johnson BK: Cortical evoked potentials on stimulation of pudendal nerve in women. Urology 21:590, 1983
15. Hassan NF, Rossini PM, Cracco RQ, Cracco JB: Unexpected motor cortex excitation by low voltage stimuli. In Morocutti C, Rizzo PA (eds): Evoked Potentials: Neurophysiological and Clinical Aspects, p 107. Amsterdam, Elsevier, 1985
16. Heisenberg W: Uber den anschaulichen inhalt der quanten theoretischen kinematik and mechanik. J Physik 43:172, 1927
17. Herron LD, Trippi AC, Gonyeau ML: Intraoperative use of dermatomal somatosensory evoked potentials in lumbar stenosis surgery. Spine 12:379, 1987
18. Jasper HH: Report of Committee on Methods of Clinical Examination in EEG. Appendix: The ten-twenty electrode system of the International Federation. Electroencephalogr Clin Neurophysiol 10:371, 1958
19. Jones SJ, Howard L, Shawkat F: Criteria for detection and pathological significance of response decrement during spinal cord monitoring. In Ducker TB, Brown RH (eds): Neurophysiology and Standards of Spinal Cord Monitoring, p 201. New York, Springer-Verlag, 1988
20. Katifi HA, Sedgwick EM: Somatosensory evoked potentials from posterior tibial nerve and lumbosacral dermatomes. EEG Clin Neurophysiol 65:249, 1986
21. Katifi HA, Sedgwick EM: Evaluation of the dermatomal somatosensory evoked potential in the diagnosis of lumbo-sacral root compression. J Neurol Neurosurg Psychiatry 50:1204, 1987
22. Keith R: Personal communication, 1989
23. Kellaway P: An orderly approach to visual analysis. Parameters of normal EEG in adults and children. In Klass D, Daley DD (eds): Current Practice of Clinical Electroencephalography, p 73. New York, Raven Press, 1979
24. Levy WJ, McCaffrey M, York DH, Tanzer F: Motor evoked potentials from transcortical stimulation of the motor cortex in cats. Neurosurgery 15:214, 1984
25. Levy WJ, York DH: Evoked potentials from the motor tracts in humans. Neurosurgery 12:422, 1983
26. Lubicky JP, Spadoro JA, Yuan HA, et al: Variability of somatosensory cortical evoked potential monitoring during spinal surgery. Spine 14:790, 1989
27. Machida M, Asi T, Sato K, et al: New approach for diagnosis in herniated lumbosacral disc. Spine 11:380, 1986
28. Machida M, Weinstein SL, Yamada T, Kimura J: Spinal cord monitoring. Spine 10:407, 1985
29. Machida M, Weinstein SL, Yamada T, et al: Dissociation of muscle action potentials and spinal somatosensory evoked potentials after ischemic damage to the spinal cord. Spine 13:1119, 1988
30. Machida M, Weinstein SL, Yamada T, et al: Monitoring of motor action potentials after stimulation of the spinal cord. J Bone Joint Surg [Am] 70:911, 1988

31. Merton PA, Morton HB: Electrical stimulation of human motor and visual cortex through the scalp. J Physiol 305:9, 1980
32. Moller AR: Evoked Potentials in Intraoperative Monitoring. Baltimore, Williams and Wilkins, 1988
33. Neuwirth MG, Nainzadeh NK, Bernstein RL: The use of pudendal nerve in monitoring lower sacral roots (S2–S4) during anterior and/or posterior spinal stabilization. Orthop Trans 13:89, 1989
34. Nuwer MR: Spinal cord monitoring. In Nuwer MR (ed): Evoked Potential Monitoring in the Operating Room, p 49. New York, Raven Press, 1986
35. Owen JH, Bridwell KH, Shimon SM, et al: Parametric studies in the neurogenic-motor evoked potential. Paper presented at the Meeting of the American EEG Society, St. Louis, MO, 1987
36. Owen JH, Bridwell KH, Shimon SM, et al: Sensitivity and specificity of somatosensory and neurogenic-motor evoked potentials in animals and humans. Spine 12:1111, 1988
37. Owen JH, Kai Y, Lenke L, Bridwell KH: Relative sensitivity of spinal versus peripheral motor evoked potentials to spinal cord ischemia. Spine (in press)
38. Owen JH, Naito M, Bridwell KH: Relationship between duration of lost evoked potentials and clinical status in animals. Spine 15:618, 1990
39. Owen JH, Naito M, Bridwell KH, Kai Y: Parametric and lesioning investigations of the neurogenic-motor evoked potential. Paper presented at the International Motor Evoked Potential Symposium, Chicago, IL, 1989
40. Owen JH, Padberg A, Holland L, et al: Clinical correlation between degenerative spine disease and dermatomal somatosensory evoked potentials in humans. Spine (in press)
41. Penfield W, Jasper H: Epilepsy and the Functional Anatomy of the Brain. Boston, Little, Brown, 1954
42. Rodriguez AA, Kanis L, Rodriguez AA, Lane D: Somatosensory evoked potentials from dermatomal stimulation as an indicator of L5 and S1 radiculopathy. Arch Phys Med Rehabil 68:366, 1987
43. Rossini PM, DiStefano E, Boatta M, Basciani M: Evaluation of sensorimotor "central" conduction in normal subjects and in patients with multiple sclerosis. In Evoked Potentials: Neurophysiological and Clinical Aspects, p 115. Amsterdam, Elsevier, 1985
44. Rossini PM, Gigli GL, Marciani MG, et al: Noninvasive evaluation of input-output characteristics of sensorimotor cerebral areas in healthy humans. Electroencephalogr Clin Neurophysiol 68:88, 1987.
45. Sabato S, Agresta C, Salzman S: Evaluation of the efficacy versus safety of spinal cord stimulation for the generation of compound muscle action potentials (CMAPs). Paper presented at the Meeting of the Scoliosis Research Society, Amsterdam, 1989
46. Salenius P, Laurent LE: Results of operative treatment of lumbar disc herniation. Acta Orthop Scand 48:630, 1977
47. Scarff TB, Dallmann DE, Toleikis JR, Bunch WH: Dermatomal somatosensory evoked potentials in the diag-

nosis of lumbar root entrapment. Surg Forum 32:489, 1981

48. Seyal M, Palma GA, Sandhu LS, et al: Spinal somatosensory evoked potentials after segmental sensory stimulation: a direct measure of dorsal medial function. Electroencephalogr Clin Neurophysiol 69:390,1988

49. Shichijo F, Gentili F, Transfeldt E, Niznik G: Neuroanatomical substrate of motor evoked potentials and cerebellar evoked potentials. Poster presentation at the Meeting of the American Academy of Neurosurgery, Toronto, 1988

50. Tamaki T, Noguchi T, Takano H, et al: Spinal cord monitoring as a clinical utilization of the spinal evoked potential. Clin Orthop 184:58, 1984

51. Tamaki T, Takano H, Inoue S, et al: The prevention of iatrogenic spinal cord injury utilizing the evoked spinal cord potential. Int Orthop 4:313, 1981

52. Tamaki T, Takano T, Takakuwa K: Spinal cord monitoring: Basic principles and experimental aspects. Cent Nerv Syst Traum 2:137, 1985

53. Williams RW: Microlumbar discectomy: a conservative approach to the virgin herniated disc. Spine 3:175, 1978

PART

II

SURGICAL APPROACHES TO THE SPINE

CHAPTER 4

Anterior Approaches to the Cervical Spine

Richard W. Maack

J. Gershon Spector

■

The treatment of diseases of the anterior cervical spine has always been challenging because of the obligatory, complex surgical exposure. The more direct posterior approach offers excellent access to the posterior spine and spinal canal, but it limits exposure of the anterior spine.

Surgeons began to implement anterior approaches to lesions of the cervical spine in the early 1950s. In 1955, Robinson and Smith were among the first to describe a safe surgical approach with dissection directed between the trachea and major vessels (carotid sheath). This was an extrapharyngeal or extravisceral technique for midcervical spinal disease.[11] Two years later, Southwick and Robinson expanded this approach to expose the anterior cervical spine from C3 to T1.[16] DeAndrade extended this approach to include the anterior occiput and skull base.[3]

Surgical exposures and techniques were refined by Cloward, who developed a retractor, drills, and other instrumentation for wider surgical exposure.[2] In 1981, Biller described a technique that offered a wide exposure of the base of the skull by means of a midline or lateral mandibulotomy.[1] There have been recent modifications of these basic approaches to the anterior spine, especially for surgery of the cervical spine above C4, a procedure often requiring the collaborative efforts of a head and neck surgeon or orthopedic surgeon and neurosurgeon.

THE LOWER CERVICAL SPINE

The extrapharyngeal anterolateral approach to the cervical spine is standard when the bodies and the interspaces of the fourth through the seventh cervical vertebra are to be exposed. The patient is anesthetized in the supine position and ventilated through a nonkinking or armored endotracheal tube, because significant mobilization of the tracheo-esophageal visceral complex is required during the operation. Normal cervical lordosis is maintained by placing a shoulder roll under the scapulae. If cervical stability is in doubt, traction devices are applied and secured with tongs to the calvarium.

The head is rotated slightly to the side opposite that for the planned incision. Smith and Robinson advocated using the left side to decrease the risk of damaging the recurrent laryngeal nerve.[14] Confined by the higher subclavian artery in the right chest, this nerve runs a longer and more horizontal course on the right side of the neck and is more vulnerable to dissection damage. Most right-handed surgeons, however, find the right side more accessible because the mandible is not an obstruction. The right-side approach also prevents damage to the thoracic duct, and the cervical esophagus is less retracted, displaced, or susceptible to perforation because of its normal anterior position on the left side of the neck.

A transverse or longitudinal incision may be used for this approach. A curvilinear transverse incision made in a skin fold usually heals in a more cosmetically appealing fashion, but it limits the surgeon in extending the exposure up or down the cervical spine more than two or three vertebrae. The incision is tailored for the specific level of the cervical spine operated upon. The angle of the mandible corresponds to C2 to C3, the hyoid bone overlies C3, and the cricoid cartilage is anterior to C6 to C7.[5] The longitudinal incision is made along the anterior border of the sternocleidomastoid muscle over the cervical spine to be exposed between the mastoid and the sternum.

After incising the skin and dividing the platysma muscle, the superficial layer of the deep cervical fascia along the sternocleidomastoid muscle is exposed. The anterior jugular vein may be retracted medially or divided. The middle layer of the deep cervical fascia bridges from the sternocleidomastoid to the anterior strap muscles of the larynx (i.e., the laryngeal depressor muscles). This fascia is incised, and the exposure is widened and deepened by blunt and sharp dissection. The omohyoid muscle, whose fibers course perpendicularly to those of the sternocleidomastoid

and is superficial to the carotid sheath (the guardian of the carotid), should be retracted or divided. The potential space between the carotid sheath and the visceral compartment is opened with blunt dissection. The carotid artery, internal jugular vein, and vagus nerve are isolated and retracted posterolaterally while the trachea, larynx, and esophagus are retracted anteromedially (Fig. 4-1).

Structures that can cause restriction of this exposure include the superior thyroid vascular pedicle and the middle thyroid vein, and these may be ligated. Avoid injury to the external branch of the superior laryngeal nerve (i.e., vocal cord tensor) by identifying and protecting this structure. It usually travels cephalad to the superior thyroid vascular pedicle (i.e., superior thyroid artery, a division of the external carotid system). The superior laryngeal nerve leaves the jugular foramen and travels deep and under the external carotid artery before joining the superior thyroid artery at the level of the greater wing of the hyoid.

At the C5 level and below, the inferior thyroid vessels may need to be divided. This is done only after the recurrent laryngeal nerve is identified and protected. The branches of the ansa hypoglossi nerve (XII) to the strap muscles usually must be sacrificed. These travel on top of the internal jugular vein and cross the potential space of the dissection to innervate the lower (infrahyoid) anterior strap muscles. Using blunt dissection, the cervical esophagus is separated from the prevertebral fascia. The deep layer of the deep cervical fascia (visceral fascia) is opened. The esophagus, larynx, and trachea are mobilized as a single unit with the

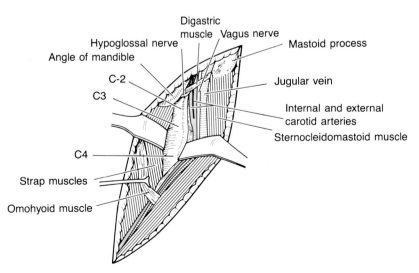

FIG. 4-1. The extrapharyngeal anterolateral approach to the cervical spine uses posterior and lateral retraction of the carotid sheath and anterior retraction of the visceral structures in the neck.

thyroid gland and strap muscles to bring the entire lower cervical spine under direct view. Protect the sympathetic neural trunk that lies on top of the prevertebral muscles just anterior to the transverse processes of the vertebrae. By confining the surgery to the midline region when operating on the vertebral bodies, injury to the cervical sympathetic chain and the vertebral arteries can be avoided. The hypoglossal nerve crosses superior and superficial to the superior laryngeal.nerve, and it usually denotes the upper limit of this surgical approach.

After the proper level has been verified radiologically, the longus colli muscles, which lie anteriorly, are sharply dissected free from the vertebral bodies and from the adherent annulus of the disc. The longus colli muscles can be divided in the midline, usually with a bovie or hot knife, to form two lateral flaps. The lateral limits of the flaps are the transverse processes of the cervical vertebrae. Occasionally, a superior or inferior U-shaped flap is used. Flaps can be sutured together with absorbable sutures at completion of surgery.

A Cloward retractor's toothed blades are placed underneath the dissected margins of the longus colli muscles to expose the anterior cervical spine. A second retractor with smooth blades may be used to maximize rostrocaudal exposure. The carotid sheath and visceral compartments are retracted manually or by self-adjusting smooth blade retractors.

The surgical approach to C7 and T1 requires further anatomic and surgical considerations. Occasionally, the prevertebral space below C6 is cramped, and it is necessary to release the tendinous sternal attachment of the sternocleidomastoid muscle to provide the necessary exposure to the prevertebral space. Carefully identify and protect the internal jugular vein. In this area, the internal jugular vein empties into the subclavian vein, and the thoracic duct enters the vein on the left side. Insertion of a gloved finger behind the sternal head, protecting the vein, is helpful before detaching the muscle from the manubrium. The fascia overlying the scalene muscles must not be entered. On the anterior scalene muscles, beneath the investing fascia, runs the phenic nerve. On the posterior edge of the anterior scalene fascia is the brachial plexus of nerves.

A modification of the exposure is advisable for the lower cervical space and the upper thoracic spine. In this approach lateral to the carotid sheath, the carotid sheath and visceral compartment are retracted medially. This retrocarotid approach provides a better ac-cess to the lower vertebra, but at a greater angle and distance.

Micheli and Hood combined the anterolateral cervical approach with a posterior transpleural transthoracic approach to provide exposure from the C3 to T9.[9] The cervical approach involves the anterior retraction of the carotid sheath with ligation of the inferior thyroid artery, which passes posterior to the carotid sheath. With this anterior carotid retraction, the dissection can be performed to the level of T1.

After the cervical wound is packed, a thoracic incision is made from the posterior margin of the axilla to the pectoral region anteriorly. Mobilization of the scapula is accomplished by releasing the serratus anterior muscle from the medial border of the scapula, leaving a cuff of muscle for reattachment for closure. The superficial muscles of the chest wall (i.e., the pectoralis major, the serratus anterior, the latissimus dorsi) are divided parallel to the third rib. The scapula is mobilized, displaced anteriorly, and rotated superiorly to expose the underlying third rib. The periosteum of the entire third rib is incised, allowing it to be removed at its attachment to the sternum and posteriorly at its attachment to the transverse process. The pleura is then incised in the bed of the third rib, exposing the first, second, and third thoracic vertebrae and discs. If lower exposure is required, osteotomy of the posterior part of the fourth and fifth rib can be performed. Operative exposure down to T9 has been obtained using this combined anterolateral cervical and posterior transpleural thoracic technique.[9]

THE MIDDLE AND UPPER CERVICAL SPINE

Two surgical approaches are commonly used to expose C3 to C1 anteriorly. One approach involves a continuation of the transcervical retroesophageal exposure superiorly toward this upper cervical region with retraction of the carotid artery posteriorly.[15] The more traditional approach involves exposure of the upper cervical spine posterior to the carotid sheath after its retraction anteriorly. With either approach, a tracheostomy must be considered if airway obstruction may be precipitated by the combination of surgical technique and pathologic conditions.

When approaching the cervical spine above C4, several significant structures prevent easy development of the potential space between the contents of the carotid sheath and the pharynx. In this region, the external carotid artery propagates the superior thyroid, lingual, and facial branches. These arteries pass anteriorly and medially, preventing posterior retraction of the carotid artery. An anterior approach to the carotid sheath contents can also damage the hypoglossal and superior laryngeal nerves, which cross directly through this area. The hypoglossal nerve passes superficially, and the superior laryngeal nerve crosses deep to the carotid artery. To prevent damage to these structures, approach the upper cervical spine posterior to the contents of the carotid sheath as described by Sherk and Pratt.[13]

An 8- to 10-cm skin incision is made along the anterior border of the sternomastoid muscle, beginning near the mastoid process. It may be necessary to detach this muscle from the mastoid tip in patients with short, stout necks. This is accomplished with a C-shaped extension of the incision posteriorly over the mastoid process. The lateral mass of the atlas lies just beneath the anterior border of the sternomastoid muscle and is easily palpated. The posterior belly of the digastric muscle crosses obliquely and passes beneath the angle of the mandible. The posterior belly of the digastric muscle is the guardian of this area, because all vital structures (e.g., hypoglossal nerve, facial nerve, carotid sheath and contents) lie beneath it. The internal jugular vein is identified and separated from the anterior surface of the atlas. This maneuver clears the

anterior surface of the atlas of the internal jugular vein, internal carotid artery, the vagus nerve, and the hypoglossal nerve. The hypoglossal nerve lies on top of and the vagus beneath the internal jugular vein. The spinal accessory nerve usually lies on top of the internal jugular vein, intimately associated with the vein wall. Its course is posterior in the posterior neck triangle until it reaches the sternomastoid, trapezius, and the muscles of the shoulder girdle. Anterior retraction of these structures exposes the anterior surface of the atlas (Fig. 4-2). The styloid process should be fractured and pushed away from the field because it interferes with this approach. This exposure provides access to the anterior rim of the foramen magnum, the atlas, and C2.

If a more distal dissection is required, to C3 and below, first identify and protect the accessory nerve. This nerve passes from the base of the skull, about 4 to 5 cm below the mastoid tip. From there, the external branch of the nerve crosses under the sternomastoid muscle and exits in the posterior triangle of the neck.

The second commonly used approach to the upper cervical spine is superior extension of the anterior retropharyngeal approach. This approach, advocated by Komisar and Tubbaddor, involves posterior lateral carotid sheath retraction.[6] The incision is made from the mastoid tip to the level of the hyoid bone. The platysma and the superficial layer of the deep cervical fascia are divided. The marginal mandibular branch of the facial nerve is found with the aid of a nerve stimulator if

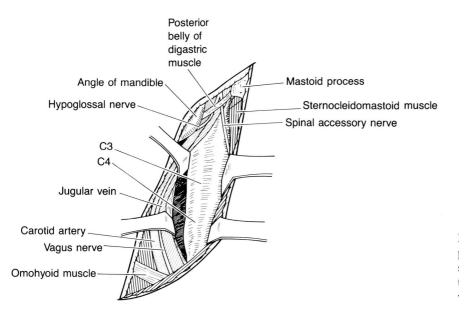

FIG. 4–2. The cervical spine approach posterior to the carotid sheath contents uses anterior retraction of the carotid artery and jugular vein.

necessary. This nerve, which is superficial to the anterior or common facial vein, is protected by keeping the dissection deep and inferior to this vein. The sternomastoid muscle is separated from the strap muscles, and the omohyoid muscle is identified and divided. The carotid vessels and the internal jugular vein and their branches are identified. The lateral retraction of these major vessels is prevented by their branches. Beginning inferiorly and progressing superiorly, ligation of the superior thyroid artery and vein, lingual artery and vein, and facial artery and vein allows lateral retraction of the carotid sheath (Fig. 4-3). The superior laryngeal nerve must be identified and protected as it crosses under the common or external carotid artery.

Unlike the low transcervical route, the retropharyngeal approach is carried out superior to the hypoglossal nerve. The styloid process may need to be fractured anteriorly if it interferes with the dissection. The submandibular gland may also require resection if further exposure is necessary. After exposure of the transverse spinal process, blunt dissection is used to mobilize the oropharynx, which is then retracted contralaterally, exposing the vertebral bodies covered by the longus colli muscles. Proper dissection is deep to the facial nerve and parotid gland.

This approach offers good exposure of C1 to C3, but it necessitates ligation of numerous branches of the external carotid artery and the internal jugular vein and risks injury to the superior laryngeal and hypoglossal nerves. In contrast, by approaching the upper spine by retracting the carotid sheath anteriorly with the laryngopharyngeal structures, a comparatively limited exposure is achieved, but the cervical sympathetic nerves are at risk for injury.

THE CLIVUS AND ATLAS

A variety of surgical approaches have been described to expose the clivus, the base of the skull, and C1. The purpose of the exposure and the extent of the surgical procedure determine the appropriate option.

The transoropharyngeal approach to the clivus, atlas, and axis is usually reserved for biopsies and drainage of infection.[8] This is performed using a Dingman or Crowe-Davis mouth retractor, which exposes the posterior pharyngeal wall (Fig. 4-4). Incision of the pharynx in the midline offers direct but limited exposure of the posterior cervical fascia and spine. This approach can be extended by dividing the soft and part of the hard palate (Fig. 4-5). Generally, a midline incision is used to divide the soft palate. The hard palate can be removed with rongeurs or high speed drills. At least one greater palatine artery (a division of the internal maxillary artery from the external carotid) must be protected for the palate to survive. The U-shaped flap is the most common variation of palatal flaps. If both palatine arteries are mobilized from their bony canals and the hook of the hamulus is resected and mobilized, this offers better exposure of the clivus and more room for some manipulation of instruments on the anterior cervical spine. A few procedures, such as removal of hypertrophic osteophytes and limited resection or drainage of osteomyelitis, can be per-

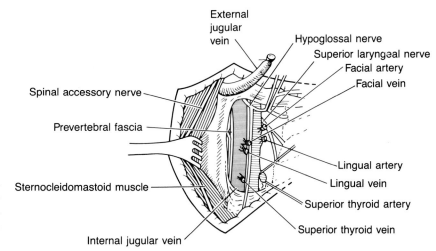

FIG. 4–3. The branches of the carotid artery and internal jugular vein are ligated to allow mobilization of the carotid sheath laterally as the hypopharynx is mobilized medially.

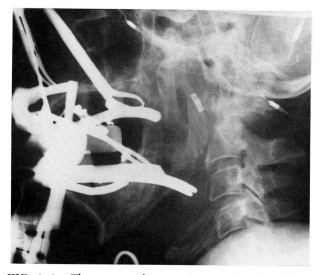

FIG. 4–4. The transoropharyngeal approach with a Dingman retractor is used to approach C2, which is partially subluxed and shows osteomyelitis.

formed with this direct approach.[12] It can also be used for limited resection of small clivus chordomas, nasopharyngeal masses, and marsupialization of craniopharyngiomas.[17]

To gain wider access and closer working distances from the clivus to C2 than either the transoral or retropharyngeal approaches, a "median labiomandibular glossotomy" approach should be used.[10] Although reference to the use of this technique in head and neck cancer surgery can be found dating back to the early nineteenth century, it was redescribed as an approach

to the upper cervical spine by Hall and for the clivus by Wood in the late 1970s.[4, 19]

A standard tracheostomy is performed and general anesthesia is continued by means of a cuffed tracheostomy tube. A midline incision splitting the lower lip is made through the chin and upper neck to the level of the hyoid bone. The incision is staggered around the lateral aspect of the chin to produce a more aesthetic scar (Fig. 4-6). It is carried through labial mucosa and gingiva to the periosteum, which is sharply incised and reflected. An oscillating power saw is used to make a stair-step anterior mandibulotomy (Fig. 4-7). In some cases, a lower central incisor must be removed to facilitate the bone cut. Taking care to prevent injury of the apexes of the anterior central incisors, four drill holes for wire closure can be made before the mandibulotomy (Fig. 4-8). The soft tissue incision is continued through the midline of the floor of the mouth, by way of the central lingual raphe and tongue back to the level of the epiglottis, and down to the hyoid bone (Fig. 4-9). Divide the hyoid bone if necessary for greater exposure. If the cervical spine is to be approached at a superior level, the soft palate can also be divided in the midline. The mandible and soft tissues are then widely retracted by means of self-retaining retractors for the spinal procedure (Fig. 4-10). The posterior pharyngeal wall can be opened in the midline, but it is usually incised as an inferiorly based apron flap with a cauterizing or hot knife.

After completing the procedure, the posterior pharyngeal wall is closed with resorbable sutures. The tongue and floor of mouth are closed in layers. The

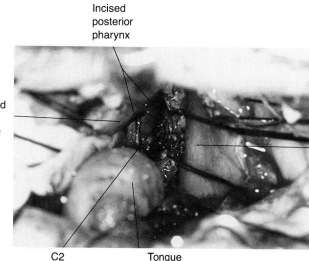

Incised posterior pharynx

Incised soft palate

Anterior tonsillar pillar

C2

Tongue

FIG. 4–5. Division of the soft and hard palate extends the cervical exposure with the transoropharyngeal approach.

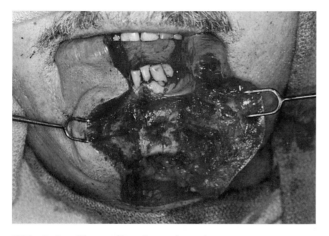

FIG. 4–6. The midline lower lip splitting incision is staggered around the lateral aspect of the chin to produce a more esthetic scar.

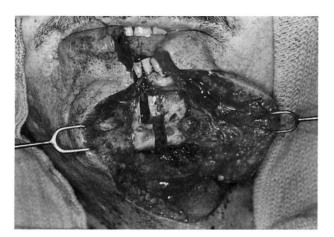

FIG. 4–7. A stair-step anterior mandibulotomy is made with an oscillating power saw.

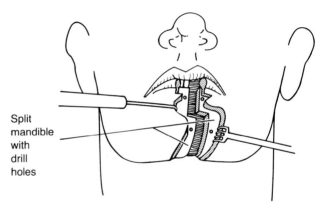

Split mandible with drill holes

FIG. 4–8. Drill holes for wire closure should be made before the mandibulotomy.

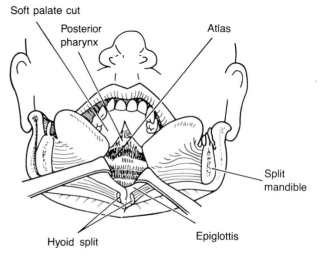

Soft palate cut

Posterior pharynx

Atlas

Split mandible

Hyoid split

Epiglottis

FIG. 4–9. The midline mandibulotomy incision is carried through the midline floor of the mouth and tongue to the epiglottis and hyoid bone.

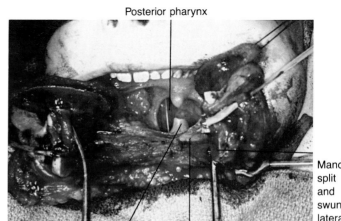

Posterior pharynx

Mandible split and swung laterally

Epiglottis   Split Hyoid bone

FIG. 4–10. The posterior pharyngeal wall is exposed with wide retraction of the soft tissues and a split hyoid.

73

mandibular osteotomy is reapproximated with stainless steel wire (24 gauge) through the previously drilled holes or with a compression bone plate. A drain is brought out through the submental region. If the mandible is wired, arch bars for intermaxillary fixation for 4 to 6 weeks ensure proper occlusion and speed mandibular union. Tube feedings are used for 7 to 10 days. The tracheostomy tube may be removed after the laryngeal edema resolves and the airway is patent, usually 7 to 10 days.

The transmandibular transcervical approach using a midline mandibulotomy as described by Biller provides the widest exposure to the midline components of the skull base, nasopharynx, clivus, anterior foramen magnum, and the upper cervical spine.[1, 4] After a tracheostomy is performed, a curvilinear incision is made extending from the mastoid tip, passing 4 to 5 cm below the mandible just above the hyoid bone, and reaching the submental region. The marginal nerve is identified and protected. The digastric tendon and styloid muscle are released from their hyoid attachments and reflected superiorly with the submandibular gland. The common and internal carotid arteries, internal jugular vein, and cranial nerves X through XII are identified and preserved. The external carotid artery is ligated and divided distal to the superior thyroid artery. The neck skin incision is then extended to include the lip-splitting incision. The mandibulotomy is made as previously described. Occasionally, a lateral osteotomy of the mandible may be used, but the lingual nerve is usually sacrificed.

The tongue is retracted contralaterally, and an incision is made in the floor of the mouth in the gingivoglossal sulcus extending toward the anterior tonsillar pillar (Fig. 4-11). The lingual nerve is identified and preserved, except for its postganglionic fibers to the submandibular and sublingual glands, which are divided. The oral and neck incisions are connected, and the hemimandible is swung laterally to create one surgical space (Fig. 4-12). The oral incision may be extended onto the lateral soft and hard palate for additional exposure of the clivus and nasopharynx if necessary. The entire oropharynx and nasopharynx is retracted contralaterally, maintaining its circumferential integrity. The pharynx is then pushed to the contralateral side, and the anterior surface of the clivus through C3 is exposed (Fig. 4-13). The closure is the same as described for the median labiomandibular glossotomy approach. A cricopharyngeal myotomy is performed to avoid prolonged swallowing difficulties.

COMPLICATIONS

Serous otitis media is a common complication after any of the transoral or transmandibular procedures. It also occurs with trauma to the lateral fossa of Rosenmüller. Insertion of a ventilation tube may be required. Prolonged dysphagia, neuromuscular incoordination in swallowing, and recurrent aspirations are rare complications. Few of these patients require a temporary gastrostomy tube or nasogastric tube. Orocervical

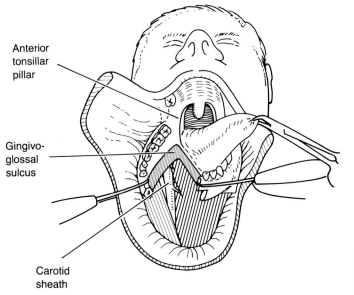

Anterior tonsillar pillar

Gingivoglossal sulcus

Carotid sheath

FIG. 4–11. The transmandibular transcervical approach continues through the gingivoglossal sulcus toward the anterior tonsillar pillar.

FIG. 4–12. The oral and neck incisions are connected with the transmandibular transcervical approach, creating one surgical space after the hemimandible is swung laterally.

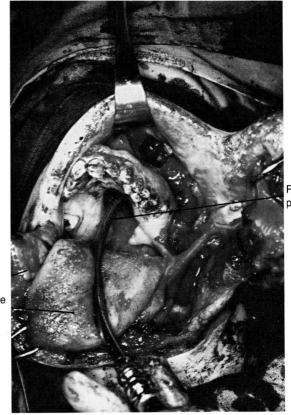

Posterior pharynx

Tongue and split mandible swung laterally

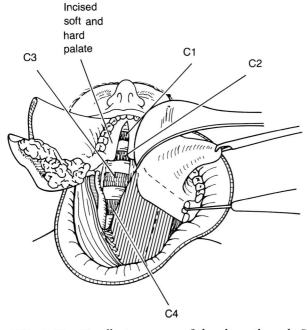

Incised soft and hard palate

C3 C1 C2

C4

FIG. 4–13. Excellent exposure of the clivus through C3 with room for surgical manipulation is achieved with the transmandibular transcervical approach.

fistulas, mandibular malunion, parapharyngeal abscesses, and vagal, accessory, or hypoglossal nerve deficits are other complications.

Theoretically, transoral approaches to the upper cervical spine carry a higher risk of infection than extrapharyngeal approaches, but the true incidence of complications has not been demonstrated. No well-designed study has substantiated the incidence of oral contamination.[10] Those familiar with performing major surgical procedures using a transoral approach recognize that infection is rarely a problem if appropriate perioperative antibiotics are used in conjunction with sound surgical technique and meticulous hemostasis.

Complications from the standard anterior retropharyngeal approaches to the cervical spine are uncommon if neurovascular structures are identified and protected during the exposure. The major complications of these procedures are neural injury, esophageal and pharyngeal perforation, hemorrhage, and airway obstruction. In employing the upper cervical approach, airway obstruction can be caused by traumatic edema, hemorrhage, or venous congestion of the upper pharynx and larynx after vigorous retraction. This can be avoided by an elective tracheostomy or prolonged nasotracheal intubation in high-risk patients. Perforation of the pharynx or esophagus can be avoided by diligent operative technique. When it happens, primary repair or reconstruction of the damaged structure must be done immediately. Nasogastric feeding is used for 7 to 10 days to allow healing.

The most commonly injured nerve in the upper cervical approach is the superior laryngeal nerve.[18] The nerve lies deep to the carotid artery and crosses the operative field diagonally at the level of C2 and C3. The major postoperative symptom is hoarseness. The recurrent nerve is at risk in the lower cervical approach. The right nerve is more often damaged; the left recurrent nerve is more resistant to stretching because of its greater length. Neural injuries can be prevented by identifying and protecting the nerves before proceeding with dissection in an area. Other neural injuries are rare, but there are occasional injuries to the cervical nerve roots, the hypoglossal, phrenic, vagus, and the sympathetic chain. Thoracic duct injury on a left-sided lower cervical approach may cause external chylorrhea. Vertebral artery injury can be avoided by delineating the midline and not proceeding beyond the lateral cervical processes before exposing the vertebral bodies.

Highly selective approaches are available for the exposure of the entire anterior cervical spine. The choice is determined by the location of the cervical body to be exposed, the necessary extent of exposure, the procedure to be performed, and the experience of the surgeon with the procedure. Careful attention to identifying and protecting vital structures in the neck during the exposure procedure usually prevents unnecessary complications. Meticulous attention to detail is a must, and cooperation between the orthopedic surgeon or neurosurgeon and an experienced head and neck surgeon can enhance the successful performance of these procedures.

References

1. Biller HF, Shugar JM, Krespi YP: New techniques for wide field exposure of the base of skull. Arch Otolaryngol 107:698, 1981

2. Cloward RB: The anterior approach for removal of ruptured cervical disks. J Neurosurg 15:602, 1958

3. DeAndrade JR, McNab I: Anterior occipito-cervical fusion using an extrapharyngeal exposure. J Bone Joint Surg [Am] 51:1621, 1959

4. Hall JE, Denis F, Murray J: Exposure of the upper cervical spine for spinal decompression by a mandible and tongue-splitting approach. J Bone Joint Surg [Am] 59:121, 1977

5. Hoff JT, Wilson CB: Microsurgical approach to the anterior cervical spine and spinal cord. Clin Neurosurg 26:523, 1979

6. Komisar A, Tubbaddor K: Extrapharyngeal (anterolateral) approach to the cervical spine. Head Neck Surg 6:600, 1983

7. Krespi YP, Gady H: Surgery of the clivus and anterior cervical spine. Arch Otolaryngol Head Neck Surg 114:73, 1988

8. McAfee PC, Bohlman HH, Riley CH, et al: The anterior retropharyngeal approach to the upper part of the cervical spine. J Bone Joint Surg [Am] 69:1371, 1987

9. Micheli LJ, Hood RW: Anterior exposure of the cervicothoracic spine using a combined cervical and thoracic approach. J Bone Joint Surg [Am] 65:992, 1983

10. Moore LJ, Schwartz HC: Median labiomandibular glossotomy for access to the cervical spine. J Oral Maxillofac Surg 43:909, 1985

11. Robinson RA, Smith G: Anterolateral cervical disc removal and interbody fusion for cervical disk syndrome. Bull Johns Hopkins Hosp 96:223, 1955

12. Saffouri MH, Ward PA: Surgical correction of dysphagia due to cervical osteophytes. Ann Otol Rhinol Laryngol 83:65, 1974

13. Sherk HH, Pratt L: Anterior approaches to the cervical spine. Laryngoscope 93:168, 1983

14. Smith GW, Robinson RA: The treatment of certain cervical-spine disorders by anterior removal of the intervertebral disc and interbody fusion. J Bone Joint Surg [Am] 40:607, 1958

15. Sobel SM, Rigual NR: Anterolateral extrapharyngeal approach for cervical osteophyte-induced dysphagia. Ann Otol Rhinol Laryngol 93:498, 1984

16. Southwick WO, Robinson RA: Surgical approaches to the vertebral bodies in the cervical and lumbar regions. J Bone Joint Surg [Am] 35:631, 1957

17. Spector JG: Management of juvenile angiofibromata. Laryngoscope 98:1016, 1988

18. Tew JW, Mayfield FH: Complications of surgery of the anterior cervical spine. In the Proceedings of the Clinical Congress of Neurosurgeons, Atlanta, 1975, p 424. Baltimore, Williams & Wilkins, 1976

19. Wood JE, Sadar ES, Levine HL, et al: Surgical problems of the base of the skull. Arch Otolaryngol 106:1, 1980

CHAPTER
5

■ ■ ■ ■

Anterior Exposure of the Thoracolumbar Spine

Ronald L. DeWald

■

The spine serves as a two-column supporting structure for the body. The posterior column, which resists tension loads, consists of the lamina, pedicles, facet joints, ligamentum flavum, and interconnecting ligaments. The anterior column, which resists compression, consists of vertebral bodies, discs, and anterior longitudinal ligaments. Stability of the spine means that both columns are functional and stable.

Pathologic changes in the spine frequently begin in the vertebral bodies, and disease, trauma, or deformity of the spine may occur anterior to the spinal cord and nerve roots. To treat these pathologic conditions, the direct anterior approach is preferred.

The development of anterior spinal surgery reflects the course of surgery in general. Improvements of anesthesia, blood banking, radiographs, and antibiotics have enabled the experienced spinal surgeon to undertake previously constrained procedures.

Arthur Hodgson introduced the value of anterior surgery for spinal conditions to the orthopedic world.[5] His work began with tuberculosis while he was the colonial surgeon in Hong Kong. Tuberculosis of the spine was common in Hong Kong, and before 1955 it was treated with antitubercular drug therapy and the usual method of immobilization in plaster beds, drainage of cold abscesses, and posterior spine fusion. Hodgson and F. E. Stock, a chest surgeon, designed a treatment program using two principles: radical excision of all diseased tissues and stabilization of the remaining spine with anterior interbody bone grafts. This work generated various approaches to the spine.[1, 2, 4, 6–8]

SURGICAL TECHNIQUE

Exposure of Thoracic Vertebra 1 to Thoracic Vertebra 4

Third-rib resection is used for the transthoracic approach to the area from T1 to T4. Resection of the third rib allows greater spreading of the intercostal space than resection of the second rib. The cephalad extension of the exposure is enhanced if there is a kyphosis deformity. Additional ribs up or down may be removed to facilitate the exposure.

The patient is placed in the lateral decubitus position with the appropriate side up. The side of the surgery depends on the presenting complaints or the appearance of the abnormality on the CT scan. It may be helpful to prepare and drape the entire upper ex-

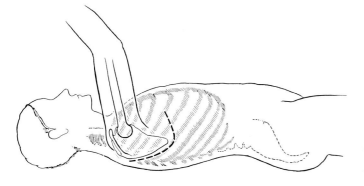

FIG. 5–1. The patient is in the lateral decubitus position. The arm is prepared and draped out of the field. A free arm drape may be used to help position the arm and use it as a retractor. The skin and subcutaneous tissue are incised between the vertebral border of the scapula and the spine at approximately T2. The incision is brought down, around the scapula, under the axilla, and anteriorly to the costal margin of the third rib.

tremity on the side of the exposure to facilitate scapula retraction and position (Fig. 5-1).

The skin is incised from the paraspinous area at T1 distally along the medial border of the scapula and under the tip of the scapula at the seventh rib. The incision continues under the axilla to the costal cartilage of the third rib.

Each muscle layer is divided down to the level of the rib. The muscles that are partially sectioned are the trapezius, latissimus dorsi, the rhomboid major, and the serratus posterior. Careful dissection and electrocautery minimize muscle bleeding and allow exposure of the periosteum of the third rib.

After the muscles are divided, the scapula is retracted cephalad and medially using a scapular retractor (Fig. 5-2).

The first rib is somewhat inside the second rib, and this is important for locating the correct rib by count-

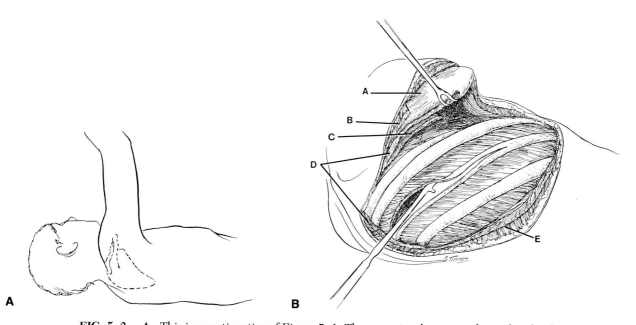

FIG. 5–2. **A.** This is a continuation of Figure 5–1. The trapezius, latissimus dorsi, rhomboid major, and posterior serratus are divided with electrocautery. **B.** Find the ribs and count down from the first rib, remembering that the first rib sits inside the second rib. The periosteum of the third rib is incised. The scapula is retracted with the scapular retractor, and work is done in the acute angle of the muscle attachment to the rib. The rib is stripped from posterior to anterior on the cephalad side of the rib and from anterior to posterior on the inferior portion of the rib. Figure labels: A, scapula; B, trapezius; C, posterior serratus; D, rhomboid major; E, latissimus dorsi.

FIG. 5–3. The rib is removed from its chondral junction to its attachment to the spine. If desired, the posterior portion of the rib can remain attached to the spine, and the rib can be severed at the vertebral transverse process. The chest spreader is inserted and the chest cavity inspected. The parietal pleura is incised to the midvertebral body and incised superiorly and inferiorly at that level. The segmental vessels are dissected and ligated.

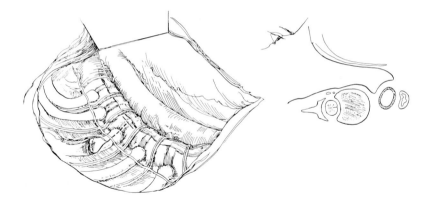

ing. The first rib is frequently identified by palpating the attachment of the scalenus anticus or medius on the second rib.[3]

The periosteum of the third rib is incised and stripped, and the rib is excised from its angle to the costocartilage. The elevator should always be placed in the acute angle of insertion of the intercostal muscle. Because the rib bed is open and a retractor is inserted, the strip is performed posterior to anterior on the superior surface and anterior to posterior on the inferior surface. The aorta, spine, ribs, pleura, and veins are inspected (Fig. 5-3).

The parietal pleura is incised by extending the incision of the pleura to the midvertebral body. The pleura is then incised superiorly and distally for the length of the wound, permitting identification of the white tissue of the intervertebral disc. Between each intervertebral disc lies the intervertebral body, and in the middle of the body are the intercostal artery and vein (Fig. 5-4). These can be dissected, ligated, and severed, allowing full dissection of the vertebral bodies. Use of a double-lumen endotracheal tube enables the surgeon to collapse the lung on the side of dissection.

Exposure from Thoracic Vertebra 2 to Lumbar Vertebra 2

The type of abnormality and its location dictates which rib is used as the entry point to the chest. In treating scoliosis, the entry should always be on the convex side of the curvature. For infection, the rib cephalad to the diseased area gives adequate proximal exposure for the lesion, and it is much easier to work down than up. For example, removal of the sixth rib provides access to the vertebral bodies from T6 to T12.

If the patient's ribs are horizontally oriented, the surgeon can usually reach the vertebrae above the excised rib, but if the ribs are sloping, it may only be possible to reach the vertebrae below (Fig. 5-5).

If direct access is needed to the spinal canal, remove the rib that leads to the disc space at the involved level. In the lower thoracic spine, the rib articulates on the facet joints of the vertebral body above and below the disc. This is a useful landmark for entering the spinal canal (Fig. 5-6).

The patient is oriented in a straight, lateral decubitus position. The appropriate holders fix the pelvis by compression between the symphysis pubis and the sacrum. A sandbag stabilizes the patient's position, and tape is used to secure the patient. The pelvis should be just distal to the break in the standard operating table

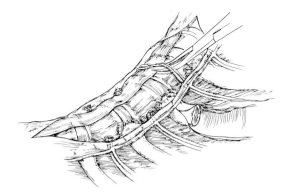

FIG. 5–4. The vessels are best dissected using a Mixter clamp. The bundle is mobilized, and a ligature is passed under the bundle and tied. The clamp is placed proximally, the vascular bundle is severed, and the clamp is tied. In this manner, the vessels can be ligated up and down the spine. Sometimes there is a small osseous branch from the segmental artery, and bone wax is needed to control this bleeding.

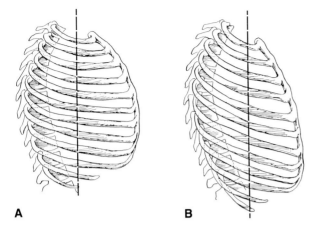

FIG. 5–5. Sloping ribs may cause selection of the incorrect rib for exposure. If it is not necessary to enter the neural canal, the rib to be removed is chosen by selecting the one opposite the vertebral body in the mid axillary line when viewing a lateral chest x-ray film. A better rule of thumb is to select the rib to the vertebra one level above the lesion. It is always easier to work down than up. If it is necessary to enter the canal, the rib that articulates at the appropriate disc space is used.

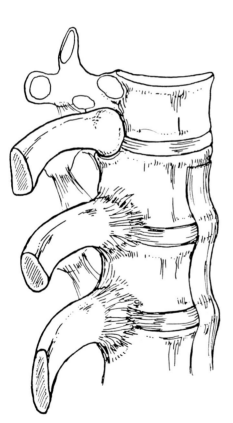

FIG. 5–6. In the lower spine, the ribs articulate with the superior portion of the corresponding vertebral body. Therefore, rib 12 articulates at the 11–12 disc space. This illustration reveals that articulation and the heavy transverse process rib ligaments. In tuberculosis and pyogenic problems, one can usually disarticulate the rib and open the abscess cavity simultaneously.

(Fig. 5-7). The table is flexed to allow more room for the surgical procedure and unflexed when closing the wound.

The skin is incised from the lateral border of the erector spinal muscles to the sternochondrocostal junction over the rib to be resected. The incision can then extend down the abdomen 3 to 5 cm medial to the anterior iliac spine, depending on how much of the lumbar spine must be exposed. It is possible to reach the sacrum through this approach (Fig. 5-8). The latissimus dorsi, trapezius, and rhomboid major and minor muscles of the back are incised as necessary. After the exposure of the chest wall, all the ribs can be counted, up from the twelfth rib and down from the first rib.

The periosteum of the rib is incised with electrocautery, and the periosteum is stripped, as previously described (see Fig. 5-8). My colleagues and I use a curved-tip rib elevator to strip the superior and inferior border of the rib. We try to maintain an intact periosteum. A doyen elevator is used to elevate the inner periosteum of the under surface of the rib.

The rib is cut with a rib cutter as far posteriorly as possible, being careful not to leave any sharp points. We then pack the rib bed with a sponge that has been soaked in a 1:500,000 solution of adrenalin. Bone wax at the end of the rib is indicated for nonthoracic surgeons. The periosteum of the rib bed is incised and opened with the Metzenbaum scissors, and the lung is packed. Pleural adhesions can be gently dissected; they are usually avascular. The lung is retracted and protected, and a chest spreader (e.g., Zielke chest spreader) is used. After a T-shaped incision of the parietal pleura, the intervertebral discs and vertebral

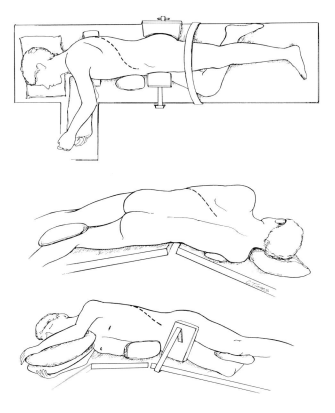

FIG. 5–7. These illustrations reveal how the patient is positioned for a thoracophrenolumbotomy. The same position is used for operating above or below the diaphragm if the surgeon wishes the patient to be in the complete lateral position. Having the patient in the full lateral position allows the surgeon to remain oriented while performing work on the neural canal. The pelvis is fixed firmly with the Siemens holders. A large sandbag is placed next to the abdomen. The incision begins at the paraspinal area at the appropriate level. The appropriate level depends on the pathology of the spine. For the lower thoracoabdominal approach, we generally use rib 10. One can remove rib 5 and continue down the spine by transecting the costochondral cartilages of ribs 6, 7, 8, 9, and 10 and by proceeding down the abdomen. This allows exposure of the spine from T4 to S1. If one removes the 10th rib, the costochondral junction is incised. The periosteum is identified by blunt dissection.

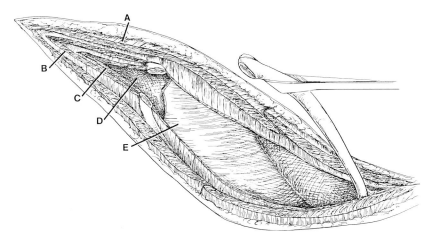

FIG. 5–8. This illustration identifies the rib, the lung, the diaphragm, the peritoneum, and the abdominal muscles. The keystone to the procedure is the costochondral cartilage. These two pieces of cartilage help the surgeon find the peritoneum, which is directly below. The costochondral cartilage is also the key landmark for closure of the wound. It divides the chest from the abdomen. The abdominal muscles are divided separately after the peritoneum is dissected free. If the affected area of the spine is T12 or above, it is possible to stay above the diaphragm. If it is T12, L1, or L2, it is sometimes possible to stay below the diaphragm, but the exposure is limited, and we prefer to transect the diaphragm for exposure to the T12, L1, or L2 area. Figure labels: **A,** external oblique; **B,** internal oblique; **C,** transversalis; **D,** peritoneum; **E,** diaphragm.

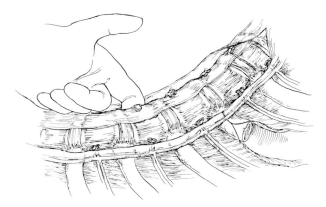

FIG. 5–9. The vessels are ligated in the middle to allow for lateral circulation at the neural foramen. This illustration depicts the spine in the midthoracic area. After the vessels are ligated, it is possible to dissect the entire spine ventrally to the opposite neural foramen. Avoid the opposite vascular bundle. The surgeon's finger is completely around the spine.

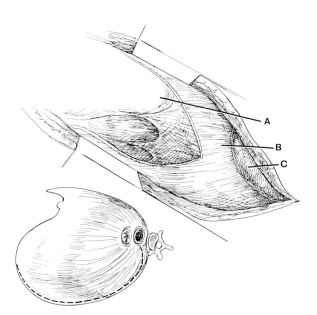

FIG. 5–10. The diaphragm is innervated by the phrenic nerve, which courses from the midline. Peripheral transection of the diaphragm avoids denervation of the posterior portion. Figure labels: **A**, peritoneum; **B**, diaphragm; **C**, lung.

bodies are identified. The artery and vein at the middle of the vertebral body are identified, ligated, and severed. The dissection is best accomplished by using a Mixter clamp and dissecting above and below the artery and vein. The clamp then scoops under the vessels, and a ligature is passed. The parietal pleura is then dissected medially and laterally. The surgeon can place his or her finger around the vertebral body (Fig. 5-9).

Segmental vessels are tied and ligated in the middle of the vertebral body to preserve the collateral circulation between the segmental arteries at the intervertebral foramen. Spinal cord monitoring is performed during the ligation of the vessels to ensure the maintenance of the vascular system of the spinal cord.

To approach the spine below T12, it is necessary to perform a thoracophrenolumbotomy. The positioning of the patient is exactly the same as above. The abdominal incision follows the course of the tenth rib, divides the costochondral junction in two equal parts, and proceeds down the external oblique fascia (see Fig. 5-8). This exposure allows access as far as the sacrum.

It is possible to stay below the diaphragm by selecting a twelfth-rib extrapleural retroperitoneal approach. The wound, however, is small, and major reconstruction is a problem. It is preferable to approach this area by removing the tenth rib, dividing the diaphragm, and incising down the abdomen.

The preferred site of transection of the diaphragm is 10 to 15 mm from the peripheral costal insertion

(Fig. 5-10). Transection of the diaphragm sections the superior and inferior diaphragmatic arteries and the motor branches for the phrenic nerves. Peripheral transection is less time consuming and avoids denervation of part of the posterior diaphragm.

Before transection of the diaphragm, find the retroperitoneal space at the area of the divided costochondral junction and gently sweep the peritoneal contents away from the undersurface of the diaphragm. Gently dissect the peritoneal contents away from the quadratus lumborum and the iliopsoas muscle. The ureter is easily identified on the posterior portion of the peritoneum. After the peritoneum is mobilized and visualized, transection of the diaphragm and of the internal oblique and transversalis muscles can commence. Because the peritoneum tends to thin out medially, start the dissection laterally (Fig. 5-11).

Segmental vessels are identified, ligated, and severed. The spine can be inspected from as high as T6 to as low in the abdomen as necessary (Fig. 5-12). The key to closing this wound is to close the costochondral cartilages, because this step aligns all intervening tissues. Use interrupted silk for closing the diaphragm. The chest tube is placed in the anterior axillary line so the patient cannot lie on it.

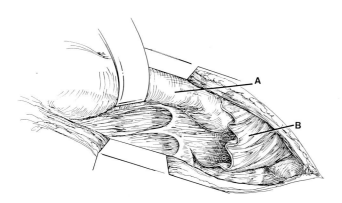

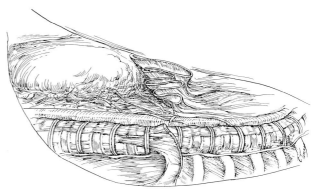

FIG. 5–11. After the diaphragm is transected, the peritoneum can be laterally to medially dissected. Because the peritoneum is thin medially, the dissection should begin laterally. The ureter lies on the posterior aspect of the peritoneum and should always be identified. Figure labels: **A,** peritoneum; **B,** diaphragm.

FIG. 5–12. The illustration reveals how the spine from T4 to S1 may be exposed by a thoracophrenolumbotomy approach.

References

1. Dwyer AF: Experience of anterior correction of scoliosis. Clin Orthop 93:192, 1973
2. Dwyer AF, Newton NC, Sherwood AA: An anterior approach to scoliosis. Clin Orthop 62:192, 1969
3. Goss CM (ed): Gray's Anatomy of the Human Body, 29th ed. Philadelphia, Lea & Febiger, 1973
4. Hodgson AR, Rau ACM: Anterior surgical approaches to the spinal column. In Apley AG (ed): Recent Advances in Orthopedics. Baltimore, Williams & Wilkins, 1964
5. Hodgson AR, Rau ACM: Anterior approach to the spinal column. Recent Adv Orthop 9:289, 1969
6. Louis RL: Surgery of the Spine. Berlin, Springer-Verlag, 1982
7. Riceborough EJ: The anterior approach of the spine for correction of the axial skeleton. Clin Orthop 93:207, 1973
8. Watkins RG (ed): Surgical Approaches to the Spine. New York, Springer-Verlag, 1983

CHAPTER

6

Paramedian Retroperitoneal Approach to the Anterior Lumbar Spine

Brent T. Allen
Keith H. Bridwell

■

TECHNIQUE

The patient is placed in the supine position. After the induction of anesthesia, the lateral edge of the left rectus abdominal muscle is identified by palpation 4 to 6 cm lateral to the midline. A vertical incision along the lateral edge of the rectus is made from the costal margin to the pubis (Fig. 6-1). The plane is deepened through the subcutaneous fat to the abdominal wall fascia. The lateral border of the rectus muscle is again palpated, and an incision is made in the anterior rectus sheath along the extreme lateral edge of the muscle. The fibers of the rectus muscle are slightly retracted medially to visualize the posterior rectus fascia and the arcuate line. The muscle should not be mobilized enough to expose the inferior epigastric vessels under the midportion of the muscle belly. However, if these vessels are inadvertently damaged, they may be safely ligated.

Above the arcuate line, the abdominal wall deep to the rectus consists of the posterior rectus fascia and transversalis fascia. Inferior to the arcuate line, the abdominal wall deep to the rectus consists of transversalis fascia. The most direct way of entering the preperitoneal space is to incise the fibers of the arcuate line and the underlying transversalis fascia (Fig. 6-2). Immediately deep to the transversalis fascia is the peritoneum. A finger can be inserted into the preperitoneal plane between the transversalis fascia and the peritoneum, and a space can be developed superiorly under the posterior rectus fascia. As this plane is enlarged, the posterior rectus and/or the transversalis fascia are divided superiorly and inferiorly along the lateral edge of the rectus muscle, exposing the peritoneum throughout the length of the incision. If the peritoneal sac is inadvertently entered, the defect is repaired with 3-0 chromic suture.

The peritoneal envelope is swept medially, and the dissection is carried into the left iliac fossa. The peritoneum is bluntly dissected off the psoas muscle, identifying the genitofemoral nerve on the anterior aspect of the psoas muscle. As the peritoneum is lifted off the posterior abdominal wall and retracted toward the midline, the ureter, gonadal vein, iliac vessels, sympathetic chain, and aorta are seen (Figs. 6-3 and 6-4). The peritoneum is mobilized medially to the midline off the posterior abdominal wall from the inferior edge of the left kidney to the sacrum.

Exposure of the lumbar spine is best started on the

(text continues on page 88)

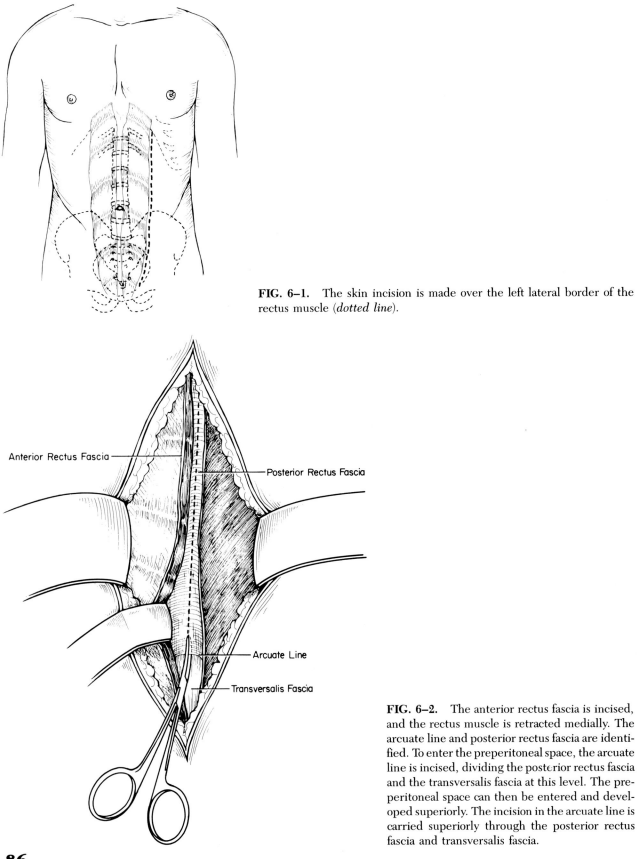

FIG. 6–1.   The skin incision is made over the left lateral border of the rectus muscle (*dotted line*).

Anterior Rectus Fascia

Posterior Rectus Fascia

Arcuate Line

Transversalis Fascia

FIG. 6–2.   The anterior rectus fascia is incised, and the rectus muscle is retracted medially. The arcuate line and posterior rectus fascia are identified. To enter the preperitoneal space, the arcuate line is incised, dividing the posterior rectus fascia and the transversalis fascia at this level. The preperitoneal space can then be entered and developed superiorly. The incision in the arcuate line is carried superiorly through the posterior rectus fascia and transversalis fascia.

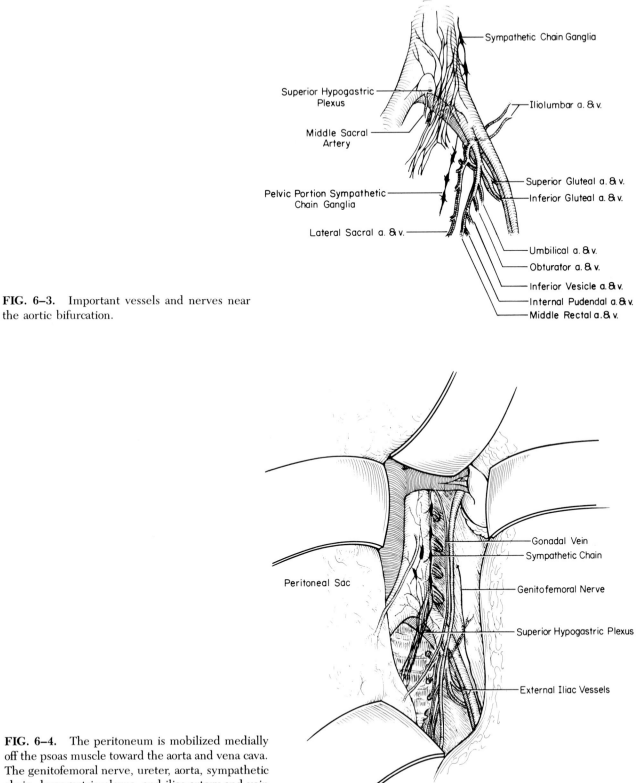

FIG. 6–3. Important vessels and nerves near the aortic bifurcation.

FIG. 6–4. The peritoneum is mobilized medially off the psoas muscle toward the aorta and vena cava. The genitofemoral nerve, ureter, aorta, sympathetic chain, hypogastric plexus, and iliac artery and vein are identified.

medial side of the psoas muscle proximal to the aortic bifurcation at the level of L4. The vertebral bodies are palpated deep to the medial edge of the psoas muscle and are exposed with a Cobb elevator, moving the psoas muscle laterally off the vertebral bodies. As the vertebral bodies are exposed, the left segmental lumbar arteries and veins are identified anterior to the vertebral body. These vessels should be individually ligated close to the aorta with 2-0 silk ties. After ligation of the lumbar vessels, the vertebral body can be clearly visualized, and a plane can be developed with a Cobb elevator between the vertebral body and anterior longitudinal ligament, exposing the entire anterior surface of the vertebral body.

CASE NO. 1—A. D.

A 56-year-old woman with diabetes presented at an outside hospital with multiple-level spinal stenosis. Preoperatively, she had normal disc height at L4–L5 and very slight degenerative spondylolistheses at L3–L4 and L2–L3. Postoperatively, she developed a three-level spondylolisthesis at L2–L3, L3–L4, and L4–L5 after spinal stenosis decompressions at those levels. This caused instability and amplified her back and leg pain. She was subsequently treated with posterior contoured Steffee plates from L2 to the sacrum, yielding partial reductions of the spondylolistheses at those three levels. After posterior pedicular fixation and transverse process fusions from L2 to the sacrum with right autogenous iliac bone graft, she had an anterior fusion. The anterior fusion was performed by way of the paramedian approach with anterior interbody fusions using fresh frozen tricortical iliac bone at L2–L3, L3–L4, and L4–L5. She has an apparent solid fusion 1 year after surgery and has had relief of back and leg pain.

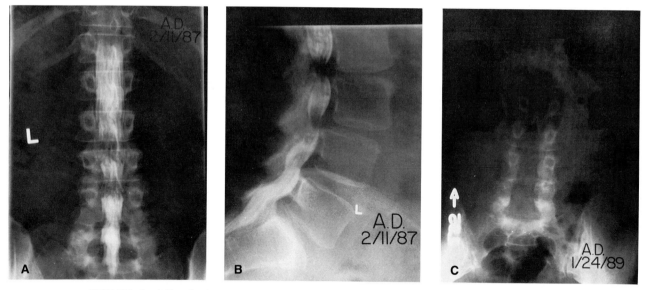

CASE NO. 1—A.D.   **A.** Anteroposterior myelogram film showing multilevel spinal stenosis.   **B.** Lateral myelogram film showing a relatively normal sagittal contour with small degenerative spondylolistheses at L2–L3 and L3–L4.   **C.** An anteroposterior upright spine x-ray film several months after her spinal stenosis decompression, which extended from L2 to the sacrum.   **D.** Standing lateral x-ray film of the lumbar spine on presentation to the author. Her spondylolistheses had increased at L2–L3 and L3–L4 and spondylolisthesis had developed at L4–L5.   **E, F.** Standing anteroposterior and lateral x-ray films 1 year after the circumferential fusion and posterior segmental instrumentation. The anterior interbody fusions from L2 to L5 were performed through the paramedian retroperitoneal approach. Instrumentation performed posteriorly to the sacrum was necessary to control the spondylolistheses from L2 to L5. It was not necessary to instrument any segments proximal to the spondylolistheses.

(continued)

CASE NO. 1—A. D. (*continued*)

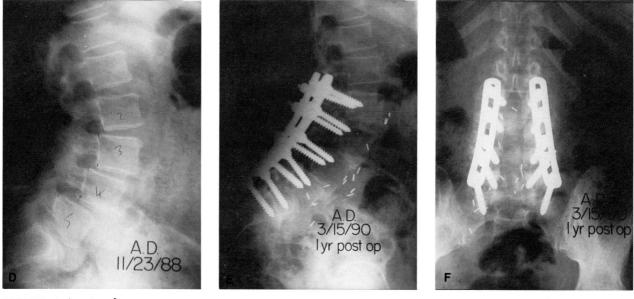

CASE NO. 1 (*continued*)

The dissection is continued superiorly to L2 and inferiorly to the sacrum. Exposure of L2 is facilitated by retracting the lower pole of the kidney superiorly. There is an inconstant lumbar vein, sometimes arising from the posterior aspect of the renal vein, that must be ligated and divided before the kidney is retracted to prevent tearing of the vein. The aorta, gonadal vein, and ureter are retracted medially throughout the procedure. The sympathetic chain is preserved if possible. Safe retraction of the ureter requires mobilization of the ureter to avoid excessive trauma. The ureter crosses anterior to the iliac vessel bifurcation as it enters the pelvis. If medial mobilization of the ureter produces unacceptable tension or limits exposure of L2, the ureter can be retracted laterally. Ureteral mobility is best performed by including a generous portion of periureteric tissue to avoid compromising the ureter's blood supply.

If exposure above L2 is necessary, the skin incision can be curved proximally in an oblique fashion to the end of the tenth, eleventh, or twelfth ribs. After entering the retroperitoneum, upper lumbar exposure is achieved by rotating the kidney medially.

Exposure of the spine distal to the aortic bifurcation demands caution and gentle technique because of the fragile left iliac vessels and their branches, which lie over the lower lumbar spine and sacrum. These vessels must be completely mobilized to gain satisfactory exposure of the lower spine. The common iliac artery and vein are generally free of small branches or tributaries and can be mobilized as a unit down to the iliac bifurcation. The superior hypogastric nerve plexus is anterior to the origin of the left iliac artery and should be preserved in males to avoid sexual dysfunction.[2] This plexus contains primarily sympathetic fibers and may lead to retrograde ejaculation and subsequent sterility in males (3–5%) if damaged. The parasympathetic fibers responsible for penile erection arise from the S2 to S4 segments and are carried in the inferior hypogastric plexus.[1] These fibers extend to the prostate, the bladder, and the base of the penis, and they usually are inferior to the operative field.

The L5–S1 disc and sacrum can usually be exposed below the aortic bifurcation after ligation of the middle sacral artery without mobilization of the iliac vessels. However, for extensive exposure from L2 to the sacrum, the bifurcation of both the common iliac artery and vein located just above the L5–S1 disc must be completely mobilized to allow a clear view of the

(*text continues on page 92*)

CASE NO. 2—M. P.

A 61-year-old woman presented with a normal-looking spine and disc spaces at L4–L5 and L5–S1 in 1983. She subsequently had three surgeries on her spine consisting of laminectomy from L4 to the sacrum and discectomy at L4–L5. By January of 1990, she had developed a painful and progressive deformity at L4–L5. The L5–S1 level was unchanged. She was, therefore, treated with a two-stage, single-anesthesia, same-day procedure, which consisted of a transverse process fusion at L4–L5 posteriorly with right autogenous iliac bone grafts placed anterior and posterior to the transverse processes at L4–L5 and single-level Steffee plates with some corrective force applied across the disc space. After the posterior pro-

cedure, the patient was repositioned supine and had an anterior interbody fusion performed at L4–L5 through a paramedian approach. The bone graft used anteriorly consisted of two bicortical iliac struts, which were harvested from the dorsal wing of the right ilium during the posterior procedure. The morbidity, blood loss, and anesthetic time for both an anterior and a posterior approach to the spine using one anesthetic is comparable to that of simultaneously performing a posterior lumbar interbody fusion (PLIF) and posterior transverse process fusion with posterior pedicle fixation in a patient who has extensive anterior canal epidural scarring from previous surgery.

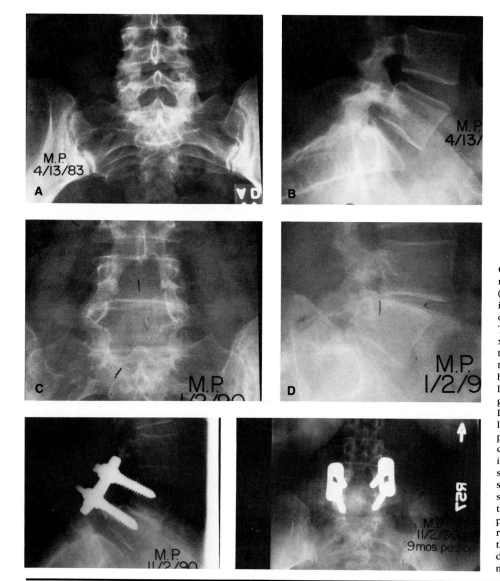

CASE NO. 2—M.P. A, B. Normal-appearing anteroposterior (AP) and lateral x-ray films showing relatively normal disc heights on this patient in 1983. C, D. The patient's AP and lateral spine x-ray films 7 years later, after three laminectomies and a discectomy at L4–L5 with a resultant hyperextension deformity, collapse of the disc space, and degenerative spondylolisthesis at L4–L5. E, F. Standing AP and lateral x-ray films in the early postoperative period after circumferential reconstruction showing partial restitution of the disc space and partial reduction of the spondylolisthesis. Subsequent fusion and maintenance of reduction has ensued. The anterior paramedian approach provides direct access to the midline front of the spine so that the surgeon does not have to fight the psoas muscle.

CASE NO. 3—C. D.

An adolescent male presented with a high-grade spondylolisthesis. He was treated with partial reduction and posterior pedicle fixation and transverse process fusion from L4 to the sacrum. Interbody fusion was refused by the parents. After subsequent non-union and recurrence of the deformity at L5–S1, he was salvaged with another reduction of the spondylolisthesis with Edwards instrumentation. After posterior reinstrumentation and new bone grafting, the patient was treated anteriorly. Through an anterior paramedian approach, autogenous iliac bone grafting was performed at the L5–S1 disc. The anterior paramedian approach makes it possible to approach the L5–S1 disc directly through the midline under the bifurcation of the great vessels without having to enter the peritoneum. The sympathetic chain usually lies to the left of the midline. Electrocautery is not used over the spine in this area. The sympathetic chain is gently swept over to the left. A subperiosteal approach is performed at L5–S1 after incising the periosteum slightly to the right of the midline to stay away from the sympathetic chain. The patient progressed to a solid fusion. Initial indications for reduction in adolescents continue to be widely debated among spinal surgeons.

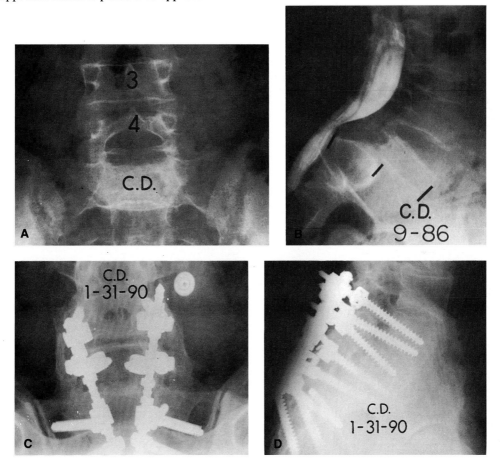

CASE NO. 3—C.D.   **A, B.** Anteroposterior and lateral x-ray films showing the high-grade spondylolisthesis.   **C, D.** The anteroposterior and lateral x-ray films after circumferential reconstruction. The advantage of a separate anterior approach is that the bone grafts can be contoured and the bed created for lordosis (greater disc height anteriorly than posteriorly). This is not possible with a flank approach at L5–S1. The principal disadvantage is the separate incision and the potential for injury to the sympathetic plexus.

lumbosacral junction. This allows the lumbosacral spine to be approached either medially or laterally to the iliac vessels. Mobilization of iliac artery bifurcation usually requires ligation of several branches of the internal iliac artery, including the iliolumbar and lateral sacral arteries (Fig. 6-5). These vessels should be ligated and divided close to their origins. If necessary, the main trunk of the internal iliac artery can usually be safely ligated and divided unilaterally, but individual branch ligation is preferred. Excessive traction on the diseased, calcified arteries often found in elderly patients should be avoided to prevent fracture of an atherosclerotic plaque and possible arterial thrombosis.

Mobilization of the internal iliac vein is challenging because of its numerous small venous tributaries. Gentle division of the investing fascia about the common iliac vein facilitates mobilization and identifies the origins of the external and internal iliac veins. There may be one or two low lumbar veins that empty into the external iliac vein, but the internal iliac vein receives

the majority of the pelvic venous flow. Exposure of the superior sacrum requires careful elevation of the internal iliac vein off the lateral aspect of the sacrum. The tributaries of the internal iliac vein are covered by the presacral fascia. This fascia firmly tethers the internal iliac vein in the pelvis and must be incised for safe identification of the tributaries and mobilization of the vein. Mobilization requires ligation and division of the iliolumbar, lateral sacral, and presacral venous tributaries as they enter the internal iliac vein (see Figs. 6-3 and 6-5). The presacral veins form a plexus over the sacrum and must be handled gently. If the tributaries are torn, they can be controlled by suture ligation. Ligation of the internal iliac vein should be avoided because it may increase venous pressure in the pelvis and promote venous oozing.

Throughout the procedure, care must be taken not to compress the iliac arteries or veins for prolonged periods to avoid thrombosis of the vessels. Because of potential trauma associated with extensive venous mo-

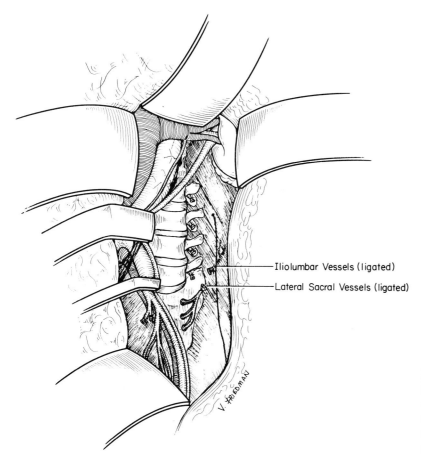

—Iliolumbar Vessels (ligated)
—Lateral Sacral Vessels (ligated)

FIG. 6–5. The aorta and vena cava are mobilized by ligating and dividing the lumbar veins. The iliac vessels are mobilized by dividing the lateral sacral and iliolumbar arteries and veins as they join the internal iliac artery and vein.

bilization during this procedure, a pneumatic compression hose may help reduce perioperative venous thrombosis.

SUMMARY

There are several advantages of the paramedian approach over a flank approach: direct anterior approach to the vertebral bodies from L2 to the sacrum, avoiding division of the lateral abdominal muscles, and not having to contend with the psoas muscle.

References

1. Flynn JC, Price CT: Sexual complications of anterior fusion of the lumbar spine. Spine 9:5:489, 1984
2. Johnson RM, McGuire EJ: Urogenital complications of anterior approaches to the lumbar spine. Urogenital Complications 154:114, 1981

PART
III

DEFORMITY: SCOLIOSIS

CHAPTER
7

Idiopathic Scoliosis

Keith H. Bridwell

Techniques for correction of idiopathic scoliosis and fusion of the spine have evolved rapidly in the past 35 years.[7, 31, 36, 112, 134] In the 1960s, Harrington instrumentation became popular for correction and fusion of spinal deformities.[51–53, 68, 74, 76, 85, 90, 92, 93, 111] In the 1970s, anterior instrumentation for lumbar and thoracolumbar curves was introduced.[23, 37, 38, 49, 57, 58, 63, 68, 69, 76, 91, 94, 99, 100, 110, 115, 146] In the early 1980s, segmental spinal instrumentation was introduced in the form of sublaminar wires and intraspinous wires.[2, 3, 16, 22, 32, 34, 46, 55, 77, 78, 95, 96, 104, 109, 119, 125, 128, 130, 144] Later in that decade, segmental instrumentation in the form of multiple hooks and rods was introduced.[8, 10, 12, 27, 30, 39, 84, 114, 116, 136, 141]

Idiopathic scoliosis is a three-dimensional deformity associated with alterations in surface contour, rotation, and the sagittal plane.[29, 123] Segmentalization of spinal fixation continues to appear desirable, but no system is universally successful in correcting all components of the deformity. For example, the routine use of sublaminar wires for idiopathic adolescent scoliosis is not as popular now as it was 5 to 10 years ago for many reasons.[61, 142] The emphasis on certain instrumentation systems in this chapter is intended as a reflection of the author's practice, the current popularity of the systems, and the extent of published data. Harrington instrumentation remains the gold standard, but anterior and posterior segmental instrumentation in the form of multiple screws, rods, and hooks appears to be the wave of the future. As always, a solid spinal fusion is mandatory for lasting results.[18, 56, 70, 92]

INDICATIONS FOR SURGERY

Surgery is usually considered when a curve approaches 40°, but the Cobb number should not be emphasized. There is really no difference between a 38° curve and a 42° curve in most instances. If the patient has two balanced 40° to 45° curves, the deformity may not be severe. Usually, the more segments that are involved in a curve, the greater the deformity. The amount of rotation and rib hump is important as well. Marked restriction of the chest cage and pulmonary functions usually does not occur until the coronal curve approaches 65° to 75°.[44, 121, 124] However, significant reductions in the pulmonary function results are possible with smaller curves if there is a severe thoracic lordotic component.[1, 20, 145] Therefore, the sagittal component may be a factor in determining indications for surgery.[118]

The patient's balance should be considered.[40] If the top and the bottom of the curve fall within the center sacral line and if C7 is centered on the sacrum, the patient is, by definition, well-compensated regardless of the curve size. Patients may show significant decompensation without terribly large curves. Significant decompensation may be seen with lumbar or thoracolumbar curves with Cobb measurements as small as 33° or 34°. Therefore, a small percentage of patients with lumbar curves less than 40° or 45° may be candidates for surgical treatment if the patients are significantly decompensated and the curves do not respond to bracing.

The patient's proximity to skeletal maturity is an important factor. If the patient is younger than 10 or 11 years old and has not started menstrual periods yet, a curve of 40° or 45° may not be an indication for immediate surgery. It may be better to try to brace the patient and allow the spine to grow before doing a definitive instrumentation and fusion. In certain instances, the curve may be permanently corrected if the patient is braced at a very young age. If it is not, perhaps the curve can be controlled until the patient reaches an older age. On the other hand, if the patient progresses beyond 40° despite bracing and significant growth is expected, instrumentation and fusion should be considered because the patient's condition will probably worsen without the surgical procedure.[73] A 40° or 45° curve in a skeletally immature patient has different implications than in a patient who is skeletally mature. At worst, a 40° to 45° curve in a skeletally mature patient progresses very slowly into adulthood.[139, 140]

FUSION

Posterior Spinal Fusion

For posterior spinal fusion, the patient is usually positioned on a four-poster frame with his or her abdomen free.[14, 56] The abdomen should not be held up by a blanket or a sheet in any way. During positioning, it is important that the upper two posts do not irritate the brachial plexus and that the shoulders are not flexed forward too far. They should not be hyperabducted beyond neutral. The elbows should not be flexed beyond 90°, and they should be placed on a soft cushioned surface. There is a small incidence of brachial plexus

stretch with positioning on the four-poster frame. Somatosensory potential monitoring of the upper extremities during the procedure may reduce the likelihood of this complication. In positioning the lower two posts, the most common complication is a lateral femoral cutaneous nerve palsy. The posts should be well cushioned, and perhaps a donut should be placed on the posts to relieve the area around the anterior superior iliac spine, where the lateral femoral cutaneous nerve traverses. For instrumentations to the middle and lower lumbar spine, the hips should be hyperextended and the knees should be flexed to extend the pelvis and the lower lumbar spine.[14] Having the hips flexed, as for a lumbar disc operation, tends to flatten lumbar lordosis.

For spinal fusions, I usually use some form of hypotensive anesthesia.[80, 87, 108] I usually do not inject with epinephrine before the skin incision, because most of the skin bleeders stop after the self-retaining retractors are placed. Then subperiosteal dissection of the musculature off the spine out to the tips of the transverse processes is important: make use of all the posterior bony structures for a fusion, and dissect all the way out to the transverse processes both in the thoracic and the lumbar spine. The spine is then cleaned of all soft tissues with a curet, and the interspinous ligaments are resected with a luxell down to the ligamentum flavum.

The next part of the fusion, the facet joint extirpation, is probably the most important step in the procedure for an idiopathic scoliosis patient.[28] All the exposed posterior elements of the spine that are not directly holding the instrumentation are decorticated. Packing the decorticated bone with autogenous bone graft can be done before or after placement of the instrumentation, as long as the bone graft is placed on the exposed decorticated bleeding bone. There usually is ample room around the instrumentation. The usual sources of autogenous bone are the posterior ilium or ribs that are harvested during a thoracoplasty. For decortication using either a curved gouge or a curved osteotome and raising as many osteal flaps as possible is the most thorough method of decortication.

Many patients with idiopathic scoliosis have enough osteogenic potential that, with good facet joint extirpation and decortication, the spine will fuse with only bank bone or no added bone.[4, 11, 33] However, I prefer the use of autogenous bone. In the idiopathic adolescent population, the morbidity from harvesting bone graft is very low. The spine seems to heal faster and with a thicker fusion with autogenous bone. With the use of allograft bone, there is always some risk of infection of the patient with either hepatitis or HIV virus, even if the bone and the donor have been tested. In this population of patients, the risks seem to outweigh the benefits of using bank bone. Paralytic patients and adults with scoliosis probably benefit from a combination of autogenous and allograft fresh frozen bone.

Anterior Spinal Fusion

The anterior approach to the spine in idiopathic adolescent scoliosis is commonly chosen for a lumbar or thoracolumbar curve and is made through a thoracoabdominal approach, which allows exposure from T10 to the sacrum.[37, 38] The convex side is positioned up, with the patient in the lateral decubitus position. The skin incision parallels the tenth rib. Dissection is carried out down through the external oblique and latissimus dorsi muscles to the tenth rib, which is subperiosteally dissected and removed.

After resection of the rib, the chest is entered through the bed of the tenth rib. The cartilage of the tenth rib is incised, and with Metzenbaum scissors, the retroperitoneal fat is developed below the diaphragm. The peritoneum is swept off the undersurface of the transversus abdominus and internal oblique muscles from a posterolateral to anteromedial position. The deep abdominal muscles are incised parallel to the skin incision. The peritoneum is swept off the undersurface of the diaphragm, and the diaphragm is incised in a radial fashion, leaving roughly a 1.5-cm peripheral cuff. The diaphragm is incised to the vertebral body. The curvilinear cut in the diaphragm extends from an anteromedial to a lateral to a posteromedial position, which denervates only a small portion of the diaphragm.

The lumbar fascia overlying the lumbar vertebral bodies is dissected with the Metzenbaum scissors, and the pleura overlying the thoracic vertebral bodies is incised after being spread with the scissors first to develop the interval between the segmental vessels and the pleura or fascia to be incised. Using a peanut and a Mixter clamp, the crossing segmental vessels at each level are identified, dissected, and tied with silk sutures and incised at each level. The segmental vessels cross at the foramen at each level.

An extraperiosteal or a subperiosteal dissection is performed to expose the vertebral bodies. An extraperiosteal dissection is somewhat easier. It is helpful to grab the segmental vessels anteriorly with a DeBakey pick-up and bluntly develop the interval between these segmental vessels and the vertebral bodies, exposing the anterior vertebral bodies. Posterior vertebral body exposure is achieved by using the Cobb elevator or a peanut, lifting up the posterior segmentals to dissect back posteriorly to the posterior border of the vertebral bodies.

After the vertebral bodies are exposed, the discs are resected at each level to the posterior longitudinal ligament. If the discectomies are being done for kyphosis, it is particularly important to resect all the anterior longitudinal ligament. If they are being done for scoliosis, it is more important to consider preserving some of the anterior longitudinal ligament, but also getting over to the concave side and back to the posterior longitudinal ligament. After cleaning the disc space with a combination of osteotomes, curets, luxells, and pituitary rongeurs, the bone graft is placed in the disc spaces. Using chunks of the autogenous rib works well. For a lumbar scoliosis, the grafts are usually placed in the anterior half of the disc space, and instrumentation is applied.

With Zielke instrumentation, the apical screws are started more posteriorly than the end screws, and the apical screws should point more anteriorly.[57] Thus, with engaging the rod into the screws, some element of "derotation" will occur. Using the lordosator-derotator forces the spine into some degree of additional lordosis. The lordosator is applied after engaging all of the nuts into the appropriate screws but before applying the compression forces on each of the screws. After the Zielke instrumentation has been applied and the spine corrected to the appropriate degree, the derotator is removed and the rods are cut short. A radiograph at this point can confirm that the spine is neither undercorrected nor overcorrected. Overcorrection can easily occur with this system in an adolescent lumbar spine. If there is remaining bone graft, raise osteal-periosteal flaps anteriorly on the vertebral bodies and pack additional bone graft into these flaps.

After the bone grafting and application of the instrumentation, a chest tube is inserted between the eleventh and twelfth ribs at the posterior axillary line. First, the diaphragm is repaired with interrupted sutures, followed by closure of the deep abdominal musculature with interrupted sutures. Repair the deep abdominal muscles to the diaphragm anteriorly with multiple interrupted sutures or with a single purse-string type suture. The intercostals and tenth rib bed are closed with interrupted sutures, followed by closure of the external oblique and latissimus dorsi muscles. Before placement of the chest tube, it is helpful to place either an Allis or Babcock clamp on the latissimus dorsi muscle distal to the skin incision and pull it up so that the chest tube will not tether the latissimus dorsi muscle. The latissimus dorsi muscle has a tendency to retract both proximally and distally during the exposure, so it is important to clearly identify its margins and to repair it at the end of the closure.

Anterior and Posterior Fusion

There are several indications for both anterior and posterior surgery in a patient with idiopathic scoliosis: severe thoracic lordosis (see Case No. 4); structural curves that measure over 80° (see Case No.19) and correct to less than 50° after flexibility maneuvers; or a rare pattern in which both thoracic and lumbar curves must be fused and applying Zielke instrumentation anteriorly allows stopping at L4 instead of L5 (see Case No. 13).

Postoperative Care

For the first 2 to 4 days after surgery, pain relief is best provided by a patient-controlled analgesia system with an intravenous narcotic. Patients accept the system and appreciate having control over their analgesia. The patient-controlled analgesia system allows continuous, consistent analgesia without additional "sticks." It is safe because the analgesic medicine is given in small doses. A percentage of patients experience nausea from morphine. It is helpful to continue with an indwelling Foley catheter in the bladder and to maintain an arterial catheter for the first 3 or 4 days. The arterial catheter allows monitoring of arterial blood gas, hemoglobin, leucocyte count, and electrolytes. Usually the nasogastric tube is not necessary after a posterior spinal fusion in an adolescent idiopathic scoliosis patient. However, after an anterior fusion, maintain a nasogastric tube intraoperatively and postoperatively for the first 2 days.

An ileus can occur after anterior and posterior fusions, but the ileus usually lasts longer after the anterior fusion. Superior mesenteric artery syndromes may occur, presenting as nausea, vomiting, and an inability to keep down food or liquids between the fifth and tenth postoperative day. Usually, the upper gastrointestinal tract recovers first, and the lower gastrointestinal tract recovers last. With a resolving ileus, there is abdominal distention, and the patient has a limited ability to pass flatus. A prolonged ileus is best treated with tincture of time, rectal tubes as needed, and increasing activity. Superior mesenteric artery syndrome often requires nasogastric suction and intravenous fluids for several days before it resolves. Although superior mesenteric artery syndrome is more likely in thin patients with dramatic correction of curves or with correction of kyphosis, these factors are not consistent. The syndrome can occur in idiopathic scoliosis patients with modest curves and modest correction.

After a transthoracic or thoracoabdominal approach, the chest tube is usually continued for 48 to 72 hours after surgery. It is removed when the drainage decreases to less than 50 ml for two consecutive 8-hour shifts. Hemovac drains are placed posteriorly in all areas of dead space and maintained for 2 or 3 days, until drainage is less than 25 ml per shift.

The incidence of pulmonary embolus is extremely small in this age group. Nonetheless it is helpful to have the physical therapist exercise the patient's arms and legs at the bedside starting the first postoperative day. These exercise sessions seem to improve the patient's motivation and perception of care by the nursing and physician staff. Pneumatic stockings may be helpful in this group of patients, but they are rarely required. Pharmacologic anticoagulation is not routinely necessary.

Usually by the third to fifth postoperative day, the patient is comfortable enough that the head of the bed can gradually be elevated. By the fourth to sixth postoperative day, the patient can sit on the edge of the bed and dangle legs. Between the fifth and seventh postoperative day, the patient can usually stand and walk.

Adolescents treated with the standard Cotrel–Dubousset tray usually have stable enough fixation that they do not require postoperative casting or bracing. For anterior Ventrale Derotations-spondylodese (VDS) instrumentation, some form of postoperative protection is advisable. Although anterior VDS fixation is very stable, it is not as rigid as Cotrel–Dubousset instrumentation because the compression rod used for the Zielke system is relatively small. Therefore, for patients treated exclusively with anterior VDS, I mold them for a two-piece thoracolumbar sacral (TLSO) as soon as their chest tube is removed. Within 48 hours they have their brace and can be standing and walking 7 to 8 days after surgery. I then continue the bracing for 4 to 7 months with the two-piece custom-molded clamshell TLSO.

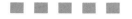

Color Section One

IDIOPATHIC SCOLIOSIS

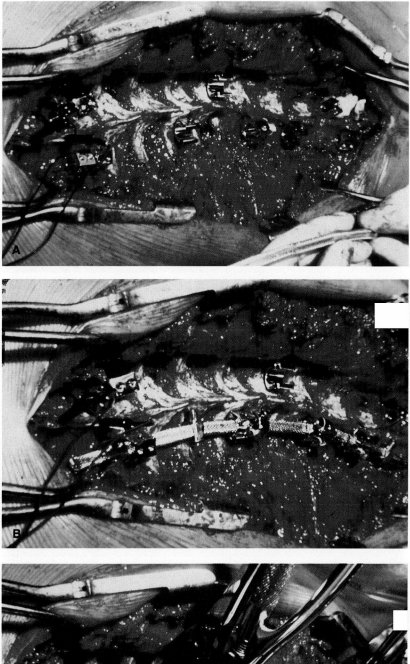

COLOR PLATE 1. Cotrel–Dubousset derotation maneuver. **A.** Placement of the 6 concave, left-sided hooks and 4 convex, right-sided hooks for a right thoracic curve.

Vertebra	L	R
T4	⌐⌐ Crosslink	⌐⌐
T7	⌐	
T8		⌐
T10	⌐	
T12	⌐ Crosslink	
L1	⌐	⌐

B. Engagement of the precontoured rod into the 6 hooks on the left side. Kyphosis is contoured from T4 to T12, and lordosis from T12 to L1. **C.** Application of the rod holders used for the rod rotation maneuver.

(continued)

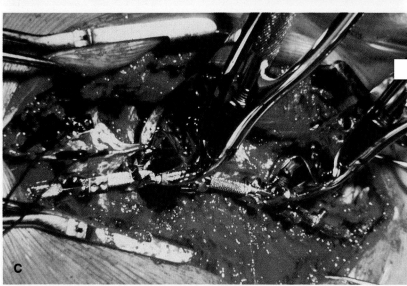

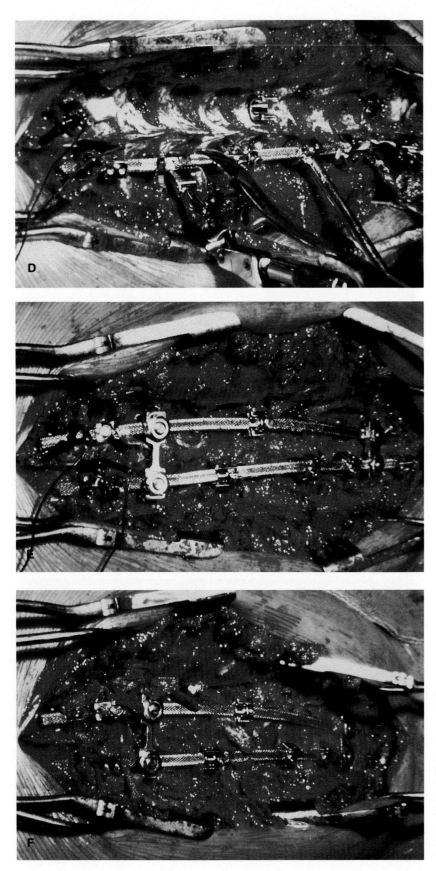

COLOR PLATE 1. (*continued*) **D.** Notice the position of the rod holders and the rod after the rod rotation maneuver. The C clamps keep the blockers engaged into the open hooks. **E.** The appearance of the spine after decortication, application of the convex rod, and application of the Texas Scottish Rite Crosslinks. In this case, the apical concave hooks were placed three segments apart. **F.** The appearance of the spine after instrumentation and application of the bone graft.

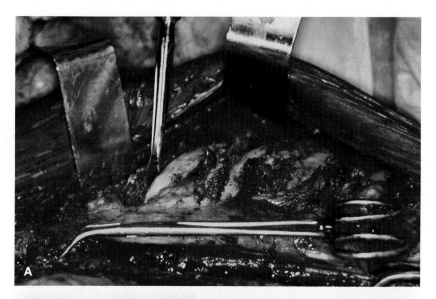

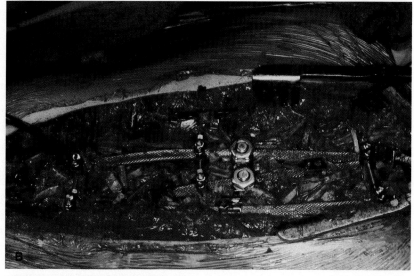

COLOR PLATE 2. Thoracoplasty.
A. Exposure of the apical convex ribs in a subperiosteal fashion and dissection of the ribs away from the underlying pleura. The towel clip is on midline spine musculature. The lower Hibbs retractor is retracting the midline spine fascia. The upper Hibbs retractor is holding the scapula. The exposure is performed through the single midline incision.
B. Appearance of the spine after instrumentation and placement of the rib bone graft harvested during the thoracoplasty. (See also Fig. 7-7.)

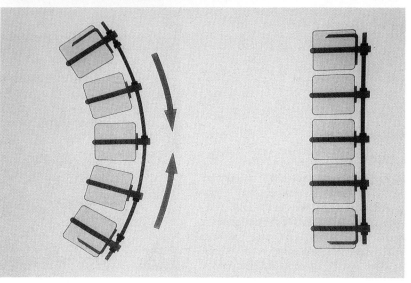

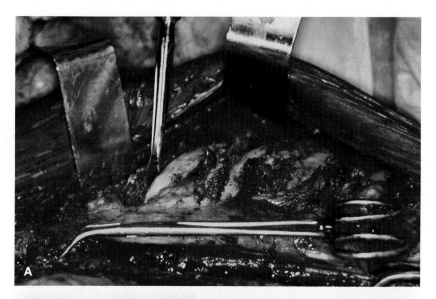

COLOR PLATE 3. Principle of compression on the convex side: shortening of the section of the spine that requires instrumentation.

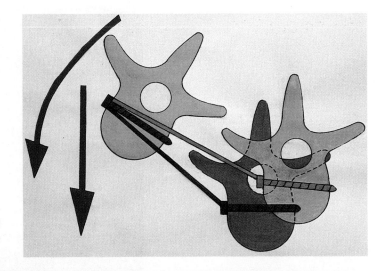

COLOR PLATE 4. Principle of derotation: the apical vertebra (*below*) is moved ventral (lordosation) between the two end vertebrae (*above*) and simultaneously derotated (*arrows*).

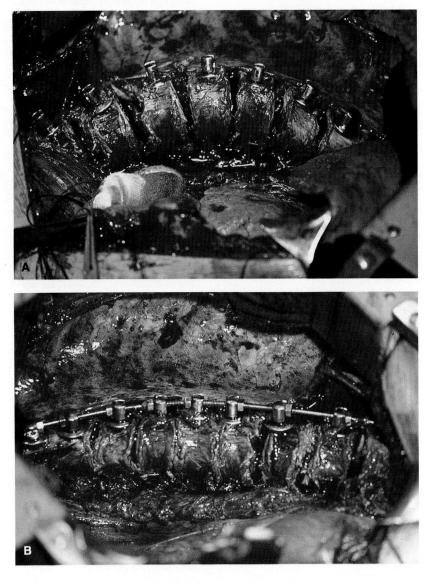

COLOR PLATE 5. Site of the operation. **A.** The discs have been removed and the screws inserted in T3–L3. The top disc (*right*) remains untouched. **B.** Completed instrumentation: bone grafting the disc spaces in the lumbar region and compression of the endplates in the thoracic region. The spine has been straightened, and derotation can be recognized by the direction of the screws.

Those smaller patients instrumented with the 5-mm Cotrel–Dubousset system probably should be protected with a postoperative brace. The custom-molded clamshell TLSO seems to work well. Not only is the 5-mm system smaller than the standard 7-mm Cotrel–Dubousset instrumentation system, but the patients on whom it is employed usually have significantly more fragile posterior elements, so early hook cut-out from the posterior elements is a concern.

If a posterior spinal fusion is performed to T4 or T5, a standard underarm two-piece clamshell TLSO with a generous chest or abdominal window is sufficient. If the instrumentation is carried higher into the thoracic spine, then it is often advisable to include shoulder straps with the brace or a low cervical component to the brace. With the use of Harrington instrumentation without any segmentalization, it appears advisable to place the patient in 23-hour-a-day casting or custom-molded bracing for the first 4 to 7 months after surgery. However, with the addition of sublaminar wires or Wisconsin wires, it may not be necessary in all cases; bracing a patient when upright for the first 3 to 4 months may be sufficient. In some cases, it may not be necessary to brace the patient at all if he or she is trustworthy. The same considerations hold true with the use of Luque instrumentation. Although it was initially believed that postoperative bracing was not necessary with this system, there have been reports suggesting that the incidence of wire breakage, rod migration, and loss of correction is less with some protective postoperative bracing.[16, 125]

By the time of discharge from the hospital, the adolescent patient has been gradually reduced from intravenous narcotics to oral narcotics to medicine comparable to propoxyphene. Usually by 4 to 6 weeks after discharge from the hospital, the adolescent's discomfort from the surgery is 95% gone.

Parents and the patient have questions about allowable postoperative activities. With the usual adolescent spine fusion, regardless of the instrumentation, the adolescent can perform light physical activities, such as swimming, bicycling, throwing a baseball, or shooting a basketball by 7 months postoperatively. By 12 months, participation in noncontact competitive athletics that involve running, jumping, or changing directions suddenly is allowable. At 2 years after the surgery, the spine fusion should reach maximal maturity, and in certain cases, it may be possible to return to certain forms of contact sports. These guidelines are rather arbitrary and need to be individualized for each case. If the fusion mass is not progressing according to

the usual expectations or if there is a hook or rod disengagement or obvious pseudarthrosis, the patient's allowable activities should be modified.

The need for postoperative and intraoperative bank blood transfusions can be reduced by cell saver recovery and preoperative autologous blood donation.[5, 129] The use of preoperative hemodilution and controlled hypotension reduces intraoperative blood loss but may not reduce total (preoperative and postoperative) blood loss. Thorough preoperative screening of prothrombin time, partial thromboplastin time, platelets, and bleeding time is advisable because some patients with idiopathic scoliosis have bleeding tendencies.[60, 62, 72] Most patients develop an inappropriate antidiuretic hormone syndrome postoperatively, which causes fluid retention and reduced urine output for the first 24 to 36 hours after surgery, followed by significant urinary diuresis.[6, 83]

CURVE PATTERNS

Type II Thoracic Curves

The Type II curve refers to a "false" double-major curve.[64, 65] Generally the stable vertebra for this type of curve is T11, T12, or L1. The lumbar curve below deviates from the plumb line somewhat and has some rotation to it. King and co-workers used the flexibility index to distinguish a Type II curve from a double-major curve. However, further experience showed that factors other than flexibility must also be considered.[65, 84] The lumbar curves usually are more flexible than thoracic curves if they are equal in Cobb measurements and if true double-major patterns exist. However, if the thoracic curves are bigger and more structural than the lumbar curves, they often can be selectively instrumented. To be considered a false double-major curve, the thoracic curve must be larger, have more rotation to it, and deviate farther from the plumb line than the lumbar curve. The thoracic curve should be the curve producing most of the deformity with a symmetrical waistline and a minimal lumbar "hump" on forward bending.

A desirable outcome for any scoliosis fusion and the Type II curves in particular is one in which the distally fused segment is bisected by the center sacral line and is perfectly centered on the sacrum, with C7 directly over the sacrum with normalized sagittal curves. A thoracolumbar kyphosis sometimes exists preoperatively. The sagittal curve from T12 to L2 should be in slight lordosis.[9] Therefore, kyphosis from T12 to L2 (especially if greater than +10° by lateral Cobb measurement) is pathologic and should be considered in the instrumentation of this curve pattern.

Instrumentation

King and colleagues described instrumentation to the "stable vertebra."[65] The stable vertebra is defined as the one that is bisected by the center sacral line. The center sacral line is drawn perpendicular to a line drawn horizontally connecting the top of the pelvis on a standing x-ray film and bisecting the sacrum (Fig. 7-1). With Harrington instrumentation, the likelihood of overcorrecting a thoracic curve to more than a lumbar curve can compensate for is relatively low, but there is always some chance of producing decompensation (see Case No. 3). If selective instrumentation and fusion is performed on the thoracic curve in a skeletally immature patient, it is always possible that the lumbar curve will continue to progress with age. Therefore, bracing the child's curves until skeletal maturity before surgery or after surgery to protect the lumbar curve may be advisable.

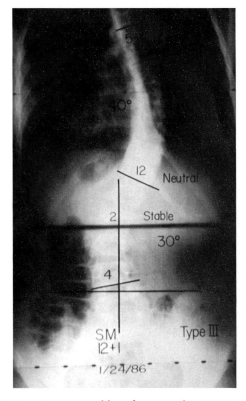

FIG. 7–1. Center sacral line drawn on this 12 + 1-year-old girl. It bisects the pedicles of L2 ("stable" vertebra). T12 is the vertebra with the least amount of rotation, and it is therefore the "neutral" vertebra.

With Cotrel–Dubousset instrumentation, there is the potential for addressing the thoracolumbar kyphosis.[12, 15, 27] However, there is also added potential for decompensation. Several researchers have reported a high incidence of decompensation with Type II curves treated with Cotrel–Dubousset instrumentation.[84, 113, 141] This has occurred most often with instrumentation down to the stable vertebra at T12 or L1 that placed all the hooks in a distraction mode on the

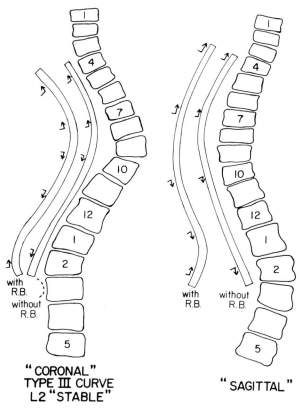

FIG. 7–2. The rod and arrows on the rod with reverse bend (RB) or lordotic bend show the correct contour of the rods, with reversal of rod bend and reversal of hook orientation on the left-sided rod between T12 and L2. On the left-sided rod (assuming a right thoracic curve), the hooks are placed to apply a distractive force where kyphosis is desired and where the disc spaces are collapsed. They are placed to apply compression where lordosis is desired and where the disc spaces are opened up. Using the hook orientation and rod contour depicted in the rod without a reverse bend will cause some kyphosing of the upper lumbar spine from T12 to L2 and is therefore not as desirable. It may also translate the stable vertebra to the left. (McAllister JW, Bridwell KH, Betz R, et al: Coronal decompensation produced by Cotrel–Dubousset derotation maneuver for idiopathic right thoracic scoliosis. Orthop Trans 13:79, 1989)

left-sided rod.[84] This may be a result of correcting the thoracic curve beyond what the lumbar curve can accommodate, because there seems to be more overall correction with Cotrel–Dubousset instrumentation than with the Harrington system.

The first solution is to reverse the bend (i.e., apply a lordotic bend) and reverse the hook orientation between the neutral and stable vertebra (Fig. 7-2; Case No. 1). The second solution is to stop the instrumentation one level above the stable vertebra. The third solution, for the larger thoracic curves, is to employ a three-rod technique (Fig. 7-3; Case No. 2) in which

CASE NO. 1—M.S.

In a 14 + 9-year-old girl with an apparent Type II thoracic curve pattern, the thoracic curve is significantly larger than the lumbar curve and deviates from the plumb line and center sacral line more than the lumbar curve. The lumbar curve is far more flexible than the thoracic curve. Although I cannot disagree with the spinal surgeon preferring to consider this a double-major curve pattern and to instrument and fuse both curves, in this case the choice was to treat it as a false double-major curve pattern. Reversal of the rod bend and reversal of hooks on the left-sided rod was accomplished between the neutral and stable vertebrae on the left-sided derotation rod. This is important for both coronal and sagittal

balance. It provides the initial lordosis in the lumbar spine, and experience has shown that placing all the hooks in the left-sided rod in a distraction mode down to the stable vertebrae leads to a much higher incidence of coronal decompensation.[84, 113] In fact, immediately after surgery, the patient became quite decompensated! However, over the course of several months, she gradually recompensated. No brace treatment was used postoperatively. The initial result was quite disturbing but the 1-year follow-up result is acceptable. Should this patient have been instrumented down to L3 or L4? This is a point of great controversy, and no surgeon has a definitive answer.

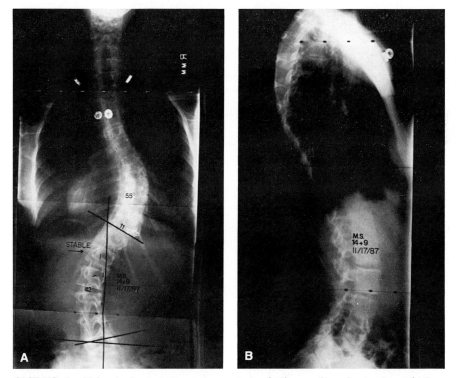

CASE NO. 1—M.S. **A.** Preoperative anteroposterior (AP) x-ray film of a standing 14+9-year-old girl. The thoracic curve is larger than the lumbar curve and has more rotation and deviates farther from the center sacral line. This represents a false double-major curve instead of a true double-major curve. **B.** Preoperative lateral x-ray film of the standing patient.

(continued)

CASE NO. 1—M.S. (*continued*)

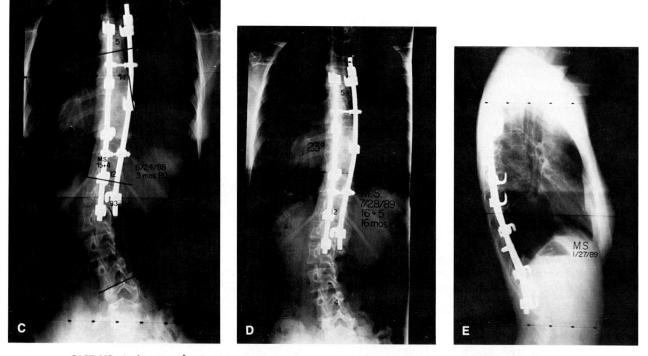

CASE NO. 1 (*continued*) **C.** The patient 3 months postoperatively is significantly decompensated to the left. The standing AP x-ray film shows the thoracic curve corrected to 14°, which is more than the lumbar curve can accommodate. This occurred despite the reversal of rod bend and hook orientation between the neutral and stable vertebra on the left side. **D.** AP x-ray film of the standing patient 16 months postoperatively. She had lost some correction of the thoracic curve and was clinically and radiographically well-balanced. No cast or brace was used postoperatively. **E.** Standing lateral x-ray film of the patient postoperatively.

selective distraction, compression, or translation are employed, rather than rod rotation. If there is not any preexisting thoracolumbar kyphosis between T12 and L2, there should be no problem in stopping the instrumentation at T12 if it is stable. This does not create kyphosis below it if the T11–T12 segment is not selectively overdistracted.[15] However, if there is a kyphosis measuring greater than +5° to +15° between T12 and L2, it may be desirable to extend the instrumentation distally and to apply initial compression and lordosing forces between T12 and L2. However, avoid stopping instrumentation at or close to the apex of the lumbar curve. If controlling a thoracolumbar kyphosis requires

fusion to the apical lumbar vertebra, then instrumenting both thoracic and lumbar curves is preferable, and the fusion should stop at L3 or L4, the distally stable lumbar vertebra.

What is good for sagittal balance is usually beneficial for coronal balance with Cotrel–Dubousset instrumentation. On the derotation rod, hooks are placed in a distraction mode where the discs are closed down and in a compression mode where they are opened up according to the standing anterior-posterior radiograph, which corresponds to the direction that the discs open up or close down on the bending films.

(*text continues on page 108*)

CASE NO. 2—L.S.

An adolescent girl had an apparent Type II false double-major curve. This case is somewhat controversial because many surgeons would predict that the long-term result would be superior with instrumentation to L3 or L4. However, this did fit the qualifications for a Type II curve, and it was treated as such. Because the thoracic curve was very large and somewhat rigid, it was not amenable to treatment with a simple derotation maneuver. There was concern that a derotation maneuver might correct the thoracic curve beyond what the lumbar curve could accommodate. Therefore, a three-rod tech-

nique was used in which selective corrective and translational forces were used. The final result is quite acceptable, with excellent coronal and sagittal balance postoperatively. In this case, there was no problem with stopping the instrumentation at T12 becaue there was no preoperative thoracolumbar or upper lumbar kyphosis. If there had been a significant upper lumbar kyphosis, extending the instrumentation distally might have been advisable, but the instrumentation should never stop at the apex of the lumbar curve!

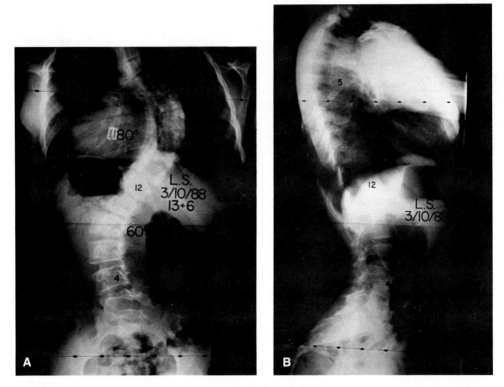

CASE NO. 2—L.S. A. Standing anteroposterior (AP) x-ray film showing large thoracic and lumbar curves in a 13 + 6 year old. Both curves significantly deviate from the center sacral line. The thoracic curve is larger and has somewhat more rotation to it. **B.** Lateral x-ray film of the standing patient. There is no thoracolumbar kyphosis. The spine is in lordosis from T12 to L2. **C.** AP x-ray film of the standing patient 1 year postoperatively. A stacked rod technique was used on the thoracic spine rather than attempting to perform a single rod rotation maneuver. This probably limited correction of the thoracic curve and therefore allowed the lumbar spine to accommodate. The spine was well-balanced at all times postoperatively. Fusion was performed to the stable vertebra because there was no thoracolumbar kyphosis. A one-segment compression claw was applied on the right side between T11 and T12 before seating the T12 hook on the left side. This prevents overdistraction of the distal segment. **D.** The postoperative lateral x-ray film of the standing patient. The lumbar spine remains in lordosis from T12 down to the sacrum.

(continued)

CASE NO. 2—L.S. (*continued*)

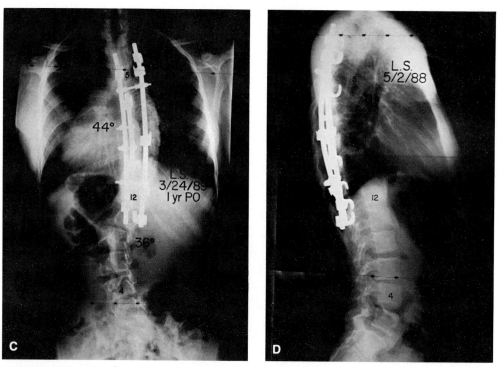

CASE NO. 2 (*continued*)

CASE NO. 3—D.G.

In a 15 + 0-year-old female with a Type II curve pattern, very acceptable correction was achieved with Harrington instrumentation of the thoracic curve. Using sublaminar wires or Wisconsin wires is satisfactory.[34, 46, 128, 144] The thoracic curve was not corrected beyond the capacity of lumbar curve to compensate. There have been reports of neurologic injury associated with sublaminar wires.[61, 142] I have had no such complication but have abandoned sublaminar wires in routine idiopathic scoliosis cases because of the medical-legal risks.

CASE NO. 3—D.G. **A.** An apparent Type II false double-major curve pattern is demonstrated by this preoperative anteroposterior x-ray film of the standing patient. The thoracic curve is larger than the lumbar curve and deviates farther from the plumb line. **B.** Lateral x-ray film demonstrating a somewhat flat spine but no thoracolumbar kyphosis. **C.** The patient was treated with contoured square Harrington instrumentation with sublaminar wires and convex Luque rod. There was no decompensation problem after surgery. The thoracic curve probably would have been corrected a great deal more with Cotrel–Dubousset instrumentation. The more limited correction with Harrington instrumentation results in fewer decompensation problems in the Type II curves. Fusion and instrumentation was performed to the stable vertebra. **D.** Lateral x-ray film of the patient 27 months postoperatively. There was no thoracolumbar kyphosis.

(*continued*)

CASE NO. 3—D.G. *(continued)*

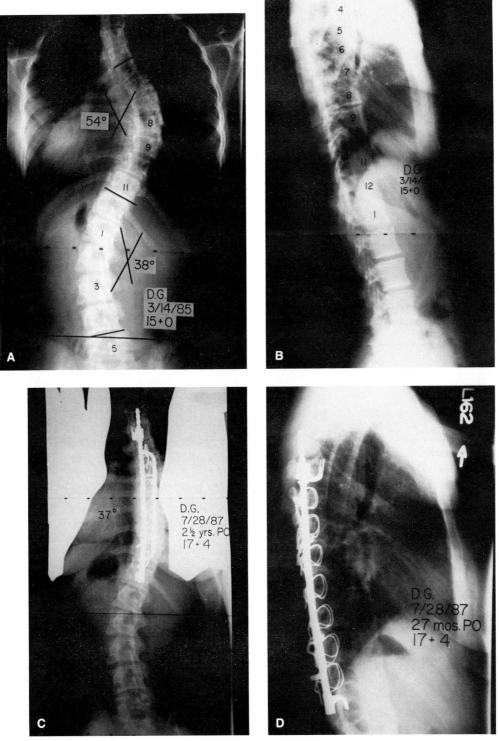

CASE NO. 3 *(continued)*

Type III Thoracic Curves

In the King classification, this type of thoracic curve is not associated with much rotation of the distal lumbar segments.[65] The stable vertebra is usually L1 or L2, most commonly L2. It is uncommon to see a thoracolumbar kyphosis with this curve pattern. However, one must be aware of the possible existence of an associated high left thoracic curve.

Instrumentation

In Type III curves, the instrumentation should usually extend a little farther down into the lumbar spine than with a Type II curve. Although a small amount of kyphosis can be tolerated in the upper lumbar spine, it is best to start the upper lumbar spine in lordosis. With either Harrington or Cotrel–Dubousset instrumentation, fusion should usually be carried to the stable vertebra. Anterior VDS is another option for thoracic scoliosis, but this has never gained popularity in North America.[50] If Harrington instrumentation is used, it is important not to overdistract the last segment (usually L1 or L2). This may be accomplished by placing a very short compression rod on the right side between T12 and L2 or by wiring together the posterior elements of L1 and L2 before applying the distractive force as described by Winter.[14, 143]

With Cotrel–Dubousset instrumentation, it is best to place a reverse bend and reversal hooks between T12 and L2 (see Fig. 7-2) or L1 and L2 on the left-sided derotation rod (assuming a right thoracic curve). This provides a better sagittal contour than placing all of the hooks on the left side in the same distraction mode.

Derotation Maneuver for a Type III Right Thoracic Curve

For the derotation maneuver for a Type III curve from T4 to L2, the open intermediate hooks on the derotation rod are centered on the apical segments, usually three segments apart if it is a flexible curve (see Color Plate 1). Assuming an apex at the T8–T9 disc, an open pedicle hook is placed at T7 on the left side, and an open lumbar hook is placed on the top side of T10 on the left side. Because the rod is pulling up on the spine at T7 and T10 during the rod rotation maneuver, it is possible and safe to use an open lumbar hook at T10 rather than an open thoracic hook.[116] The laminotomy does not need to be as big as for a standard Harrington hook. Taking a little bit of bone off the undersurface of T9 facilitates placement of the hook.

At T4 on the left side a "closed claw" is placed, which is a closed pedicle hook on T4 and closed lumbar hook on the transverse process of T4. Placing the hook on the transverse process of T4 keeps the proximal end of the rod from migrating medially and inadvertently pushing the proximal pedicle hook into the spinal canal during rod rotation. At T12 on the left side, an open lumbar or open thoracic hook is placed. Be sure it is not displaced into the spinal canal as it is being pushed down during the rod rotation. At L2 on the left side, a closed lumbar laminar hook is placed on the downside of L2 so that the T12 and L2 hooks are facing each other in compression. The hooks placed on the caudal side of the lumbar vertebrae can generally be inserted between the ligamentum flavum and the posterior elements without formally exposing the epidural space.

Careful separation with a curette and testing with the "laminar developer" is helpful. Before placement of the hooks on the thoracic transverse processes, use the sharp "transverse process developer" to divide the soft tissues and ligaments between the transverse process and the rib to facilitate placement of the closed lumbar hooks. If the transverse process hook and pedicle hook do not align, the taller body lumbar hook is sometimes appropriate for the transverse process. Hooks on the right side should include a closed claw at T4, an open pedicle hook at T8, an open hook somewhere between T10 and T12, and a closed lumbar laminar hook on the topside of L2.

The derotation rod is placed first. Kyphosis is contoured into the rod from T4 to T12 and lordosis from T12 to L2. The rod is then engaged into all the hooks. The hook-rod approximator is used to place the T10 hook inside the rod so the appropriate blocker can be engaged. If the other two open hooks cannot fit into the rod initially, bringing the rod to the hook at T10 usually aligns them. All three open hooks are engaged with their respective blockers by applying just enough force to seat them, and C-clamps are placed to prevent the blockers from sliding out. None of the bolts on the hooks are tightened down.

Using rod holders or Schlein clamps, the rod is then rotated 90° in a counterclockwise direction. The bolts on the C-clamps should initially be facing far to the right, because after the rod rotation maneuver, they will be facing far to the left. After the rod rotation maneuver is complete, the bolts are tightened down, the C-clamps are removed, and final selective distraction and compression forces are applied to seat appropriately all the hooks.

The rod is then contoured for the right side with

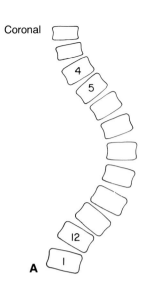

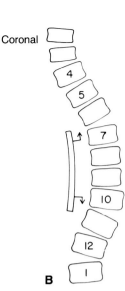

A

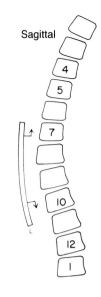

B

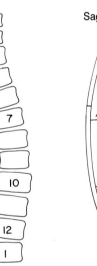

C

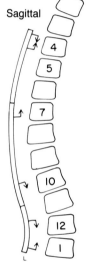

D

FIG. 7–3. Correction of 85° right thoracic curve with limited flexibility. **A.** T4 is the proximal neutral vertebra, and L1 is the distally stable vertebra. T5 to T11 measures 85° to 90° in this Type III curve. **B.** Distractive force is applied between T7 and T10 on the left side. **C.** Distractive force is applied between T4 and T12 on the left side with compression between T12 and L1. **D.** Translational forces applied through the devices for transverse traction pull the two rods together and achieve further correction. **E.** Application of the right-sided rod. This technique is helpful when the curve is too stiff for a simple derotation maneuver. See Case Nos. 18 and 19.

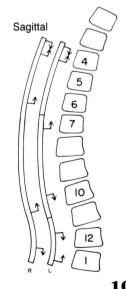

E

CASE NO. 4—K.S.

In this 15 + 8-year-old girl, the right thoracic scoliosis is associated with a very significant thoracic lordosis. The average thoracic kyphosis in this age group is roughly 30° to 35°, and the sagittal Cobb measurement in this patient is 40° to 45° from the norm. Significant diminution of pulmonary function exists. The deformity is rather rigid, and it is very unlikely that, even with a Cotrel—Dubousset derotation maneuver, thoracic kyphosis could be restored. Therefore, the patient was treated with a

two-stage procedure. Stage one consisted of anterior discectomies and posteriorly based wedges through the vertebral bodies. The second procedure consisted of placing bilateral, square Harrington rods, which were contoured into kyphosis. Sublaminar wires were passed at each level, and the spine was brought to the instrumentation, creating thoracic kyphosis, as described by Bradford.[13] Today this is best done under one anesthesia.

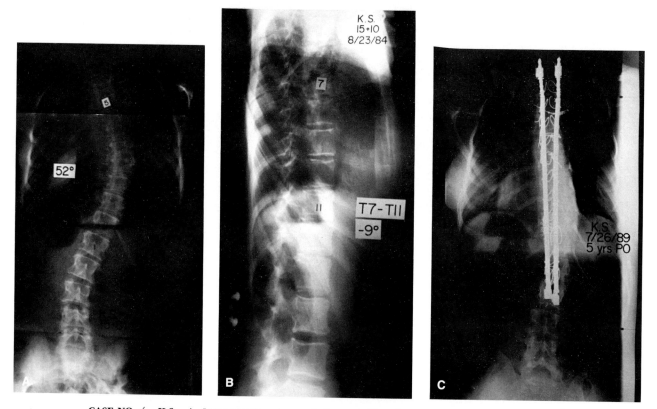

CASE NO. 4—K.S. A. Long-cassette anteroposterior x-ray film of a 15 + 8-year-old-female with the long, sweeping Type III right thoracic curve. **B.** A preoperative lateral x-ray film of the standing patient demonstrates thoracic lordosis. **C.** The patient 5 years postoperatively. She was treated with anterior osteotomies and posteriorly with bilateral square Harrington distraction rods, contoured for the desired sagittal plane and supplemented with sublaminar wires. There is some separation of the right-sided rod from the hook and some residual tilt at L2–L3. **D.** Postoperative lateral x-ray film of the standing patient showing a significant improvement in the sagittal Cobb measurement of the thoracic spine from T7 to T11. There was a 31° improvement. **E.** A close-up of the thoracic spine and the sagittal plane 5 years postoperatively.

(continued)

CASE NO. 4—K.S. *(continued)*

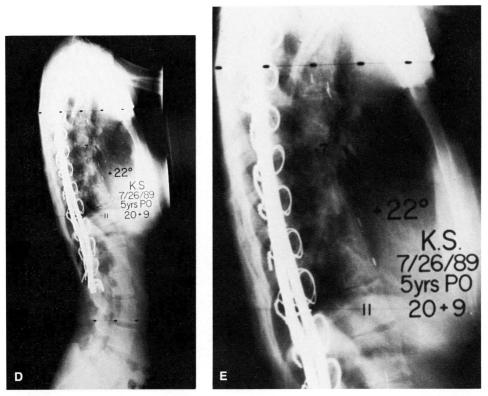

CASE NO. 4 *(continued)*

kyphosis from T4 to T12 and lordosis from T12 to L2. Generally, the surgeon attempts to contour a little less kyphosis into this rod than the rod on the left side. On the right-sided rod, compression forces are applied from T4 to T10, T11, or T12 and distraction forces from T10, T11, or T12 to L2 (Case No. 5).

For all thoracic curves corrected with Cotrel–Dubousset instrumentation, I make a point of having a two-segment compression claw at the distal end on one side or the other to be certain the distal segment is not overdistracted.[15] This principle helps to start the upper lumbar spine in lordosis and prevent the occurrence of junctional kyphosis. Devices for transverse traction are then placed on the proximal and distal quarters of the construct after all hooks are seated with the appropriate selective distraction and compression forces.

I usually perform the facet joint extirpations at the same time I place the hooks from the proximal to distal direction, working side to side. Initial decortication of the posterior elements is performed just before placing the rod on each side. After all the instrumentation is placed, additional decortication is followed by application of the bone graft. There is generally ample room under and around the instrumentation to place bone graft. I usually place the bone graft before the devices for transverse traction, although the order of these steps is arbitrary.

CASE NO. 5—A.W.

For this 13 + 8-year-old boy with a Type III curve, reversal of hook and rod orientation on the left-sided rod was advisable in the upper lumbar spine. This provided upper lumbar lordosis and the best coronal balance by placing hook in a distraction mode where the discs are narrowed and a compression mode where the discs are opened up.

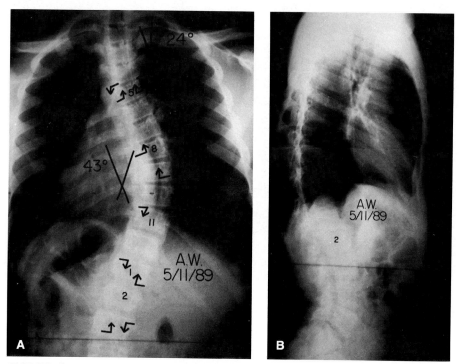

CASE NO. 5—A.W.   **A.** Preoperative standing anteroposterior (AP) x-ray film. L3 is the stable vertebra. The orientation of the disc spaces changes from L1 to L3. **B.** Preoperative lateral x-ray film.   **C.** Postoperative standing AP x-ray film.   **D.** Postoperative standing lateral x-ray film.

(continued)

Type IV Thoracic Curves

Type IV curves are thoracic curves that extend down to L4, which is the stable vertebra.[65] Because the apex is T10, it is considered to be a thoracic curve. A certain percentage of the Type IV curves have a sagittal malalignment, which consists of a severe thoracic lordosis and a thoracolumbar kyphosis. Others have a smoother sagittal contour from the top to the bottom of the curve. With Harrington instrumentation, it is manda-

tory to instrument to the stable vertebra, which is usually L4. To preserve lumbar lordosis, it is important to place a compression rod on the right side (assuming a right thoracic curve) from L1 to L4 or L2 to L4. Contouring a square Harrington rod is not enough, even with the use of Wisconsin wires or sublaminar wires, to preserve lumbar lordosis.[21]

With Cotrel–Dubousset instrumentation, two techniques are possible, depending on the sagittal contour and the flexibility of the curves. If there is no

CASE NO. 5—A.W. (*continued*)

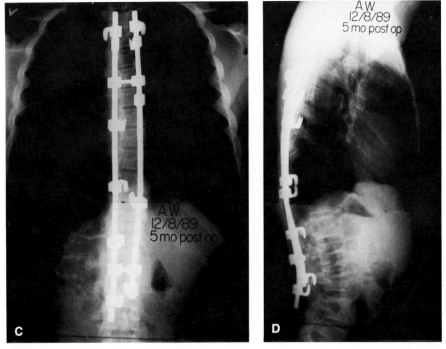

CASE NO. 5 (*continued*)

thoracolumbar kyphosis, one or two levels may be saved if several criteria can be met: on the left side bender (assuming a right thoracic curve), L2 falls within the center sacral line, and all the segments from L2 to the sacrum derotate and level off; the thoracic curve is flexible enough for derotation maneuver; the most caudal segment instrumented (L1, L2, or L3) is neutral in rotation; and there is no thoracolumbar kyphosis.

Using Cotrel–Dubousset instrumentation to L2 for a right thoracic curve, there are three steps (Fig. 7-4) : First, place the four hooks in a distraction mode on the left-sided derotation rod and perform the derotation maneuver. The top three hooks are fastened down and engaged. The fourth hook is left loose. Second, with the right-sided rod, apply the appropriate forces, being sure to apply compression forces between T12 and L2 to ensure that lumbar lordosis is maintained and preserved. Third, after fixing down the right-sided rod, attend to the left rod, and apply the final corrective forces for seating between the last two hooks on the left side. I have used this technique in 7 patients who have been followed from 1 to 3 years, but probably a 5-year follow-up is mandatory before this technique can be definitely recommended. The preliminary results are encouraging; in each case, the patient has remained compensated, L2 has been pulled within the stable zone, and lumbar lordosis from L1 to L5 and from T12 to L2 has been maintained and preserved (Case No. 6).

If there is significant thoracolumbar kyphosis and thoracic lordosis, the two sagittal curves must be addressed separately. The sagittal malalignment between T12 and L2 mandates carrying the instrumentation (Fig. 7-5) down to L4 (the stable vertebra). The first step is to apply a left-sided derotation rod from T4 to

(*text continues on page 117*)

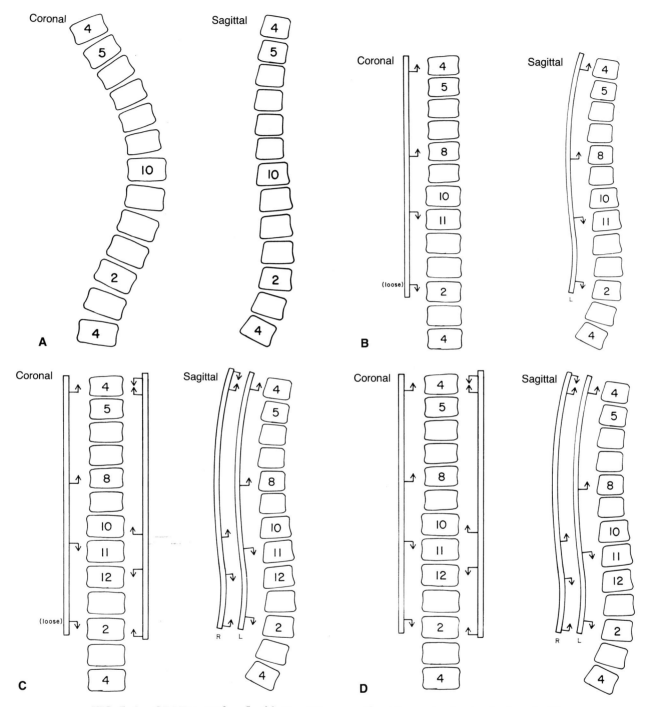

FIG. 7–4. CDI T4 to L2 for a flexible Type IV curve without thoracolumbar kyphosis. **A.** The spine preoperatively. **B.** The first step of performing the derotation maneuver but not seating down the hook at L2. **C.** Application of the right-sided convex rod and compression lordosing force between T12 and L2. **D.** The final seating of the hooks and rods in the anteroposterior and lateral planes.

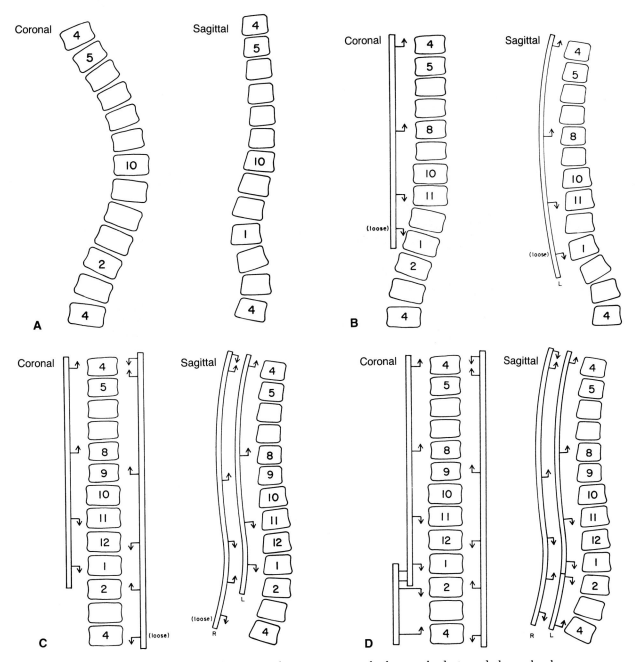

FIG. 7–5. Reduction of Type IV thoracic curve with thoracic lordosis and thoracolumbar kyphosis. **A.** Preoperatively, the spine is in lordosis from T4 to L1, in kyphosis in the upper lumbar spine, and in lordosis in the lower lumbar spine. T10 is the apical vertebra, and L4 is tilted into the curve in the coronal plane. **B.** A derotation maneuver for the thoracic spine converts thoracic lordosis to kyphosis. The hook at L1 is left loose. **C.** On the opposite side, place a right-sided rod and apply compression forces between T12 and L2 to achieve upper lumbar lordosis. Once this is achieved, the left L1 hook can be seated. **D.** Then apply compression forces on the left side again, between L2 and L4, to preserve lumbar lordosis. These are the initial forces necessary to achieve the maximal coronal and sagittal correction. The hooks on the right side from L2 to L4 are not seated until the compression lordosing force is applied on the left.

CASE NO. 6—M.R.

An 11 + 10-year-old girl with a Type IV curve and significant decompensation to the right does not have any gross sagittal malalignment. There is no pathologic thoracolumbar kyphosis. With Harrington instrumentation, it would be necessary to carry the fusion to L4, but by using the Cortel–Dubousset derotation maneuver, it is possible to save two lumbar levels. On the left side bending radiograph on this patient, L2 levels off to the pelvis.

The distal hook on the left-sided rod was not seated until compression forces were applied along the right-sided rod from T12 to L2, saving lumbar motion segments and preserving upper lumbar lordosis. Early results in this case are encouraging. Probably a 5-year follow-up is necessary to be sure that additional lumbar segments do not require a distal extension of the fusion.

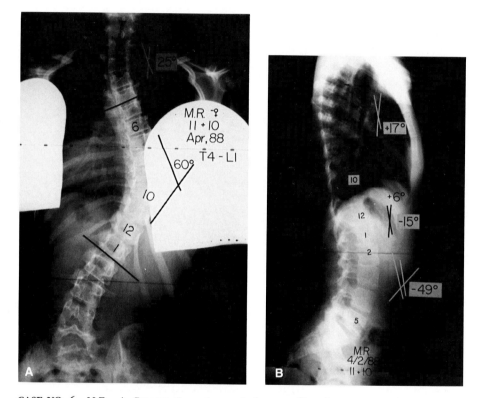

CASE NO. 6—M.R.   A. Preoperative anteroposterior x-ray film of an 11 + 10-year-old patient standing. She is significantly decompensated to the right. This is a Type IV curve, with L4 being the stable vertebra.   **B.** Preoperative lateral x-ray film of the standing patient.   **C.** Instrumentation and fusion performed down to L2. L2 is slightly to the right of the center sacral line. The patient is well-balanced, and C7 is centered clinically and radiographically on the sacrum.   **D.** Postoperative lateral x-ray film of the standing patient showing excellent lordosis from T12 down to L5. On the right-sided rod, the two-segment-compression lordosing claw was applied and performed from T12 to L2 before the final seating of the L2 hook on the left side. Upper lumbar lordosis is maintained.

(continued)

CASE NO. 6—M.R. *(continued)*

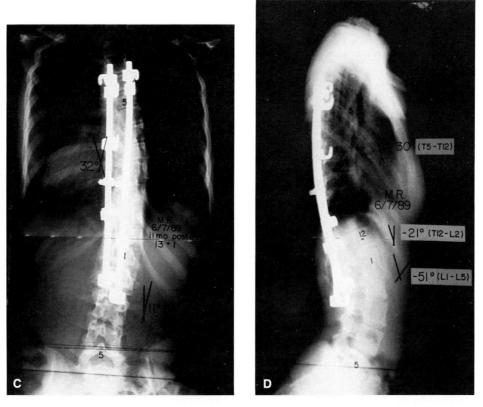

CASE NO. 6 *(continued)*

T12 or L1 and to perform a derotation maneuver to address the thoracic lordosis. In the second step, the longer, right-sided rod should be placed from T4 to L4, being sure to contour lordosis and apply compression-lordosing forces between T12 and L2 to address the thoracolumbar kyphosis. Third, on the left-sided rod, either with a domino extending the instrumentation down to L4 with hooks in a compression mode from L2 to L4 or by replacing the rod on the left side from T4 to L4, place hooks in a distraction mode from T4 to T12 and in a compression mode from L2 to L4. It is important that compression forces are applied between T12 and L2 on the right side before any force is placed between T12 and L2 on the left side to correct the thoracolumbar kyphosis. Compression forces should be applied between L2 and L4 on the left before any distraction force is applied. The initial force applied seems to determine the ultimate sagittal contour. To preserve lumbar lordosis, initially apply compression forces to the spine (Case No. 7).

CASE NO. 7—K.G.

An adolescent female with a Type IV curve pattern has a noticeable midthoracic lordosis and thoracolumbar kyphosis. Complicating matters further, she also has a structural high left thoracic curve of 36°. Treatment of this curve with Cotrel–Dubousset instrumentation is somewhat complicated. The first step was to perform a derotation maneuver with a left-sided rod from T5 to L1 to improve the thoracic lordosis. Then a rod was added on the top to correct the high left thoracic curve. A long rod was placed on the right side from T2 to L4. On this right-sided rod, compression forces were applied across the thoracolumbar junction to address the thoracolumbar kyphosis. After these forces were applied, an additional rod was added on the left side by means of a domino attachment to carry the left-sided instrumentation down to L4, applying compression and lordosis from L2 to L4. This produced good coronal and sagittal balance that would not have been possible with other instrumentation. The long spinal fusion was unavoidable in this case.

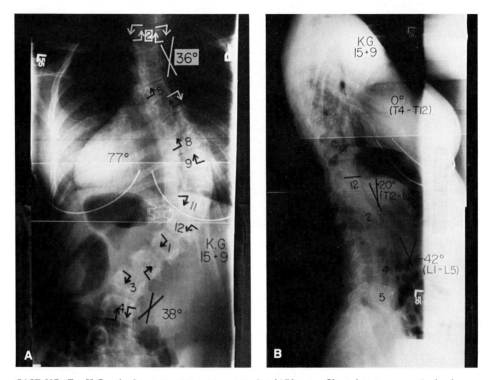

CASE NO. 7—K.G.   **A.** Long-cassette anteroposterior (AP) x-ray film taken preoperatively showing a Type IV thoracic curve pattern with the apex at T10 and L4 tilted. There is also a high left thoracic curve.   **B.** Long-cassette lateral x-ray film showing a thoracic lordosis and a thoracolumbar kyphosis.   **C.** Long-cassette AP x-ray film taken postoperatively showing satisfactory coronal alignment.   **D.** Long-cassette lateral x-ray film taken postoperatively showing some normalization of the sagittal thoracic and thoracolumbar deformities.

(continued)

Type V Thoracic Curves

Type V is the King classification for the double thoracic curve.[65] For a Type II or Type III curve, the proximal junctional neutral vertebra is T4. For the double thoracic curve, the proximal junctional neutral vertebra is more likely to be T5 or T6. On clinical examination, if it is the usual high left thoracic, low right thoracic curve pattern, the patient's left shoulder is level to the right shoulder or slightly higher, and a small high left rib hump appears on forward bending. If the first rib is higher on the left side than on the right side on the

CASE NO. 7—K.G. *(continued)*

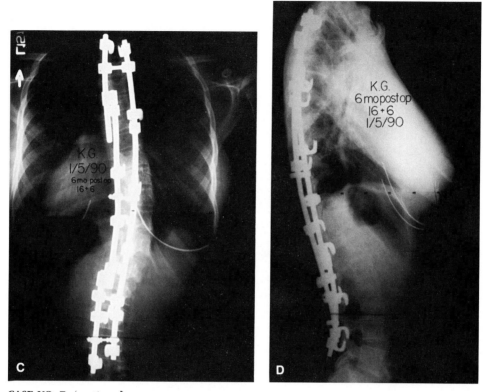

CASE NO. 7 *(continued)*

standing anterior-posterior radiograph, this indicates a double thoracic curve pattern. Rotation of the thoracic segments from T2 to T5 on the standing anterior-posterior radiograph and incomplete correction and derotation of this upper curve on the (left) side-bending radiograph are also clues. The principal cosmetic deformity created by the upper thoracic curve is shoulder asymmetry. Usually there is not as much of a rib hump associated with the high left thoracic curve as with the lower right thoracic curve because the high curve involves fewer segments. The upper thoracic curve tends to be hyperkyphotic, and the lower right thoracic curve tends to be hypokyphotic.

Instrument both curves if doing so levels the shoulders. The instrumentation should be carried up to the proximal neutral vertebra of the high thoracic curve, which is usually T2 but may be T1. Include the upper left thoracic curve if the Cobb measurement of the upper thoracic curve on the standing radiograph exceeds the anticipated Cobb angle after correction or if

the left shoulder is higher than the right shoulder. It is easy to overlook the contribution of the upper thoracic curve and focus in on the lower thoracic curve, which is usually a larger curve and creates a greater chest cage deformity. The consequence is unbalanced shoulder heights.

Instrumentation

Using Harrington instrumentation, a single dollar-sign rod works satisfactorily. It may be supplemented with Wisconsin wires or sublaminar wires and contouring of the rod.[33, 77, 78] Placing a short compression assembly on the transverse processes of the posterior elements on the convex side may reduce the kyphosis in the high thoracic curve.

With Cotrel–Dubousset instrumentation, the two curves should be treated separately because of the difference in the sagittal curves. Assuming a high left and lower right thoracic pattern (Fig. 7-6*A*, *B*), the

(text continues on page 122)

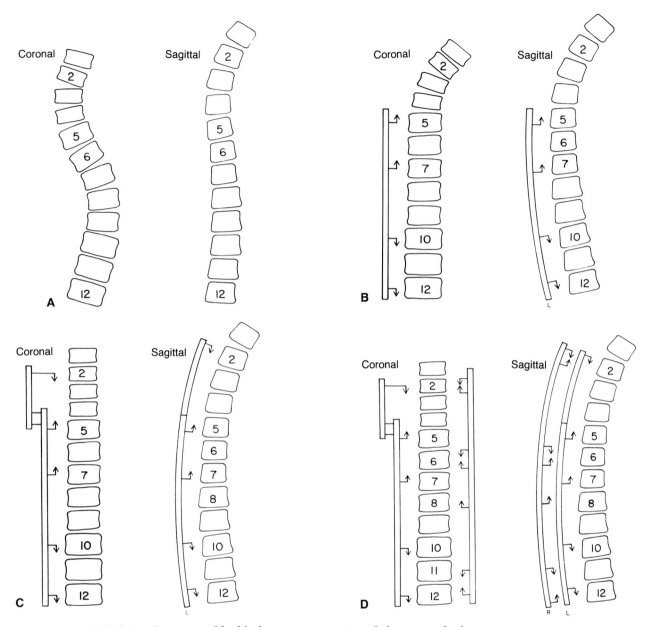

FIG. 7–6. Correction of double thoracic curve. **A.** Left thoracic–right thoracic curve pattern with T5 as the transitional vertebra. Slight hyperkyphosis from T2 to T5 and hypokyphosis from T5 to T12. **B.** Correction of the right thoracic curve and a slight kyphosing of the spine from T5 to T12. **C.** Correction of the upper left thoracic curve from T2 to T5, reducing the hyperkyphosis by applying compression forces. This rod linked to the other one with a domino. **D.** Application of the right-sided rod.

CASE NO. 8—T.B.

In a 16 + 10-year-old girl with a double thoracic curve pattern, the junctional neutral vertebra between the thoracic curves is T6. There is rotation of the vertebral segments from T2 to T6. The first rib is higher on the left side than the right side. These are all indications of a double thoracic curve pattern requiring instrumentation of both curves to provide symmetrical shoulder heights.

The instrumentation is performed by first performing the derotation maneuver for the lower right thoracic curve and then applying compression forces between T2 and T5 on the left side using the domino attachment to add on to the previous rod. The long rod on the right side is placed. The hooks are in the distraction mode between T2 and T6 on the right side. They are in a compression mode between T2 and T5 on the left side. The initial force applied to the spine with Cotrel–Dubousset instrumentation seems to be the most important for ultimate coronal and sagittal correction. Therefore, first applying compression to the left side of the upper left thoracic curve makes sense for correcting the hyperkyphotic deformity that exists.

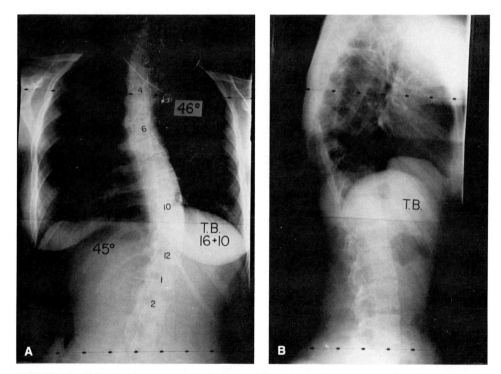

CASE NO. 8—T.B. **A.** Anteroposterior (AP) x-ray film of a standing patient with a double thoracic curve. The first rib is higher on the left side than the right. T6 and T7 are the junctional neutral vertebrae. The curve from T2 to T6 measures 46° and has rotation to it. On the side-bending x-ray film, this curve corrected less than the lower right thoracic curve did. **B.** Lateral x-ray film of the standing patient. **C.** Postoperative AP x-ray film on the standing patient. After performing a derotation maneuver from T6 to L2 with a left-sided rod, the domino attachment was placed, and an additional rod was placed from T2 to T6, applying compression forces on the convex side of the upper thoracic curve. **D.** Postoperative lateral x-ray film of the standing patient.

(continued)

CASE NO. 8—T.B. *(continued)*

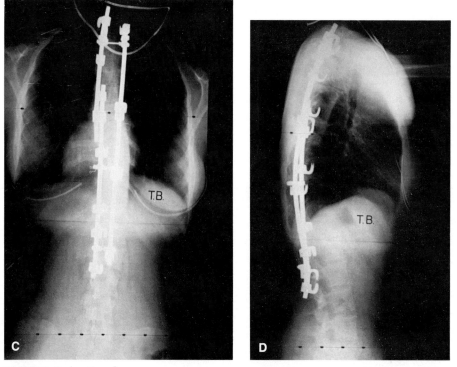

CASE NO. 8 *(continued)*

standard derotation maneuver should be performed on the lower right thoracic curve. On the left side, place short instrumentation from (usually) T2 to T5, and apply compression. This corrects the kyphotic component and the scoliotic component. Derotation is not that much of a concern for the upper thoracic curve. Fixation on T2 may be achieved by placing either a "CPT claw" (i.e., closed pedicle hook in T2 and closed lumbar laminar hook on the transverse process of T2) or by performing a laminotomy on the top side of T2 to place a closed lumbar hook facing caudally. By contouring the desired sagittal curve into the short rod and hooking it to the longer, lower concave rod at the level of the pedicle hook at T5 with a closed-closed domino, the instrumentation can be extended. Application of compression forces between T2 and T5 can be accomplished by bolting down the hooks at T2 or on the domino and applying a compression force just above T2 or just below the domino. If the domino is used, make

sure that the derotation rod used for the lower right thoracic curve is a little longer than is usually needed so that the domino can be placed above the T5 hook. It is advisable to place the domino on the rod before performing that derotation maneuver.

If dominos are not available, perform the derotation maneuver for the lower right thoracic curve, and on the right side, place long instrumentation from T2 to the distally fused segment. On the right side, a pedicle hook is best placed at T2, an open lumbar hook should be placed on the transverse process, and open pedicle hook should be placed on the pedicle of T6 (an open claw). A selective distraction force is then applied between T2 and T6 on the right side. After fixing the rod to all hooks on the right side, remove the temporary left-side derotation rod and place a single, long rod on the left side, applying the appropriate distraction and compression forces to reseat all the hooks. There is usually some loss of correction of the right thoracic curve associated with changing the rods. Generally three transverse traction devices or cross-links are placed after the instrumentation is complete (Case No. 8).

Thoracolumbar Curves

Thoracolumbar curves have an apex at T11, T12, or L1.[14] They are amenable to correction with anterior Zielke (VDS) instrumentation or posterior segmental instrumentation.[23, 49, 57, 69, 91, 94, 98, 146] With anterior Zielke instrumentation, it is usually possible to save several lumbar levels, and fusion below L3 is rare. With anterior VDS, the surgeon fuses only those discs tilted into the curve on the side bending radiograph, assuming the fractional lumbosacral curve is flexible. In some cases, it is possible to stop at L2 or L1 with this instrumentation system (Case No. 11).

Thoracolumbar curves have a tendency to be

CASE NO. 9—E.F.

For an adolescent girl with a primary thoracolumbar curve and secondary thoracic curve, the options of treatment include Cotrel–Dubousset instrumentation of both curves or Zielke instrumentation of only the thoracolumbar curve. Anterior Zielke instrumentation of the thoracolumbar curve could probably be stopped at L2. Harrington instrumentation would have to include both

curves and would probably necessitate instrumentation to L4. In this case, Cotrel–Dubousset instrumentation can be stopped at L3, because it is neutral and falls within the center sacral line on right side bending. That option was chosen; notice the upper lumbar lordosis provided by the instrumentation.

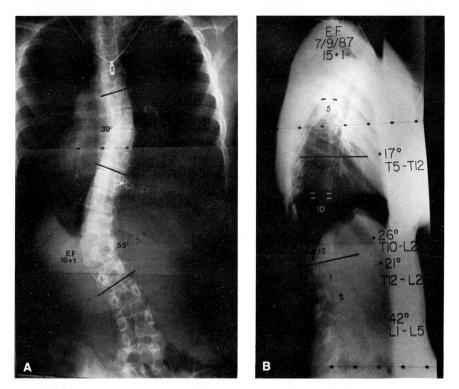

CASE NO. 9—E.F. **A.** Preoperative long-cassette anteroposterior (AP) x-ray film showing decompensation to the left. L4 is the stable vertebra. L3 is slightly to the left of the stable zone and is only minimally rotated. **B.** Preoperative lateral x-ray film of the standing patient showing a thoracolumbar kyphosis. **C.** Postoperative AP x-ray film showing a well-balanced spine in the coronal plane and L3 centered on the center sacral line. **D.** Long-cassette lateral x-ray film taken postoperatively showing correction of the thoracolumbar kyphosis and restoration of upper lumbar lordosis.

(continued)

CASE NO. 9—E.F. *(continued)*

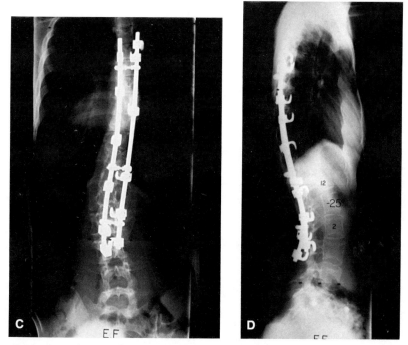

CASE NO. 9 *(continued)*

slightly hyperkyphotic. In adolescents, the sagittal deformity usually is not too bad. The more severe cases of rotatory kyphosis and hyperkyphosis occur more often in adults with scoliosis. However, any degree of kyphosis at the thoracolumbar junction caused by the curve is important in deciding whether to treat the curve anteriorly with Zielke instrumentation or posteriorly with posterior segmental instrumentation. Posterior instrumentation may be better for correcting the kyphotic component if it is a true kyphosis.

Although Harrington instrumentation can be used across the thoracolumbar junction, a surgeon should always think about applying compression-lordosing forces to the spine as instrumentation is carried into the lumbar segments. In this respect Cotrel–Dubousset instrumentation has certain advantages.

In applying Cotrel–Dubousset instrumentation for a thoracolumbar curve, it is always important to apply the instrumentation to the convex side of the curve and to apply compression forces and rod rotation forces initially. Usually the apical hooks are placed only two segments apart. For example, if the apical segments are T12 and L1, the apical hooks are placed facing each other on the posterior elements of T12 and L1. After completing the rod rotation on the left side (assuming a left thoracolumbar curve), the right side is addressed by placing hooks in a distraction mode. This can be accomplished with Harrington instrumentation by applying a compression construct on the convex left side followed by a distraction with wire construct on the right side. Applying the segmental compression construct first offers the best chance of preserving lumbar lordosis (Case Nos. 9 and 10).

(text continues on page 128)

CASE NO. 10—K.B.

A 19 + 6-year-old female with a 42° right thoracolumbar curve and significant right coronal decompensation would usually be an excellent candidate for anterior VDS, but she was not a candidate for postoperative bracing for a variety of psychosocial reasons. Therefore, Cotrel–Dubousset instrumentation alleviated the need for postoperative protection. A longer fusion was required than anticipated with anterior VDS. Notice the excellent preservation of lumbar lordosis.

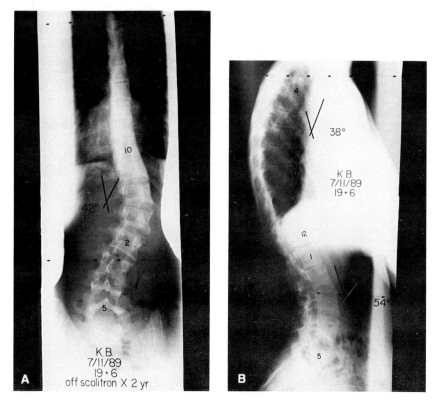

CASE NO. 10—K.B.   **A.** 19 + 6-year-old female with a 42° thoracolumbar curve from T10 to L2 and a 22° curve from L2 to L5. Although the curve sizes are not large, she is significantly decompensated to the right side.   **B.** Preoperative lateral x-ray film on the standing patient showing slightly exaggerated thoracic kyphosis and lumbar lordosis. **C.** The standing patient's anteroposterior x-ray film taken postoperatively. The hooks were arranged to apply a distractive force where the discs were collapsed and for compression where the discs were open. To preserve lordosis, the compression and lordosing forces are always applied before the distraction forces. Alternatively, the patient probably could have been treated with anterior VDS from either T12 to L2 with slight overcorrection or from T11 to L3. However, the patient's behavioral pattern was not conducive to postoperative protection with a cast or brace.   **D.** A long-cassette lateral x-ray film taken postoperatively showing excellent preservation of lumbar lordosis. Junctional kyphosis may develop at the top of this instrumentation, which stops in the lower thoracic spine.

(*continued*)

CASE NO. 10—K.B. *(continued)*

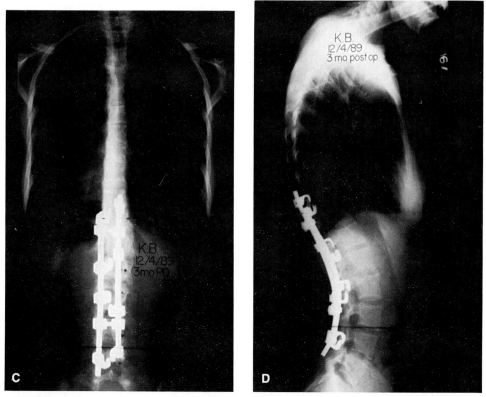

CASE NO. 10 *(continued)*

CASE NO. 11—J.L.

This is a 12 + 11-year-old girl who has developed a 40° thoracolumbar curve despite aggressive bracing. She is still skeletally immature. Although the Cobb measurement is not excessive, there is considerable rotation to the curve, and she is decompensated to the right. In the sagittal plane, she has relatively normal sagittal contour with good lumbar lordosis and no thoracolumbar ky-phosis. With Harrington instrumentation, fusion down to L4 would have been required. With Cotrel–Dubousset instrumentation, perhaps the fusion could have been stopped at L3. In her case, anterior VDS instrumentation was performed from T11 to L2 with good derotation and preservation of the sagittal contour. Notice her curve pattern is very similar to Case No. 10.

CASE NO. 11—J.L.   A. Preoperative anteroposterior x-ray film of standing patient showing coronal decompensation to the right.   **B.** Normal sagittal contour.   **C.** Anterior Zielke instrumentation and solid anterior spinal fusion from T10 to L2 taken 25 months postoperatively.   **D.** Preservation of the sagittal contour of the patient. The curve pattern is almost identical to Case No. 10.

(continued)

CASE NO. 11—J.L. (*continued*)

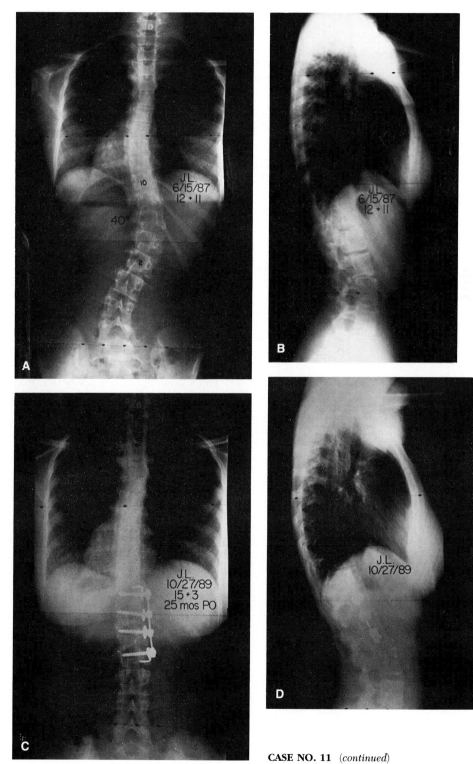

CASE NO. 11 (*continued*)

Double-Major Curves

In the double-major curve pattern, both the lumbar and thoracic curves have roughly equivalent Cobb measurements, with equal amounts of rotation and deviation from the plumb line and the center sacral line. Even if the lumbar curve is slightly bigger than the thoracic curve, it is not uncommon that the lumbar curve will be more flexible on the side-bending maneuver, but that should not fool the surgeon into thinking that it is a false double-major (King Type II) curve pattern.

The greatest concerns in treating double-major curves are preserving as many lumbar segments as

CASE NO. 12—S.M.

This is a 13 + 7-year-old girl with a very large left lumbar curve. Although this technically may not be considered a double-major curve because the lumbar curve is bigger, it is included in this section because the thoracic spine also requires fusion. There is quite a bit of tilt to L4, which is outside of the stable zone, and it has significant rotation to it. L4 levels off incompletely on the right side-bending maneuver. It seems impossible to pull L4 to within the stable zone, level it off, and derotate it with a posterior fusion and instrumentation alone. Therefore, anterior releases and interbody fusions are performed first, followed by the posterior instrumentation to L4. The postoperative result is a good lordosis, but there is a disappointing amount of derotation and translation of the apical vertebra to the center sacral line. The spine appeared quite flexible at the time of posterior instrumentation, and the derotation maneuver on the spine occurred very smoothly, but this case illustrates that in a lumbar spine, placing hooks on the posterior elements is not as mechanically efficient as it is in the thoracic spine. Hooks are not as efficient as vertebral body screws placed either anteriorly in the vertebral bodies or through the pedicles for correcting the translational and rotatory lumbar deformity.

CASE NO. 12—S.M. **A.** Standing preoperative anteroposterior (AP) x-ray film. Notice the tremendous tilt at L4–L5. L4 lies to the left of the center sacral line. **B.** Standing lateral x-ray film taken preoperatively. Notice the apparent thoracolumbar kyphosis.

(continued)

CASE NO. 12—S.M. *(continued)*

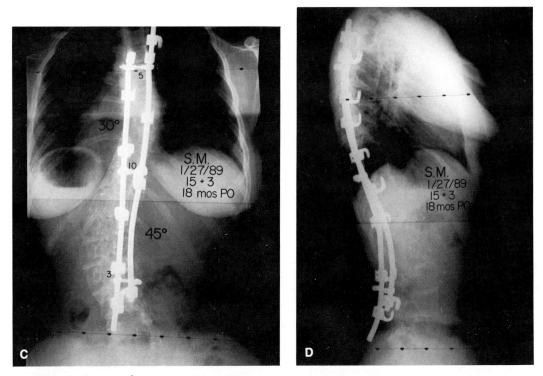

CASE NO. 12 *(continued)* **C.** Long-cassette AP x-ray film of the standing patient taken 18 months postoperatively. L4 is well within the stable zone and level to the pelvis. However, there is considerable residual rotation to the lumbar curve. In retrospect, an additional hook on the left-sided rod at L1 facing caudad and an additional hook on the right-sided rod at L2 should have been used and might have resulted in better correction. **D.** Lateral x-ray film of the standing patient taken 18 months postoperatively showing apparent correction of the thoracolumbar kyphosis.

possible and maintaining the patient's lordosis. Many studies have strongly suggested that degenerative problems in later years are more likely after using Harrington instrumentation for the more distal lumbar spine.[24, 42, 45] We do not know to what extent the results are influenced by the iatrogenic lumbar kyphosing effect of Harrington distraction instrumentation or by the loss of mobile segments below.[75] Michel and coworkers suggested that the lumbar vertebral bodies below a long fusion changed morphologically with time, resulting in a normal lordosis.[89, 90] However, we prefer to stop all instrumentation at L3 or higher, with L3 perfectly centered on the center sacral line and with a physiologic lumbar lordosis across the instrumented segments. At the thoracolumbar junction from T12 to L2, the average patient has approximately $-5°$ of lor-

dosis. From L1 to L5, the average patient has approximately $-45°$ of lordosis.

With Harrington instrumentation for double-major curves, the fusion is usually extended to L4. The distally fused segment should be the stable segment (i.e., that segment bisected by the center sacral line). If Harrington instrumentation is used, some kind of compression assembly should be initially applied to the lumbar spine on the convex side before applying the concave distraction force. Compression forces must be applied to the convex side of the lumbar curve first to preserve lordosis. A contoured square Harrington rod should be used in addition to wire fixation with Wisconsin or sublaminar wires. However, simply contouring a square Harrington rod with or without wires does not preserve lumbar lordosis.[21]

CASE NO. 13—R.J.

This is a 17 + 4-year-old girl with a curve pattern similar to the previous case. The lumbar curve is larger than the thoracic, but both curves require fusion. She has the same dilemma of an uncharacteristically stiff and low left lumbar curve in which instrumentation to L4 posteriorly probably will not center L4 perfectly over the sacrum and will leave a residual lumbosacral curve from L4 to the sacrum. Therefore, Zielke instrumentation is performed anteriorly, followed by posterior Cotrel–Dubousset instrumentation. With the anterior Zielke procedure, the derotator-lordosator is heavily relied on. The amount of compression force applied across the disc spaces is discreet, and bone graft is packed into the anterior disc spaces to preserve lumbar lordosis. The Cotrel-l–Dubousset instrumentation posteriorly is further

contoured and placed to preserve lordosis. Intentionally, no effort is made to kyphose the thoracic spine with a derotation maneuver because lumbar lordosis has been fixed by anterior VDS, and the sagittal plumb line must be maintained just posterior to S1. This technique may not provide as much lumbar lordosis as in the previous case, but it more effectively pulls the apical lumbar vertebral body to the center sacral line and does a better job of leveling off the distally fused segment. In this respect, anterior VDS Zielke instrumentation appears to be superior to Cotrel–Dubousset instrumentation in the lumbar spine. Technically it would have been preferable to place the distal lumbar screws from a more posterior starting point in the bodies.

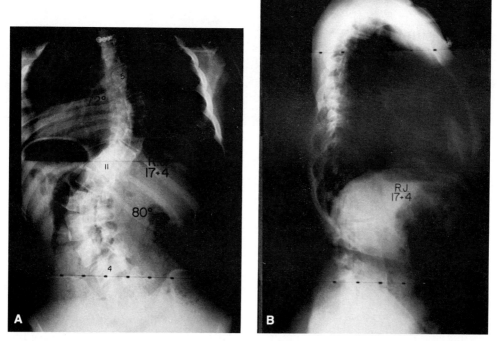

CASE NO. 13—R.J. **A.** Preoperative anteroposterior x-ray film of a standing patient demonstrates a 72° thoracic curve from T5 to T11 and an even larger lumbar curve from T11 to L4. The curve from L4 to the sacrum does not completely level off on the right side bender, but it does improve by approximately 70%. **B.** Preoperative lateral x-ray film of the standing patient. **C.** Postoperative x-ray film of the standing patient. She was treated with anterior VDS from T12 to L4 and Cotrel–Dubousset instrumentation from T4 to L4. Notice the excellent correction of the rotation in the lumbar spine and the excellent centralization of the apical lumbar vertebra to the center sacral line. There is still a slight coronal tilt at L4–L5. **D.** Lateral x-ray film of the standing patient shows a somewhat flat lumbar spine despite placing a bone graft in the anterior half of the disc space and using the derotator. The apical Zielke screws were placed posteriorly in the vertebral bodies and appear to lie more anteriorly now because of the derotation maneuver created by the Zielke derotator.

(continued)

CASE NO. 13—R.J. (*continued*)

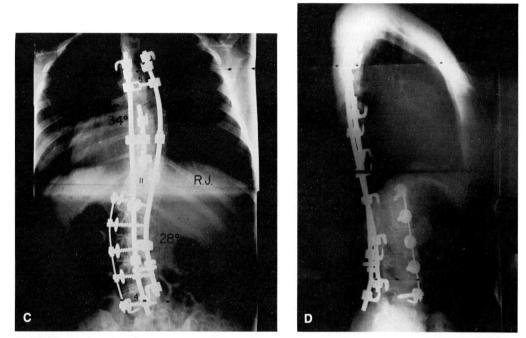

CASE NO. 13 (*continued*)

With Cotrel−Dubousset instrumentation, it may be possible to stop at L3 in very selected cases in which Harrington instrumentation would have to be carried to L4, but excellent scoliosis surgeons have failed to accomplish this feat. My experience has been that the instrumentation can be stopped at L3 only if L3 is neutral (or within 10° of neutral by Pedriolle template) and intersected, if not bisected, by the center sacral line on the standing radiograph. The curve from L3 to the sacrum must be totally flexible (e.g., it bends out completely on the right side-bending film for a left lumbar curve). Probably only a minority of double-major curves can be stopped at L3 instead of L4 with Cotrel−Dubousset instrumentation. The spine after instrumentation and fusion should ideally show the distally fused segment bisected by the center sacral line and within 10° of being neutrally rotated.

The technique of Cotrel−Dubousset instrumentation for double-major curves consists of applying the hooks (on the left-sided rod) in the thoracic spine as one would for a thoracic curve with hooks in the distraction mode from T4 to T12 and with the lumbar spine having four hooks on the convex side, all in a compression mode. The two apical lumbar hooks should be facing each other, open and only one segment apart. For example, if the instrumentation is being carried from T4 to L3, the distal four hooks on the left convex side should be placed at T12, L1, L2, and L3, assuming that the instrumentation can be stopped at L3 and assuming that the apical disc is the L1−L2 disc. If the apical

CASE NO. 14—M.C.

In this adolescent girl with a double-major curve pattern and a Grade I isthmic spondylolisthesis at L5–S1, the thoracic and lumbar curves are equally structural (Cobb measurement and rotation). The goals are to preserve lumbar lordosis and to leave as many unfused segments above the spondylolisthesis as possible. With the Harrington system, the instrumentation would have to extend to L4. With Cotrel–Dubousset instrumentation, L3 is close to being neutral, permitting the surgeon to stop there. In this case, further effort toward leveling off L3 and L2 is accomplished by placing Zielke screws through the pedicles at L3, L2, and L1 and applying compression forces across them and through the Cotrel–Dubousset hooks. This provides a good lordosis and leveling off at L3. This is a modification of Klaus Zielke's "Harrington-Royale" procedure.

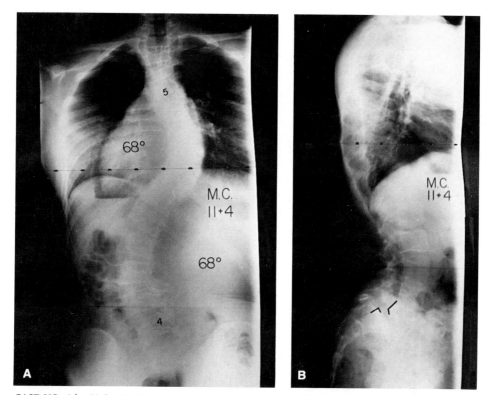

CASE NO. 14—M.C. **A.** Long-cassette anteroposterior x-ray film taken preoperatively shows a double-major curve pattern because the thoracic and lumbar curves deviate equally from the plumb line and have equal amounts of rotation to them. Although the lumbar curve is more flexible than the thoracic on the side-bending maneuvers, this is not a false double-major curve pattern. **B.** Long-cassette lateral x-ray film taken preoperatively shows an isthmic spondylolisthesis at L5–S1. **C.** Long-cassette x-ray film of the patient taken postoperatively shows instrumentation with Cotrel–Dubousset fixation and posterior VDS, which applies compression and lordosing forces from L1 to L3 in an effort to pull up L3. A 5-year follow-up is mandatory to know if L3 will stay within the stable zone. **D.** Long-cassette lateral x-ray film of the patient taken postoperatively shows preservation of lumbar lordosis and two motion segments between the end of the fusion mass and the spondylolisthesis.

(continued)

CASE NO. 14—M.C. *(continued)*

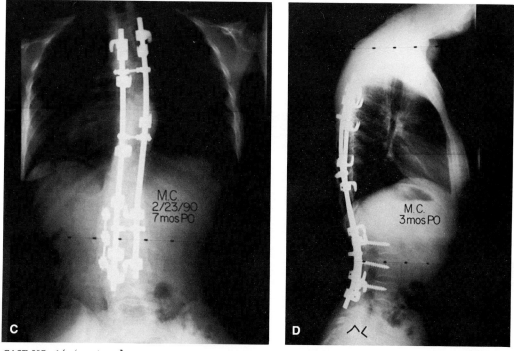

C

D

CASE NO. 14 *(continued)*

disc is L2–L3, it is necessary to fuse to L4. After performing the rod rotation maneuver and applying the appropriate forces to the rod on the left side, the right-sided rod is placed with hooks in the compression mode on the right side from T4 to T12 and in the distraction mode from T12 to L4 on the right side. The use of Cotrel–Dubousset instrumentation in adolescents provides excellent preservation of lumbar lordosis (Case Nos. 12 and 15).[15]

Instrumentation and fusion below L4 in adolescent patients is rare, but there are lumbar and thoracolumbar curves in which L5 is the stable vertebra and L4 is outside of the center sacral line with considerable rotation.[14] The apex of these curves is usually either the L3 vertebral body or the L3–L4 disc. For these curves, it may be advisable to perform an anterior Zielke instrumentation to allow the instrumentation and fusion to stop at L4 rather than having to fuse posteriorly to L5 with Harrington instrumentation (Case No. 13).[68] A disadvantage of anterior Zielke instrumentation to L4 is that it does somewhat reduce lumbar lordosis.[98] If the curve is particularly supple and flexible, it may be possible to stop at L4 with Cotrel–Dubousset instrumentation if the surgeon also places Zielke VDS pedicle screws posteriorly in L4, L3, L2, and perhaps L1 and applies compression forces through these pedicle screws on the convex side. Placing screws in the pedicles seems to provide a more efficient and corrective moment arm on the lumbar vertebrae than do laminar hooks in my experience (Case No. 14).

CASE NO. 15—L.R.

In this 12 + 7-year-old girl with a double-major curve pattern, notice that L3 is neutral and the curve from L3 to the sacrum bends out on the right side-bending maneuver. Therefore, she is a candidate for stopping the instrumentation at L3. This provided good sagittal and coronal alignment.

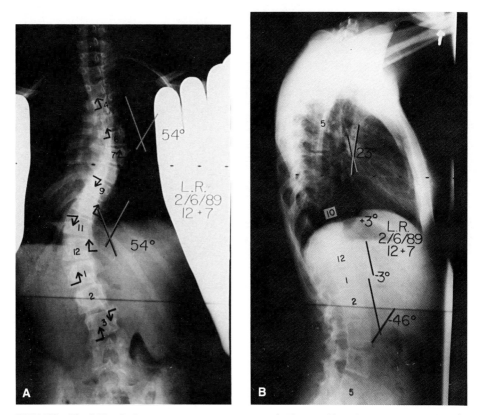

CASE NO. 15—L.R. A. Long-cassette anteroposterior (AP) x-ray film taken preoperatively. L4 is the stable vertebra. L5 is sacralized. **B.** Long-cassette lateral x-ray film showing relatively normal thoracolumbar and lumbar lordosis. **C.** Long-cassette AP x-ray film taken postoperatively showing excellent coronal balance and in this case excellent centralization of the lumbar curve. **D.** Long-cassette lateral x-ray film showing excellent sagittal contour.

(continued)

Lumbar Curves

For lumbar curves, it is important to make every effort to fuse as few segments as possible and to maintain lumbar lordosis.

The instrumentation systems most commonly employed as of 1989 are Cotrel–Dubousset instrumentation and anterior Zielke VDS instrumentation.[49, 57,] [58, 63, 98, 146] The Zielke instrumentation can save more lumbar levels and provides better curve correction, better derotation, and better translational correction. In my hands, the displacement of the apical vertebrae from the center sacral line is much less after treatment with anterior Zielke instrumentation than with Cotrel–Dubousset instrumentation for most lumbar and thoracolumbar curves. The derotational effects of Cotrel–

CASE NO. 15—L.R. (*continued*)

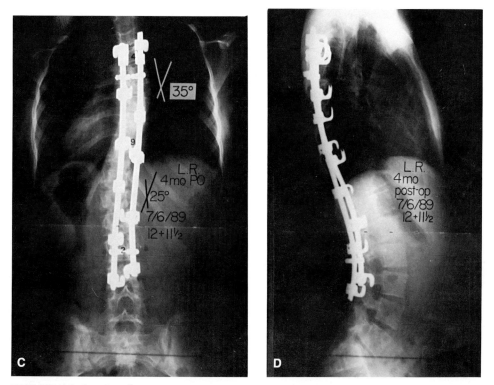

CASE NO. 15 (*continued*)

Dubousset instrumentation on the lumbar spine are somewhat disappointing because they do not bring the apical vertebrae as close to the center sacral line as anterior Zielke instrumentation does. Cotrel–Dubousset instrumentation can be used to save levels in the lumbar spine in a few selected cases, and it is excellent for preserving and even enhancing lumbar lordosis.[15] Zielke instrumentation has a tendency to reduce lumbar lordosis even if the derotator is used and even if bone graft is packed into the anterior disc spaces (Case Nos. 16 and 17).[98]

All these factors must be weighed in deciding which system to use for treating lumbar curves. Both are excellent, safe techniques with very high rates of

solid fusion.[23, 49, 98–100] Zielke instrumentation requires more postoperative protection because it is less rigid than Cotrel–Dubousset instrumentation, but it is an excellent method for achieving solid fusion because bone grafts are placed in a vascular bed (the vertebral bodies) and are placed under compression by the instrumentation system. Advantages of the Zielke system over the Dwyer system are that greater forces can be placed on the spine, the instrumentation is somewhat more rigid, and the use of the VDS lordosator-derotator allows additional derotation of the spine and better preservation of lumbar lordosis.[37, 38, 76]

Tricks to preserve lumbar lordosis with anterior VDS include placing bone graft in the anterior half of

CASE NO. 16—J.J.

An adolescent girl had a primary lumbar and secondary thoracic curve. This is a King Type I curve. It can be considered a false double-major curve, with the lumbar curve being the primary curve and the thoracic curve the secondary one. The lumbar curve is bigger, has more rotation, and deviates further from the plumb line than the thoracic curve. This could be treated with Harrington instrumentation including both curves and fusing from T4 to L4. Perhaps with Cotrel–Dubousset instrumentation, the fusion could be stopped distally at L3. Instead of these methods, a very short instrumentation was performed from T12 to L2 because of the extreme flexibility of the left lumbar curve.[91] This resulted in marked cosmetic improvement for the patient. Although the thoracic curve measures a Cobb angle close to 40°, the cosmetic appearance of the thoracic curve is satisfactory. This patient has excellent coronal and sagittal compensation, with only two fused motion segments of her spine. Notice that the segments fused are shorter than the lumbar curve and are overcorrected intentionally.

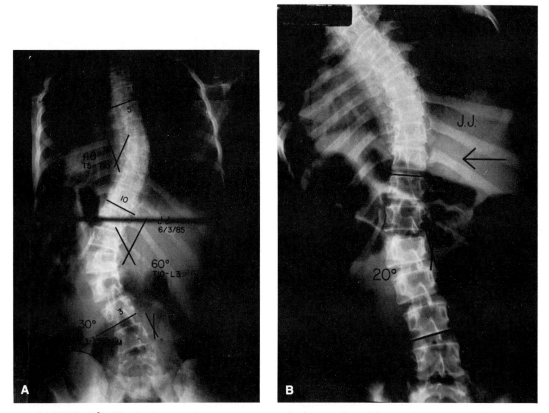

CASE NO. 16—J.J. **A.** Preoperative anteroposterior (AP) x-ray film of the standing patient. The lumbar curve from T10 to L3 deviates farther from the plumb line and has more rotation to it than the thoracic curve from T5 to T10. **B.** Notice that on the left side bender that the lumbar curve is quite flexible. The only discs that do not open up are the T12–L1 and L1–L2. **C.** The thoracic curve is quite flexible, and the lumbosacral curve from L3 to the pelvis bends out completely. **D.** An AP x-ray film of the standing patient taken 4 years postoperatively. There is excellent coronal balance, and L2 is centered perfectly on the sacrum. **E.** Standing lateral x-ray film taken 4 years postoperatively shows a mild thoracolumbar kyphosis, which was not clinically apparent.

(continued)

CASE NO. 16—J.J. *(continued)*

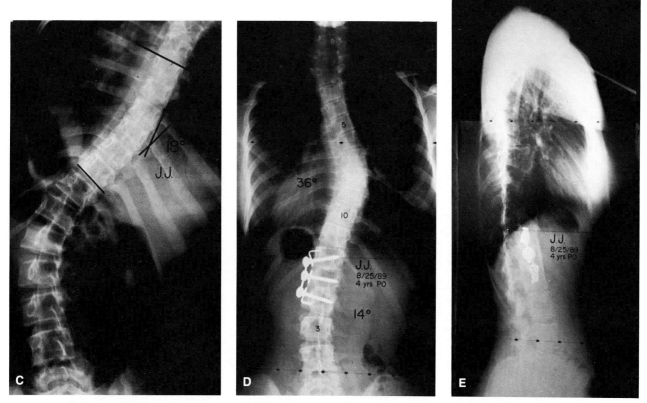

CASE NO. 16 *(continued)*

the disc space, starting all of the screws in the vertebral bodies an equal distance from the pedicle (i.e., starting the apical screws more posteriorly and aiming them more anteriorly), and using the lordosator. Alignment of the screws may be the most critical point, because with screw-rod engagement, the apical vertebral bodies are brought anteriorly, producing derotation and lordosis. However, applying compression forces anteriorly across the disc spaces reduces lordosis. In reviewing cases with Dr. Michael Neuwirth, we found that lordosis was enhanced with anterior VDS in some cases and reduced in others, but with an overall slight reduction in lumbar lordosis across the instrumented segments that was demonstrated by radiographic analysis but not appreciated clinically.[98] The use of Cotrel–Dubousset instrumentation for lumbar curves probably better preserves lordosis, but it requires fusion of more segments. An occasional complication of Cotrel–Dubousset instrumentation and other posterior systems for lumbar curves that I have never seen with anterior VDS is an increased kyphosis above the top of the instrumentation, which can be cosmetically displeasing. This is seen in patients for whom the instrumentation ended cranially between T8 and T12.

CASE NO. 17—N.R.

An 11 + 11-year-old girl with a 45° left lumbar curve from T11 to L3, which caused decompensation to the left, progressed to this point despite aggressive Boston bracing. She was treated with anterior spinal fusion and Zielke instrumentation from T12 to L3. Two years and 8 months postoperatively, at age 14 + 11, she had excellent coronal and sagittal balance. Notice that from T12 to L3, there is a slight kyphosing effect from the Zielke instrumentation.

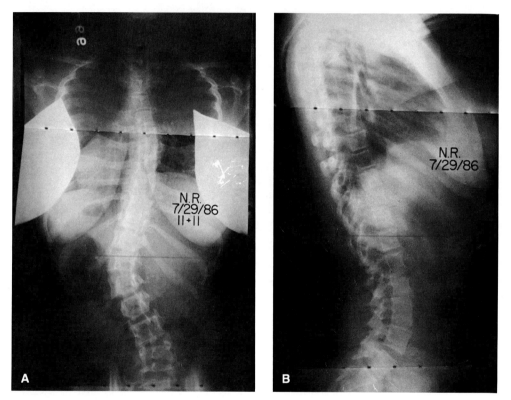

CASE NO. 17—N.R.   **A.** Preoperative anteroposterior (AP) x-ray film of the standing patient.   **B.** Preoperative lateral x-ray film of the standing patient.   **C.** Standing AP x-ray film 2 + 8 years postoperatively. With Harrington instrumentation, posterior fusion would have been necessary from T9 to L4.   **D.** Postoperative lateral x-ray film of the standing patient.

(continued)

THORACOPLASTY

For the patient with a thoracic curve of 70° or greater, the instrumentation does not correct the residual distortion of the rib cage.[10, 133, 138] For these patients, resecting some of the convex apical ribs is reasonable.[122]

Thoracoplasty does not improve pulmonary function.[10] In fact, it causes a temporary reduction that should recover after the ribs heal. Therefore, thoracoplasty for cosmetic reasons should only be considered for patients who have satisfactory pulmonary function tests preoperatively. Usually 5-cm segments of the ribs are

CASE NO. 17—N.R. (*continued*)

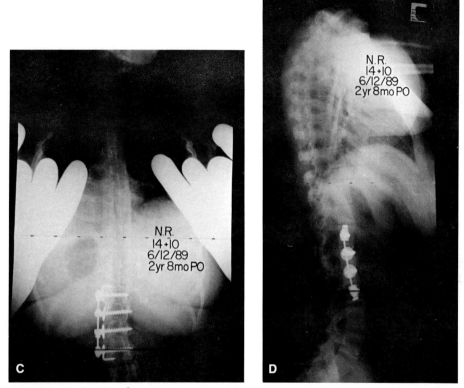

CASE NO. 17 (*continued*)

resected on the convex side through the apical five or seven ribs, as necessary, to level off the rib hump (Fig. 7-7; see also Color Plate 2). The most common error is not resecting enough ribs and not resecting the ribs medially enough (Case No. 18; Fig. 7-7).

In the adolescent patient, it is usually possible to subperiosteally dissect the ribs without entering the pleural cavity. If the pleural cavity is entered, it may be possible to repair the pleural rent. If it is a large, irregular rent, it may be necessary to place a chest tube.

The thoracoplasty can be performed through the midline posterior spine incision by retracting the fascia and working under it and the latissimus dorsi or through a separate parallel vertical incision centered over the rib hump. It is easier to access the medial rib through the midline subfascial approach and easier to access the lateral rib through the separate incision.

It may be helpful to place the adolescent patient in a TLSO brace for the first 3 months after surgery to protect the chest cage while the ribs regenerate. The ribs that are harvested during thoracoplasty usually provide adequate bone grafting for the fusion, obviating supplementation with autogenous iliac bone graft.[2]

(*text continues on page 142*)

CASE NO. 18—P.F.

In a 14 + 8-year-old girl with an 84° right thoracic curve and a very significant right thoracic rib hump, the curve was too big and too stiff to be treated by a single derotation maneuver. Instead a three-rod technique was employed, and it was supplemented with a thoracoplasty. Several of the apical convex ribs were resected and used for the bone graft instead of using autogenous iliac bone. Additional correction might have been possible with multiple concave rib osteotomies.[81]

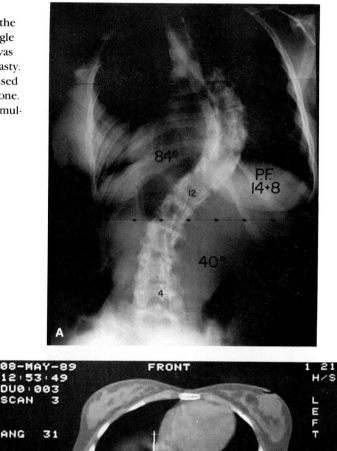

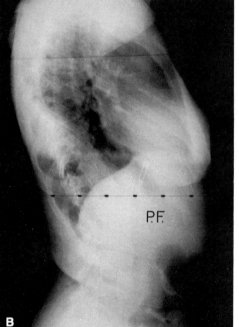

CASE NO. 18—P.F. **A.** The thoracic curve measures 84°, and the lumbar curve is 40°. This is a Type III curve. **B.** Lateral x-ray film of the patient taken preoperatively. **C.** A CT scan of the apex of the deformity of the patient taken preoperatively. Even with complete derotation of the spine, if it were possible, the patient would continue to have a significant residual rib hump. Notice the distortion of the rib cage on the right side, which is partially independent of the rotational deformity. **D.** Postoperative anteroposterior x-ray film of the standing patient. A stacked-rod technique was used because the right thoracic curve only corrected to 65° on the right side bender. The osteotomies through the convex right ribs were done as a thoracoplasty technique. The rib graft was used as the bone graft. **E.** Postoperative lateral x-ray film of the standing patient.

(continued)

CASE NO. 18—P.F. (*continued*)

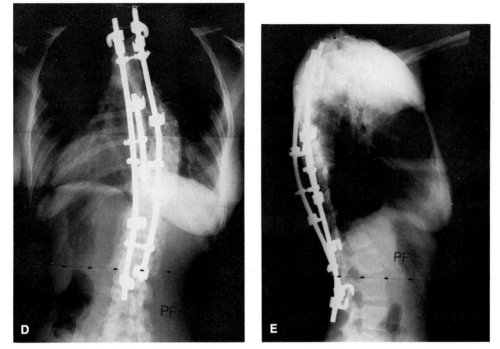

CASE NO. 18 (*continued*)

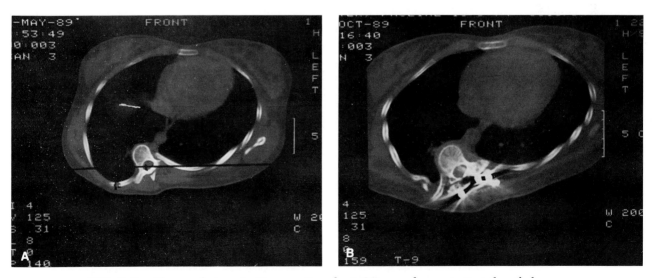

FIG. 7–7. Thoracoplasty. **A.** Preoperative chest CT scan demonstrating the rib hump. **B.** Chest CT scan demonstrating the rib hump 4 months postoperatively. The result would have been better had an additional 2 cm of rib been resected medially at this level. (See also Color Plate 2.)

ASSOCIATED CONDITIONS

With idiopathic scoliosis, the literature states that the adolescent patient should not be complaining of pain, but at least 20% of the adolescent patients do complain of some type of back pain on presenting to the physician. Most back pain is very mild, mechanical in nature, and perhaps brought on by the patient's anxiety about his or her scoliosis. However, if a patient complains of severe or unrelenting pain or of a consistent, boring pain, the complaints should be taken seriously. Any complaint of night pain should heighten suspicion. The patient may have an osteoid osteoma or an osteoblastoma.[43] If not apparent on plain films, a bone scan is an excellent way to identify these lesions. The bone scan can be supplemented by tomograms, magnetic resonance imaging (MRI), or computed tomography (CT) to further delineate the lesion. If the deformity is very small and very flexible, resecting the osteoid osteoma or osteoblastoma may be all that is necessary. On the other hand, if a deformity is large and structural and does not bend well on the flexibility maneuvers, it may be necessary to resect the lesion and to treat the scoliosis (see Case No. 20).

Examination of the patient with idiopathic scoliosis should also include a careful neurologic examination of upper and lower extremities and the 12 cranial nerves. There is an association between apparent idiopathic scoliosis and syringomyelia and Arnold Chiari malformation in certain instances and an association between left thoracic scoliosis and tumors (e.g., neuroblastoma, osteoblastoma) and intraspinal pathology.[14, 26, 47] Therefore, any left thoracic curve and any curve that is not a typical pattern for idiopathic scoliosis should heighten suspicion (Case Nos. 20, 21, and 22). Diastematomyelia and distal spinal cord tethers can exist with idiopathic scoliosis curve patterns, although they are

(text continues on page 149)

CASE NO. 19—J.K.

A 14 + 9-year-old girl presented with a 138° right thoracic curve. Presentation of such a large curve at such an early age is very unusual. A curve of this magnitude and stiffness should arouse suspicion of an underlying neuromuscular disorder or association with some form of spinal cord stretch, such as a Chiari malformation, a syringomyelia, or tethered cord. However, this patient's neurologic examination was entirely normal. There were no family histories of dysplastic hereditary conditions or neuromuscular conditions. Her myelogram performed from occiput to coccyx was normal.

This curve was very stiff on side-bending and prone push maneuvers. Although most idiopathic scoliosis in 1989 that is considered "operative" does not significantly reduce pulmonary functions, this curve did. The preoperative forced expiratory volume (FEV_1) was 1.33 L, and the preoperative forced vital capacity (FVC) was 1.25 L.

The patient was treated initially with halo traction and then a right-sided thoracotomy with several discectomies in the thoracic spine. The apical three vertebral bodies were decancellated, and the posterior vertebral body shells were resected. She received additional halo traction and was treated with a posterior instrumentation and fusion with the Cotrel–Dubousset system. Trying to perform a simple derotation maneuver was not very practical with such a large curve. Instead, selective distraction and compression forces were applied. A three-rod technique was used in which a selective distraction force was applied through the apical intermediary segments and then through the end segments. The apical segments were translated to the end segments with the use of the devices for transverse traction. Then the third convex rod was placed. Bone graft was taken from the right ilium, and the residual anterior bone graft (rib and vertebral body bone) was used posteriorly as well. Immediately postoperatively the patient's halo was removed. She was upright within a week postoperatively. She gained 5 inches (12.7 cm) in standing height. Her postoperative FEV_1 was 1.90 L and FVC was 1.82 L 6 months after surgery.

CASE NO. 19—J.K. **A.** Preoperative standing anteroposterior (AP) x-ray film showing a 138° right thoracic curve. **B.** Preoperative standing lateral x-ray film. **C.** The standing long-cassette AP x-ray film 2 years after surgery. **D.** The standing long-cassette lateral x-ray film 2 years after surgery. **E.** The patient's rib hump before surgery. **F.** The patient's clinical preoperative appearance. **G.** The patient's clinical appearance 5 days postoperatively. **H.** The patient's clinical appearance from the right side 5 days postoperatively. **I.** The patient's clinical appearance 2 years postoperatively.

(continued)

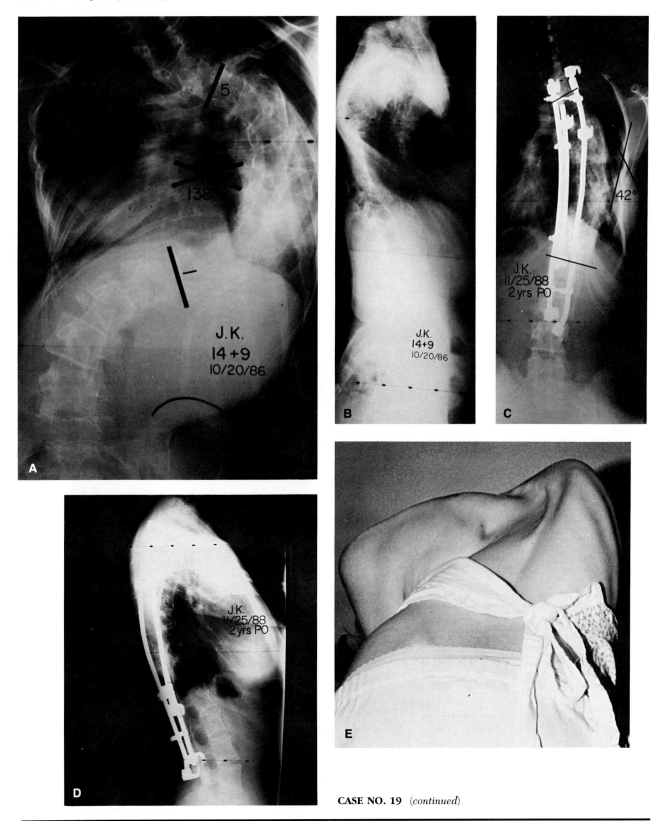

A

J.K.
14 + 9
10/20/86

B

J.K.
14+9
10/20/86

C

J.K.
11/25/88
2 yrs PO

42°

D

J.K.
11/25/88
2 yrs PO

E

CASE NO. 19 (*continued*)

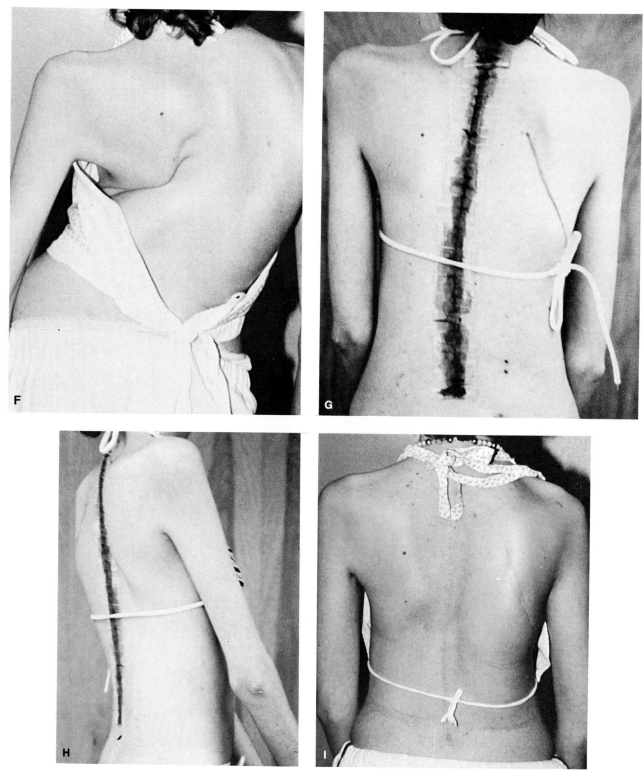

CASE NO. 20—R.R.

A 13 + 6-year-old girl presented with a left thoracic scoliosis. She was neurologically normal and had mild complaints of chest pain. A left thoracic scoliosis is somewhat unusual and should arouse suspicion of other underlying conditions. Work-up revealed a "hot" right eighth rib on a bone scan. A CT scan of this area revealed what appeared to be an osteoblastoma. Sometimes resection of the offending lesion resolves the spinal de-

formity, but this case of spinal deformity was quite structural. Therefore, during the same operation, the rib was resected through a posterior approach and a posterior fusion and Cotrel–Dubousset instrumentation was performed. Because of the stiffness of the curve, the concave apical hooks were placed five segments apart instead of the usual three segments apart.

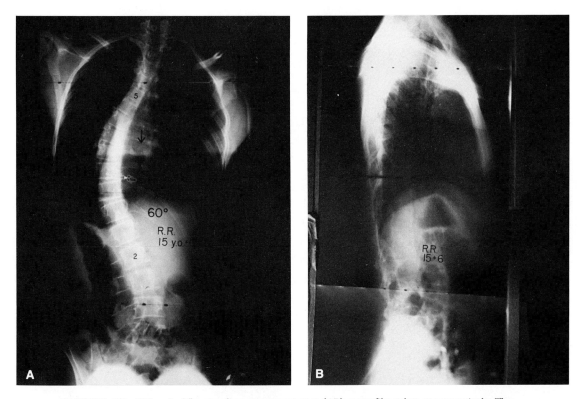

CASE NO. 20—R.R. **A.** The standing anteroposterior (AP) x-ray film taken preoperatively. The arrow points to the expansile mass at the base of the ninth rib. **B.** The preoperative lateral x-ray film of the standing patient. **C.** CT scan showing the osteoblastoma at the base of the right ninth rib. **D.** The standing patient's AP x-ray film 1 year postoperatively. The right ninth rib was resected at the time of the posterior spinal fusion and instrumentation. Usually with Cotrel–Dubousset instrumentation, the apical hooks of the derotation rod are placed only three segments apart. In this case, they were placed five segments apart because the patient had a very stiff curve as determined by the preoperative bending films. **E.** The standing lateral x-ray film 1 year postoperatively.

(continued)

CASE NO. 20—R.R. (*continued*)

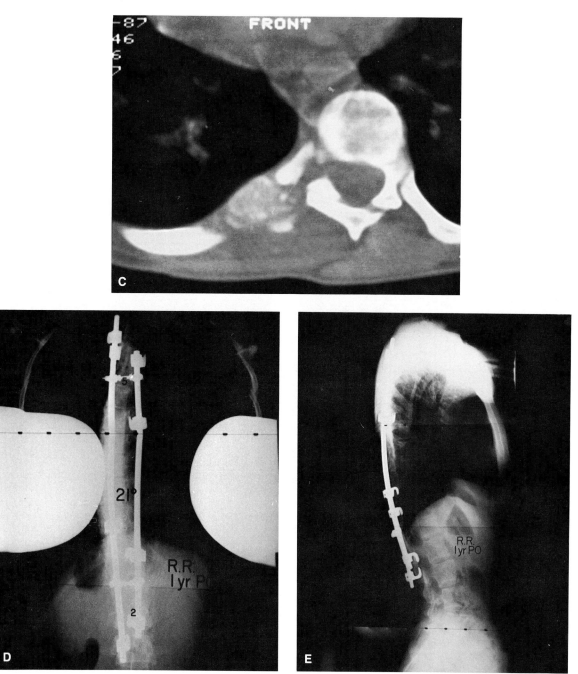

CASE NO. 20 (*continued*)

CASE NO. 21—M.H.

An 18-year-old boy with a very large left cervical-thoracic curve had no discernible connective tissue disorder. He did not have neurofibromatosis, and there was no congenital deformity. He presented with quadraparesis, which is very unusual for scoliosis without a significantly kyphotic component. A myelogram from skull to coccyx showed the patient had no Chiari malformation, syrinx, diastematomyelia, or tethered cord. However, his spinal cord was being stretched across the apical pedicles. Although the patient's spine did not clinically appear kyphotic and the sagittal radiograph did not show any kyphosis, there was a rotatory kyphosis in that the con-

cave pedicles rested significantly more anteriorly than the convex pedicles, and the resultant rotation meant that the pedicles stretching the spinal cord were somewhat anterior to it. Is this idiopathic scoliosis? It does not look like idiopathic scoliosis, but there is no other diagnosis that can be attached to this patient. He was treated with a modified Hyndman-Schneider procedure with resection of the apical pedicles and heads of ribs, resulting in a spinal cord transposition that provided total neurologic recovery. Posterior spinal fusion was performed in situ.

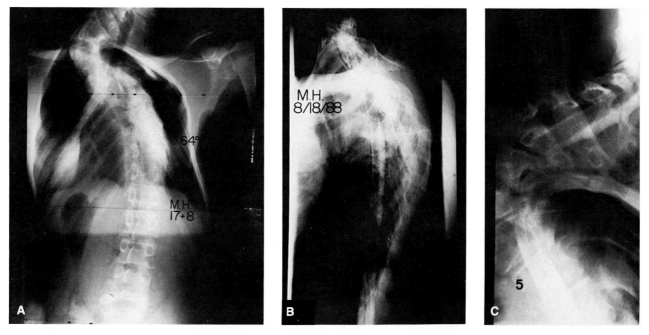

CASE NO. 21—M.H. **A.** The standing anteroposterior (AP) x-ray film of a 17 + 8-year-old boy. Notice the very large and sharp angular deformity at the cervical thoracic junction. **B.** The lateral x-ray film of the patient with myelogram dye in place. Notice that the spine does not appear to be particularly kyphotic. The block on the myelogram is not very apparent because the shoulder girdle obscures detail. Dye was injected from above and below. **C.** Notice the attenuation of the dye column across the apical three segments at the cervical-thoracic junction. **D.** Notice the very small, stretched spinal cord in the corner of the spinal canal on this axial image at the apex of the curve. The spinal cord appears to be stretched by the apical concave pedicle(s). **E.** Status after the resection of the apical pedicles and ribs on the concave side. The transposed spinal cord appears to be of normal size and configuration. This cut corresponds to the previous one. The postoperative study was performed to ensure that the decompression was complete. **F.** Postoperative AP x-ray film showing the resection of the apical pedicles and medial ribs on the concave side. The patient attained a full neurologic recovery. This presentation is distinctly atypical for idiopathic scoliosis. The trach was removed shortly after this x-ray.

(continued)

CASE NO. 21—M.H. (continued)

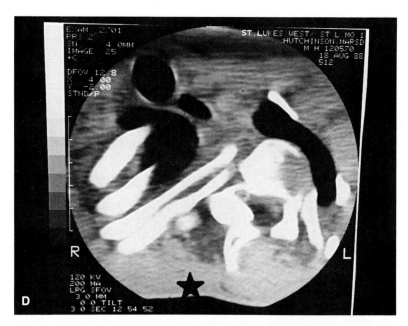

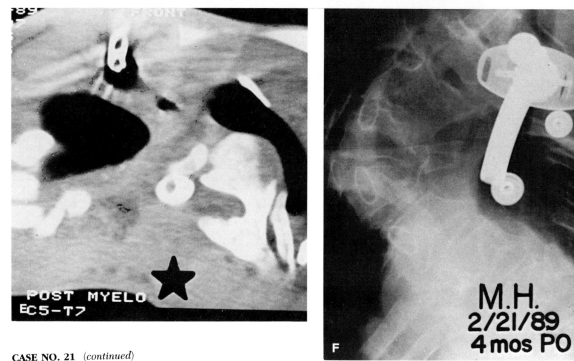

CASE NO. 21 (continued)

CASE NO. 22—S.H.

A 9 + 7-year-old girl with a left thoracic curve was neurologically normal, but left thoracic curves always arouse suspicion. An MRI scan demonstrated a syringomyelia.

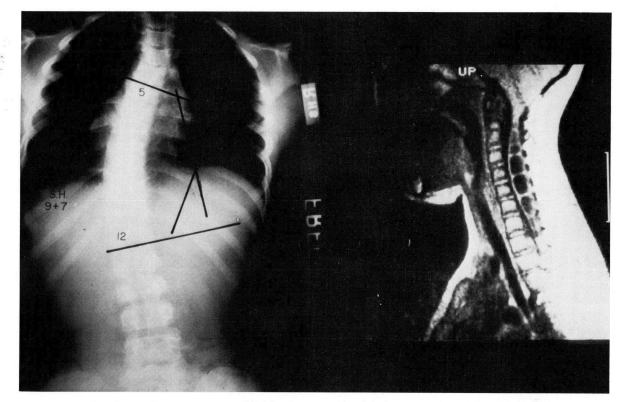

CASE NO. 22—S.H. A 9 + 7-year-old girl presenting with a left thoracic scoliosis and a syringomyelia as demonstrated on the lateral MRI.

less common than in the congenital cases.[14] These conditions may co-exist if the patient complains of significant pain or has neurologic anomalies or atypical curves.

Idiopathic scoliosis is really a diagnosis of exclusion. We say that a patient has idiopathic scoliosis only when we have ruled out all of the other possible causes.

INFANTILE AND JUVENILE SCOLIOSIS

Idiopathic scoliosis is classified as "infantile" if the patient is under the age of 3.[25, 86, 88, 131] Juvenile scoliosis is defined as between age 3 and age 10 or the "onset of adolescence."[14, 82, 135] It is desirable to brace as many of these patients as possible, but progression may occur

CASE NO. 23—M.S.

A 9 + 1-year-old boy had a structural 64° left thoracic curve and a 71° right thoracolumbar curve that progressed despite aggressive bracing. Unfortunately, there was no choice but to perform a long spinal fusion from T3 to L4. His spine is too small for standard Harrington or Cotrel−Dubousset instrumentation. It would be amenable to the 3/16-in Luque rods and 18-gauge sublaminar wires. Instead, the 5-mm "pediatric" Cotrel−Dubousset instrumentation system provided reasonable correction and preservation of lumbar lordosis.

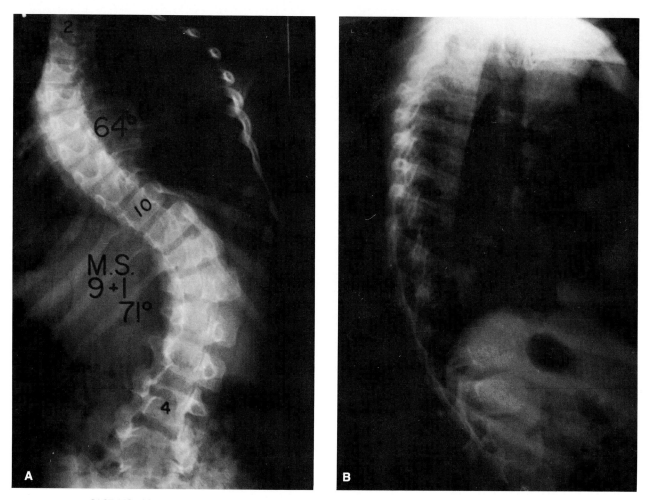

CASE NO. 23—M.S. **A, B.** Preoperative anteroposterior (AP) and lateral x-ray films. **C, D.** AP and lateral x-ray films of standing patient 16 months postoperatively demonstrating a solid posterior spinal fusion after instrumentation with the "pediatric" 5-mm CDI tray.

(continued)

despite bracing. Bracing should be performed with a custom-molded TLSO or a Milwaukee brace (CTLSO), which can be modified with a custom molded pelvis. In bracing a very young patient, there is always concern about causing rib cage distortion. Although the physician would prefer an orthosis with total contact, total

CASE NO. 23—M.S. *(continued)*

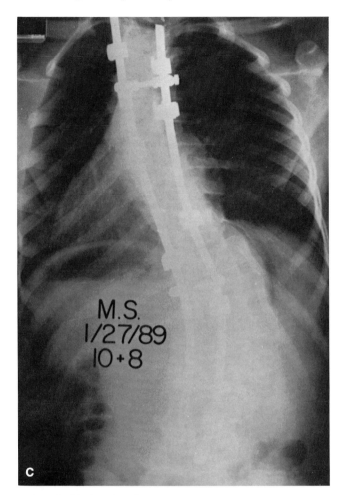

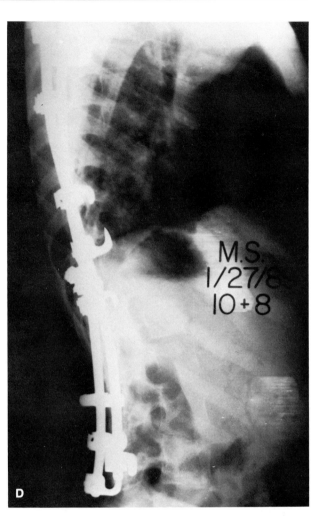

CASE NO. 23 *(continued)*

contact can squeeze the rib cage and create a "tooth-paste" effect.

If casting or bracing is not effective in controlling the deformity, surgical treatment may be mandatory.[67, 71] The curves with the higher angles between rib and vertebra (rib–vertebral angle) and the greater amount of rotation and rib hump are least likely to respond to bracing.[25, 88, 131]

For these patients, the first line of surgical attack is a subcutaneous rod technique.[93, 127] This consists of placing the hook at the top and the bottom of the curve and gradually lengthening the spine. The surgeon and patient return to the operating room every 6 to 9 months to further lengthen the rod to control the deformity while the spine grows. There are innumerable complications associated with this method of treatment. Quite often the rods cannot be contoured easily for the sagittal curves of the patient. Not uncommonly the posterior elements are so thin that the hooks easily fracture through them. After two or three exposures of the spine, the proximal and distal hook purchase sites hypertrophy and do eventually hold hooks.

The "Luque trolley" has been applied to some of these infantile and juvenile deformities.[77, 78] This consists of performing an extraperiosteal exposure of the spine, not disturbing the facet capsules, placing sublaminar wires at every level, and placing a "Luque U" on the spine, leaving the "U" long on either the top or the bottom so that the spine can continue to grow around the wires. However, this technique has not been entirely satisfactory. Quite often, multiple wires break and many of the segments of the spine spontaneously fuse anyway. Reoperating and redoing a Luque trolley is more formidable than revising a subcutaneous rod technique. Therefore, we do not currently have a consistently good system for surgically instrumenting the spine without a fusion to allow growth in the young patient.

If these techniques are not successful and the patient's spine continues to deform, definitive instrumentation and fusion should be considered. It is better to have a short, straight spine than a short, crooked spine. In general, early instrumentation and fusion of the thoracic spine is not as cosmetically displeasing as early instrumentation and fusion of the lumbar spine. Despite a posterior fusion of the thoracic spine, the chest cavity continues to grow in the horizontal and axial planes but not vertically.

The addition of the 5-mm Cotrel–Dubousset instrumentation tray with the smaller hooks has improved our ability to instrument the spine in patients between age 5 and age 10 who are quite small and require instrumentation and fusion. The 5-mm system is much harder to use than the standard 7-mm Cotrel–Dubousset instrumentation system. The 5-mm rod is considerably more flexible, and the rod rotation maneuver is not as impressive as with the 7-mm rod.

Nonetheless, this system does afford satisfactory fixation with the ability to apply selective distraction and compression forces and to achieve segmental fixation (Case No. 23).

At a very early age there is a potential for a "crankshaft" phenomenon.[35, 54] This refers to the vertebral bodies continuing to grow despite a solid posterior spinal fusion, with worsening of the deformity and "bending" of the posterior fusion due to vertebral body growth. Exact indications for performing a circumferential fusion on a patient under the age of 10 have never been clearly delineated. However, the surgeon should consider a circumferential fusion if the patient is particularly young or has a particularly large deformity that is not entirely correctable with the instrumentation available.

COMPLICATIONS

Pseudarthrosis

Pseudarthrosis can occur with any spinal condition requiring fusion.[4, 11, 14, 70] The incidence among adolescent patients is relatively small, certainly under 10% and maybe as low as 2% with modern segmental instrumentation and the use of autogenous bone graft. Pseudarthrosis seems to occur most often at the thoracolumbar junction and at the most distally fused segment. The more rigid and sturdy the instrumentation, the longer it may be before pseudarthrosis is apparent.

Diagnosis of the pseudarthrosis may be made by oblique radiographs, by a broken rod, or by tomograms or a bone scan and tomogram study. There are significant false negatives associated with the bone scans, the oblique radiographs, and the tomograms. In my expe-

---

CASE NO. 24—C.G.

A 19-year-old man presented 3.5 years after Harrington instrumentation for idiopathic scoliosis from T4 to L4. He was well compensated preoperatively and immediately postoperatively. However, postoperatively, he complained of significant right leg pain. A laminectomy at L5 was performed in search of a "dermoid" tumor. His right leg pain persisted. He presented to me with significant decompensation and continuing right leg pain.

A CT scan and myelogram study revealed that the hook

at L4 was through the dura and inside the thecal sac. The posterior instrumentation was removed, and the dura was repaired at L4. His right leg pain resolved. At the time of exploration, pseudarthroses were found at T11–T12 and L3–L4. The solid fusion at the other lumbar segments prevented him from recompensating. He subsequently required circumferential osteotomies to repair the pseudarthroses and to rebalance him in the coronal plane.

(continued)

CASE NO. 24—C.G. (*continued*)

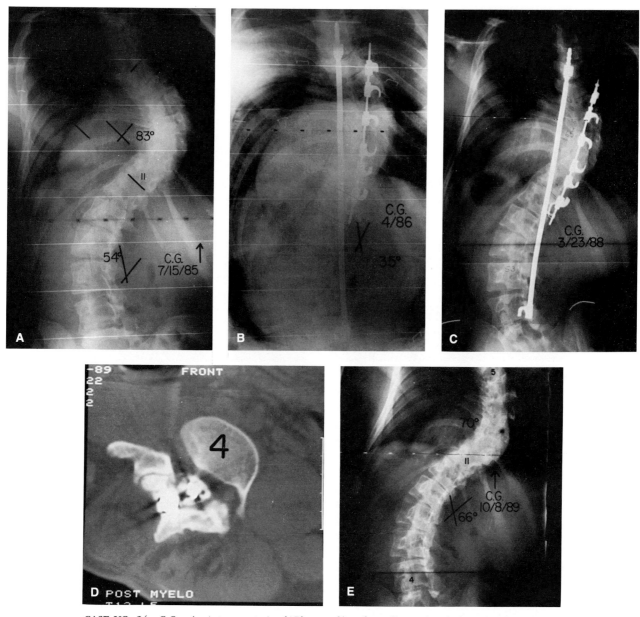

CASE NO. 24—C.G. **A.** Anteroposterior (AP) x-ray film of standing patient before treatment showing excellent coronal balance. **B.** Standing AP x-ray film immediately after the Harrington instrumentation showing excellent coronal balance. **C.** Presentation 3 years later showing the patient decompensated almost 12 cm to the right. **D.** Axial CT scan slice with myelogram dye showing the hook inside the thecal sac at L4. **E.** Long-cassette AP x-ray film showing the patient after removal of the instrumentation. He was unable to recompensate himself. **F.** AP x-ray film of patient after circumferential osteotomies, instrumentation, and repair of the pseudarthroses. Coronal balance was restored. **G.** Long-cassette lateral x-ray film of standing patient after reconstruction.

(*continued*)

CASE NO. 24—C.G. *(continued)*

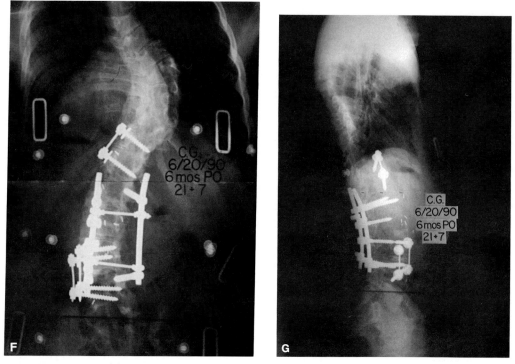

CASE NO. 24   *(continued)*

rience, the most practical method for detecting pseudarthrosis, other than seeing a broken rod, is to study the oblique radiographs that profile the pseudarthrosis. In the patient who is skeletally immature at the time of fusion and instrumentation, pseudarthrosis may be seen as a "fat" disc space. If the patient has a fusion at an early age, the vertebral bodies anteriorly continue to grow at the expense of the disc space, and the posterior fusion prevents additional vertical growth. Therefore, if one disc looks particularly wide, this suggests there is not a posterior fusion at this level, and the vertebral bodies are not growing at the expense of the disc space at this level.

If a pseudarthrosis exists at the most distally fused segment, perhaps not all of these "terminal segment" or "end segment" pseudarthroses need to be reoperated, regrafted, and fused. Reoperation is necessary if the patient becomes symptomatic or if the distally fused segment develops recurrent deformity. If the deformity does not change beyond the immediate postoperative status, often the segments can be left alone.

However, if pseudarthrosis is at the apex of the deformity or at the thoracolumbar junction, it almost always requires reoperation and repair.

Upon reoperation, it is helpful to add more bone graft to the pseudarthrosis and to reinstrument the spine, preferably applying compression across the pseudo.[70] A mistake that the surgeon can make is to explore a fusion, find the pseudarthrosis at the apex, remove the instrumentation, and apply bone graft without any reinstrumentation of the spine. This can lead to the development of an increasingly kyphotic deformity because the spinal extensor muscles have been rendered somewhat incompetent by the previous surgery. If there are multiple pseudarthroses in the lumbar spine, the surgeon may elect to instrument the spine anteriorly with Zielke instrumentation. An anterior pseudarthrosis after Zielke instrumentation may be repaired by applying posterior segmental instrumentation with autogenous bone grafts so long as the anterior instrumentation has not failed in such a way as to cause visceral or vascular perforation. However, the surgeon should always be concerned about leaving behind broken anterior instrumentation.

Wound Infection

The incidence of wound infection in the previously unoperated adolescent idiopathic patient is less than 1%.[14] If it does occur and is caused by a *Staphylococcus* species, it is often possible to debride the wound, evacuate the hematoma, irrigate the wound, and close over tubes successfully. If the infection is caught later or is caused by a somewhat more aggressive microorganism, it may be necessary to debride the wound, pack it open, return to the operating room, and close over tubes secondarily. If gram-negative organisms such as *Pseudomonas* or *Escherichia coli* infect the wound and gross purulence occurs, it may be necessary to let the wound granulate from the bottom up. In North America, it is a commonly accepted practice to place the patient on prophylactic antibiotics before the surgery and for the first 24 to 48 hours after surgery to reduce the likelihood of wound infection.[102] A cephalosporin agent is used unless the patient has some preexisting susceptibility to a more aggressive organism or a history of a previous wound infection.

Coronal Malalignment

Fusion to the stable vertebrae with Harrington instrumentation has withstood the test of time.[7, 22, 31, 34, 51–53, 65, 76, 90, 92, 109, 119] The two curve types in which coronal decompensation is most likely to occur are Type II false double-major curves and double thoracic curve patterns in which the surgeon has failed to recognize the severity of the upper thoracic curve. With Cotrel–Dubousset instrumentation, coronal malalignment problems have been accentuated somewhat.[84, 113, 141] This is probably because the overall correction with Cotrel–Dubousset instrumentation is slightly greater than with Harrington instrumentation. As a consequence, the instrumentation is less forgiving of the compensatory curves. With Cotrel–Dubousset instrumentation for a right thoracic curve, it also helps to place a reversal of the rod bend and a reversal of hooks between the neutral and stable vertebrae. There are some double thoracic curve patterns for which the surgeon can use Harrington instrumentation for only the lower right thoracic curve, but with Cotrel–Dubousset instrumentation, it is more likely that both curves must be fused and instrumented.

The senior editors of this work have seen patients who have presented with significant coronal decompensation after posterior Harrington instrumentation in which the distal hook was inadvertently placed into the lumbar thecal sac through the dura (Case No. 24).

Sagittal Malalignment

One of the most serious criticisms of Harrington instrumentation is that it reduces lumbar lordosis and can lead to flat-back deformities (Case No. 25).[7, 14, 21, 132] Unfortunately, even with contouring of the square Harrington rod and the use of Wisconsin wires or sublaminar wires, there is a tendency to reduce lumbar lordosis if a distraction force is applied to the spine posteriorly. This can only be prevented by applying some compression force (by hooks or wires) to the lumbar spine before applying the distraction force.[143] This can be accomplished with Harrington instrumentation by applying a compression rod on the convex side from L1 or L2 to L4 before placement of the concave Harrington distraction rod. One of the advantages of Cotrel–Dubousset instrumentation is that it relies in part on rod rotation and in large measure on applying compression forces to the lumbar spine first.[27, 116] Preliminary results suggest that the Cotrel–Dubousset instrumentation may be helpful in preserving lumbar lordosis.[15, 116]

Thoracic hypokyphosis is often associated with right thoracic curves.[29, 101, 103, 104] Hypokyphosis has been associated with reduced pulmonary function and mitral valve prolapse.[120] There is no instrumentation system that can consistently correct rib cage distortion and restore normal thoracic kyphosis in hypokyphotic patients.[15, 22, 34, 50, 59, 133, 138, 144] Harrington instrumentation without any segmental fixation does not restore kyphosis at all.[1, 7, 14, 138] The use of Wisconsin wires and sublaminar wires with Harrington rods contoured into kyphosis may improve the sagittal deformity somewhat.[2, 3, 32, 77, 78, 117, 144] Cotrel–Dubousset instrumentation may improve thoracic kyphosis, although it is not always successful. During the Cotrel–Dubousset rod rotation maneuver, the rod can flatten and bend to the spine, rather than the spine bending with the rod. The other common sagittal deformity seen with double thoracic curves is kyphosis of the upper left thoracic curve. This is not usually a serious cosmetic deformity, but it is one to which the surgeon should pay attention.

Thoracolumbar kyphosis can occur in double-major curves and Type II thoracic curves. If a significant thoracolumbar kyphosis does exist, instrumentation to

CASE NO. 25—L.C.

A 29 + 11-year-old woman had Harrington instrumentation and posterior fusion as an adolescent from T4 to L5. L5 is sacralized. She had a thoracolumbar kyphosis, a significant sagittal flat-back syndrome. Her sagittal vertical axis lies significantly anterior to the sacrum. A plumb line dropped from C7 should intersect the back end of the S1 vertebral body. She also has a pseudarthrosis at L4–L5. She required circumferential osteotomies to restore her sagittal vertical axis to normal and to repair the pseudarthrosis.

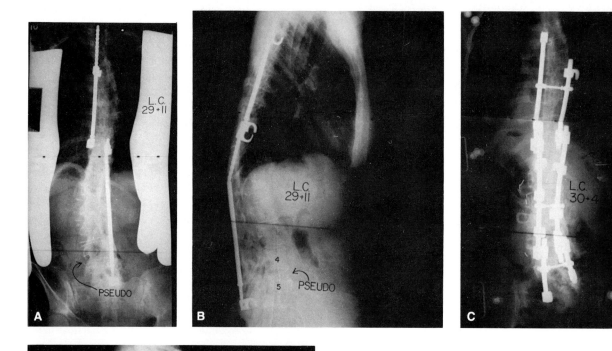

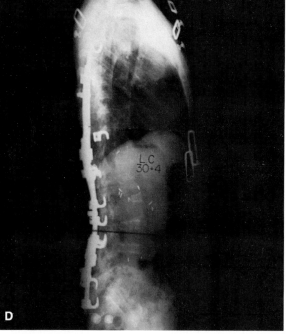

CASE NO. 25—L.C. **A.** Anteroposterior (AP) x-ray film of standing patient showing the Harrington instrumentation and the pseudarthrosis at L4–L5. L5 is sacralized. **B.** Standing lateral x-ray film showing the flat back deformity. Notice the pseudarthrosis at L4–L5. **C.** Long-cassette AP x-ray film taken postoperatively. **D.** Long-cassette standing lateral x-ray film taken postoperatively showing the normalization of the sagittal vertical axis.

T12 may worsen the deformity, but if no preexisting pathologic thoracolumbar kyphosis exists, instrumentation is not likely to cause this problem unless the T11 to T12 segment is overdistracted. If thoracolumbar kyphosis does exist, it probably is advisable to carry the Cotrel–Dubousset instrumentation further into the lumbar spine to control the sagittal deformity. The ability to reverse a thoracolumbar kyphosis to its physiologic curve depends on the inherent flexibility of the spine and the correct placement of the instrumentation.

Iatrogenic Paralysis

The Scoliosis Research Society Morbidity and Mortality Committee and MacEwen have reported an incidence of iatrogenic paralysis with idiopathic scoliosis surgery of 0.7%.[79] Therefore, it is currently accepted practice in most spinal centers to perform some form of spinal cord monitoring during the operative procedure to reduce the likelihood of irreversible paralysis.[17, 19, 41, 97, 105–107, 142] The clinical tests used are the Stagnara wake-up test and the Hoppenfeld clonus test.[48]

More sophisticated spinal cord monitoring techniques are also evolving. Somatosensory potential monitoring of the spinal cord has been universally accepted for several years as a useful adjunct. However, there is some concern that somatosensory potentials seem to monitor principally the posterior columns and that they occasionally produce false-negative results.[106] Therefore, several techniques for monitoring of the motor tracts are being developed.[105–107, 126, 137] The goal of any form of spinal cord monitoring is to identify evidence of early paresis while the surgeon still has the opportunity to modify the instrumentation to restore neurologic function.

The two most common causes of iatrogenic paralysis are an unrecognized, underlying spinal cord tether or other anomaly and an inadvertent displacement of a hook or rod into the spinal canal. With Cotrel–Dubousset instrumentation, the initial incidence of paralysis reported to the Scoliosis Research Society Morbidity and Mortality Committee appeared to be higher than the incidence for Harrington instrumentation. Theoretically, the apical hooks on the left-sided derotation rod at T7 and T10 should not pose any problem because they are being pulled by the maneuver posteriorly away from the spinal cord. Placement of an open lumbar hook under the T10 lamina has been suggested as a safe technique to reduce the likelihood of the hook

pulling through the posterior element.[116] The surgeon must be careful in placing such a large hook in the spinal canal during the assembly of the instrumentation. The hooks that are more likely to displace into the spinal canal during the rod rotation are the hooks on the ends, at T4 and T12 or L1, where these hooks can be pushed down anteriorly into the spine during derotation. A helpful strategy involves placing the most proximal hook on the transverse process at T4 to keep the closed pedicle hook from displacing medially and anteriorly.

In applying forces on hooks and deciding on rod rotation maneuvers, the surgeon must assess the flexibility of the spine. Applying a corrective force across a localized rigid kyphosis can be disastrous. Trying a simple rod rotation maneuver on a very large, stiff curve is flirting with disaster. Not all curves are amenable to simple rod rotation maneuvers unless they are "released" by one method or another.

No matter how experienced and careful the spinal surgeon is, there will always be a possibility of an accidental slip of an osteotome or a hook, bruising the spinal cord. All efforts should be made to eliminate this source of iatrogenic paralysis or paresis.

Alterations in the patient's blood pressure may also render the spinal cord more susceptible to ischemia. Usually the average, healthy spinal cord is not affected by a systemic mean blood pressure of 60. However, if uncontrolled hypotension occurs significantly below this level, the spinal cord may be more susceptible to stretching or irritation by correction of the spinal deformity.[66]

SUMMARY

The diagnosis of idiopathic scoliosis remains one of exclusion. Most idiopathic scoliosis requires no treatment, but a small percentage of these patients benefit from bracing, and an even smaller percentage require surgery

In 1990, Cotrel–Dubousset instrumentation is very popular for the surgical treatment of idiopathic scoliosis, but it is in no way comprehensive. It is being modified as shortcomings are identified. Other multiple hook, rod, and cross-link systems (e.g., The Texas Scottish Rite Hospital [TSRH] system) are being developed and used clinically. The amount of derotation provided by these systems is currently being studied and debated. Our abilities to accurately and reproducibly measure rotation, derotation, and chest cage dimensions are crude at best. It is impressive that spinal surgeons are trying to achieve three-dimensional correction, but their success is yet unproven.

My perception is that the degree of derotation achieved with Cotrel–Dubousset instrumentation is very small, although apical translation, overall Cobb correction, and sagittal preservation may be superior to other systems. Derotation in lumbar and thoracolumbar curves exists with Dwyer and Zielke instrumentation, but often at the expense of some loss of lumbar lordosis. The spinal surgeon should keep an open mind about these systems and recognize the applications and limitations of each.

Acknowledgment

Thanks to Adam S. Fenichel, M.D., for his work on the step-by-step Cotrel–Dubousset diagrams.

References

1. Aaro S, Ohlund C: Scoliosis and pulmonary function. Spine 9:220, 1984
2. Allen BL Jr, Ferguson RL: The Galveston experience with L-rod instrumentation for adolescent idiopathic scoliosis. Clin Orthop 229:59, 1988
3. Allen BL Jr, Ferguson RL: The Galveston technique for L-rod instrumentation of the scoliotic spine. Spine 7:276, 1982
4. Aurori BF, Weierman RJ, Lowell HA, et al: Pseudarthrosis after spinal fusion for scoliosis. A comparison of autogeneic and allogeneic bone grafts. Clin Orthop 199:153, 1985
5. Bailey TE Jr, Mahoney CM: The use of banked autologous blood in patients undergoing surgery for spinal deformity. J Bone Joint Surg [Am] 69:329, 1987
6. Bell GR, Gurd AR, Orlowski JP, Andrish JT: The syndrome of inappropriate antidiuretic-hormone secretion following spinal fusion. J Bone Joint Surg [Am] 68:720, 1986
7. Benson DR: Idiopathic scoliosis. The last ten years and state of the art. Orthopedics 10:1691, 1987
8. Bergoin M, Bollini G, Hornung H, et al: Is the Cotrel–Dubousset really universal in the surgical treatment of idiopathic scoliosis? J Pediatr Orthop 8:45, 1988
9. Bernhardt M, Bridwell KH: Segmental analysis of the sagittal plane alignment of the normal thoracic and lumbar spines and thoracolumbar junction. Spine 14:717, 1989
10. Betz RR, Huss GK, Clancy M: Indications for rib resection with Cotrel–Dubousset instrumentation for correction of adolescent idiopathic scoliosis. Orthop Trans 13:179, 1989
11. Bialik V, Piggott H: Pseudarthrosis following treatment of idiopathic scoliosis by Harrington instrumentation and fusion without added bone. J Pediatr Orthop 7:152, 1987
12. Birch JG, Herring JA, Roach JW, Johnston CE: Cotrel–Dubousset instrumentation in idiopathic scoliosis. A preliminary report. Clin Orthop 227:24, 1988
13. Bradford DS, Blatt JM, Rasp FL: Surgical management of severe thoracic lordosis. A new technique to restore normal kyphosis. Spine 8:420, 1983
14. Bradford DS, Lonstein JE, Moe JH, et al: Moe's Textbook of Scoliosis and Other Spinal Deformities, 2nd ed. Philadelphia, WB Saunders, 1987
15. Bridwell KH, Betz RR: Sagittal plane analysis in idiopathic scoliosis patients treated with Cotrel–Dubousset instrumentation. Presented at the annual meeting of the North American Spine Society, Quebec City, Quebec, July 1989
16. Broadstone P, Johnson JR, Holt RT, Leatherman KD: Consider postoperative immobilization of double-L rod S.S.I. patients. Orthop Trans 8:171, 1984
17. Brown RH, Nash CL, Berilla JA, Amaddio MD: Cortical evoked potential monitoring: A system for intraoperative monitoring of spinal cord function. Spine 9:256, 1984
18. Bunch WH: Posterior fusion for idiopathic scoliosis. Instr Course Lect 34:140, 1985
19. Bunch WH, Scarff TB, Trimble J: Current concepts review: Spinal cord monitoring. J Bone Joint Surg [Am] 65:707, 1983
20. Burke SW, Seago R, French HG, et al: Thoracic lordosis and pulmonary function in idiopathic scoliosis. Orthop Trans 9:484, 1985
21. Casey MP, Asher MA, Jacobs RR, Orrick JM: The effect of Harrington rod contouring on lumbar lordosis. Spine 12:750, 1987
22. Cataletto, M, Flawn L, Levine D: Intralaminar wire fixation with Harrington instrumentation in idiopathic scoliosis. A preliminary report of 100 consecutive cases in children. Orthop Trans 10:466, 1986
23. Chan, DP: Zielke instrumentation. Instr Course Lect 32:208, 1983
24. Cochran T, Irstam L, Nachemson A: Long-term anatomic and functional changes in patients with adolescent idiopathic scoliosis treated by Harrington rod fusion. Spine 8:576, 1983
25. Conner AN: Developmental anomalies and prognosis in infantile idiopathic scoliosis. J Bone Joint Surg [Br] 51:711, 1969
26. Conrad RW, Richardson WJ, Oakes WJ: Left thoracic curves can be different. Orthop Trans 9:126, 1985
27. Cotrel Y, Dubousset J, Guillaumat M: New universal instrumentation in spinal surgery. Clin Orthop 227:10, 1988
28. Court-Brown CM, Stoll JE, Gertzbein SD: Thoracic facetectomy and bone grafting in the surgical treatment of adult idiopathic scoliosis. Spine 12:992, 1987
29. Deacon P, Dickson RA: Vertebral shape in the median

sagittal plane in idiopathic thoracic scoliosis. A study of true lateral radiographs in 150 patients. Orthopedics 10:893, 1987

30. Denis F: Cotrel–Dubousset instrumentation in the treatment of idiopathic scoliosis. Orthop Clin North Am 19:291, 1988
31. Dickson RA: Idiopathic scoliosis. Br Med J 298:906, 1989
32. Dickson RA, Archer IA: Surgical treatment of late-onset idiopathic thoracic scoliosis. The Leeds procedure. J Bone Joint Surg [Br] 69:709, 1987
33. Dodd CAF, Fergusson CM, Freedman L, et al: Allograft versus autograft bone in scoliosis surgery. J Bone Joint Surg [Br] 70:431, 1988
34. Drummond DS: Harrington instrumentation with spinous process wiring for idiopathic scoliosis. Orthop Clin North Am 19:281, 1988
35. Dubousset J, Herring JA, Shufflebarger H: Inevitable progression of scoliosis following posterior fusion alone in the immature spine. The Crankshaft phenomenon. Orthop Trans 13:116, 1989
36. Dunn HK: Spinal instrumentation. Part I. Principles of posterior and anterior instrumentation. Instr Course Lect 32:170, 1983
37. Dwyer AF: Experience of anterior correction of scoliosis. Clin Orthop 93:191, 1973
38. Dwyer AF, Schafer MF: Anterior approach to scoliosis: Results of treatment in fifty-one cases. J Bone Joint Surg [Br] 56:218, 1974
39. Ecker ML, Betz RR, Trent PS, et al: Computer tomography evaluation of Cotrel–Dubousset instrumentation in idiopathic scoliosis. Spine 13:1141, 1988
40. Engler GL: Preoperative and intraoperative considerations in adolescent idiopathic scoliosis. Instr Course Lect 38:137, 1989
41. Engler GL, Spielholz NI, Bernhard WN, et al: Somatosensory evoked potentials during Harrington instrumentation for scoliosis. J Bone Joint Surg [Am] 60:528, 1978
42. Fabry G, Van Melkebeek J, Bockx E: Back pain after Harrington rod instrumentation for idiopathic scoliosis. Spine 14:620, 1989
43. Fakharani-Hein M, Griss P, Ludke A, Bittinger A: Rapidly developing scoliosis in an adolescent due to spinal osteoblastoma. A case report. Arch Orthop Trauma Surg 107:259, 1988
44. Gagnon S, Jodoin A, Martin R: Pulmonary function test study after spinal fusion in young idiopathic scoliosis. Spine 14:486, 1989
45. Ginsburg H, Goldstein L, Chan D, Jensen M: Longitudinal study of back pain in postoperative idiopathic scoliosis: Long-term follow-up, phases I, II, and III. Orthop Trans 11:125, 1987
46. Guadagni J, Drummond D, Breed A: Improved postoperative course following modified segmental instrumentation and posterior spinal fusion for idiopathic scoliosis. J Pediatr Orthop 4:405, 1984
47. Haher TR, Abouzeid JM, Rondon D, Thelmo W: Briefly noted: Neuroblastoma presenting as a paraver-

tebral mass and painful scoliosis in a 21-year-old woman. Spine 11:489, 1986
48. Hall JE, Levine CR, Sudhir KG: Intraoperative awakening to monitor spinal cord function during Harrington instrumentation and fusion. Description of procedure and report of three cases. J Bone Joint Surg [Am] 60:533, 1978
49. Hammerberg KW, Rodts MF, DeWald RL: Zielke instrumentation. Orthopedics 11:1365, 1988
50. Hammerberg KW, Zielke K: V.D.S. instrumentation for idiopathic thoracic curvatures. Orthop Trans 9:439, 1985
51. Harrington PR: Surgical instrumentation for management of scoliosis. J Bone Joint Surg [Am] 42:1448, 1960
52. Harrington PR: Treatment of scoliosis: correction and internal fixation by spine instrumentation. J Bone Joint Surg [Am] 44:591, 1962
53. Harrington PR, Dickson JH: An eleven-year clinical investigation of Harrington instrumentation. Clin Orthop 93:113, 1973
54. Hefti FL, McMaster MJ: The effect of the adolescent growth spurt on early posterior spinal fusion in infantile and juvenile idiopathic scoliosis. J Bone Joint Surg [Br] 65:247, 1983
55. Herring JA, Wenger DR: Segmental spinal instrumentation: a preliminary report of 40 consecutive cases. Spine 7:285, 1982
56. Hibbs RA: A report of 59 cases of scoliosis treated by the fusion operation. J Bone Joint Surg [Am] 6:3, 1924
57. Horton WC, Holt RT, Johnson JR, Leatherman KD: Zielke instrumentation in idiopathic scoliosis: Late effects and minimizing complications. Spine 13:1145, 1988
58. Jackman KV, Highland TR, Chan DPK: Spinal effects of VDS instrumentation. Orthop Trans 9:486, 1985
59. Jefferson RJ, Weisz I, Turner-Smith AR, et al: Scoliosis surgery and its effect on back shape. J Bone Joint Surg [Br] 70:261, 1988
60. Johnson JR, Holt RT, Horton W, et al: Abnormal bleeding tendency due to defective platelet function in patients with idiopathic scoliosis. Orthop Trans 12:244, 1988
61. Johnston CE, Hoppel LT, Norris R, et al: Delayed paraplegia complicating sublaminar segmental spinal instrumentation. J Bone Joint Surg [Am] 68:556, 1986
62. Kahmann RD, Rao GH, White JG, Bradford DS: Platelet function in adolescent idiopathic scoliosis. Orthop Trans 13:99, 1989
63. Kaneda K, Fujiya N, Satoh S: Results with Zielke instrumentation for idiopathic thoracolumbar and lumbar scoliosis. Clin Orthop 205:195, 1986
64. King HA: Selection of fusion levels for posterior instrumentation and fusion in idiopathic scoliosis. Orthop Clin North Am 19:247, 1988
65. King HA, Moe JH, Bradford DS, Winter RB: The selection of fusion levels in thoracic idiopathic scoliosis. J Bone Joint Surg [Am] 65:1302, 1983
66. Kling TF, Fergusson NV, Leach AB, et al: The influ-

ence of induced hypotension and spine distraction on canine spinal cord blood flow. Spine 10:878, 1985

67. Koop SE: Infantile and juvenile idiopathic scoliosis. Orthop Clin North Am 19:331, 1988

68. Korovessis P: Combined VDS and Harrington instrumentation for treatment of idiopathic double-major curves. Spine 12:244, 1987

69. Kostuik JP, Carl A, Ferron S: Anterior Zielke instrumentation for spinal deformity in adults. J Bone Joint Surg [Am] 71:898, 1989

70. Lauerman WC, Bradford DS, Transfeldt EE, et al: The management of pseudarthrosis after spinal fusion for idiopathic scoliosis. Orthop Trans 13:116, 1989

71. Leatherman KD, Johnson JR, Holt RT, Hoffman G: Surgical treatment of progressive juvenile idiopathic scoliosis. Orthop Trans 9:127, 1985

72. Liebergall M, Wachtfogel YT, Colman RW, et al: Platelet abnormalities in idiopathic scoliosis. Orthop Trans 12:244, 1988

73. Lonstein JE, Carlson JM: The prediction of curve progression in untreated idiopathic scoliosis during growth. J Bone Joint Surg [Am] 66:1061, 1984

74. Lovallo JL, Banta JV, Renshaw TS: Adolescent idiopathic scoliosis treated by Harrington-rod distraction and fusion. J Bone Joint Surg [Am] 68:1326, 1986

75. Luk KDK, Lee FB, Leong JCY, Hsu LCS: The effect on the lumbosacral spine of long spinal fusion for idiopathic scoliosis. A minimum 10-year follow-up. Spine 12:996, 1987

76. Luk KDK, Leong JCY, Reyes L, Hsu LCS: The comparative results of treatment in idiopathic thoracolumbar and lumbar scoliosis using the Harrington, Dwyer, and Zielke instrumentations. Spine 14:275, 1989

77. Luque ER: Segmental spinal instrumentation: a method of rigid internal fixation of the spine to induce arthrodesis. Orthop Trans 4:391, 1980

78. Luque ER, Cardoso A: Segmental correction of scoliosis with rigid internal fixation. Orthop Trans 1:136, 1977

79. MacEwen GD, Bunnel WP, Sriram K: Acute neurological complications in the treatment of scoliosis. J Bone Joint Surg [Am] 57:404, 1975

80. Malcolm-Smith NA, McMaster MJ: The use of induced hypotension to control bleeding during posterior fusion for scoliosis. J Bone Joint Surg [Br] 65:255, 1983

81. Mann DC, Nash CL Jr, Wilham MR, Brown RH: Evaluation of the role of concave rib osteotomies in the correction of thoracic scoliosis. Spine 14:491, 1989

82. Mannherz RE, Betz RR, Clancy M, Steel HH: Juvenile idiopathic scoliosis followed to skeletal maturity. Spine 13:1087, 1988

83. Mason RJ, Betz RR, Orlowski JP, Bell GR: The syndrome of inappropriate antidiuretic hormone secretion and its effect on blood indices following spinal fusion. Orthop Trans 13:99, 1989

84. McAllister JW, Bridwell KH, Betz R, et al: Coronal decompensation produced by Cotrel–Dubousset derotation maneuver for idiopathic right thoracic scoliosis. Orthop Trans 13:79, 1989

85. McLean TE, Denis F, Winter RB, Lonstein JE: Treat-

ment of idiopathic scoliosis greater than 100° (a review of 69 cases). Orthop Trans 13:87, 1989

86. McMaster MJ, Macnicol MF: The management of progressive infantile idiopathic scoliosis. J Bone Joint Surg [Br] 61:36, 1979

87. McNeil JW, DeWald RL, Kuo KN, et al: Controlled hypotensive anesthesia in scoliosis surgery. J Bone Joint Surg [Am] 56:1167, 1974

88. Mehta MH: The rib-vertebra angle in the early diagnosis between resolving and progressive infantile scoliosis. J Bone Joint Surg [Br] 54:230, 1972

89. Michel CR, Lalain JJ, Caton J, Bernard J: The long-term development of the lumbar curve after Harrington instrumentation for idiopathic thoracic or double-major scolioses. Orthop Trans 9:585, 1985

90. Michel CR, Lalain JJ: Late results of Harrington's operation. Long-term evolution of the lumbar spine below the fused segments. Spine 10:414, 1985

91. Millis MB, Hall JE, Emans JB: Short (3 segment) anterior instrumentation and fusion for progressive thoracolumbar scoliosis. Orthop Trans 9:438, 1985

92. Moe JH: A critical analysis of methods of fusion for scoliosis: An evaluation in two hundred and sixty-six patients. J Bone Joint Surg [Am] 40:529, 1958

93. Moe JH, Kharrat K, Winter RB, Cummine JL: Harrington instrumentation without fusion plus external orthotic support for the treatment of difficult curvature problems in young children. Clin Orthop 185:35, 1984

94. Moe JH, Purcell GA, Bradford DS: Zielke instrumentation (VDS) for the correction of spinal curvature. Analysis of results in 66 patients. Clin Orthop 180:133, 1983

95. Moore SV, Eilert RE: Segmental spinal instrumentation: Complications, correction and indications. Orthop Trans 7:413, 1983

96. Nasca RJ: Early experience with segmental spinal instrumentation. Orthop Trans 8:207, 1984

97. Nash CL, Lorig RA, Schatzinger LA, Brown RH: Spinal cord monitoring during operative treatment of the spine. Clin Orthop 126:100, 1977

98. Neuwirth MG, Bridwell KH, Capelli A: Coronal and sagittal balance and correction of compensatory coronal and sagittal curves after anterior VDS instrumentation for idiopathic lumbar/thoracolumbar scoliosis. Presented at the annual meeting of Scoliosis Research Society, Amsterdam, The Netherlands, September 1989

99. Ogiela DM, Chan DPK: Ventral derotation spondylodesis. A review of 22 cases. Spine 11:18, 1986

100. Ogilvie JW: Anterior spine fusion with Zielke instrumentation for idiopathic scoliosis in adolescents. Orthop Clin North Am 19:313, 1988

101. Ogilvie JW, Schendel MJ: Calculated thoracic volume as related to parameters of scoliosis correction. Spine 13:39, 1988

102. Ogilvie JW, Wilson M: Blood levels of antimicrobial prophylaxis in spine surgery. Orthop Trans 13:93, 1989

103. Ohlen G, Aaro S, Bylund P: The sagittal configuration and mobility of the spine in idiopathic scoliosis. Spine 13:413, 1988

104. Osebold WR, Yamamoto S, Merkel C, Hurley JH: Ef-

fect of segmental spinal instrumentation on scoliosis, vertebral rotation, and torso decompensation. Orthop Trans 13:179, 1989

105. Owen JH, Jenny A, Bridwell KH: Effects of spinal cord lesioning on somatosensory and neurogenic-motor evoked potentials in animals and humans. Orthop Trans 13:83, 1989

106. Owen JH, Laschinger J, Bridwell KH, et al: Sensitivity and specificity of somatosensory and neurogenic-motor evoked potentials in animals and humans. Orthop Trans 12:225, 1988

107. Owen JH, Naito M, Bridwell KH, Oakley D: Relationship between duration of spinal cord ischemia and post-operative neurological deficits in animals. Presented at the annual meeting of the North American Spine Society, Amsterdam, The Netherlands, September 1989

108. Patel NJ, Patel BS, Paskin S, Laufer S: Induced moderate hypotensive anesthesia for spinal fusion and Harrington-rod instrumentation. J Bone Joint Surg [Am] 67:1384, 1985

109. Phillips WA, Hensinger RN: Wisconsin and other instrumentation for posterior spinal fusion. Clin Orthop 229:44, 1988

110. Puno RM, Johnson JR, Ostermann PA, Holt RT: Analysis of the compensatory thoracic and lumbosacral curves following Zielke instrumentation for primary thoracolumbar curves. Orthop Trans 13:87, 1989

111. Renshaw TS: The role of Harrington instrumentation and posterior spine fusion in the management of adolescent idiopathic scoliosis. Orthop Clin North Am 19:257, 1988

112. Resina J, Alves AF: A technique of correction and internal fixation for scoliosis. J Bone Joint Surg [Br] 59:159, 1977

113. Richards BS, Birch JG, Herring JA, et al: Frontal and sagittal plane balance following Cotrel–Dubousset instrumentation. Orthop Trans 13:78, 1989

114. Richards BS, Johnston CE 2d: Cotrel–Dubousset instrumentation for adolescent idiopathic scoliosis. Orthopedics 10:649, 1987

115. Schafer MF: Dwyer instrumentation of the spine. Orthop Clin North Am 9:115, 1978

116. Shufflebarger HL, Ellis RD, Clark CE: Cotrel–Dubousset instrumentation in adolescent idiopathic scoliosis: Minimum 2 year follow-up. Orthop Trans 13:79, 1989

117. Shufflebarger HL, Kahn A, Rinsky LA, Shank M: Segmental spinal instrumentation in idiopathic scoliosis: a retrospective analysis of 234 cases. Orthop Trans 9:124, 1985

118. Shufflebarger HL, King WF: Composite measurement of scoliosis: A new method of analysis of the deformity. Spine 12:228, 1987

119. Silverman BJ, Greenbarg PE: Idiopathic scoliosis posterior spine fusion with Harrington rod and sublaminar wiring. Orthop Clin North Am 19:269, 1988

120. Smith MK, Kavey RE, Lubicky JP: Idiopathic scoliosis and mitral valve prolapse. J Fam Pract 19:229, 1984

121. Smyth RJ, Chapman KR, Wright TA, et al: Pulmonary function in adolescents with mild idiopathic scoliosis. Thorax 39:901, 1984

122. Steel HH: Rib resection and spine fusion in correction of convex deformity in scoliosis. J Bone Joint Surg [Am] 65:920, 1983

123. Stokes IAF, Armstrong JG, Moreland MS: Spinal deformity and back surface asymmetry in idiopathic scoliosis. J Orthop Res 6:129, 1988

124. Szeinberg A, Canny GJ, Rashed N, et al: Forced vital capacity and maximal respiratory pressures in patients with mild and moderate scoliosis. Pediatr Pulmonol 4:8, 1988

125. Taddonio RF, Weller K, Appel M: A comparison of patients with idiopathic scoliosis managed with and without postoperative immobilization following segmental spinal instrumentation with Luque rods: A preliminary report. Orthop Trans 8:172, 1984

126. Tamaki T, Tsuji H, Inoue S, Kobayashi H: The prevention of iatrogenic spinal cord injury utilizing the evoked spinal cord potential. Int Orthop 4:313, 1981

127. Tavares JM, Wong RZ: Subcutaneous Harrington rods in the treatment of juvenile scoliosis. Orthop Trans 13:179, 1989

128. Thometz JG, Emans JB: A comparison between spinous process and sublaminar wiring combined with Harrington distraction instrumentation in the management of adolescent idiopathic scoliosis. J Pediatr Orthop 8:129, 1988

129. Thompson JD, Callaghan JJ, Savory CG, et al: Prior deposition of autologous blood in elective spinal surgery. J Bone Joint Surg [Am] 69:320, 1987

130. Thompson GH, Wilber RG, Shaffer JW, et al: Segmental spinal instrumentation in idiopathic scoliosis. A preliminary report. Spine 10:623, 1985

131. Thompson SK, Bentley G: Prognosis in infantile idiopathic scoliosis. J Bone Joint Surg [Br] 62:151, 1980

132. Thompson JD, Renshaw TS: Analysis of lumbar lordosis in posterior spine fusions for idiopathic scoliosis. Orthop Trans 12:539, 1988

133. Thulbourne T, Gillespie R: The rib hump in idiopathic scoliosis: Measurement, analysis, and response to treatment. J Bone Joint Surg [Br] 58:64, 1976

134. Tolo VT: Surgical treatment of adolescent idiopathic scoliosis. Instr Course Lect 38:143, 1989

135. Tolo VT, Gillespie R: The characteristics of juvenile idiopathic scoliosis and results of its treatment. J Bone Joint Surg [Br] 60:181, 1978

136. Transfeldt EE, Bradford DS, Coscia M, et al: Changes in segmental coupling in vertebral rotation following Cotrel–Dubousset for idiopathic scoliosis. Orthop Trans 13:80, 1989

137. Transfeldt EE, Niznik G, Shichijo F, et al: Motor and sensory spinal tract activation following epidural electrical stimulation in the cat. Orthop Trans 13:82, 1989

138. Weatherley CR, Draycott V, O'Brien JF, et al: The rib deformity in adolescent idiopathic scoliosis. A prospective study to evaluate changes after Harrington distraction and posterior fusion. J Bone Joint Surg [Br] 69:179, 1987

139. Weinstein SL: Idiopathic scoliosis: Natural history. Spine 11:780, 1986

140. Weinstein SL, Ponseti IV: Curve progression in idiopathic scoliosis. J Bone Joint Surg [Am] 65:447, 1983

141. West JL, Boachie-Adjei O, Bradford DS, Ogilvie JW: Decompensation following CD instrumentation: A worrisome complication. Orthop Trans 13:78, 1989

142. Wilber RG, Thompson GH, Shaffer JW, et al: Postoperative neurological deficits in segmental spinal instrumentation. A study using spinal cord monitoring. J Bone Joint Surg [Am] 66:1178, 1984

143. Winter RB: Harrington instrumentation into the lumbar spine. Technique for preservation of normal lumbar lordosis. Spine 11:633, 1986

144. Winter RB, Anderson MB: Spinal arthrodesis for spinal deformity using posterior instrumentation and sublaminar wiring. A preliminary report of 100 consecutive cases. Int Orthop 9:239, 1985

145. Winter RB, Lovell WW, Moe JH: Excessive thoracic lordosis and loss of pulmonary function in patients with idiopathic scoliosis. J Bone Joint Surg [Am] 57:972, 1975

146. Zielke K, Stunkat R, Beaujean: Derotation and fusion: Anterior spinal instrumentation. Orthop Trans 2:270, 1978

CHAPTER

8

Zielke Procedures in Scoliosis Correction

Johannes P. Giehl
Klaus Zielke

■

INTRODUCTION

The Universal Spinal Instrumentation System (USIS) has developed from the Ventrale Derotations–Spondylodese (VDS) system, which I designed in 1974. It has become popular worldwide for anterior surgery in scoliosis. With the popularization of transpedicular surgery, Prof. Harms and I found that this system, with some supplements introduced by the former, had a place in posterior spinal surgery. Thus the field of possible surgical activities with this instrumentation system has enlarged. My former colleagues and residents, who are now accomplished spinal surgeons in their own right, have separate chapters on special indications, giving a complete overview of the possibilities of USIS in *anterior* and *posterior* spinal surgery. The reader is referred to the subchapter of Chapter 19, "Correction of Long, Curved Deformities in Ankylosing Spondylitis," by Hehne and Zielke; Chapter 22, *Surgical Treatment of Spondylolisthesis: The Harms Technique*, by Boehm and Harms; Chapter 31, *Surgical Treatment of Failed Back Syndrome*, by Colemont and Zielke; and Chapter 39, *Zielke Pedicle Screw Systems for Thoracic and Lumbar Spine Fractures*, by Harms.

K.Z.

Operative correction of scoliosis is a broad field. There are many techniques, some antiquated, some that have stood the test of time, and some that are still at the developmental stage. Because each method has its own features, no one procedure is ideal for correcting all types of curves. The best treatment can be offered by a surgeon who has broad experience and who can therefore employ the most suitable technique for each patient.

The Harrington method of applying corrective force, with its clear rules and very good results, is still the method we use most often. Modification by Stagnara widened the procedure's indications to include severe kyphoscoliosis.[27a] In our opinion, the Luque system should only be used for patients with neurologic deficits because of the high neurologic risk involved (i.e., four times greater than for the Harrington procedure).[8a]

The most "topical" technique is Cotrel–Dubousset (CD) instrumentation. In our practice, we have ob-

163

served that the amount of derotation achieved is relatively small. The neurologic risk is greater than that of the Harrington operation,[8a] although this may reflect the relative newness of the CD procedure. The stability gained without the use of orthoses is an advantage of this procedure.

The correction of lumbar compensatory curves by means of pedicle screws (the "Harrington-Royale"procedure, according to Zielke) is an extension of the time-tested Harrington procedure. The lumbar sagittal profile of the spine is normalized by lordosation. This procedure enables the surgeon to achieve an excellent correction including only a few segments in most patients with considerable lumbar kyphosis or compensatory curves.

Scoliosis is a three-dimensional deformity. In many cases, the ventral Zielke technique corrects all three components: the frontal plane, the sagittal profile, and the rotation. The lack of a risk of neurologic damage from applying distraction force, the short fusion necessary, and the low degree of trauma resulting from the ventral approach are important factors. The patients recover quickly and are happy with the cosmetic results. The more exacting technique is not too high a price for the experienced surgeon to obtain such excellent results. Ventral and dorsal Zielke procedures have the basic aim of correcting all three curve components, and the goal is the restoration of a physiologic form to the spine.

VENTRAL ZIELKE INSTRUMENTATION

History and Principles

The instrumental correction of scoliosis can be carried out in principle by dorsal or ventral instrumentations. According to the laws of mechanics, a curved spine can be straightened in three ways: by traction at both ends or distraction force applied in the longitudinal direction, by compression on the convex side, or by pressure or traction on the apex—that is, transverse forces.

The easier dorsal approach to the spine led to dorsal instrumentations and procedures that applied forces to the laminae. The dorsal approach was first generally adopted in the operative correction of scoliosis (Harrington procedure).[15] The three types of corrective forces were realized dorsally: corrective force applied to the concave side, compression (Harrington's compression device) on the convex side (see Color Plate 3),

and traction at the apex (Cotrel's "depositif de traction transversal," i.e., transverse traction device). Dwyer, referring to studies by Roaf, initiated the application of corrective forces on the ventral side.[4] The convexity of the curve is shortened by the implants. They are inserted directly into the solid and form-giving vertebral bodies, contrasting with the indirect exertion of force on the laminae. The basic advantages of the Dwyer procedure lie in the better possibility of correction due to the removal of discs, in the lower neurologic risk because shortening of the spine is achieved, in the short fusion, and in the more satisfactory segmental stabilization.[5, 6, 24, 25, 27]

Essential shortcomings of the Dwyer procedure became known: kyphosis caused by compression without derotation on the convex side alone, pseudarthrosis as a consequence of cable fractures, and the insufficient fixation of the cable in the screw heads.[18, 21, 35]

Zielke and Stunkat developed the "Ventrale Derotations-spondylodese" (VDS), which included the basic principle of the ventral compression on the convex side in the Dwyer operation, but which also offered the possibility of derotation and lordosation or kyphosation (see Color Plate 4).[32–34] The implants and instruments of the VDS procedure have been described in numerous publications.[28, 29, 31, 39]

Preoperative Considerations and Technique

Preoperative planning concentrates on the characteristics of the major and compensatory curves. Standardized films of the whole spine in two planes and side-bending films are necessary. Instrumentation is then planned from end- to end-vertebra based on the x-ray film of the anterior-posterior view of the standing patient. The lowest vertebra to be instrumented may not be tilted more than 15° to the pelvis on the bending film (right bender for a left lumbar curve), and it may not be rotated more than 20% (Nash/Moe). Deviations in the profile can be recognized in the sagittal plane. Kyphosation is achieved by not using bone grafts in the disc spaces, and lordosation is achieved by derotation of the curve into the sagittal plane and by the use of bone grafts (e.g., autologous rib or iliac crest) in the disc spaces.

Correction of the major curve requires the absence of posterior bars. In the preoperative assessment, great care should be taken to rule out posterior bars, because they could lead to a minimal correction or to an unbalanced spine after VDS. If detected, they require an osteotomy before undertaking any other procedure.

The corrective behavior of the compensatory curves is especially important; a considerable horizontalization of the lowest instrumented vertebra must be possible, and if the upper compensatory curve cannot be completely corrected, the major curve does not have to be completely corrected either. If these guidelines are not followed, the result will be an unbalanced spine, or gaping of nontused lumbar discs will occur on the convex side. The ventral approach to the thoracic and lumbar spine has been described in many publications.[2, 4, 14, 19, 23, 27]

After resection of the discs, the screws are inserted from the convex side into those vertebral bodies determined preoperatively (see Color Plate 5A). The position of the screws corresponds to the rotation of the vertebra. After insertion of the threaded rod (diameter of 3.2 mm), which is completed by check nuts at both ends, the nuts are moved into the screw heads, and the Maquet table is unflexed, partially straightening the scoliotic curve. The lateral curve is then turned into the sagittal plane with the derotation instrument (Fig. 8-1). In this way, lordosation and derotation of the single vertebrae are achieved. Simultaneously, compression on the convex side, beginning at the apex, effects a further scoliosis correction.

The art of the correction procedure lies in the best possible combination of compression on the convex side, derotation, and the different sizes of the bone grafts in the disc spaces.

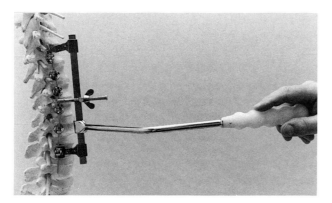

FIG. 8–1. Derotation device on the model shows the apex drawn into the sagittal plane by a special screw; both end vertebrae are fixed points. The spinous processes and the intervertebral foramina illustrate derotation.

After the correction, the screws at both ends are secured with check nuts; the instrumented section of the spine must be mechanically stable (see Color Plate 5B).

Tricks and Pitfalls

The uppermost screw has to withstand the greatest corrective force, although it is inserted in the weakest vertebra.[31] The instrumentation of the next cephalad segment without correction is recommended to distribute the forces. Despite this, any retraction of the cranial screw during the correction should be carefully observed. If necessary, stop the correction. The disc space is filled with a rib graft. We recommend that the bore holes of osteoporotic vertebrae be filled with methylmethacrylate to ensure a safe anchoring of the screws.

In more severe curves, the rod at both ends occasionally springs out of the screw heads. This can be avoided by the use of screw heads with lateral slits facing the ventral direction. The eccentric course of the rod in the slit of the screw head sometimes makes it difficult for the nut to click into place; after fixation of the screw head by a clamp, the nut can be screwed into the opening of the screw head (Fig. 8-2).

In contrast to thoracic instrumentation, a relative or absolute overcorrection is possible in thoracolumbar and lumbar curves. This leads to an unbalanced spine or to a gaping (i.e., discs opened up significantly more on one side than the other in the coronal plane) of the nonfused distal lumbar discs. The correction of the thoracolumbar or lumbar curves may only be carried out as far as the bending result of the thoracic compensatory curve, which will produce a maximal spontaneous correction of the thoracic curve. Overcorrection is avoided by convex-sided insertion of bone grafts into the disc spaces.

Rehabilitation

Postoperatively, patients must be nursed in an intensive care unit. After a few days, they can be transferred to a normal ward. A week after the operation, the patient is provided with a Stagnara brace or with a plaster body jacket in which he or she is remobilized and then discharged. The fusion is usually consolidated within 4 months. After conventional tomography in the frontal plane documents this, the brace is removed.

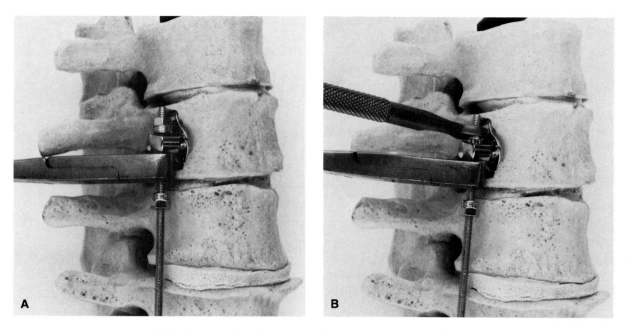

FIG. 8–2. A, B. The seating of a nut into the screw head.

Indications

In principle, all scoliotic curves can be corrected and stabilized by means of VDS instrumentation as long as the instrumentation does not extend cranially to T4 and does not include S1 caudally. In each case, carefully consider whether the technically more exacting procedure would make a better correction or a shorter fusion possible than a dorsal instrumentation or whether a combined ventrodorsal procedure permits saving the lumbar motion segments in double-major curves. A certain mobility is necessary, because ankylosing facet joints in adults can impair the correction, and preceding dorsal osteotomies may be necessary. If the operating surgeon is not experienced in this method, he or she must consider whether a Harrington procedure with a somewhat less ideal correction would be a safer method for the patient suffering from a congenital curve or adult scoliosis.

VDS is very helpful in cases with deficient posterior elements, in paralytic scoliosis, and in thoracolumbar and lumbar curves because of the excellent correction and the short fusion, which means that lumbar motion segments can be preserved. Lumbar kyphosis in cases of lumbar major curves can often be corrected by means of VDS. After instrumentation of the major curve in false double-major curves, the lumbar or thoracic compensatory curve usually partially corrects itself. The excellent possibility of derotation and the

corresponding cosmetic improvement are strong arguments for using VDS for young patients.

The VDS procedure is not indicated for complex congenital curves, for severe (i.e., more than 100° according to Cobb) and rigid thoracic kyphoscoliosis, or for bone destruction of the vertebral bodies (e.g., by neurofibromatosis). Long C-shaped paralytic curves sometimes require instrumentation of 10 or more segments; superior operative skill is necessary.

Anterior VDS should not be carried out if lung function is bad (i.e., vital capacity less than 1000 ml), because breathing insufficiency can sabotage the postoperative course.

Idiopathic Scoliosis
Thoracolumbar and lumbar single curves are appropriate domains of the VDS procedure.[8, 10] The instrumentation is very short, and it preserves valuable lumbar motion segments. A pathologic kyphosis can often be corrected (Fig. 8-3A–D), and the cosmetically conspicuous waist-line asymmetry is improved by derotation. The thorax deformity in thoracic curves is nicely corrected by this procedure. In thoracic lordoscoliosis, kyphosation is possible.[30] Double-major curves require a very long fusion, usually as far as L4 or L5, if only treated posteriorly. Lumbar VDS can horizontalize L2 or L3 satisfactorily; the lower hook of the Harrington rod can be inserted here (Fig. 8-4A–C). If a combined ventrodorsal technique is used, an average

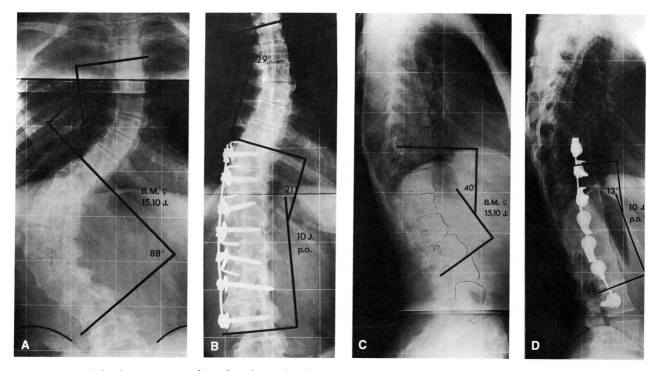

FIG. 8–3. **A, C.** Idiopathic thoracolumbar kyphoscoliosis. **B, D.** Result after 10 years: stable correction of kyphosis and scoliosis, with slight gaping of the L4–L5 disc because of relative overcorrection.

FIG. 8–4. A. Idiopathic double-major curve. The Harrington instrumentation would have included L4. **B.** By means of VDS of T10–L2, L2 is horizontalized. **C.** After Harrington correction, both major curves have been corrected to a large extent. The spine is balanced, saving two further lumbar motion segments.

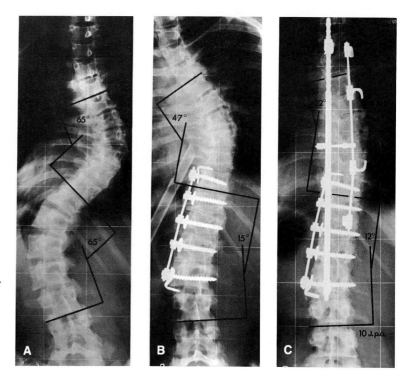

of 1.5 more lumbar motion segments can be saved than with the Harrington "dollar-sign" instrumentation.[9]

Congenital Scoliosis

Congenital scoliosis caused by an isolated hemivertebra can be corrected and stabilized by resection of the hemivertebra and VDS instrumentation (Fig. 8-5A–C). This method eliminates the risk of distraction inherent in the dorsal technique. In complex deformations of the vertebrae, VDS should be considered if a regional pathologic lordosis can be corrected by a ventral epiphysiodesis.

Neuromuscular Scoliosis

Myelodysplasia, cerebral palsy, myopathy, and poliomyelitis are the most frequent causes of neuromuscular scoliosis. Morphologically, these are mostly C-shaped curves with pathologic kyphoses. VDS provides excellent correction in the frontal and sagittal planes (Fig. 8-6A–E). VDS is able to correct a pelvic obliquity. This improves the patient's balance and ability to sit and reduces soft tissue problems (e.g., ulceration of the skin).[20]

VDS is particularly helpful when the patient suffers from deficient posterior element formation. Rotational kyphosis or pathologic lordosis, which frequently occur, can also be corrected.

In paralytic scoliosis, we regularly carry out dorsal instrumentation (i.e., Harrington, Luque, or pedicle screws) after ventral correction of the deformity; by these means, further correction and stability are achieved, often making orthoses unnecessary.

Results

Up to 1989, more than 700 VDS procedures have been performed in the German scoliosis centers in Bad Wildungen and in Tübingen. Besides Zielke and his colleagues, numerous physicians in other parts of the world have reported their results.[12, 13, 16, 26, 36–38] With only five exceptions (those who had moved to an unknown address or who were abroad), all 215 patients with idiopathic scoliosis who had been operated on up to 1982 were reexamined afterwards, and the follow-up ranging from 5 to 12 years was analyzed.

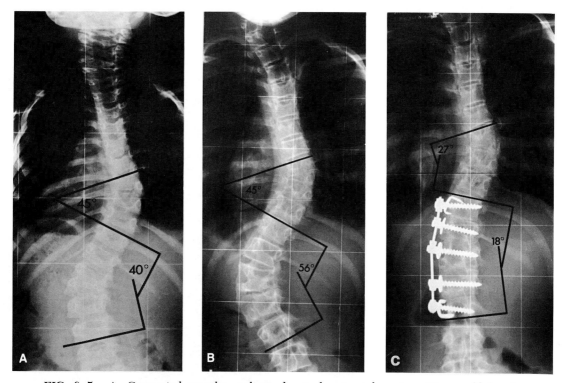

FIG. 8–5. A. Congenital complex scoliosis due to hemivertebrae in a 10-year-old female patient. **B.** Progression of the lumbar curve over 2 years. **C.** Resection of the hemivertebra and VDS of T11–L3; spontaneous correction of the congenital thoracic curve.

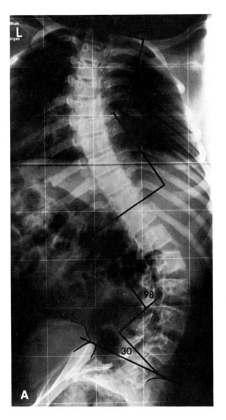

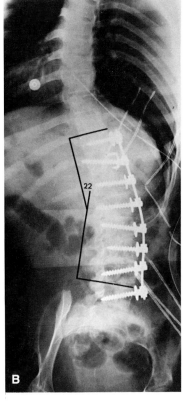

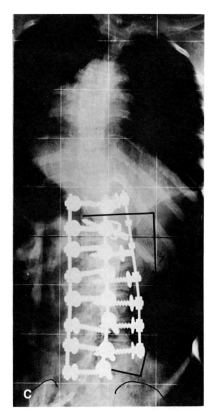

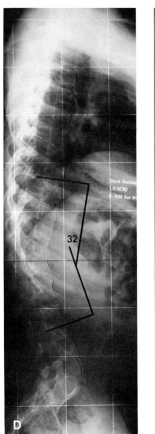

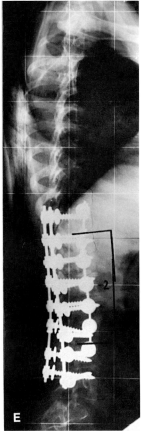

FIG. 8–6. A. A long lumbar paralytic curve into the pelvis with coronal decompensation (16-year-old female patient with poliomyelitis). **B.** VDS of T10–L5: excellent scoliosis correction and almost complete correction of the pelvic obliquity and decompensation. **C.** Additional stabilization by means of pedicle screw instrumentation for T10–L5 and fusion. Notice the loosening of the threaded rod in the region of the VDS screws at T11 and T12 due to dorsal correction. **D.** Preoperative film of the spinal profile of the same patient: thoracolumbar kyphosis. **E.** After ventral and dorsal correction, satisfactory lumbar lordosis is achieved.

The average age of patients at the time of operation was 19.2 years (range, 10.1–55.5 years). When first used in 1974, the operation lasted almost 4 hours; in 1986, it took only 2.5 hours. Loss of blood during the operation averaged 850 ml in the beginning; in a comparable group in 1986, the average blood loss was only 400 ml. Both improvements are due to experience with this technique and to arterial hypotension, which has been carried out intraoperatively since 1983.

The subjective satisfaction of the patients who were operated on corresponds with the excellent cosmetic improvement. Rib hump correction amounted to 60% on average. Lumbar asymmetry correction was almost complete. Usually patients feel that the limited mobility of the spine after fusion is not of great importance, particularly after thoracic and thoracolumbar instrumentation. Although the mobility of the scoliotic spine is limited preoperatively, a fusion that is as short as possible is important.

Preoperatively, we found mild, subjective pain complaints in 17% of the cases with double-major curves and in 76% of cases with other curve patterns. A year after surgery, most patients had no complaints; 5 to 10 years after surgery, the proportion of patients with complaints was the same as the preoperative rate. We were unable to find any correlation with the extent of the curves or the corrections, technical failures, or pseudarthroses.

Cobb Angle

The correction of the Cobb angle (Fig. 8-7A) averaged 64% in thoracic curves, 67% in thoracolumbar curves, 62% in lumbar curves, and 67% in double-major curves. The long-term correction was stable, with the

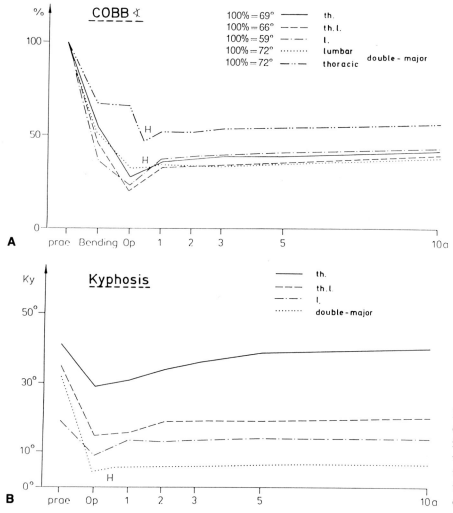

FIG. 8–7. **A.** Average correction of the Cobb angle during long-term follow-up. **B.** Kyphosis (average values) during the period of observation. **C.** Average rotation correction. **D.** Average vital capacity during long-term follow-up.

exception of those patients with pseudarthroses, delayed fusion (with rod fractures), or instrumentations of wrong levels.

As a consequence of relative overcorrection, the caudal end vertebra is often shifted caudally in lumbar and thoracolumbar curves. The disc space adjacent to the instrumentation then gapes on the convex side, and the quality of the correction in the frontal plane is not adequtely reflected in the improvement of the Cobb angle. Therefore, we defined the tilt index (TI) as the average tilt of the discs in the lower half of the lumbar curve, measured when the patients were standing: the number of mobile segments in this half of the curve was stated (Fig. 8-8A,B). A large angle is then disadvantageous, and a large number of segments is favorable. The improvement in the TI was 48% in double-major

curves (i.e., VDS and Harrington procedures) and 32% in lumbar instrumentation (Table 8-1). The actual improvement in the static condition is thus smaller than would be assumed on the grounds of a curve correction of 70%.

Kyphosis

The assessment of the correction in the sagittal plane is complex because exact normal figures are not defined. VDS has had a favorable influence on thoracic kyphosis that is either too severe or too slight.[30] The average thoracolumbar kyphosis (Fig. 8-7B) was reduced from 35° to 14°. The thoracolumbar rotational kyphosis in double-major curves was corrected by the ventrodorsal method (VDS and Harrington procedure). The improvement amounted to 80%.

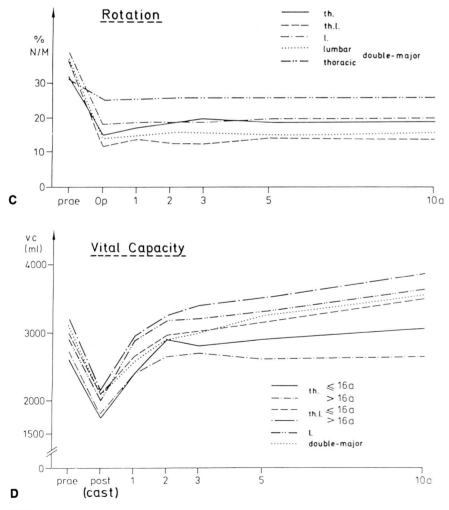

FIG. 8–7. (continued)

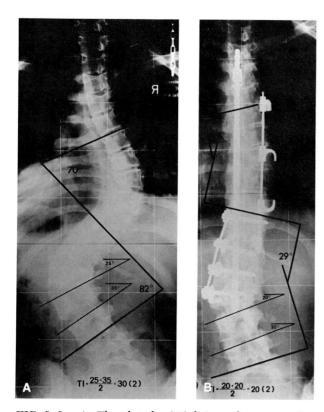

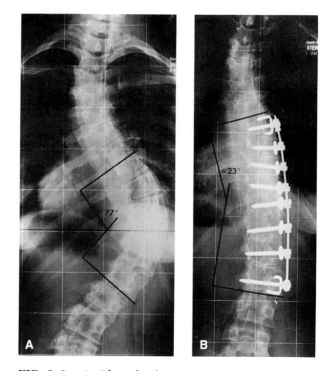

FIG. 8–8. A. The tilt index (TI) denotes the average slant of the discs in the lower half of the lumbar curve when patients are standing. **B.** Postoperatively, L2–L3 and L3–L4 gape due to relative overcorrection by VDS; the lower-end vertebra is now L4. The VDS correction of approximately 65% is not reflected in the result. The TI improved by only 33%. The result would have been better with VDS to L3.

FIG. 8–9. A. Idiopathic lower thoracic curve. **B.** After VDS for T8–L3, major and compensatory curves are balanced with no gaping.

Rotation

Rotation correction relative to the initial condition, when measured at the apex vertebra according to Nash/Moe (percentage figures), was 44% in the thoracic curves (Fig. 8-10); in curves localized elsewhere, the correction rate was 60%. Although it was often

possible to carry out complete corrections, they sometimes were not done because it would cause an overcorrection relative to the compensatory curves above and below.

The small derotation effect of the CD technique has been reported by Ecker and Drummond.[7] In 1986, we treated 71 idiopathic thoracic and thoracolumbar curves and assessed the achieved derotation in comparative groups (i.e., VDS and CD instrumentation) according to Aaro's criteria.[1] The correction of the sagittal rotational angle (RA_{SAG}) after VDS was 48% in thoracic cases, 56% in the thoracolumbar cases, and 7% in thoracic CD cases (Figs. 8-9 through 8-12).

Vital Capacity

The vital capacity (Fig. 8-7D) returned to its initial value on average in the second postoperative year and exceeded this value later by 10%.

Complications

General Problems

Intraoperative and postoperative problems are rare (Table 8-2). Serious, irreversible disturbances did not

TABLE 8-1. Tilt Index and Cobb Angle

Curves	Tilt index	Cobb angle
Lumbar scoliosis (n = 40)	21.0 → 14.2° (2.0 s) (1.2 s)	59.0 → 22.4°
Correction	32.4%	62.0%
Double-major (lower curve) n = 72	21.7 → 11.3° (2.4 s) (1.6 s)	72.0 → 23.8°
Correction	48.1%	67.0%

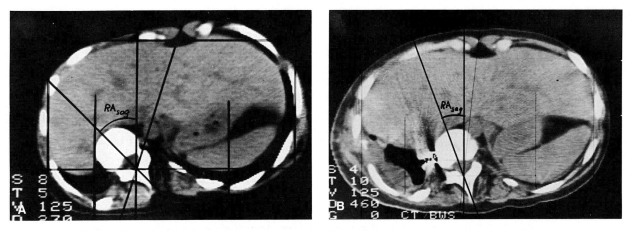

FIG. 8–10. This is the same patient shown in Figure 8–9. The RA$_{SAG}$ of the apex vertebra, which is independent of the improvement in the Cobb angle, has been corrected from 45° (**A**) to 20° (**B**).

FIG. 8–11. This is the same patient shown in Figure 8–9, illustrating tangential projection of the rib hump. Preoperative asymmetry (**A**) has been corrected to a great extent after the operation (**B**).

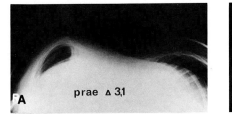

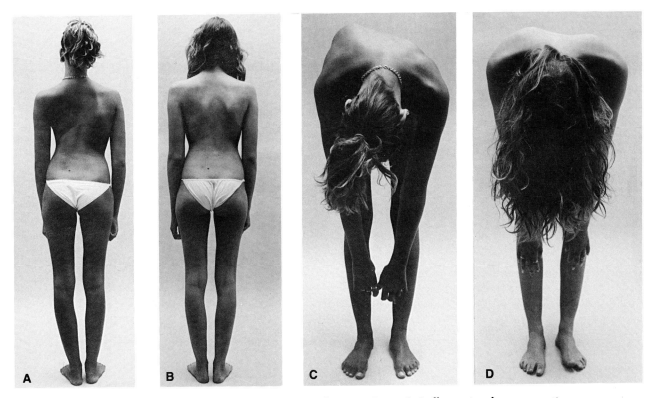

FIG. 8–12. Dorsal view of the same patient shown in Figure 8–9, illustrating the preoperative (**A**) and postoperative (**B**) conditions. **C, D.** Examination of the rib hump before the operation and after correction.

TABLE 8-2. VDS Complications (1975–1982)

Complications	Thoracic and Thoracolumbar (n = 103)	Lumbar (n = 40)	Double-Major (lower curve) (n = 72)
Death			
Motor/sensory deficit			
Deep infection			
Hemothorax	4		
Chylothorax	1		
Thrombosis		1	
Sympathectomy syndrome		4	3

occur. Our patients appreciated a shorter period of convalescence than that after dorsal spine surgery.

In principle, all the surrounding structures can be injured when the spinal column is exposed ventrally. A detailed description of the possible problems and their management was given by Hack and colleagues.[39] The experienced spine surgeon usually can avoid these complications by a careful operative technique.

Technical Mistakes

Technical mistakes were frequent (10%) in the first 50 VDS operations (Table 8-3).[37] Most problems were caused by screws that were too short and became loose, by an instrumentation of the wrong segments, or by an overcorrection. Technical mistakes occurred in 6.5% of all cases operated on before 1982; in a comparable group in 1986, technical mistakes occurred in 4% of the cases; neither ventral nor dorsal reoperations were necessary.[8] The significant decrease in technical problems was due to longer experience with the VDS system.

Implant Failures

Implant failures occurred in 11.6% of the 215 cases treated before 1982 (Table 8-4). Lumbar instrumenta-tions were proportionally over-represented. Implant fractures (including three screw fractures) occurred exclusively in the cranial and caudal end segments. Most implant fractures occurred during the year after stabilization by orthosis. In 50% of the cases, these were accompanied by a loss of correction and delayed fusion. In 3 cases, a dorsal fusion ensued; in 3 other cases, fusion could not be verified. We observed that all implant fractures occurred in absolute or relative over-correction or in instrumentations that did not include the end vertebra. After learning to avoid this mistake, we have seen no more implant fractures.

"HARRINGTON-ROYALE" ACCORDING TO ZIELKE

History and Principles

The correction of a thoracolumbar kyphosis at the end of a thoracic curve has just recently attracted attention. The kyphosis can be found in the form of a rotational kyphosis between two major curves or between a thoracic major curve and a lumbar minor curve. Thoracic VDS achieves only a partial normalization of the profile if there is severe kyphosis outside of the instrumenta-

TABLE 8-3. VDS Technical Failures (1975–1982)

Complications	Thoracic and Thoracolumbar (n = 103)	Lumbar (n = 40)	Double-Major (lower curve) (n = 72)
Chylothorax		1	
Vertebral fracture	1		
Screw/staple in disc space		1	2
Overcorrection		3	1
Wrong segments	1	1	
Screw loosening	2	1	

TABLE 8-4. VDS Implant Failures (1975–1982)

Complications	Thoracic and Thoracolumbar (n = 103)	Lumbar (n = 40)	Double-Major (lower curve) (n = 72)
Rod dislocation		1	
Rod/screw fracture (including cases with loss of correction)	6 (3)	15 (10)	4 (0)

tion. Applying Harrington distraction force causes an additional kyphosis in the lowest segment that is instrumented.[11] A consequence of thoracolumbar and lumbar kyphosis is a lower lumbar hyperlordosis, which may lead to degenerative, painful back syndromes and symptomatic retrolistheses.[3, 22]

After the establishment of pedicle-screw instrumentations, Zielke initiated the correction of thoracolumbar kyphosis in thoracic scoliosis and double-major curves by means of dorsal compression using pedicle screws (Fig. 8-13A,B). There was also some correction of the lower compensatory curve.

The instruments consist of a Harrington rod with a threaded lower part. The end of the rod fits into the screw head and guarantees a right-angle fixation (Fig. 8-14A–C). In the area of the threaded part either compression or distraction can be exerted on each separate segment, just as it can be by contralateral pedicle-

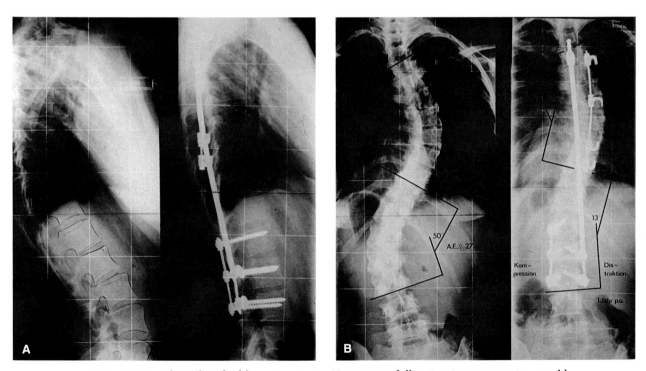

FIG. 8–13. Idiopathic double-major curve. Harrington dollar-sign instrumentation would have to include L4. Harrington-Royale instrumentation only involves L3. Normalization of the lumbar profile (**A**) and nearly perfect correction of the lumbar curve (**B**).

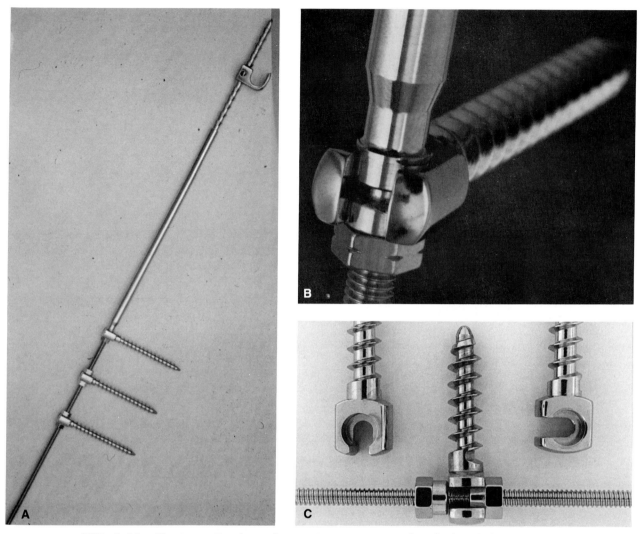

FIG. 8–14. Harrington-Royale implants. **A.** Distraction rod with threaded lower part. **B.** The end of the rod fits into the pedicle-screw head. **C.** The hexnuts do so as well. Both connections guarantee a right-angle fixation.

screw instrumentation. Thus, both a correction of the thoracolumbar kyphosis and of the lumbar curve can be carried out.

Preoperative Considerations and Technique

Planning for the operation is concentrated on the study of the caudal curve. Bending films are mandatory. The pedicle-screw instrumentation is carried out from the upper-end vertebra of the caudal curve to the segment below which all the discs can level off (Fig. 8-15). Experience has shown that the lower half of the compensatory curve corrects itself spontaneously.

The dorsal preparation of the spinal column corresponds to that of the Harrington procedure. Pedicle screws are placed on both sides in the area of the cranial half of the compensatory curve. A correction of the curve is carried out by distraction on the concave side by means of a separate threaded rod. Compression on the threaded part of the rod effects lordosation. Both

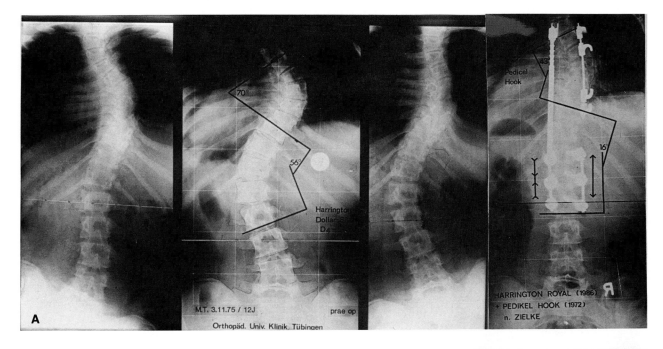

FIG. 8–15. False double-major curve. Harrington dollar-sign instrumentation would have included L3. Bending films show a nonstructural part of the lumbar curve caudal to L2. **A.** Segmental curve correction between T12 and L2 yields a correction of the whole lumbar curve. **B.** Normalization of the profile is very good.

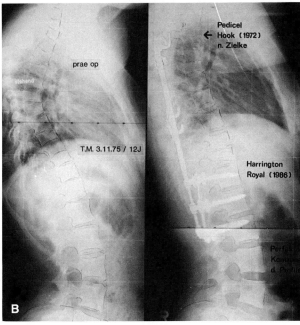

processes can be correspondingly varied according to individual requirements (see Fig. 8-13A,B). The thoracic major curve is corrected in the usual way by means of distraction. The operation is finished by a usual facet fusion and wound closure.

Follow-Up Treatment

Postoperative care and rehabilitation are the same as after the Harrington procedure, and a more detailed description is not necessary.

Indications

Thoracolumbar Kyphosis

False double-major curves with a lumbar minor curve and thoracolumbar kyphosis are ideal indications. The kyphosis is corrected by means of dorsal segmental compression. A normal physiologic sagittal profile and a partial correction of the lower compensatory curve result (Fig. 8-16A,B)

False Double-Major Curve

The correction of the lumbar curve is carried out by means of pedicle screws in the upper area of the curve. Compared with the dollar-sign instrumentation, several more lower lumbar motion segments can be saved.

Double-Major Curves

The Harrington dollar-sign instrumentation often must include L5 in correcting a severe lumbar curve. Insuf-ficient horizontalization of the lumbosacral vertebrae and only one remaining motion segment below the long fusion predispose the patient to chronic degenerative problems. The segmental pedicle-screw correction guarantees a superior lumbar correction and horizontalizes L4. The thoracolumbar rotation kyphosis is corrected, and an almost normal profile of the spine can be achieved (Fig. 8-17A,B).

Miscellaneous Corrections

Segmental correction also enables the surgeon to create a kyphosis in pathologic lordosis (Fig. 8-18A,B).

Results

More than 70 Harrington-Royale instrumentations have been carried out in Tübingen and Bad Wildungen since 1987. Although a statistical evaluation of the re-

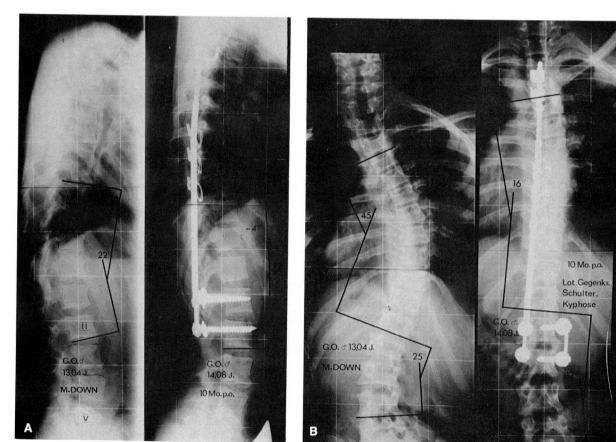

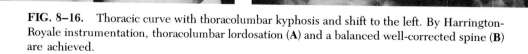

FIG. 8–16.   Thoracic curve with thoracolumbar kyphosis and shift to the left. By Harrington-Royale instrumentation, thoracolumbar lordosation (**A**) and a balanced well-corrected spine (**B**) are achieved.

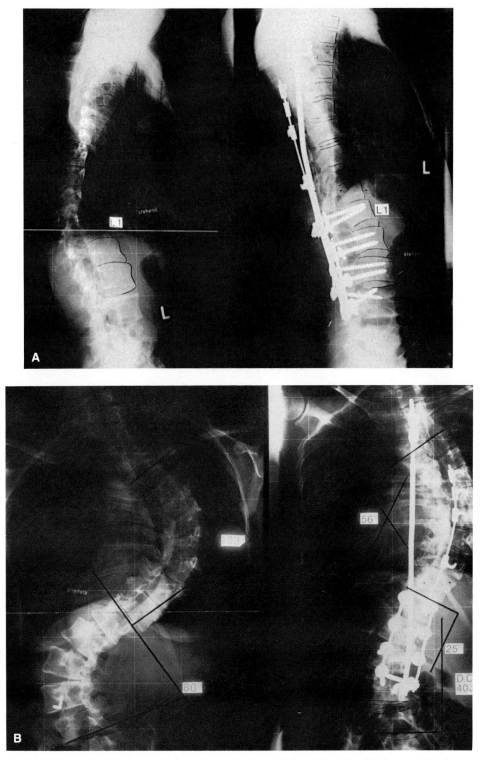

FIG. 8–17. Adult scoliosis with severe curves and thoracolumbar kyphosis. Harrington correction would have been necessary to L5. Segmental pedicle-screw instrumentation down to L4 results in a reasonable profile (**A**) and curve correction (**B**).

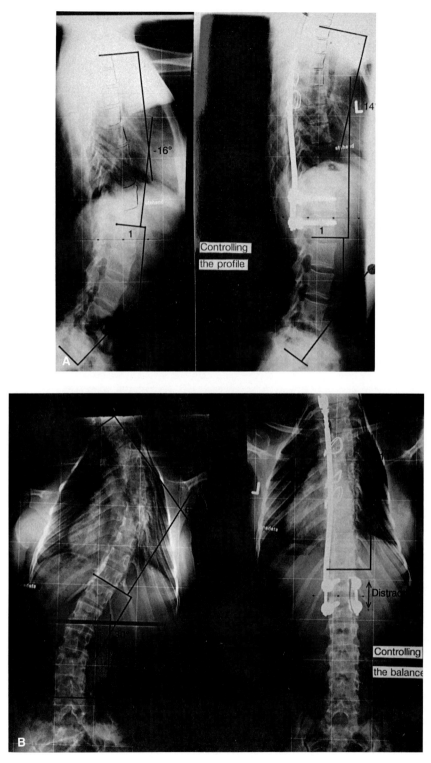

FIG. 8–18. Thoracic scoliosis, severe lordosis, and thoracic dysplasia corrected by Harrington-Royale between T1 and L1. Notice the improved sagittal profile (**A**) excellent curve correction, and balancing of the spine (**B**).

sults has not yet been made, we can ascertain that a normalization of the thoracolumbar and lumbar profile of the spine was almost always possible. The rate of correction of the lumbar curve in cases of false double-major curves was usually more than 80%; in cases of double-major curves it was more than 60%, although only the upper part of the curve had undergone instrumentation and fusion. This method usually preserved 1 or 2 more low lumbar motion segments than the dollar-sign instrumentation. The correction of the curve by pedicle screws is accompanied by a considerable derotation; clinically, the asymmetry of the lumbar region usually disappeared.

PROBLEMS AND CONCLUSIONS

Formerly we used a 3.2-mm Harrington rod with a threaded lower part; several rod fractures occurred where the upper part of the rod meets the threaded lower part. Pseudarthroses were not found. After switching to the 4-mm rod, we had no more implant failures. The positioning of pedicle screws in the scoliotic spine is technically exacting. Although nerve root lesions are conceivable, we saw none in our cases. Expert mastery of the pedicle screw technique is necessary if neurologic lesions are to be avoided.

The Harrington-Royale procedure is a valuable addition to the methods available to a surgeon dealing with the spine. It combines the reliable principle of Harrington distraction with the possibility of correcting a pathologic thoracolumbar or lumbar kyphosis. We see it as an alternative to thoracic VDS if a sufficient spontaneous correction of a more severe lumbar scoliosis or kyphosis cannot be expected. The Harrington-royal procedure corrects this deformity by including only a minimum of motion segments. In double-major curves, the fusion is much shorter than in the dollar-sign instrumentation, saving additional lumbar motion segments while obtaining a well-compensated result.

References

1. Aaro S, Dahlborn M: Estimation of vertebral rotation and the spinal and rib cage deformity in scoliosis by computer tomography. Spine 6:460, 1981
2. Bradford D, Winter RB, Lonstein JE, Moe JH: Techniques of anterior spinal surgery for the management of kyphosis. Clin Orthop 128:129, 1977
3. Casey MP, Asher MA, Jacobs RR, Orrick JM: The effect of Harrington rod contouring on lumbar lordosis. Spine 12:750, 1987
4. Dwyer AF, Newton NC, Sherwood AA: An anterior approach to scoliosis—a preliminary report. Clin Orthop 62:192, 1969
5. Dwyer AF: Experience of anterior correction of scoliosis. Clin Orthop 93:191, 1973
6. Dwyer AF, Schafer MF: Anterior approach to scoliosis. Results of treatment in 51 cases. J Bone Joint Surg [Br] 56:218, 1974
7. Ecker ML, Betz RR, Trent PS, et al: Computer tomography evaluation of Cotrel-Dubousset instrumentation in idiopathic scoliosis. Spine 13:1141, 1989
8. Giehl JP, Zielke K: Idiopathic thoracic and thoracolumbar scoliosis. Early and long-term results after VDS and CD with special regard to rotational correction. Paper XVII, S 43. Meeting SICOT, München, 17 August 1987, Kongresband. Demeter, Gräfelfing
8a. Lowe TG: Scoliosis Research Society, Morbidity and Mortality Committee, 1987 report
9. Giehl JP, Zielke K: Idiopathische kombinierte Skoliose; Erhaltung lumbaler Bewegungssegmente durch die Kombination der VDS nach Zielke mit der Harrington-Distraktionsspondylodese—Langzeitergebnisse. Paper 36. Jahrestagung der Vereinigung Süddeutscher Orthopäden e.V., Baden-Baden, 28 April 1988
10. Giehl JP, Zielke K: Idiopathische lumbale Skoliose—Langzeitergebnisse der VDS nach Zielke. Paper 6. Deutsch-Japanische Orthopädentagung, Homburg/Saar, 15 und 16 September 1988
11. Giehl JP: Kontrolle der Profile der lumbalen Krümmung mit dem "Harrington-royal" nach Zielke. Paper presented at the International Symposon on the Lumbar Profile in Spine Surgery, 6–7 November 1989, Bad Wildungen, W. Germany
12. Giehl JP, Zielke K, Hack HP: Die Ventrale Derotationsspondylodese nach Zielke. Orthopäde 18:101, 1989
13. Griss P: Kritische Analyse von 60 VDS-Operationen bei Skoliose (1979–1983). In Bauer R (ed): Der vordere Zugang der Wirbelsäule, S 116. Stuttgart, Thieme, 1983
14. Hall JE: The anterior approach to spinal deformities. Orthop Clin North Am 3:81, 1972
15. Harrington P: Treatment of scoliosis. J Bone Joint Surg 44:591, 1962
16. Heine J, Matthias HH: Erste Ergebnisse mit der ventralen Derotationsspondylodese. In Bauer R (ed): Der vordere Zugang zur Wirbelsäule, S 121. Stuttgart, Thieme, 1983
17. Hopf CH, Matthias HH, Heine J: Erste Ergebnisse der operativen Behandlung der Skoliose mit dem CD-Instrumentarium. Z Orthop 125:347, 1987
18. Hsu LS: Dwyer instrumentation in the treatment of adolescent idiopathic scoliosis. J Bone Joint Surg [Br] 64:536, 1982
19. Louis R: Surgery of the Spine. Berlin, Springer-Verlag, 1983
20. Metz P, Zielke K, Hack HP: Operative management of scoliosis in neuromuscular diseases. Semin Orthop 2:192, 1987

21. Michel CR, Onimus M: Complications de l'operation de Dwyer. In Bauer R, Zielke K (eds): Wirbelsäule in Forschung und Praxis, Bd 72. Stuttgart, Hippokrates Verlag, 1978

22. Michel CR, Lalain JJ, Caton J, Bérard J: Evolution à long terme de la courbure lombaire après instrumentation de Harrington pour scoliose thoracique ou double majeure. Rev Chir Orthop 71:187, 1985

23. Morscher E: Der vordere Zugang zur Brustwirbelsäule. In Bauer R (ed): Der vordere Zugang zur Wirbelsäule, S 60. Stuttgart, Thieme, 1983

24. Onimus M, Michel CR: A propos de certaines indications de l'operation de Dwyer. Communication an 13ème congrès Mondial de la Société International de la Chirurgie Orthopédique et Traumatologique, Copenhagen, 7–12 Juli 1975

25. Onimus M: L'operation de Dwyer dans les scolioses paralytiques avec bassin oblique. In Bauer R, Zielke K (eds): Wirbelsäule in Forschung und Praxis, Bd 72, S 26. Stuttgart, Hippokrates Verlag, 1975

26. Purcell G: Zielke instrumentation (VDS) for the correction of spinal curvature. Analysis of results in 66 patients. Clin Orthop 180:133, 1983

27. Riseborough EJ: The anterior approach to the spine for the correction of deformities of the axial skeleton. Clin Orthop 93:207, 1973

27a. Stagnara P, Jouvinoux P, Peloux J, et al: Cyphoscolioses essentialles de l'adulte. Formes severes de plus de 100°. Redressement partial et arthrodese. Presented at the XI SICOT Congress, Mexico City, Mexico, 1969

28. Stürz H: Biomechanical principles of the VDS and their implications for the operative technique. Paper delivered at the 21st VDS-Symposium, Department of Orthopedics, University of Rochester, New York, 1982

29. Ulrich H: Materialbelastungsprüfung bei VDS- und Dwyer-Implantaten. In Bauer R, Zielke K (eds): Die Wirbelsäule in Forschung und Praxis, Bd 72, S116–120. Stuttgart, Hippokrates Verlag, 1978

30. Völpel J, Zielke K: VDS bei idiopathischen Thorakalskoliose. (in preparation)

31. Wörsdöfer O, Ulrich CH, Magerl F: Biomechanische Untersuchungen verschiedener Fixations- und Korrektursysteme an der Wirbelsäule. Paper 50. VDS-Operationsschulungsseminar, Bad Wildungen, 3–6 November 1986

32. Zielke K, Pellin B: Ventrale Derotationsspondylodese. Symposium on Kyphosis and Scoliosis, Belgrad, 1975

33. Zielke K, Stunkat R, Duquesne J, Beaujean F: Ventrale Derotationsspondylodese. Orthop Praxis 11:562, 1975

34. Zielke K, Stunkat R, Delatte F, Beaujean F: Traitement des scolioses par spondylodèse par voie antérieure avec l'instrumentation des dérotation et de lordosation (VDS). Paper Réunion anuelle de la groupe d'etude de la scoliose, St. Etienne, February 1976

35. Zielke K, Berthet A: Ventrale Derotationsspondylodese—vorläufiger Bericht über 58 Fälle. Beitr Orthop Traumatol 25:85, 1978

36. Zielke K: Ventrale Derotationsspondylodese, Behandlungsergebnisse bei idiopathischen Lumbalskoliosen. Z Orthop 120:320, 1982

37. Zielke K: Indikationen, Ergebnisse und Komplikationen der ventralen Derotationsspondylodese. In Bauer R (ed): Der vordere Zugang zur Wirbelsäule, S 109. Stuttgart, Thieme, 1983

38. Zielke K: Der heutige Stand der operativen Behandlung der Skoliose. Paper XXVI. Fortbildungsveranstaltung Berufsverband der Fachärzte für Orthopädie, Hamburg, 9. November 1985

39. Zielke K, Hack HP, Harms J: Spinal instrumentation. InBradford DS, Hensinger RM (eds): The Paediatric Spine, p 491. New York, Thieme, 1985

CHAPTER 9

Cotrel–Dubousset Instrumentation (CDI) for Adolescent and Pediatric Scoliosis

Daniel Chopin
Christian Morin

COTREL–DUBOUSSET INSTRUMENTATION FOR ADOLESCENT IDIOPATHIC SCOLIOSIS

DANIEL CHOPIN

INSTRUMENTATION

Cotrel–Dubousset instrumentation consists of three implant elements: the rods, the hooks and screws, and the transverse traction devices.[4, 5]

Rod

The rod is the essential part of the system. It is cylindrical and its entire surface is covered by small diamond-shaped points. The design offers the following advantages:

1. Hooks or screws can be firmly fixed into any position at any level.
2. Hooks or screws can be placed to apply distraction force or compression force.
3. The rod can be bent at any level over its entire length with no risk of losing strength. It is possible to conform the rod closely to or even restore the physiologic sagittal curve of the spine.
4. Rotation of the prebent rod within the bodies of the hooks or screws may produce movement of the instrumented vertebrae in three axes, correcting the three-dimensional deformities of scoliosis.
5. Two separated rods are used on either side of the spine, firmly locked together by the transverse traction device. They form a stable frame, often making external support unnecessary after the operation.

Hooks and Screws

To obtain segmental instrumentation, it was necessary to design closed-body implants for the end vertebrae and opened-body implants for the intermediate vertebrae (Fig. 9-1). A conoid cylindrical blocker pushed into the cavity of an opened-body hook transforms it into a closed-body implant (Fig. 9-2). A new vertebral

183

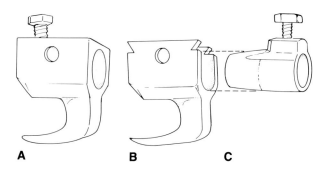

FIG. 9–1. **A.** Closed body hook. **B.** Open body hook. **C.** Conoid cylindrical blocker.

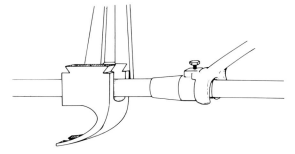

FIG. 9–2. Introduction of the blocker into an open body hook.

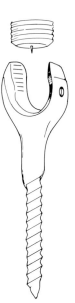

FIG. 9–3. Vertebral screw with posterior opening and its cap.

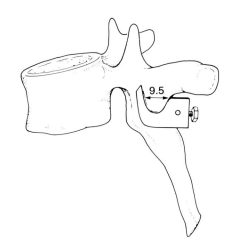

FIG. 9–4. Standard pedicular hook.

screw (tulip screw) becomes a closed-body implant by screwing a cap over the rod (Fig. 9-3).

Fixation with vertebral screws provides immediate stability. The other implants become stable only after a force has been applied. A pedicular hook or infra-laminar hook is stable only if a cephalad-directed force is applied and the implant contacts the lamina.

Hooks may be placed facing each other around a lamina as a claw. This claw will be immediately stable in relation to the vertebra without requiring any corrective or compression force.

It is convenient to describe the hooks, claws, and screws relative to the anatomic location of their insertion.

Hooks
The pedicular hook is inserted at the portion of greatest strength in the vertebra. The blade is 9 mm wide and 15 mm long. The upper rim of the blade is notched to straddle the inferior surface of the pedicle.

The anterior surface of the body of the hook is positioned against the posterior cortex of the inferior articular facet (Fig. 9-4). The standard pedicular hook

has a groove 9.5 mm wide. If the facet is narrow, it is possible to use a pedicular hook with a 6.5-mm reduced groove. If the posterior arch of the vertebra is small (e.g., cervical area), a cervical hook is preferred.

The thoracic laminar hook has a blade 5.5 mm wide and 12 mm long.

The anterior aspect of the body of the hook slopes upward from back to front; when the hook is inserted, it gradually displaces backwards as it penetrates the sublaminar space (Fig. 9-5). If hooks have to be used on both sides of the same lamina, the blade must be reduced in width (4 mm) to avoid overlapping of the two blades inside the spinal canal.

The lumbar laminar hook has a blade 7 mm wide and 14 mm long with a flat anterior surface (Fig. 9-6). In case of bilateral instrumentation on the same lamina, a blade progressively reduced in width (5 mm) should be used.

Screws

The first generation of vertebral screws were composed with opened and closed bodies. Blockers were used to change an opened screw to a closed one. The second generation (tulip screw) does not need blockers (Fig. 9-7). First- and second-generation screws are available in 5- and 6-mm diameters, from 30 mm to 50 mm long.

The sacral screws are 7 mm in diameter (Fig. 9-8). They have a hexagonal head and two kinds of necks. The short neck is for sagittal insertion and the long neck is for oblique insertion.

Claws

Claws accomplish an immediately stable and solid grip. The pediculotransverse claw is the most popular claw. It is obtained by a pedicular hook and a grip above the transverse process. A lumbar laminar hook is used for the grip above the transverse process. The claw may not be efficient if the posterior arch of the vertebra is narrow. In this case, contact between the bodies of the two hooks does not allow a good fit of the transverse hook on its bony support (Fig. 9-9). If that is the situation, the lumbar hook should be changed for a transverse hook that has the same blade but a reduced body (Fig. 9-10).

A pediculolaminar claw is used when it is impos-

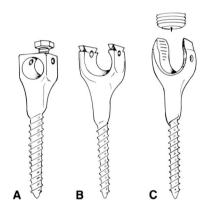

FIG. 9–7. Vertebral screws from the front: closed (**A**), open (**B**), and tulip screw (**C**).

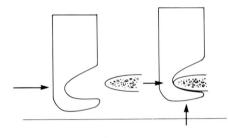

FIG. 9–5. The thoracic hook is gradually displaced away from the dura as insertion progresses.

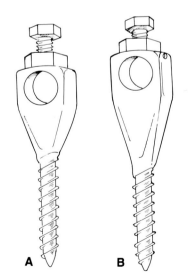

FIG. 9–8. Sacral screw with short (*left*) and long (*right*) neck.

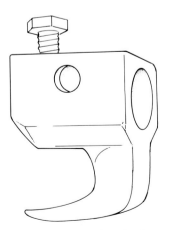

FIG. 9–6. Lumbar hook.

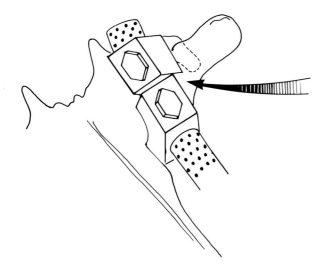

FIG. 9–9. Pediculotransverse claw with a lumbar hook on the superior rim of the transverse process. Notice the contact between the hook bodies before loading on the bony support (*arrow*).

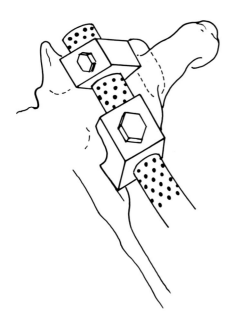

FIG. 9–10. Pediculotransverse claw with a reduced body hook.

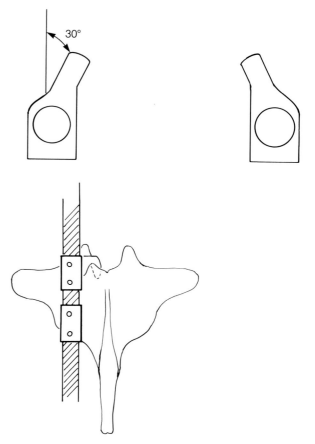

FIG. 9–11. Pediculolaminar claw.

sible to perform a pediculotransverse claw, mainly in the upper thoracic area (T1 or T2), where the transverse process is implanted too far laterally from the axis of the insertion of the pedicle hook. In this case, it is not possible to have a correct alignment of the two openings. To resolve this problem, my colleagues and I use a special thoracic hook with a reduced and displaced blade instead of a transverse hook (Fig. 9-11). Lumbar claws are produced by hooks or by a hook and screw.

To allow passage of the rod inside the supralaminar and infralaminar hooks, it is necessary to use special hooks with different body lengths if a hook claw is used on a single lamina. This is due to the obliquity of the lamina. The supralaminar hook should have a standard-length body. The infralaminar hook should be reduced. The claw is oblique, like the lamina, to optimize bony contact (Fig. 9-12). If both sides of the vertebra have to be instrumented by this kind of claw, blades should be progressively reduced in width.

A claw made with a hook and screw is difficult because the pedicle is lateral in relation to the lamina. Vertebral screws for this reason will not line up with a standard laminar hook. To introduce the rod in the vertebral screw and the laminar hook, the blade of the laminar hook needs to be more lateral in relation to the body of the hook than is the standard laminar hook.

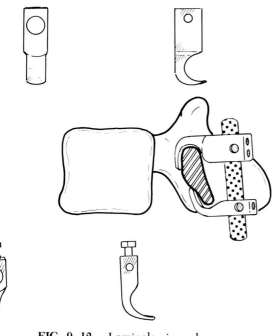

FIG. 9–12. Laminolaminar claw.

For a claw made with a vertebral screw and an infralaminar hook, the same vertebra can be instrumented if the body of the hook is reduced in height. The blade must be oblique to fit the inferior part of the lamina, which is also oblique (Fig. 9-13).

For a claw made with a vertebral screw and a supralaminar hook, the same vertebra cannot be instrumented, and the hook must be on the next cephalad vertebra. The blade should be lateral and anterior in relation to the body. This explains the special shape of the hook with its displaced body (Fig. 9-14).

Device for Transverse Traction

The device for transverse traction (DTT) is made of a threaded rod and four hooks, one fixed and three mobile. The grooves of the hooks are made so that they have a good anchorage on the closed rod when they are tightened, acting like a jaw.

One DTT at each extremity links the two rods. In

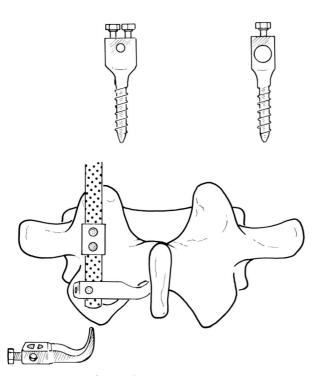

FIG. 9–13. Claw with screw and infralaminar hook.

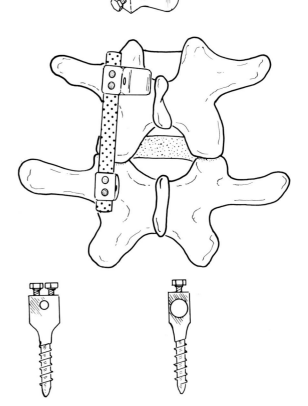

FIG. 9–14. Claw with screw and supralaminar hook.

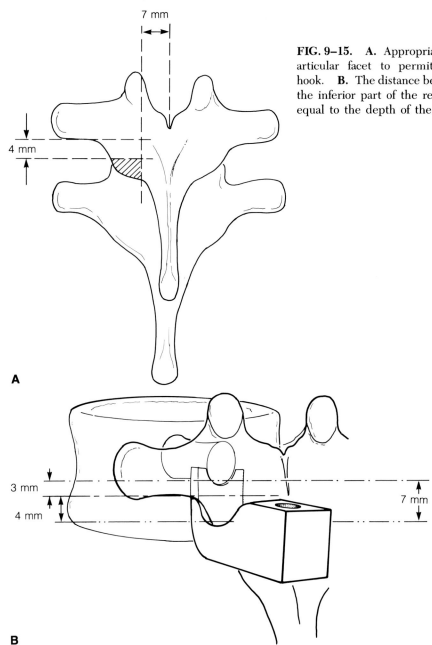

FIG. 9–15. **A.** Appropriate landmarks to remove a piece of inferior articular facet to permit adequate positioning of a pedicular hook. **B.** The distance between the inferior part of the pedicle and the inferior part of the remaining inferior articular facet must be equal to the depth of the hook blade from its base to the notch.

the lumbar area, it is best to contract the device, and in the sacral area, it is best to apply a distractive force with the device, thereby giving strong triangulation. In the thoracic area, the DTT should be neutral.

IMPLANT INSERTION
Pedicular Hook Implantation

In scoliosis a pedicular hook is used alone at the upper-end vertebra on the concave side in the mobile curve, at the upper-intermediate vertebra on the concave side, and at the apical vertebra on the convex side. Its implantation is possible from T1 to T10. Proper seating of a pedicular hook is crucial if it is to move the vertebrae in three dimensions. For example, in the frontal plane, it is possible to move the upper-end vertebra horizontally or to translate the upper-intermediate vertebra. In the sagittal plane, it is possible to move the superior intermediate vertebra on the concave side posteriorly or to push the apical vertebra on the convex side ventrally. These actions are essential to achieve derotation.

A portion of the inferior articular facet must be removed to introduce the bifid blade of the pedicular hook (Fig. 9-15). This is performed by two osteotomies, one longitudinal and one transverse. To achieve a safe implantation, it helps to remember the numbers 7 and 4.

There should be 7 mm between the longitudinal osteotomy and the axis of the spinous process. With fewer than 7 mm, one part of the blade may protrude inside the neural canal. A good point to begin the longitudinal osteotomy is usually the junction of the lamina with the inferior articular facet. This osteotomy must not be parallel to the axis of the body of the patient but to the axis of the spinous process.

Four is the number of millimeters between the transverse osteotomy and the inferior border of the transverse process. The distance between the inferior edge of the pedicle and the inferior border of the transverse process is almost constant (3 mm) at all levels. If more than 4 mm of inferior articular facet is left, the notch of the hook will not straddle the pedicle because the groove of the hook is 7 mm deep.

If more than 4 mm is removed, forward displacement of the hook's body is no longer prevented, increasing the possibility of nerve root entrapment. The transverse osteotomy must be parallel to the line joining the right angle of the longitudinal osteotomy. These two osteotomies allow the inferior end of the facet to be removed and permit visualization of the cartilage of the superior articular facet of the inferior vertebra.

The bifid pedicular elevator is then used to prepare the way of the blade toward the pedicle and to check the location (Fig. 9-16). This instrument must be used with great care. It is introduced in the interarticular space, not into the inferior articular facet. It must find its own way, sliding on the superior articular facet. If pushed in a too horizontal direction, it may bump against the inferior facet and weaken it. If pushed in a too vertical direction, it may break the upper facet and push a bony fragment in the spinal canal.

This elevator divides the anterior part of the facet joint capsule and then bumps against the pedicle. I check the grip by lateral translation (never by medial translation) of the tip of the pedicular elevator (Fig. 9-17). If the vertebra moves laterally when you translate the elevator, you are in the right place. If not, you are too far laterally or not enough inferior articular facet has been removed.

The pedicular hook is then inserted with the hook holder and the inserter. The horns of the hook are

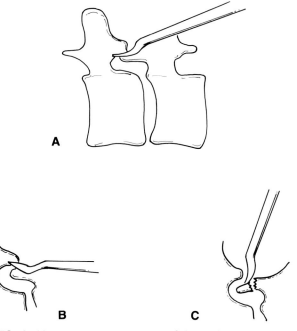

FIG. 9–16. **A.** Proper insertion of the pedicle elevator in the facet joint. **B.** Too horizontal introduction of the elevator with the risk of being inside the inferior articular facet. **C.** Too vertical introduction with the risk of breaking the superior articular facet.

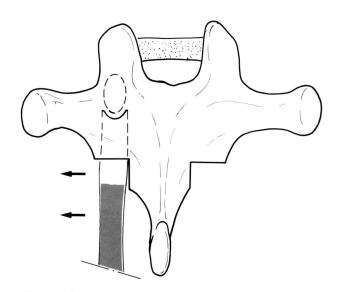

FIG. 9–17. Moving the vertebra laterally by lateral translation of the elevator tip proves that is is in place.

finally impacted into the larger posterior part of the pedicle by gentle tapping with a hammer.

Proper seating of the pedicular hook is attested to by the following points on the x-ray film (Fig. 9-18):

1. If there is no vertebral rotation, the hook is seen in the pedicle axis, and the blade is 1 or 2 mm below the image of the pedicle.
2. If there is still some vertebral rotation, the blade may be seen outside the body of the hook on the concavity or on the convexity.

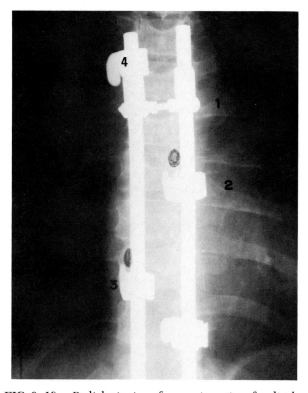

FIG. 9–18. Radiologic view of proper insertion of pedicular hook and pediculotransverse claw. Notice certain details for each hook. Hook number 1: no vertebral rotation, the hook is in the pedicle axis, and the body hides the blade. Hook number 2: remaining rotation in the concave side, the notch lies normally below the picture of the pedicle, and the blade is outside the body of the hook. Hook number 3: remaining rotation in the convex side, and as for hook number 2, the blade is outside the body of the hook. Hook number 4: in pediculotransverse claw, the body of the transverse hook protrudes medially in relation to the body of the pedicular hook, and the blade of the transverse hook is lateral to the pedicular hook.

Transverse Process Hook Implantation

A transverse hook must never be used alone. It is part of the pediculotransverse claw. In mobile scoliosis, this claw is used at the upper end on the convex side. In rigid scoliosis, if two rods on the concave side are used or if there is a kyphotic component, pediculotransverse claws must be used at the upper end on the convex and concave sides. In pure kyphosis, two claws are used on both sides and at least at two levels.

The transverse hook is inserted over the transverse process. The seat is prepared with a transverse elevator. Its sharp borders allow division of the costotransverse ligament. Room must be made with the elevator, especially medially, to provide alignment of the transverse hook with the pedicular one.

The pedicular hook is then inserted, following the same path as for an isolated implantation. Although the transverse and pedicular hooks are directed in different ways (i.e., the pedicular hook is sagittal; transverse is 30° outward), their bodies line up for the rod. The claw is obtained by approximating the two hooks using the hook compressor.

Because of the low height of the posterior arch of the vertebra, premature contact of the two body hooks sometimes occurs during the approximation, before a good loading of one hook on the bony support is obtained. In this case, a transverse hook with a reduced body should be used (Fig. 9-19).

In T1 or T2, the more lateral implantation of the transverse process does not allow transverse grip, and it must be changed for a pediculolaminar grip (i.e., the laminar hook has a reduced body and oblique blade).

On the x-ray film, the body of the transverse hook protrudes medially in relation to the body of the pedicular one, and the blade must be seen lateral to the pedicular hook (Fig. 9-18).

Laminar Hook Implantation

Laminar hook implantation can be done over the superior edge of the lamina or beneath its inferior edge, according to the direction of the forces the surgeon must apply.

Supralaminar insertion is used in scoliosis in the thoracic spine or in the lumbar spine. An infralaminar hook is used when pedicular implantation of a hook is not possible, usually below T10 on the convex side of

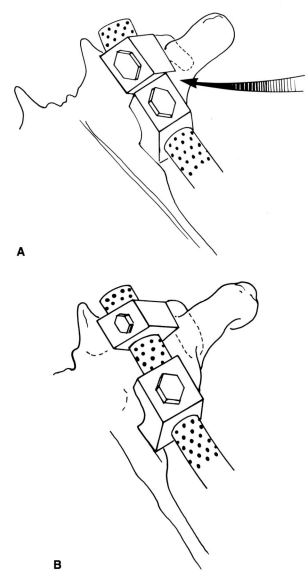

FIG. 9–19. **A.** Premature contact between pedicular and transverse body hooks, with bad contact (*arrow*) between the transverse process and the blade of the transverse hook. **B.** A reduced body transverse hook avoids this problem.

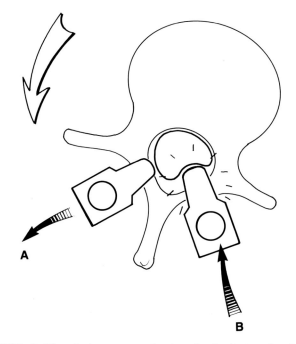

FIG. 9–20. Action on supralaminar hooks during the derotation as a function of their place on the rod. **A.** The hook is attracted backward; there is no risk. **B.** The hook is pushed forward, which can be dangerous.

any kind of curve and the inferior part of the apical claw on the convex side of a lumbar curve.

Thoracic and lumbar hooks are theoretically designed to be used at the thoracic and lumbar levels, respectively. The type of hook used depends on the action of the hook during the derotation maneuver (Fig. 9-20). Some hooks will be pulled backward (e.g., the lower intermediate vertebra on the concave side)

and present only minimal risk. A lumbar hook in this case may be sometimes used in the thoracic area. In other cases, hooks may be pushed forward with potential risk of neurologic injury from the blade of the hook in the canal. This situation may require a thoracic hook for a convex lumbar implantation.

Supralaminar insertion requires opening the ligamentum flavum. In the lumbar area, there is enough room to make the implantation without removing bone. In the thoracic area, the spinous process of the superior vertebra must be removed first. After the canal is opened, lateral extension is obtained by excising the medial part of the inferior articular facet of the superior vertebra. Removal of the superior articular facet should be avoided because it may weaken bony support of the hook.

Infralaminar insertion may lead to problems when improperly seated. Frequently, removal of one piece of the inferior border of the lamina is necessary for good positioning of the hook. Care must be taken to preserve the lateral wall of the inferior facet to avoid lateral dislodgment of the hook.

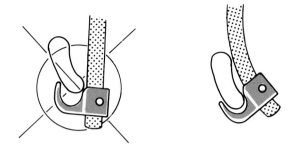

FIG. 9–21. Proper bending of the inferior part of the convex rod is needed for good positioning of the lower-end infralaminar hook.

The interspinous ligament and the facet joint capsule must be preserved when the hook is inserted on the lower-end vertebra of the curve. The inferior half of the lamina is not strictly frontal but oblique backward and downward. The blade of the hook must be parallel to this direction. If not, the tip of the blade will abut against the lamina, giving poor contact. To prevent that from happening, bending of the convex rod at its distal end is required (Fig. 9-21).

If two hooks have to be used on both sides of the same vertebra (e.g., the last vertebra in a kyphotic deformity), reduced blades must be used to avoid overlapping in the vertebral canal (Fig. 9-22).

On the lateral x-ray film, the more posterior and oblique position of the convex infralaminar hook in relation to the concave supralaminar can be seen (Fig. 9-23).

Vertebral Screw Implantation

Vertebral screws are used only in the lumbar area. Screws are immediately stable, unlike hooks that require a force. Each moment applied to the screw will

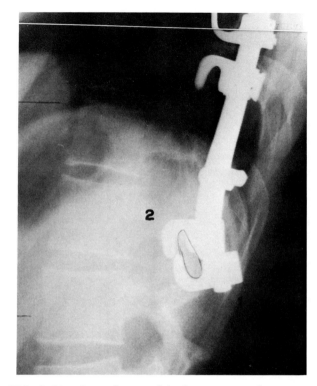

FIG. 9–23. Sagittal view of the bottom part of an instrumentation with infralaminar and supralaminar hooks. Both hooks are in contact with lamina. The infralaminar hook (1) is more posterior and oblique than the supralaminar hook (2).

be transmitted to the vertebra; this is particularly true if the vertebra is instrumented by two vertebral screws linked by an interpedicular plate (Fig. 9-24). The direction of the vertebral screw is the same as the direction of the pedicle (Fig. 9-25).

In the sagittal plane, the L3 pedicle is usually horizontal (i.e., neutral to the head and foot). The pedicle

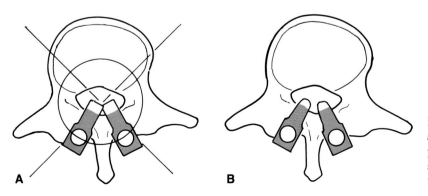

FIG. 9–22. **A.** When two laminar hooks are inserted on the same lamina, overlapping of the blade may occur if a standard size is used. **B.** This is prevented by using a reduced blade.

above is in an cephalad direction, and the pedicle below is in a caudad direction. This is confirmed by a sagittal preoperative x-ray film or, during surgery, by checking the line joining the posterior part of the superior and articular facet that is at a right angle with the pedicle.

In the coronal plane, the screws converge toward the midline, because the pedicles are oriented with an inward direction that increases from L1 to L5 (from 5° to 25°). Furthermore, when two screws on either side of the vertebra are convergent, resistance to pull-out is more than if they are parallel.

In order to give the best orientation to the screw, its point of introduction must be carefully chosen. It is on a line joining the middle of the two transverse processes at the bottom part of the superior articular facet, lateral to the interfacet joint.

A precise and safe technique for implantation is necessary to achieve good positioning of the screw, whatever the anatomic configuration of the spine. Using a motor drill to find the direction of the pedicle in a scoliotic spine is quite dangerous. The following technique gives us satisfaction in every case. A piece of cortical bone is removed from the bottom of the superior articular facet, allowing us to see the spongy bone for the point of introduction of the screw. A conical curette is manipulated very gently in the direction of the pedicle. A distinct feeling and noise made by the curette turning in the spongy bone of the pedicle and the vertebral body helps to find the way.

If any resistance to the progression occurs or if any doubt exists, we check by using a firm K wire or depth gauge, which must find bone all around and at bottom. This wire also expresses the length of the screws. The

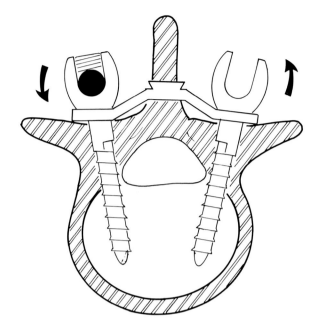

FIG. 9–24. Extremely solid grip on the vertebra by two screws linked by a plate allows better derotation.

anterior cortex of the vertebral body may be reached but should not be penetrated. The diameter of the screw is chosen before the surgery. The upper disc may be damaged if the direction of the screw is too oblique. The nerve root may be damaged if the insertion is too low or if the direction is inferior (Fig. 9-26).

Sacral Screw Implantation

Double sacral screwing is the most solid construct for implantation (Fig. 9-27). The L5 inferior facet is re-

FIG. 9–25. **A.** Screws must be convergent in the transverse plane. **B.** Points of introduction of the screws.

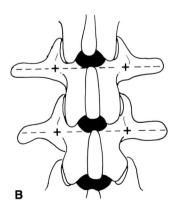

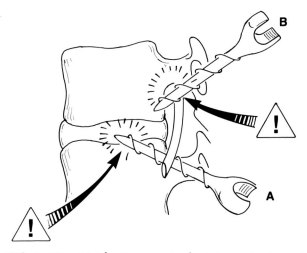

FIG. 9–26.   Mistakes in screw implantation.   **A.** Screw is too oblique upward and may damage the subjacent disc.   **B.** Screw is too oblique downward (or too low) and may damage the nerve root.

moved first to identify the sacral facet. The first screw has its point of insertion 2 mm above the middle of the cartilaginous sacral facet. The second one is introduced 7 mm below and 7 mm outward from the first screw.

In the sagittal plane, the screws are parallel to the sacral plateau. In the coronal plane, the first screw is medially directed. The second one is laterally directed, 20° to 30° outward. Too much obliquity of the second screw drives it into the sacroiliac space. The triangular construct gives better resistance to pull-out forces. A special guide allows correct positioning of the second screw after insertion of the first one and allows good alignment of the channels of the screw heads. A short-neck screw for the sagittal plane and a long-neck screw for the oblique allows proper alignment.

Iliosacral Screw Implantation

The iliosacral screw can be very useful in cases of osteoporotic bone or for a salvage procedure after a failed previous fixation using sacral screws (Fig. 9-28).

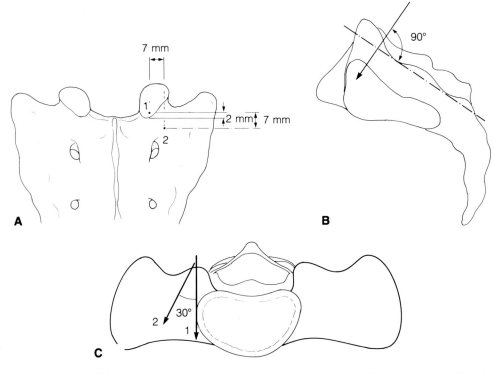

FIG. 9–27.   Double sacral screw fixation.   **A.** Point of introduction of the upper screw (1) and the lower screw (2).   **B.** Both screws are at right angles with the upper third of the sacrum.   **C.** The upper screw (1) is sagittal or slightly medial; the lower screw (2) is laterally directed.

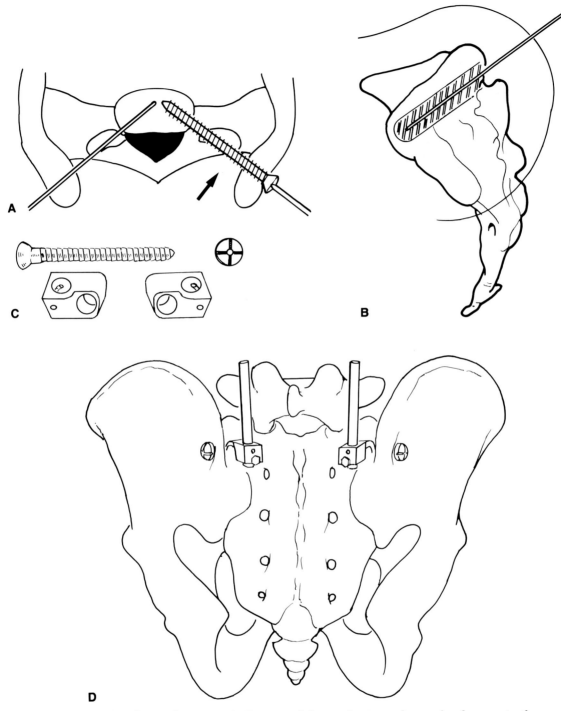

FIG. 9–28. Iliosacral screw. **A.** Position of the guidewire and cannulated screw in the transverse plane. **B.** The wire is directed slightly upward in the sagittal plane. **C.** Rod-screw connector. **D.** Rod-screw and connector in place.

Compression or distraction forces can be applied on this screw, and its lateral position is useful in cases of pelvic obliquity.

The screw, which is cannulated, is inserted on a guidewire using an x-ray film for direction. This guide is introduced on the outer cortex of the iliac wing, near the inferior linea gluteal, and is directed in such a way that it enters the sacrum at the bottom of the articular facet of S1 and is parallel or slightly converging toward the sacral plateau. Frontal and lateral x-ray films of the positioning of the wire are absolutely necessary before a trephine prepares the way for the screw. The screw penetrates the iliac wing. When the top of the screw appears in the sacroiliac space, the wire is temporarily withdrawn and a rod screw connector system is positioned before screwing continues.

IMPLANT INSERTION GUIDELINES

Most of the implants can be immediately positioned on the spine after their site of implantation has been prepared. This is not the case for intracanal hooks, which must be inserted only before rod introduction. Careful facet joint decortication must be carried out before the rod has been positioned.

The rod has to be contoured in a harmonious manner, usually according to the ideal sagittal plane. During the introduction and rotation of the rod, the im-

plants must remain in position. There is always potential danger with an intracanal hook and potential danger of breakage of the bony support if a hook becomes dislodged.

When introducing a rod in an open hook by using the rod introducer, be sure that the hook is well seated. There should be less than 10 mm between it and the rod (Fig. 9-29).

If a blocker is forced into an open forward-tilted hook, the opening may become wider and interfere with fixation. The hook must be adjusted to the blocker by means of a compressor clamp. By doing this, the hook displaces away from the bone; it should be immediately loaded again (Fig. 9-30).

No derotation maneuver should be carried out before the surgeon is sure that the rod can move freely through the implants.

Loading of the implants must be in a precise order, remembering that loading one hook unloads the ones placed in the same direction (Fig. 9-31).

Fixation and blocking of a hook on the rod is accomplished by tightening the bolt until its head breaks. This is done only after normal evoked potentials are seen or after the wake-up test. Tighten the bolt in its axis to avoid bending, premature breakage, and inefficient fixation. Bending may also occur during the spreading maneuver if care is not taken to screw the bolt on the side of the concavity of the blade first (Fig. 9-32).

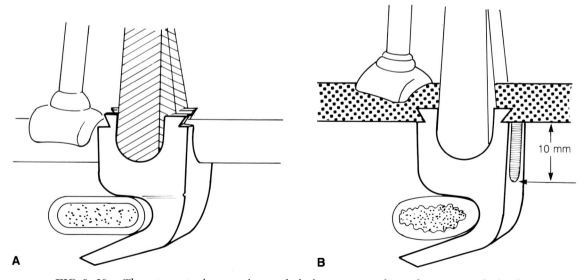

FIG. 9–29. These two mistakes must be avoided when using a rod introducer. **A.** The hook is not seated well. **B.** The distance between the rod and hook is more than 10 mm.

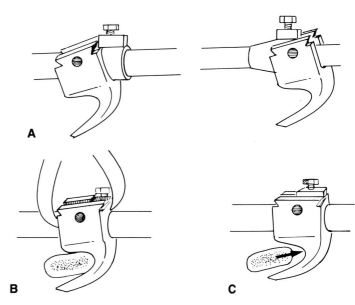

FIG. 9–30. **A.** Bad technique for forcing a blocker into an open hook. **B.** The correct way to do it, by approximation with a clamp. **C.** Do not forget to load the hook again after the maneuver.

This instrumentation gives some three-dimensional correction and a solid construct, reducing the need for external support. The long-term stability is accomplished by the fusion. The aim of the treatment is to restore a spinal balance in the frontal and sagittal planes. The surgical treatment deals with many factors:

1. Three-dimensional geometric analysis of the deformity
2. Stiffness of the main curve including structural factors such as disc, bony deformity, synostosis, and rib cage deformity
3. The forces applied with the instrumentation to correct the deformity according to the geometric analysis, limited by the structural factors
4. The new position of the corrected segment and the possibility to balance the trunk with the mobile segments
5. Frontal and sagittal balance to determine the length of the instrumented area

Principles of Instrumentation

1. Because the instrumentation acts on the posterior column, applying distraction should cause kyphosis and compression should cause lordosis.[1]
2. Rotation of the contoured rod mobilizes the apical zone medially and posteriorly to restore the kyphosis in the thoracic area and anteriorly and

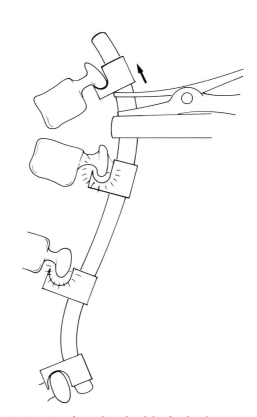

FIG. 9–31. Loading of one hook loads a hook in an opposite direction but unloads a hook in the same direction.

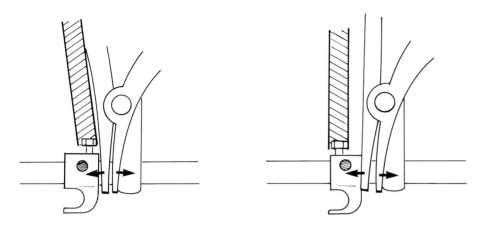

FIG. 9–32. To avoid tilting the hex screwdriver and the screw while loading the hook, first screw the bolt on the concave side of the blade.

medially in the lumbar area to restore lordosis and sagittal alignment. The rod is inserted on the concave side in the thoracic area, where a combination of distraction and posterior rotation of the rod restores kyphosis. In the lumbar area, the rod is inserted on the convex side, where a combination of compression and anterior rotation of the contoured rod restores frontal and sagittal balance.

3. Both sides of the posterior column are instrumented at end vertebrae and at the intermediate vertebra at different areas. The concave and convex rods are contoured differently to increase possibilities of correction.

4. The transverse system stabilizes the two rods on each end on the construct and increases the strength.

Determination of the Strategic Vertebrae

It is necessary only to instrument the strategic vertebrae. To determine these, we analyze the frontal and sagittal long standing films, bending films of the main and adjacent curves in the front plane, and bending films of the junctional zone in the sagittal plane (flexion, extension).[13]

Apical Zone
The apical zone is the stiffest zone of the deformity. On the convex bending film, the discs are still closed on the concave side (two or three spaces). The limits of the area are the upper and lower intermediate vertebrae. The apical vertebra is the most rotated and the most horizontal vertebra. Its lateral border is perpendicular

to the floor. In the lumbar spine, the apex may be a disc space.

End Vertebra
The first, temporary determination of the end vertebrae is made on the basis of standing and bending x-ray films, but the definitive choice is always made on the basis of sagittal films. The lower-end vertebra must be in the stable zone of Harrington on the concave bending films. The Harrington zone is that area defined by two parallel vertical lines from the lumbosacral facets. The end vertebra must be neutral on concave bending films in immature patients but can be mildly rotated in adults. The disc below the end vertebrae should be open on both sides on the bending x-ray films.

The definitive choice of the end vertebra is done with a sagittal x-ray film. If the lower vertebra determined in the frontal plane is at the apex of a junctional kyphosis, the instrumentation must be extended lower, and the hook is reversed to compress the kyphosis to restore the sagittal alignment and avoid decompensation. On the basis of a frontal x-ray film, the instrumentation is extended to the next neutral vertebra.

Upper-End Vertebra
The upper-end vertebra is the upper, neutral vertebra demonstrated on the frontal x-ray film. If there is an upper structural thoracic curve with a high shoulder and an oblique T1 to the convexity of the lower thoracic curve, the instrumentation must include this curve. In the sagittal plane, the instrumentation is extended superiorly if the upper vertebra is at the apex and hyperkyphosis exists.

STRATEGY FOR TYPICAL CASES

Thoracic Lordoscoliosis

In mobile thoracic lordoscoliosis, the concave side is instrumented first (Fig. 9-33).

1. The site of the hooks is prepared, and the inferior facets on the noninstrumented area are removed.
2. The end vertebrae and intermediate hooks in the concave area are positioned.
3. The rod is contoured according to the sagittal alignment on the instrumented area.
4. The rod is introduced in the upper and inferior closed hooks and on the intermediate hooks by means of the blockers.
5. The intermediate hooks are secured to the vertebrae by applying distraction and stabilized with a C-ring.
6. The rod is progressively rotated with gentle movements. The intermediate hooks sometimes have to be reseated.

7. The rod is rotated well past the neutral position, and the hooks are reseated by means of applying gentle distraction and secured to the rod; the C-rings are then removed.
8. This convex rod is contoured at each extremity with less contour in the intermediate zone to increase the derotating effect on the apical vertebra by pushing it forward.
9. The convex rod is introduced first in the upper pediculotransverse grip that is secured to the rod. The application of distraction on the apical hook causes a compression between the upper vertebrae and the apex.
10. The rod is pushed to the spine with the inferior hook on it. The inferior hook is pushed under the lamina with the blocker pusher. Proper bending of this rod, parallel to the inferior part of the lamina (often requiring further lordotic contouring), is important. If the rod is not parallel, progression of the hook will be stopped before its proper seating with a risk of early pull-out. Once engaged, compression can be applied on this hook. After somatosensory evoked potential monitoring and wake-up tests are done, decortication is achieved, preserving the spinous process for morphologic examination. Autogenous bone grafting from the iliac crest is applied.
11. The cross-links are applied to the system, one at each extremity. The fixed DTT hook is placed on the convex rod first, and the corresponding hooks are tightened until they are bent. The concave rod is secured in the same manner, and neutralization or slight approximation is achieved. Closure with subcutaneous aspirative drainage is performed. If there is a junctional kyphosis, the plan is different at the inferior portion of the curve (Fig. 9-34).

Lumbar Scoliosis[7]

The general principles remain the same. The convex side is instrumented first to restore the lordosis. The two intermediate convex hooks are convergent and are stabilized with the C-ring. The convex rod is rotated ventrally and medially. All the hooks are secured by means of compression. The concave rod is then inserted. An intermediate hook is not systematically used. The hooks are not in a good position to achieve

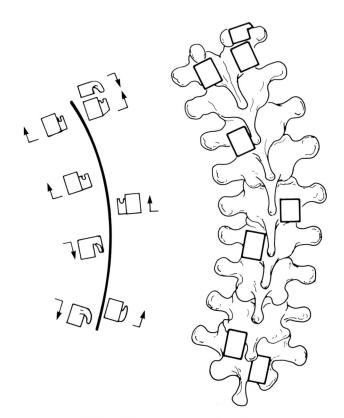

FIG. 9–33. Thoracic lordoscoliosis.

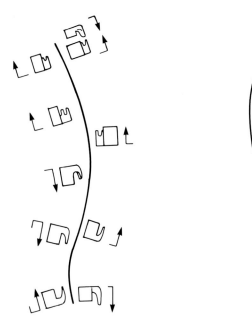

FIG. 9–34. Thoracic lordoscoliosis with junctional kyphosis, seen from the frontal plane (*left*) and the sagittal plane (*right*). The instrumentation is reversed at the bottom part of the curve.

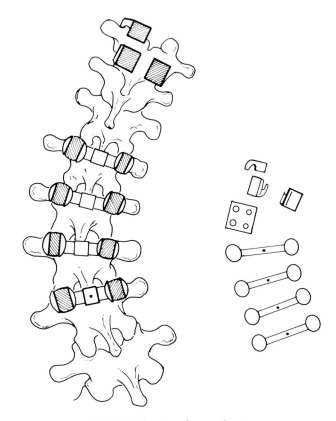

FIG. 9–35. Lumbar scoliosis.

derotation because they are too close to the spinous process, and the spine does not follow the movement of the hooks. In fact, with this instrumentation, there is a good realignment of the spine in the frontal and sagittal planes, but the rotation is not corrected and the anterior column remains laterally positioned. A better three-dimensional correction is achieved using bilateral vertebral screws with transverse plates at each lumbar level (Fig. 9-35).

With this kind of fixation, the first stage is performed on the convex side with the same rotation of the contoured rod, but this rod is fixed only on each extremity.

The concave rod is inserted in the same vertebrae and introduced to the intermediate screws with the rod introducer or double-threaded screws (Fig. 9-36). Frontal alignment is achieved with adequate compression and concave and convex corrective force at each level.

Double-Major Curves

A combination of the strategies for thoracic and lumbar areas is used with one long S-shaped rod. The rod is placed on the concavity of the thoracic curve and the convexity of the lumbar curve. It is inserted into the

closed hooks placed on the extremities, two intermediate divergent open hooks on the concave thoracic curve, two intermediate convergent hooks on the convex lumbar curve, and sometimes one hook at the transitional vertebra (Fig. 9-37).

After securing the intermediate hooks with a C-ring, the S-shaped rod is rotated, restoring thoracic kyphosis and lumbar lordosis in one maneuver (Fig.

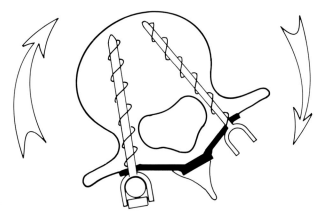

FIG. 9–36. Lumbar scoliosis (transverse plane).

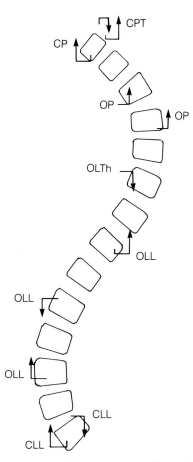

FIG. 9–37. Double-major curve (frontal plane).

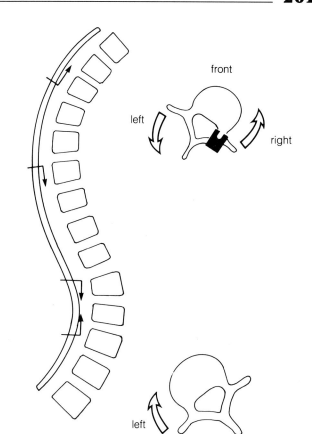

FIG. 9–38. Double-major curve viewed in the sagittal plane (*left*) and the transverse plane (*right*).

9-38). On the opposite side, the rod is placed in the instrumented vertebrae of the thoracic curve and in the junctional vertebrae between the two curves. For a long spine, three DTT must be applied, two extremes and one intermediate, the last one applying corrective force.

Double Thoracic Curves[13]

When two thoracic curves must be instrumented, it is not possible to correct the deformity by rotation of one rod.[8] In this condition, the lower curve is corrected first with a rod 2 cm longer cephalad to insert a connecting tube. The tube allows a connection with a rod inserted in a pediculotransverse grip on the convex side of the upper curve. Sometimes a common pedicular grip is used at T1 or T2.

One long rod with a proper contour is inserted in the superior hook on the concave upper thoracic curve. This rod is inserted into the pediculotransverse grip in

the vertebrae between the two curves, then the apical vertebra of the lower curve, and then the inferior convex vertebra.

If the upper thoracic curve is long, another possibility is to correct the concavity of the upper curve with the usual four hooks and rod rotation. Then connect the convexity of one curve to the concavity of the other curve with a domino.

Rigid Curves

If the curve is severe and rigid, it is not possible to correct it by rotation of a contoured rod in the thoracic area. Instead, the two-concave-rod technique may be used. It consists of mobilizing the apex by approximating between a short, concave apical rod and a long, contoured concave rod (Fig. 9-39).

The short rod is as short as possible. The three or four apical vertebrae are spanned by a rod between a closed pedicular and a closed laminar hook. There is no

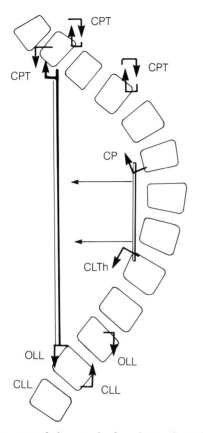

FIG. 9–39. Rigid thoracic lordoscoliosis (frontal plane).

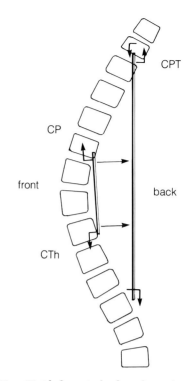

FIG. 9–40. Rigid thoracic lordoscoliosis (sagittal plane).

need to try to derotate the short rod because the amount of derotation is the same between the different vertebrae. The short rod allows the medial and posterior translation of the apical zone.

The long, concave rod is contoured according to the sagittal plane and placed straight in the frontal plane. To avoid any translation, it must be secured at the upper part with a pediculotransverse grip and in the lower part, leaving the rod long enough to abut against the spinous process. A better grip is a claw on two adjacent vertebrae. The short rod can be approximated to the long rod by two DTT. The long rod must be free to move. Gentle distraction is applied on each extremity of the long rod (Fig. 9-40).

Convex instrumentation includes two pediculotransverse grips, one for the upper vertebra and a second grip two or three levels below. The lower grip is made with a claw on two adjacent vertebrae.

There is no apical convex hook because in these cases it does not improve the correction and, because it can be pushed inside the canal, may be dangerous.

Because of the deformity, it is generally difficult to bend the rod. It is easier to prebend it partly, then insert it in the two upper grips and adapt the shape of the rod to the spine with the in situ rod benders. The elasticity of the rod is used to improve the correction at the time of the insertion of the inferior claw. Two DTT should be used to apply corrective force to the long rods on each extremity.

Severe Double-Major Curves

Severe double-major curves can be instrumented with a long S-shaped rod, using the rotation of the rod for the lumbar area with two intermediate lumbar hooks. For the thoracic, stiffest part, approximation between a short concave rod and the long rod is done. On the convex side, the upper grip is accomplished with two pediculotransverse claws in the upper thoracic, one hook in the lower thoracic, upper lumbar area and one supralaminar lumbar for the inferior grip. Proper bending of the rod is adapted to the spine with the rod benders. Three DTT connect the long rods.

Figures 9-41 through 9-48 illustrate the following
(*text continues on page 209*)

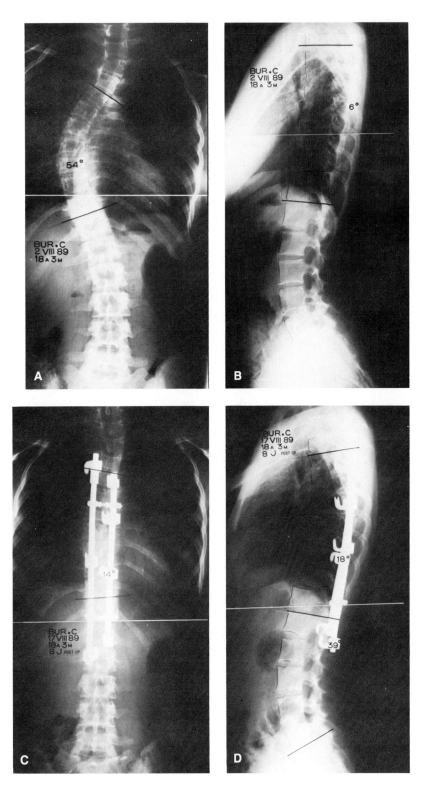

FIG. 9–41. These radiographs reveal a right thoracic lordoscoliosis of 54° and hypokyphosis of 6°. Correction in both frontal and sagittal planes with restoration of thoracic kyphosis was accomplished by rotation of the concave rod, as shown on the anterior-posterior x-ray film.

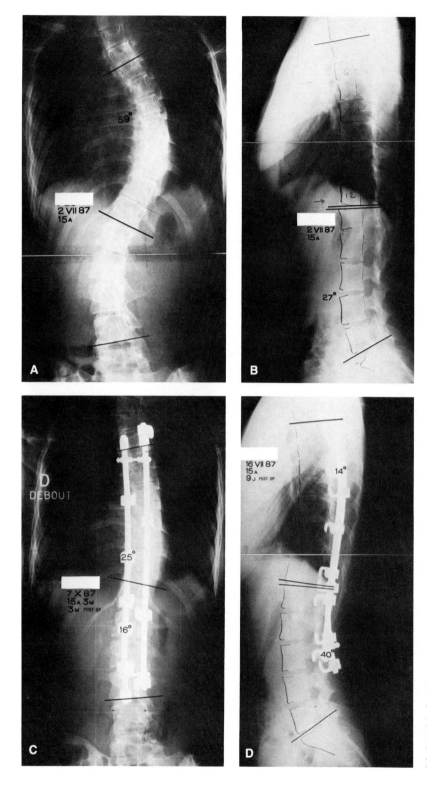

FIG. 9–42. This patient had a thoracic lordoscoliosis with a secondary structural curve and a junctional kyphosis. Fusion was performed down to L3 with reverse instrumentation in the lumbar area. Notice restoration of the sagittal alignment with thoracic kyphosis and lumbar lordosis.

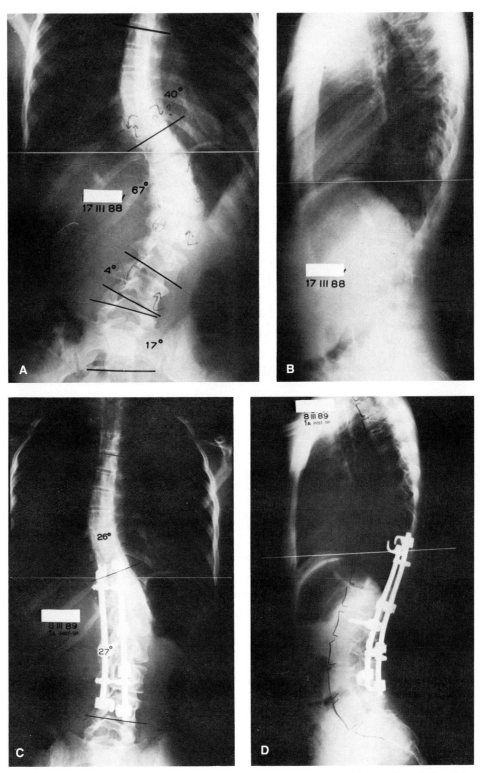

FIG. 9–43. This patient had a lumbar scoliosis of 67°. Fusion was performed from T10 to L4, with rotation of the convex rod first. Good frontal and sagittal alignment was obtained, but no correction of rotation was achieved.

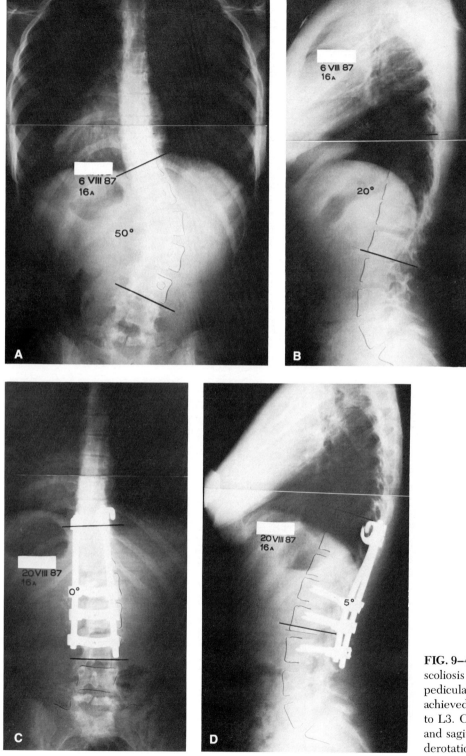

FIG. 9–44. These films illustrate lumbar scoliosis correction with screws and interpedicular plate. Better derotation can be achieved. Fusion was performed from T10 to L3. Complete correction of the frontal and sagittal plane was accomplished with derotation.

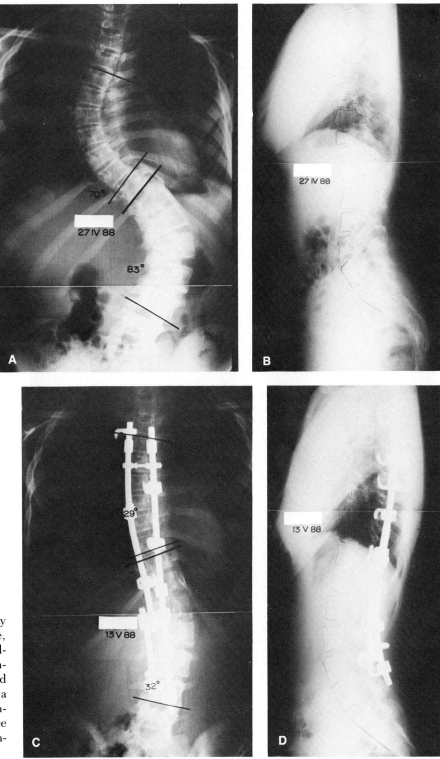

FIG. 9–45. Anterior-posterior x-ray films illustrate a double-major curve, right thoracic curve with thoracic lordosis, and left lumbar curve with lumbar kyphosis. Correction was achieved with a concave thoracic rod and then a convex lumbar rod. The concave lumbar rod is joined by a domino. Notice improvement of the sagittal alignment.

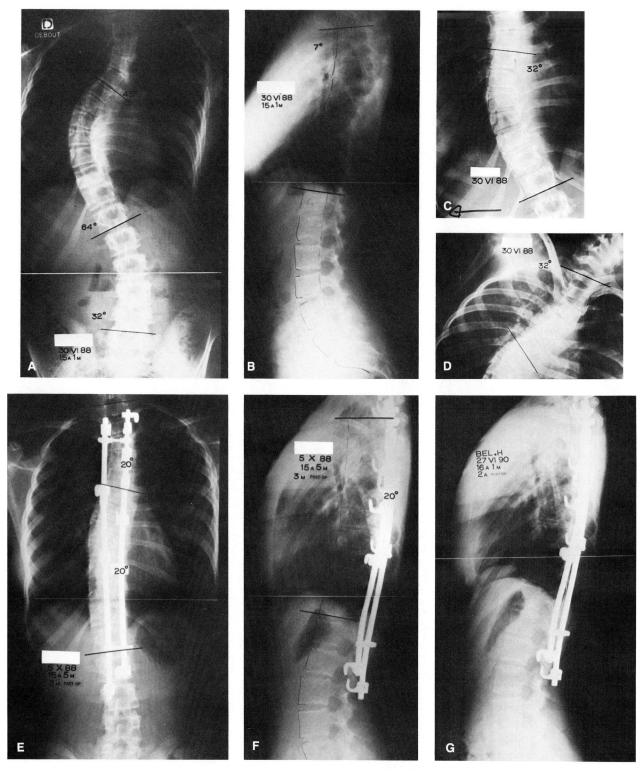

FIG. 9–46. **A, B.** Anterior-posterior view of a right thoracic lordoscoliosis and a structural left thoracic curve. **C, D.** Notice correction on the convex bending film of the two curves. **E, F.** Correction of the main thoracic curve was achieved by concave rod rotation and connection with an axial connector for the upper curve. A long contoured rod was used for both curves on the right side. **G, H.** The 2-year follow-up films.

208

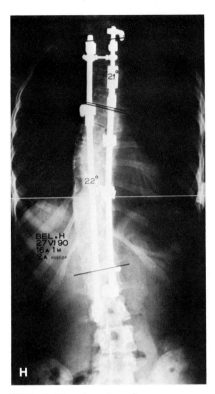

FIG. 9–46.   (*continued*)

conditions: thoracic lordoscoliosis (Fig. 9-41), thoracic lordoscoliosis with a junctional kyphosis (Fig. 9-42), lumbar scoliosis treated with and without pedicle screws (Figs. 9-43 and 9-44), double-major scoliosis (Fig. 9-45), double-thoracic scoliosis (Fig. 9-46), double-major scoliosis with thoracic lordosis and lumbar kyphosis (Fig. 9-47), and rigid, severe kyphoscoliosis (Fig. 9-48).

POSTOPERATIVE CARE

The patient should stay supine for the first hours to facilitate hemostasis. Standing is usually possible without any external support.

The adolescent patient is allowed to swim and go back to school at the end of the first month. A delay of 1 year is requested before resumption of strenuous activ-

ity. The stability of the construct allows these guidelines even for severe curves.

COMPLICATIONS

Septic Complications[12]

Difficulties with instrumentation requiring many manipulations and the dead space created by the volume of implants can increase the risk of infection. To diminish this risk, adequate preoperative planning is necessary to save intraoperative time. The bone grafting must be adequate to fill the dead space created by the implants. Subcutaneous closed drainage helps reduce hematoma.

Neurologic Complications

Neuropathy can be caused by the implants. This can happen with a supralaminar hook that is displaced into the canal. It must be secured and checked carefully until the rod stabilizes it, particularly during rod introduction. The anterior-posterior forces applied on the hook during the correcting maneuvers are important. In the thoracic area, the intermediate laminar hook is pulled backward and moves away the cord. In the lumbar area, however, this intermediate hook is pushed forward, and it is generally better to use the thoracic laminar hook to avoid any protrusion into the canal. For the same reason, the apical convex hook must always be a pedicular hook and not a laminar one.

If two adjacent laminar hooks are used on the same vertebra, one must use a reduced blade to avoid overlapping and narrowing of the canal.

During realignment of the spine, theoretically, no distraction is applied, avoiding elongation of the cord. However, during correction of the spine deformity, careful monitoring of the neurologic state, using evoked potentials and wake-up tests, is mandatory.

STRATEGIC MISTAKES

The surgeon must analyze simultaneously the frontal and sagittal plane, remembering that the final decision is determined by the sagittal plane and the instrumentation must never be stopped at the apex of a kyphosis.[1,2]

(*text continues on page 212*)

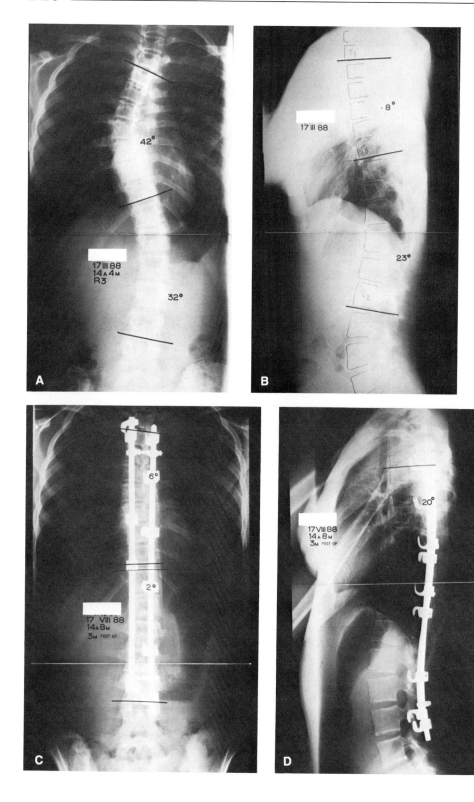

FIG. 9–47. Anterior-posterior view of moderate thoracic and lumbar curves in the frontal plane but severe thoracic lordosis and thoracolumbar kyphosis. Correction of the curves in both planes was achieved by rotation of a concave thoracic and convex lumbar rod. Notice thoracic apical correction and convex contraction.

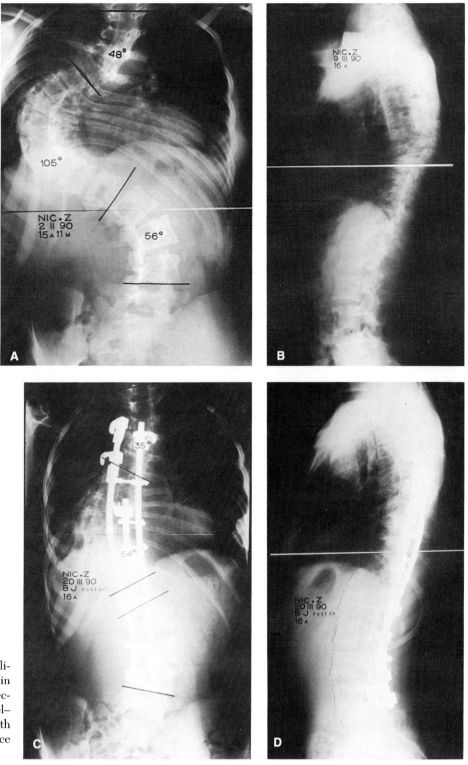

FIG. 9–48. Severe kyphoscoliosis. The surgery was performed in stages—anterior thoracic discectomies followed by posterior Cotrel–Dubousset instrumentation with the three-rod technique. No brace was used postoperatively.

PEDIATRIC COTREL–DUBOUSSET INSTRUMENTATION SYSTEM

CHRISTIAN MORIN

In some conditions, the volume of the standard Cotrel–Dubousset instrumentation is too large. Bone or soft tissue atrophy or the small size of the patients mandates reduced instrumentation—the pediatric instrumentation. The pediatric rod is 5 mm in diameter, whereas the standard rod is 7 mm. Hooks, screws, blockers, and DTT jaws are also reduced. Ancillary instrumentation must also be modified to fit the smaller implants.

Pediatric instrumentation may be used in two different ways:

1. In the definitive way, the instrumentation is associated with spinal fusion because the bone age is mature.
2. In the temporary way, instrumentation is carried out without spinal fusion and acts as an internal orthosis. Very limited subperiosteal exposure is necessary. Of course, the heads of the bolts fixing the rod and implants are not broken as in the definitive technique, so that they can be unscrewed and rescrewed after manipulations during the period of growth.

DEFINITIVE METHOD

It is quite unusual to have to use the pediatric set for an adolescent idiopathic scoliosis. Usually when the bone age is mature enough for an arthrodesis, the posterior elements of the spine and the soft tissues around them are large enough to allow the use of standard instrumentation. However, if the surgeon must use pediatric instrumentation in a case, it is better to use a special cold-drawn 5-mm rod, which has intermediate resistance between the standard and pediatric rods (Fig. 9-49).

The standard rod is more adapted than the pediatric rod to resist torsional forces during the derotation maneuver, which is the usual way to correct adolescent idiopathic scoliosis. The standard rod also better supports the weight of an adolescent. My colleagues and I use 30 kg as the upper weight limit for absolute security of the pediatric rod. This is less than the average weight of an adolescent with idiopathic scoliosis.

Bone and soft tissue atrophy in adolescents is more often seen in neuromuscular, mesenchymal, or osteochondrodystrophic disorders, especially after a very long orthopedic treatment has been carried out.

Some of these scoliosis curves are still mobile enough to be corrected by derotation. The strategy and the postoperative care in these cases are the same with pediatric instrumentation as with the standard set (Fig. 9-50).

Some cases treated with pediatric instrumentation can be much more difficult to manage. The curves are larger and stiffer. Spinal arthrodesis takes place at the end of a very long orthotic treatment. Vital capacity may be severely restricted, and preparation by halo traction may be needed. Two-rod techniques, instrumentation by claws, and postoperative protection by brace for 3 months are required in these severely deformed and osteoporotic spines (Fig. 9-51).

The versatility of Cotrel–Dubousset instrumentation allows many possibilities. It is easy to associate standard and pediatric instrumentation with special connecting systems (e.g., axial tubes or dominos). This can be helpful in neuromuscular disorders. In the lumbar and lumbosacral area, it is safer to use standard instrumentation. Soft tissue atrophy is rarely a problem at this level, where the instrumentation will be deeply located in the lordosis. In the thoracic area, we sometimes have to deal with atrophy. As the mechanical solicitation at this level is less important, it is quite possible to use pediatric instrumentation (Fig. 9-52).

TEMPORARY METHOD

The temporary method described here is investigational. The first trials were performed in 1986 at the Institut Calot in France, using the standard pediatric rod with a diamond-shaped surface. Strategic vertebrae were instrumented, taking care to expose the bony structures just enough to fit them with the implants. The rods were inserted in a transmuscular or subcutaneous way. These initial trials were disappointing, however. During the second approach 6 months later, fibrous tissue embedded the diamond-shaped rod to hold the implants; exposure was much more difficult than during the first surgery, and manipulation was quite impossible. For this reason, the pediatric rod has been modified with resin. This provides a smooth

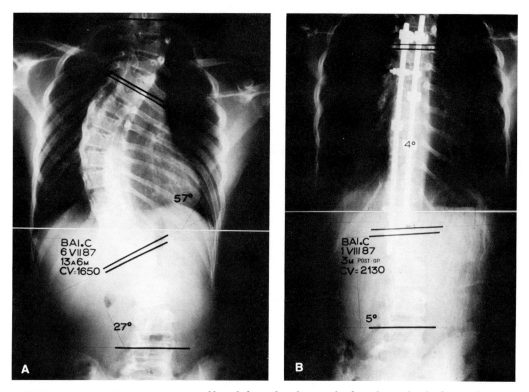

FIG. 9–49. **A.** Preoperative x-ray film of idiopathic thoracic lordoscoliosis that had never been treated in a 13 + 6-year-old boy with the same bone age. Notice the small posterior elements on the frontal x-ray film. **B.** Postoperative x-ray film showing good correction in frontal and transverse plane despite some deformity occurring in the concave rod during the derotation maneuver. It was impossible to use standard hooks.

surface to the rod without precluding strong anchorage of the hook on the rod. Even with this modification, if great care is not taken during the hook implantation, too much fibrosis may develop with time, causing a tethered effect that can be worse than the natural history of the scoliosis.

For this reason we recommend that if an indication for temporary instrumentation is present, only the hemiposterior arch of the two end vertebrae on the concave side be dissected. External orthotic support is necessary with this instrumentation. We have found two advantages for this temporary system:

1. A pediculotransverse grip at the upper part and a laminolaminar grip at the bottom part of the curve allow better stability.
2. Facility and efficiency in obtaining more tension

of the device is accomplished by means of a connecting system (Fig. 9-53).

This is a difficult technique, and many reoperations through the growth period are performed until fusion is possible. It must be reserved for patients for whom orthopedic treatment alone is inefficient or badly tolerated.

Our major concern is that even with a minimal surgical approach, scar tissue develops in the concavity of the scoliosis. As the anterior column of the spine keeps on growing, a "crankshaft" phenomenon develops, as it can after early posterior spinal fusion. To avoid this problem, the temporary instrumentation should be associated with a convex anterior epiphysiodesis.

(text continues on page 217)

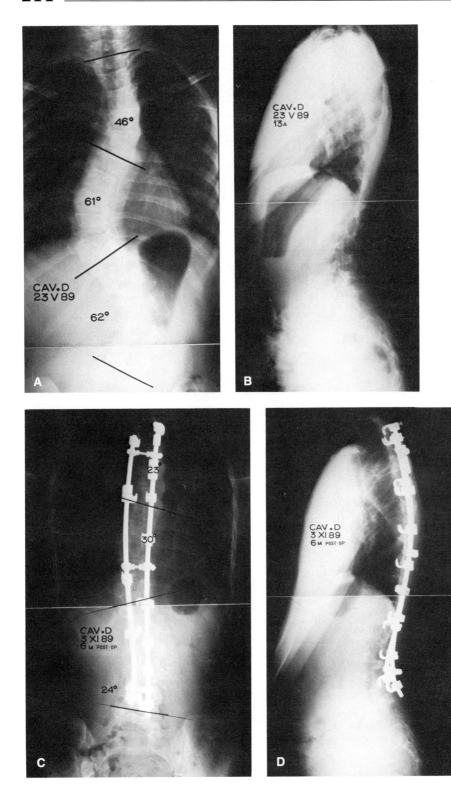

FIG. 9–50. A, B. Preoperative x-ray films of scoliosis in a patient with Ehlers-Danlos syndrome. Slight kyphosis is seen at the junction of the two major curves (low thoracic and lumbar). Shoulder sign is seen in relation to a high thoracic curve. C, D. Postoperative x-ray films showing correction obtained by posterior derotation of the low thoracic spine and anterior derotation of the lumbar spine using the same rod on the left side of the spine (concavity of the low thoracic curve and convexity of the lumbar curve). Extension to the high thoracic curve was achieved by connecting a short rod to the lower spine to correct the shoulder level. Only one rod is used on the other side to stabilize the spine.

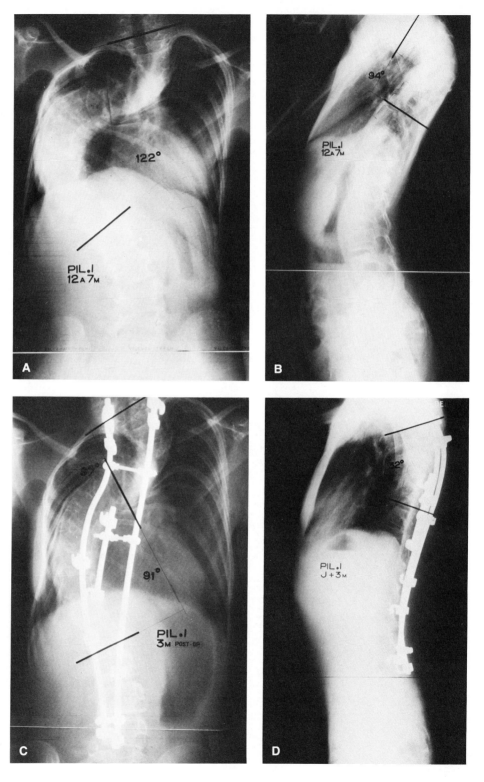

FIG. 9–51. **A, B.** Preoperative x-ray films show severe scoliosis with a high thoracic kyphosis at the junction of the two major thoracic curves after 10 years of brace treatment and 3 weeks of halo wheel chair traction. **C, D.** Postoperative x-ray films show correction obtained by translation of a small rod toward the long concave rod by means of one device for transverse traction. Notice the bilateral pediculotransverse grip at the upper part of the instrumentation because of the kyphosis. The inferior part of the instrumentation on the left side is a laminar claw to improve the balance and to add strength.

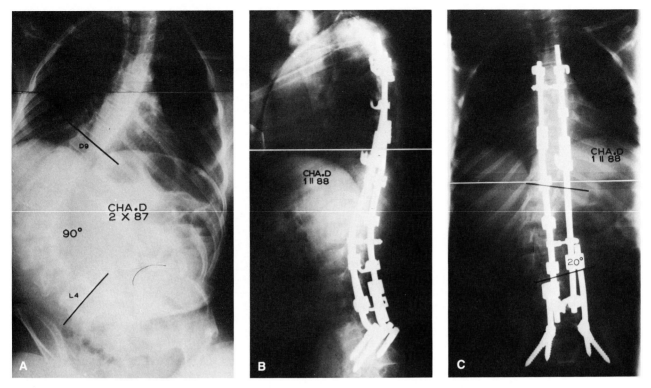

FIG. 9–52. **A.** Preoperative x-ray film showing a paralytic scoliosis with pelvic obliquity in a patient with cerebral palsy.   **B, C.** Postoperative x-ray films showing that the main part of the instrumentation is performed with the standard set. Pediatric rod and hooks are used in the upper part, and the connection is made by two axial tubes.

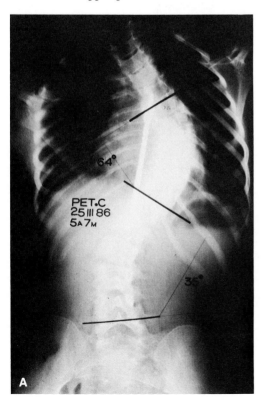

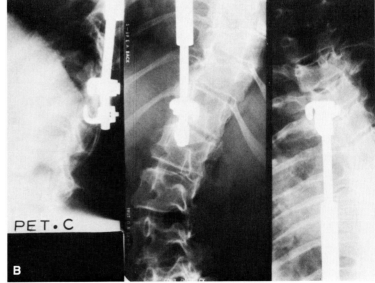

FIG. 9–53. **A.** Preoperative x-ray film showing failure of subcutaneous Harrington rod instrumentation in a case of infantile idiopathic scoliosis.   **B.** Postoperative x-ray films illustrate temporary instrumentation with two pieces of modified Cotrel rod connected with an axial tube. Pediculotransverse and laminolaminar claws grip at the two extremities of the curve.

216

References

1. Bridwell K, Capelli A, Franken C, et al: Sagittal plane analysis in idiopathic scoliosis patients treated with Cotrel–Dubousset instrumentation. Presented at Sixth International Congress on Cotrel–Dubousset Instrumentation, Monte Carlo, 1989
2. Bridwell K, Betz RR, Capelli AM, et al: Sagittal plane analysis in idiopathic scoliosis patients treatted with Cotrel–Dubousset instrumentation. Presented at Sixth International Congress on Cotrel–Dubousset Instrumentation, Monte Carlo, 1990
3. Chopin D, Plais PY, Geyer B, et al: Thoracic lordoscoliosis and Cotrel–Dubousset instrumentation. In Proceedings of the Fifth International Congress on Cotrel–Dubousset Instrumentation, pp 181–188. Montpellier, Sauramps Medical, 1988
4. Cotrel Y, Dubousset J: A new technique of spine fixation by a posterior approach in the treatment of scoliosis. Rev Chir Orthop 70:489–494, 1987
5. Cotrel Y, Dubousset J, Guillaumat M: New universal instrumentation in spinal surgery. Clin Orthop 227:10–23, 1988
6. Graf H, Hecquet J, Dubousset J: Approche tridimensionalle des deformations rachidiennes. Rev Chir Orthop 69:407–416, 1983
7. Graf H, Mouilleseaux B: La scoliose lombaire de l'adulte, pp 66–76. Paris, Masson, 1990
8. Passuti N: Cotrel–Dubousset instrumentation for high structural thoracic curves: Surgical technique and results concerning 25 cases. In Sixth International Congress on Cotrel–Dubousset Instrumentation. Monte Carlo and Montpellier, Sauramps Medical, 1990
9. Roye DP, Farcy JPC, Schwab F: Cotrel–Dubousset instrumentation and idiopathic scoliosis. In Sixth International Congress on Cotrel–Dubousset Instrumentation. Monte Carlo and Montpellier, Sauramps Medical, 1990
10. Sessa S, Dubousset J: L'instrumentation CD dans la scoliose idiopathique. Les resultats angulaires de 70 cas. Rev Chir Orthop 76:112–117, 1990
11. Shufflebarger HL, Ellis RD, Clark CE: Cotrel–Dubousset instrumentation (CDI) in adolescent idiopathic scoliosis: Mimimum two years follow-up [abstract]. Scoliosis Research Society 23rd Annual Meeting, Baltimore, October 1988
12. Shufflebarger HL, Clark CE: Complications of CD in idiopathic scoliosis. In Sixth International Congress on Cotrel–Dubousset Instrumentation, pp 241–243. Monte Carlo and Montpellier, Sauramps Medical, 1990
13. Transfeldt E, Thompson J, Bradford DS: Three-dimensional changes in the spine following Cotrel–Dubousset instrumentation for adolescent idiopathic scoliosis. In Sixth International Congress on Cotrel–Dubousset Instrumentation, pp 73–80. Monte Carlo and Montpellier, Sauramps Medical, 1990

CHAPTER
10

Texas Scottish Rite Hospital (TSRH) Instrumentation System

Richard B. Ashman
J. Anthony Herring
Charles E. Johnston II

■

DEVELOPMENT OF THE CROSSLINKS

In 1985, Johnston and Ashman began seeking a mechanical solution to the problem of rod migration in sublaminar segmental instrumentation (SSI). Although this instrumentation, introduced by Luque in the 1970s, had revolutionized the treatment of neuromuscular spinal deformity primarily because of the increased stability provided by the segmental fixation, there remained the problem of postoperative rod migration due to the sometimes tenuous rod-wire-bone interface.[1, 5, 6, 16] Loss of fixation with cyclic loading occurred, with consequent loss of correction (Fig. 10-1). Rod migration was most likely in neuromuscular cases in which osteopenia prevented the rods from being tightly secured to posterior elements by the wires and there was no meaningful linking of one rod to the other.

The concept of cross-bracing of spinal rods had been introduced by Weiler through studies of the load-carrying capacities of SSI constructs on a computer model.[22] A rigid plate implant, which is connected to a spinal rod by an eye-bolt and locking nut, now available as the Texas Scottish Rite Hospital (TSRH) Crosslink™, was developed to bring the concept of rigid cross-bracing to reality. The three-point interference clamp mechanism (Fig. 10-2), using a threaded nut that, when tightened, clamps a rod securely to the crossing plate, was first evaluated by testing calf spines with significant experimental scoliosis imposed by extreme rod contouring. The axial stiffness of an SSI construct was significantly improved by the simple addition of cross-links.[13] With the movement between rods eliminated, the increased stiffness to axial load proved a most important benefit of cross-linking, especially in severe deformities in which significant rod contouring was required because of residual deformity and which produced an alarming loss of construct stiffness.[13] Using custom implants, the first surgical case using cross-links was performed in 1985 (Fig. 10-3).

Cotrel–Dubousset instrumentation for scoliosis correction and fixation was introduced concurrently and was of interest because of the use of dynamic transverse traction (DTT) devices to cross-link the standard 7-mm knurled rods (Fig. 10-4A). The introduction of the rotational maneuver to correct scoliosis was a significant new technique in deformity surgery, and it was logical to assume that a system that used rotational correction should be tested for its ability to resist torsional loads.

219

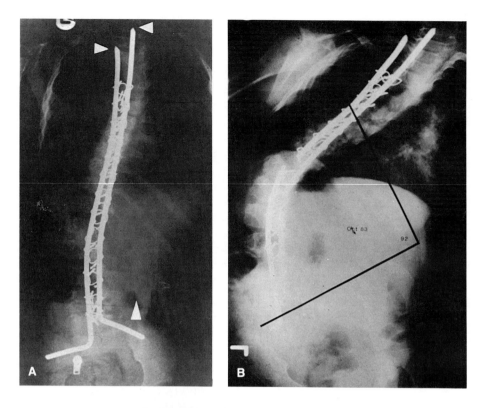

FIG. 10–1.   A. Immediate postoperative shift in sublaminar segmental instrumentation to the pelvis. The right rod has migrated cephalad in relation to the left (*arrows*), with return of pelvic obliquity. **B.** Significant loss of correction, with rod fractures, from continued cyclical rod movement and loss of fixation.

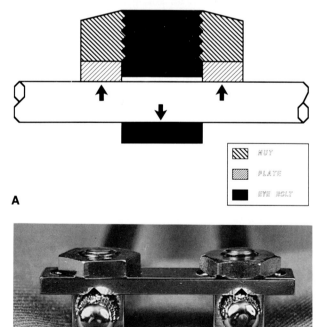

FIG. 10–2.   A. The eye-bolt in cross-section. Three points of rod contact produce the clamping mechanism. **B.** The original cross-link design (end view).

The results of torsional testing on standard Cotrel–Dubousset constructs unlinked, cross-linked with the DTT device, and cross-linked with the TSRH plate, revealed that the DTT enhanced the torsional stiffness of the construct only minimally over unlinked rods. There was very little increase in stiffness when the inter-rod distance exceeded 2.5 cm, suggesting that the small-diameter threaded rod connecting the clamps was the primary cause of this excessive flexibility (Fig. 10-4). In contrast, the torsional stiffness of a Cotrel–Dubousset construct cross-linked with the TSRH plate was greater at all inter-rod distances and increased as the spread between the rods increased (Fig. 10-4*B*).[12]

The original implant was subsequently modified (Fig. 10-5) to increase the thickness of the plate and to decrease the size of the oval holes, allowing a thicker isthmus to be placed between them. The isthmus allows contouring of the plate to accommodate rods that are not precisely parallel or are in significantly different planes owing to marked deformity, while decreasing the susceptibility to plate fracture. Although the plate was increased in thickness, it carries a low profile compared with the earlier implant and with the DTT device (Fig. 10-5) by decreasing the height of the nut.

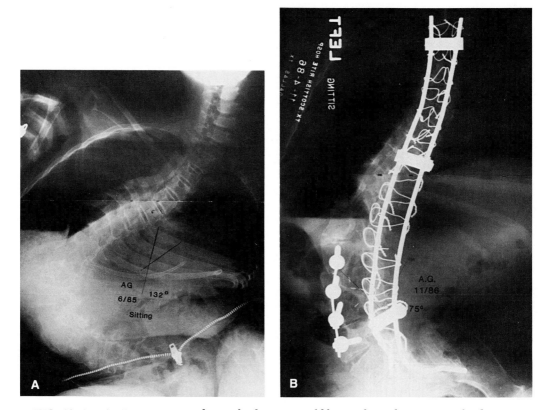

FIG. 10–3. **A.** Preoperative radiograph of a 14-year-old boy with Duchenne muscular dystrophy and a neglected spinal deformity. Bend films showed passive correction to 90°. The patient's pulmonary function was estimated to be 28% of predicted FEV_1. **B.** Simultaneous anterior and posterior corrections were performed because of the patient's expected inability to tolerate staged procedures. Correction to only 75° was achieved. One year postoperatively, no shift of rods or loss of correction is apparent. Three crosslinks have stabilized this markedly contoured, flexible construct. The patient survived for 4 years without any loss of correction.

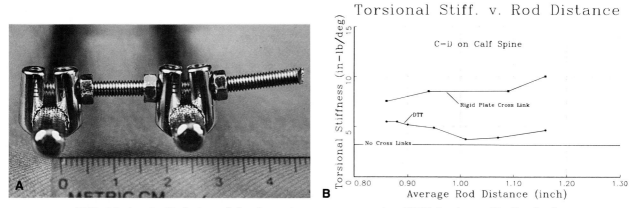

FIG. 10–4. **A.** End view of the dynamic transverse traction (DTT) implant. **B.** Graph of torsional stiffness and inter-rod distance for Cotrel–Dubousset constructs unlinked, cross-linked with DTTs, and cross-linked with TSRH implants. Torsional stiffness imparted by the TSRH Crosslinks™ increases as the inter-rod distance increases.

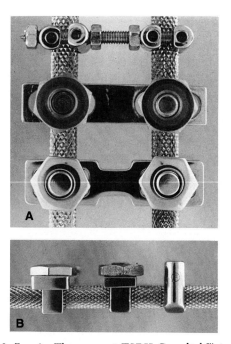

FIG. 10–5. **A.** The present TSRH Crosslink™ in profile with the obsolete first-generation implant (*middle*) and the dynamic transverse traction device. **B.** Notice the low profile of the present implant (*left*).

Clinical use of this device in over 150 cases with a minimum of 1 year of follow-up has demonstrated its utility in stabilizing all types of spinal rod systems, with a negligible incidence of loosening or failure.[14] The spiral lock thread of the eye-bolt and the necessity of tightening the nuts to 17 Nm of torque are primarily responsible for the low incidence of nut loosening.

CONSTRUCT RESEARCH

The cross-link device increases the axial stiffness of rod-wire systems in which the sole rod-to-bone connection is by a twisted wire, such as traditional SSI.[13] It is also known to increase the torsional stiffness of both rod-wire systems and rod-hook systems in which the rods are fixed to the spine by a hook, with a set screw or ratchet-jamming mechanism providing the connection between rod and hook.[12,13] However, the clinical efficacy of increased spinal construct stiffness, while appearing intuitively to be appropriate, has never been studied in terms of the participation of the construct in the process of biologic arthrodesis. Gurr and coworkers demonstrated an increased incidence of arthrodesis when spinal fusions were augmented with

implants in dogs, but the quality of the fusion mass as a function of the stiffness of the construct has never been evaluated.[10]

Preliminary results of an in vivo spinal fusion model in goats revealed that stiffer constructs do increase the axial and torsional stiffness of the ensuing fusion mass.[11] Standardized 10-segment posterior fusions using segmental wiring with Drummond button-wire implants were carried out, attempting to increase the overall construct stiffness by using rods of larger diameter and adding cross-linking. Although rod-wire slippage during cyclic loading[18] in vivo prevented significant additional axial stiffness to be imparted by rods of larger diameter or by cross-linking, 6.4-mm rods produced fusion masses significantly stiffer in axial testing than 3.2-mm rods (Fig 10-6A).

In torsional testing, the rod-wire slippage problem was apparently not critical, because both larger rod diameter and rigid cross-linking significantly increased the torsional stiffness of the ensuing fusion mass (Fig. 10-6B), as predicted by earlier experimental bench testing.[2,12,13] This offered preliminary evidence linking the quality of the fusion mass to the stiffness of the internal fixation construct, providing experimental justification for the use of stiffer spinal constructs from a purely biologic standpoint of seeking a more robust fusion mass. At the same time, the fusion mass obtained from 4.8-mm rods rigidly cross-linked (Fig. 10-6C) was just as stiff as the fusion mass associated with unlinked 6.4-mm rods (Fig. 10-6B), suggesting that smaller-diameter, more easily implanted rods, when cross-linked, provide the same stiffness as unlinked, heavier rods, which may be more difficult to contour and implant. Further studies to more thoroughly evaluate the relationship of construct stiffness and ensuing fusion mass continue, using a constrained interface between eye-bolt and pedicle screw to eliminate the rod-wire slippage problem (Fig. 10-7). Preliminary results show no significant changes in fusion mass quality by varying the stiffness of constructs in a short, three-segment fusion (unpublished data).

HOOKS, SCREWS, AND RODS

The eye-bolt three-point clamp mechanism was logically extended to attach a hook or screw rigidly to a rod (Fig. 10-8). The hooks are designed so that the rod can be attached from above (i.e., open) for easy assembly of the construct intraoperatively. Because there is a small recess on each side of the rod groove in the hook (Fig.

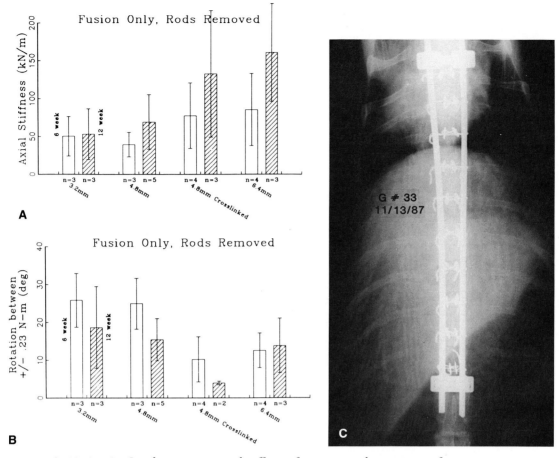

FIG. 10–6. **A.** Graph comparing axial stiffness of experimental ten-segment fusion masses, 6 or 12 weeks postoperatively, with internal fixation removed. Four different groups of constructs were used as internal fixation. **B.** Graph comparing torsional stiffness of the same spine fusions, as measured by rotation allowed between specimen ends. Decreasing rotation indicates increasing torsional stiffness. **C.** Radiograph of experimental posterior spinal fusion, using 4.8-mm rods and TSRH Crosslinks™.

10-8*A*), the eye-bolt can be tightened sufficiently to keep the rod seated in the hook, but it is still loose enough to allow compression, distraction, or rotation maneuvers to be performed without additional temporary implants or devices to keep the rod seated during these maneuvers. Hook holders are attached at the side of the hook opposite where the eye-bolt nut will be tightened, and they do not impede rod entrance into the hook from above or subsequent nut tightening (Fig. 10-8*B*).

The integrity of the clamping mechanism provided by the eye-bolt has been evaluated in pull-off studies, comparing the axial and torsional force required to loosen an eye-bolt (Fig. 10-9). For example, using one or two set screws, the axial and torsional pull-off

strength of the TSRH eye-bolt was found to be equal to or better than any of the various Cotrel–Dubousset devices. This is important because one of the perceived disadvantages of a smooth rod is that it may not be possible to attach a hook or screw without slippage. The importance of the spiral lock thread on the eye-bolt and the requirement of tightening the nut to 17 Nm of torque cannot be overemphasized.

Why should a smooth rod be used? Intuitively, there should be a minimal tendency for friction or binding between a smooth rod and hook body during a rotational maneuver. Friction between a rougher, knurled rod and hook body could prevent satisfactory rod rotation, or more seriously, it could displace a hook during the rotation maneuver if the binding is too

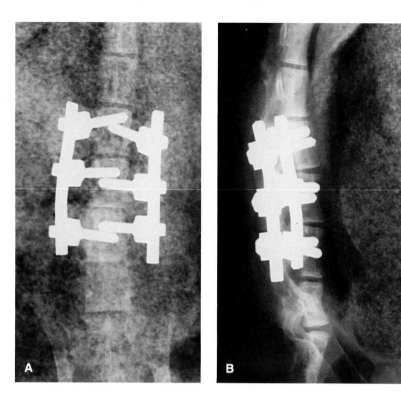

FIG. 10–7. **A.** Three-level experimental posterior fusion using pedicle screws internally fixed with a solid rod. **B.** The stiffness of this constrained system is varied by using rods of different diameters.

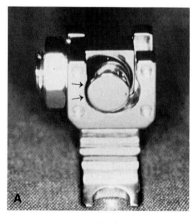

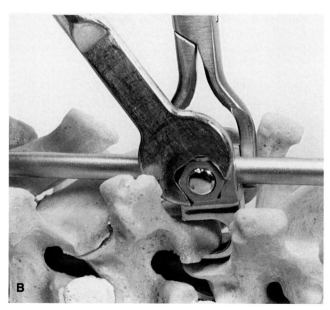

FIG. 10–8. **A.** End view of hook attached to rod by the eye-bolt mechanism. Notice recesses on each side of the groove for the rod (*arrows*). **B.** Tightening of the locking nut. Access to the nut is not impeded by the hook holder.

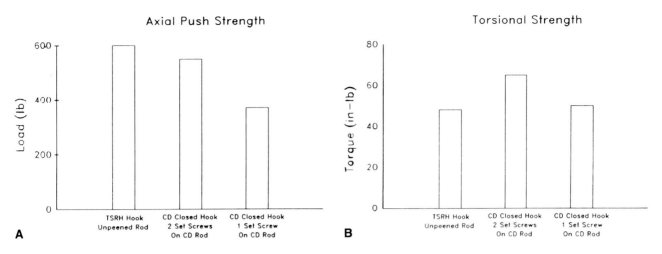

FIG. 10–9. **A.** Axial push-off strengths of TSRH hook and eye-bolt on a smooth unpeened rod, compared with a Cotrel–Dubousset (CD) closed hook with one and two set screws. **B.** Torsional strengths of same three hook and rod mechanisms.

great. Pedicle hook displacement into the spinal canal during the rotational maneuver has been suspected in some cases of neurologic injury associated with Cotrel–Dubousset instrumentation.[21] A smooth rod should have little tendency to displace pedicle hooks into the spinal canal because of the lack of binding during the rotational maneuver.

Accurate anatomic design of pedicle hooks maximizes their rotational stability. Modification from existing pedicle hooks includes widening and deepening the radius between tines, so that they may more firmly "grasp" the pedicle (Fig. 10-10A), and altering the shape of the axilla of the hook, so that the inferior laminar edge and articular process can be grasped by an anatomic, rather than circular, design (Fig. 10-10B,C). The design changes incorporated into the TSRH pedicle hook significantly improved rotational stability in each of three testing protocols in which hook contact with the pedicle or lamina surface was varied from minimal to ideal (Fig. 10-10D).[4] Additionally, the TSRH hook design allowed less intrusion into the canal should the hook still rotate off the pedicle and displace medially (Fig. 10-10E). The smooth rod prevents binding between the rod and hook during the rotational maneuver and the pedicle-hook modifications improve stability to rotational force, protecting against neurologic injury.

Study of available pedicle-screw systems, primarily focusing on the stresses responsible for the fatigue fractures of pedicle screws seen clinically, demonstrated the need for important improvements in design

of screws used in a constrained system. Ashman and colleagues have identified the root of the screw at its junction with the rod or plate in constrained systems as the point of maximal stress concentration and the predictable point of failure.[3] TSRH bone screws for use with the spinal instrumentation system have incorporated into the design a large-diameter, nonthreaded root of the screw (according to screw length requirements) to minimize stress concentration at the site of greatest vulnerability—the junction between the shank and the root of the screw where the rod and eye-bolt mechanism attaches (Fig. 10-11A). Cyclic testing to produce fatigue fractures (plus or minus 440 N axial load at 2 Hz) demonstrated that the 6.5-mm screws showed no failure at greater than 1 million cycles, similar to other constrained (e.g., AO Fixateur Interne) and nonconstrained (e.g., Luque plates, AO notched plate) systems (Fig. 10-11B). If used as a transpedicular device, the TSRH screw design is satisfactory for dealing with screw fracture at the screw-plate or screw-rod junctions, with fatigue characteristics in bench testing similar to nonconstrained systems.

The TSRH screws may also be used for anterior fixation of the spine. Both screw diameters (6.5 and 5.5 mm) have cancellous-type threads, suitable for fixation in the anterior vertebral body. This implantation is performed for anterior stabilization after vertebrectomy for decompression in acute trauma or as a late procedure for deformity or anterior cord impingement (Fig. 10-12). In certain lumbar and thoracolumbar scoliosis patterns, anterior instrumentation and fusion

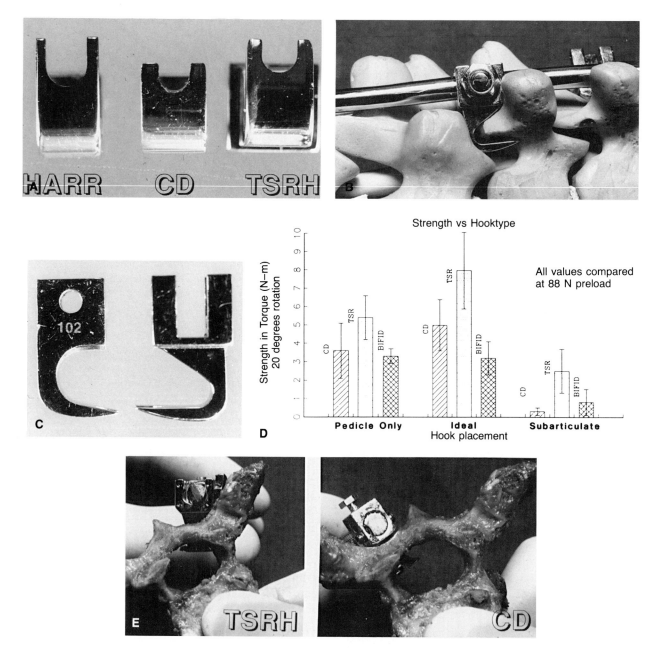

FIG. 10–10. **A.** View of the tines of various pedicle hooks. TSRH design includes a wider and deeper radius to "grasp" the pedicle rather than simply contacting it. Harrington (HARR) tines are easily deformed during insertion, and the length of the tines allows possible medial protrusion into spinal canal. **B.** Anatomic axilla of TSRH hook shoe, formed to fit the laminar surface precisely. **C.** Circular design of some pedicle hooks (*left*) do not provide the same anatomic, "press-fit" grasp of the lamina, increasing rotational instability. **D.** Graph depicting experimental rotational stability in torque of three hook designs tested. "Pedicle only" and "subarticulate" placements provide suboptimal contact between bone and hook. **E.** Amount of canal encroachment possible if pedicle hooks rotate off the pedicle medially.

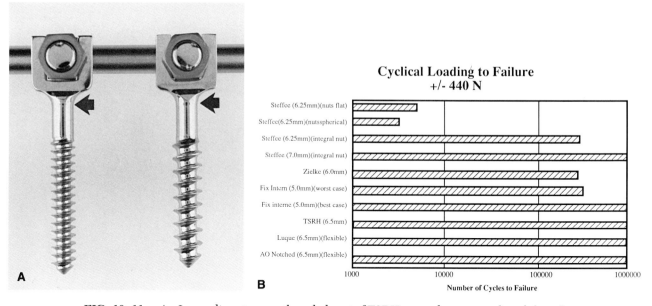

FIG. 10–11. **A.** Large-diameter, nonthreaded root of TSRH screw decreases vulnerability of the screw-rod junction to fatigue and failure by decreasing stress concentration (*arrows*). **B.** Graph of the number of cycles until failure at different eccentrically applied axial loads for various screw-rod or screw-plate devices.

is advantageous, and the TSRH instrumentation can be used as an anterior instrumentation, using vertebral screws and the 4.8-mm solid rod (Fig. 10-13). By using the hooks and screws posteriorly or the screws anteriorly, the TSRH instrumentation can be considered a universal spinal implant system.

Although preliminary studies suggest that stiffer spinal constructs produce stiffer fusion masses, using an extremely stiff rod is still controversial.[11] Rotational correction of a scoliosis requires that the rod be stiff enough that the spine conforms to the contouring of the rod and that the kyphosis that is contoured into the rod is maintained after the rotational maneuver. Many surgeons using Cotrel–Dubousset instrumentation have reported that the rod flexibility often does not produce the desired amount of kyphosis, because the rods bend intraoperatively during the rotation maneuver in response to the stiffness of the deformity. Rod flexibility provides a safety factor during the rotation maneuver in case the kyphosis countoured into the rod is excessive or the spinal deformity is too stiff to allow full rotational correction. For this reason, the TSRH instrumentation provides three levels of rod stiffness (i.e., 4.8 mm, flexible 6.4 mm, and stiff 6.4 mm). In a patient

with a severe deformity that is moderately flexible, the use of the stiffer rods on the concavity allows the surgeon to seek maximal rotational correction without loss of the contoured-rod kyphosis. If significant stiffness of the spine prevents such correction, the more flexible rod can be used, primarily for ease of implantation. The same considerations apply to the correction and internal fixation of post-traumatic or degenerative deformities. All TSRH rods have a shot-peening surface treatment that increases the fatigue life of the rods over untreated ones (Fig. 10-14).[8]

Because the hooks, screws, and cross-links use the same locking mechanism to attach these devices to the rod and eye-bolt system, the versatility of the TSRH spinal instrumentation system is perhaps its greatest advantage over other systems. The eye-bolt mechanism makes the system extremely easy to revise. The locking nut is loosened, and the system can be immediately disassembled. Because all the hooks and screws open from the top, a dislodged hook can be easily replaced, the rod reseated, and the eye-bolt tightened, without having to disassemble the entire construct and start over. In revision of previously operated cases, surgical exposure can often be limited to a local area of

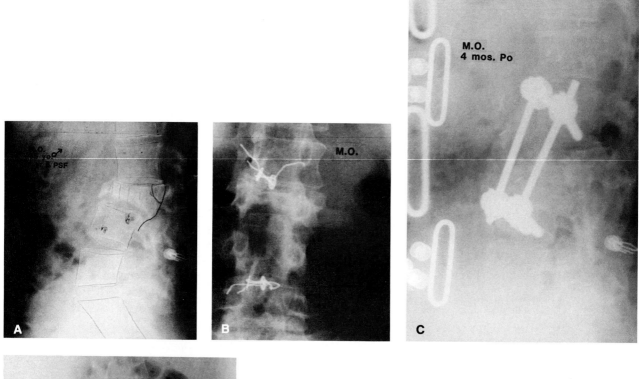

FIG. 10–12. **A.** Lateral radiograph of a standing 35-year-old man 1 year after posterior fusion and instrumentation ("instrument long, fuse short") for an L3 burst fracture with minimal neurologic deficit. Collapse into kyphosis occurred after implant removal. The fusion mass appears to extend to L5. **B.** Anterior-posterior (AP) radiograph with retained button-wire spinous process implants. **C.** Lateral radiograph 4 months after anterior vertebrectomy and instrumentation to correct kyphosis. Two 4.8-mm solid rods are used between 5.5-mm screws anchored in L2 and L4. **D.** Postoperative AP radiograph. A tricortical iliac crest graft was used to strut the L3 vertebrectomy space (*arrows*). (Case courtesy of R.S. Curtis, M.D.)

pseudarthrosis, and a reinstrumentation applied without having to remove intact instrumentation above or below the level of revision (Fig. 10-15). When necessary to extend the fusion, instrumentation can be added without disturbing the existing instrumentation (Fig. 10-16).

The routine cross-linking of separate sets of rods when performing instrumentation (i.e., TSRH-Galveston) to the pelvis in patients with neuromuscular scoliosis and pelvic obliquity makes it possible to obtain maximal correction and fixation of pelvic obliquity as a separate step in the operative procedure. This technique eliminates the extremely complex rod contours (Galveston bends) required to place a rod in the iliac wing while accommodating deformities in the lumbar and thoracic spine above (Fig. 10-17).[1,7]

(*text continues on page 234*)

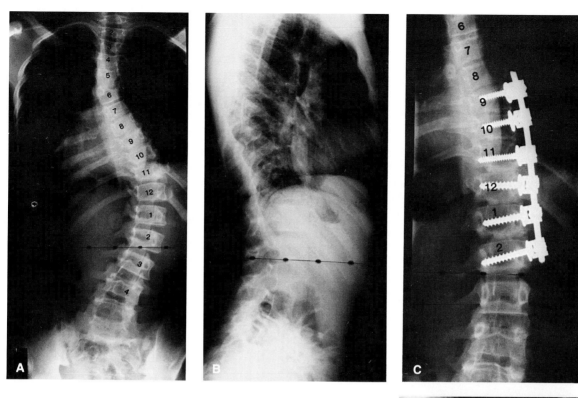

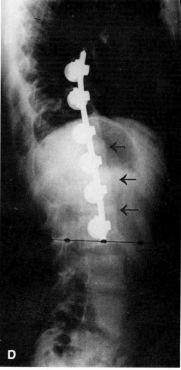

FIG. 10–13. **A.** A 14-year-old boy with an idiopathic right thoracolumbar deformity. Left bend films demonstrated leveling of L3, making short anterior fusion to L2 possible. **B.** Lateral radiograph showing an essentially straight segment of spine from T9 to L3. **C.** Anterior-posterior radiograph taken 4 months postoperatively. The residual mild lumbar curve is balanced well with the upper left thoracic (untreated) curve. **D.** Lateral radiograph. Sagittal contour shows maintenance of preoperative alignment, with no iatrogenic kyphosis at the upper lumbar area. There is also evidence of solid fusion at several disc spaces (*arrows*) only 4 months after surgery.

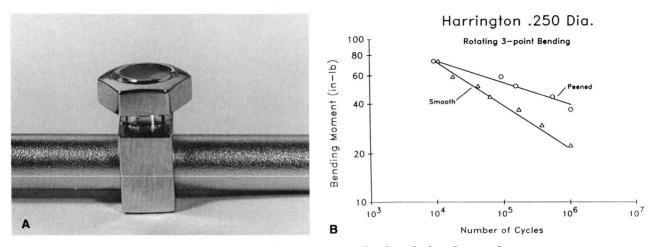

FIG. 10–14. **A.** Shot-peening surface treatment of rods, which enhances fatigue resistance. **B.** The effect of shot-peening at the ratchet-rod junction (an area notorious for fatigue fracture) on the fatigue characteristics of a Harrington rod. By this simple surface treatment, the number of cycles until failure is increased at every value of bending moment.

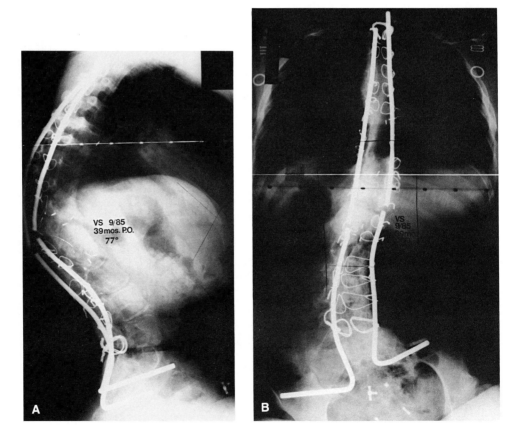

FIG. 10–15.

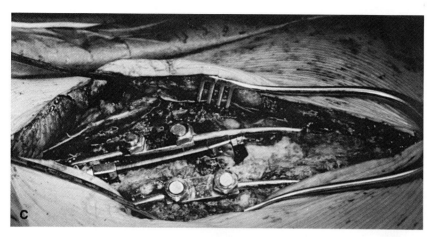

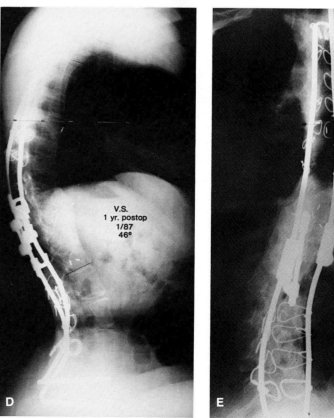

◀ **FIG. 10–15. A.** A 16-year-old paraplegic girl 3 years after a staged anterior-posterior fusion with posterior Luque sublaminar segmental instrumentation (SSI) to correct a postlaminectomy, postradiation kyphosis caused by a spinal cord astrocytoma. Recurrent deformity and pain occurred with rod fracture. **B.** AP radiograph of failed instrumentation. **C.** Intraoperative photograph of rod repair with axial plates and eyebolts and of additional short compression instrumentation across the pseudarthrosis. **D, E.** One year after surgery, the correction and fusion are maintained with only a short posterior revision and pseudarthrosis repair, without having to revise the entire previous SSI construct.

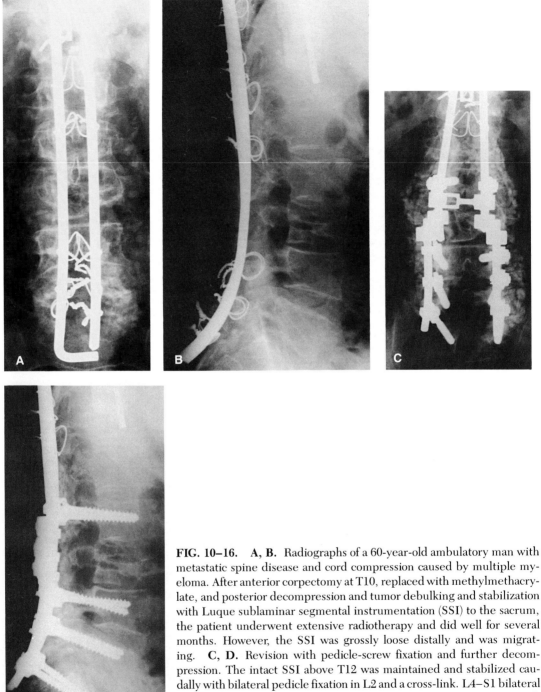

FIG. 10–16.   **A, B.** Radiographs of a 60-year-old ambulatory man with metastatic spine disease and cord compression caused by multiple myeloma. After anterior corpectomy at T10, replaced with methylmethacrylate, and posterior decompression and tumor debulking and stabilization with Luque sublaminar segmental instrumentation (SSI) to the sacrum, the patient underwent extensive radiotherapy and did well for several months. However, the SSI was grossly loose distally and was migrating.   **C, D.** Revision with pedicle-screw fixation and further decompression. The intact SSI above T12 was maintained and stabilized caudally with bilateral pedicle fixation in L2 and a cross-link. L4–S1 bilateral pedicle fixation was achieved and connected to the upper construct with the side-to-side cross-links to achieve excellent fixation with only limited lumbosacral revision. (Case courtesy of Gary Lowery, M.D.)

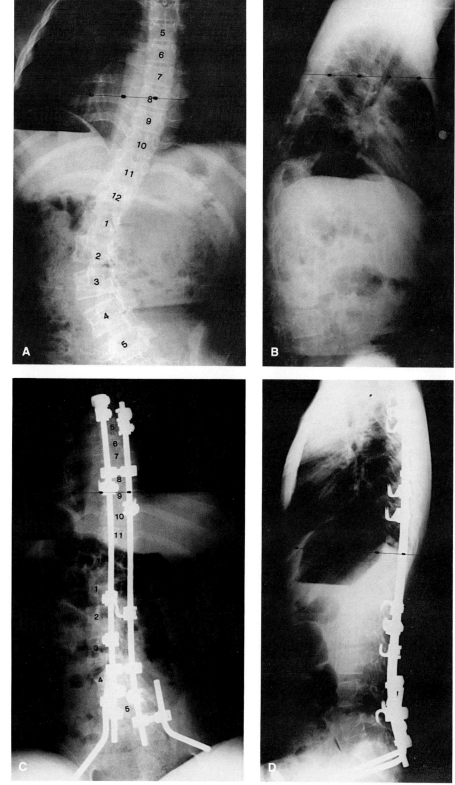

FIG. 10–17. A, B. A 14-year-old boy with Duchenne muscular dystrophy, progressive scoliosis, and pelvic obliquity. **C, D.** Postoperative correction using two sets of double rods. Instrumentation from T4 to L5 is accomplished first to obtain balance in the sagittal plane, and then it is linked to separate Galveston iliac rods with side-by-side TSRH Crosslinks™. Pelvic obliquity can be corrected as a separate step by distracting the high side of the pelvis against the long construct already locked in place and compressing on the down side.

CURRENT SYSTEM

The TSRH implant system is made of 316 LVM stainless steel of implant grade. This metal is biologically inert and is compatible with any other spinal implants made of surgical-grade 316L stainless steel. The implants consist of hooks, rods, eye-bolts, screws, and Crosslinks™. The instruments for insertion will also be described.

Hooks

All hooks attach to the rod using an eye-bolt and nut. The eye-bolt locks the hook to the rod with a three-point sheer clamp connection (see Figs. 10-2*A* and 10-8*A*). The nuts tighten down with a Spiralock mechanism that, when tight, will not loosen with repeated stress. (This nut locking technology is borrowed from the aircraft industry.) In the event of reoperation, however, all the nuts may be loosened.

The pedicle hooks are anatomically designed to encompass the pedicle without penetrating its cortex (Figs. 10-10 and 10-18). Thus the width of the opening of the hook is slightly wider than an average pedicle diameter. The edges of the hook are sharpened to allow penetration of the capsule of the joint; the notch of the hook is dull so as not to cut into the pedicle. The shoulder of the hook is buttressed to allow contact with the articular facet.

Three standard laminar hooks are used in the system. The buttressed laminar hook is the most often used (Fig. 10-19). The shoulder of the hook is buttressed to produce anatomic contact with the lamina and prevent movement of the hook toward the neural canal. This hook is usually used over the lamina and faces caudally. The large, more circular laminar hook usually faces cephalad under a lamina or over a transverse process (Fig. 10-20). The offset and smaller circular laminar hook is sometimes useful to attach a rod to the hook when the plane of the hook is more anterior than the plane of the rod (Fig. 10-21).

A special transverse process hook that has a closed top is useful as the cephalad hook on the convexity of a curve (Fig. 10-22). The closed design facilitates placement of the eye-bolt in an area where exposure is often limited. Once the rod has been threaded through the eye-bolt and closed hook, it cannot dislodge from the hook even though no nut tightening is performed, which is convenient when exposure and space are limited.

Pediatric-sized hooks are also available (Fig. 10-23). The small hooks have a single upright and may be attached to the rod on either side; they are of an appropriate size for the small patient. Along with a single pedicle hook, there are two designs of laminar hook. The eye-bolts are smaller and accommodate the 4.8-mm (³/₁₆″) rod.

The vertebral screws are available in two thread diameters, 5.5 and 6.5 mm. The former threads are

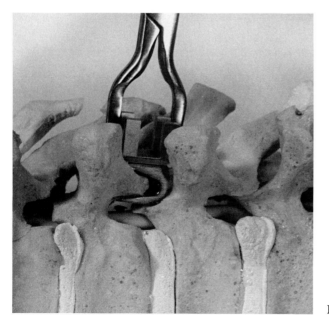

FIG. 10–18.   Pedicle hook seated against a pedicle.

fine cancellous; the latter are classic cancellous. The screws attach on either side to the rods with the eye-bolt connectors. The root of the screw has been designed for fatigue resistance (see Fig. 10-11).

Rods

Rods are available in three sizes and stiffnesses. The smallest is a 4.8-mm ($^3/_{16}$″) rod of the same size and

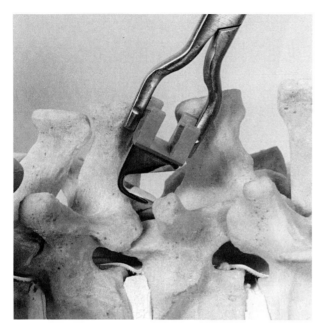

FIG. 10–19. Buttressed laminar hook.

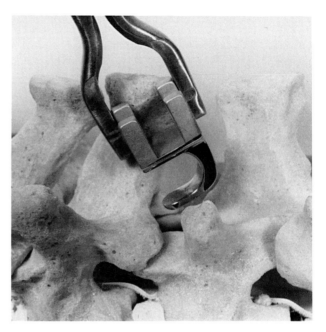

FIG. 10–20. Large circular laminar hook.

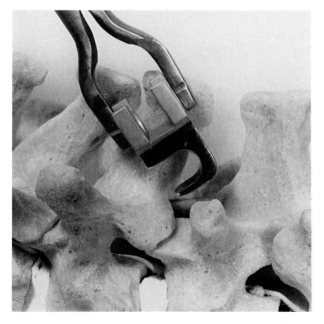

FIG. 10–21. Offset small circular laminar hook.

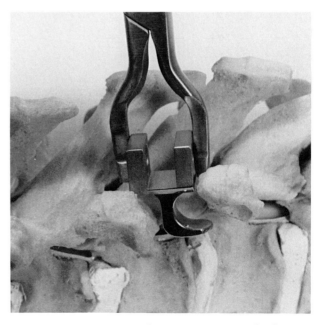

FIG. 10–22. Closed transverse process hook.

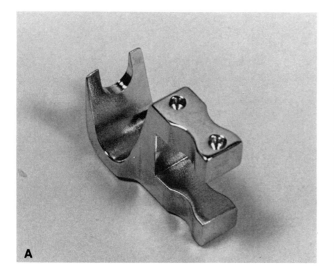

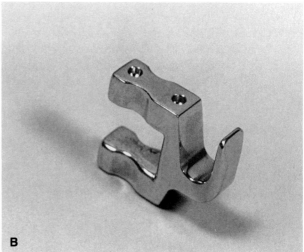

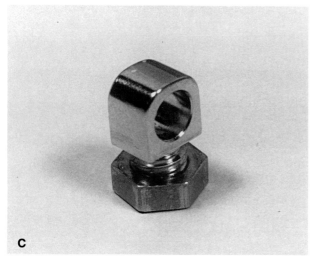

FIG. 10–23. Pediatric hooks. **A.** Pediatric pedicle hook.
B. Pediatric laminar hook. **C.** Pediatric eyebolt.

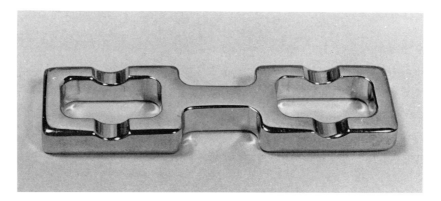

FIG. 10–24. Crosslink™ plate with grooves for the rods.

stiffness of the classic Luque rod. Two 6.4-mm (1/4") rods are available—one that is very stiff, similar to the Harrington rod, and one that is more flexible and more easily contoured.

The surface of the rod is treated with a shot peening process (see Fig. 10-14A). This imparts a certain roughness so that when the nuts are moderately tight on the eye-bolts, the hooks can be moved in distraction or compression and will then maintain their position on the rod without the use of C-clamps. At this tightness the rod can still be rotated. Subsequent tightening of the nuts will lock the rods against rotation. This feature greatly facilitates the process of distraction, compression, and rod rotation.

Crosslinks™

The Crosslink™ plates are used to rigidly connect two rods (Fig. 10-24). Mechanical testing has shown that the rod-and-hook construct is much stiffer and therefore more stable when rigidly connected together than when either unlinked or linked by a flexible connector. The Crosslink™ plates are available in sequential sizes to allow connection of rods that are varying distances apart (Fig. 10-25). When the rods are not parallel, the plates must be contoured with bending devices to align the grooves exactly perpendicular with the rods, to achieve a secure and stable connection.

Insertion Equipment

The following devices are used to insert the components of the TSRH instrumentation system.

Hook Holders. The hook holders attach to the hooks parallel to the rod entrance into the hook, a feature that allows the holders to remain on the hooks while the rod is inserted (see Figs. 10-19 to 10-22).

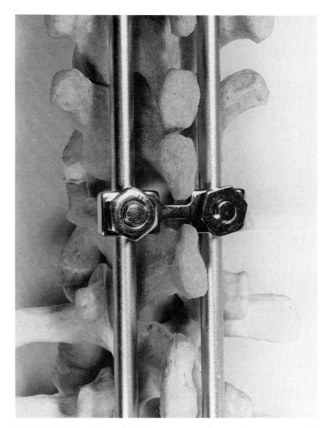

FIG. 10–25. Crosslink™ system and attachment to rod.

Hook Inserter. The hook inserter fits inside the hook to provide two-handed control during hook insertion.

Trial Hooks. The trial hooks are identical to the implants but are rigidly attached to a color-coded handle (Fig. 10-26). This design allows trial hook insertion with one hand. After the trial hook is inserted, it is not necessary to insert the implant hook until final instrumentation.

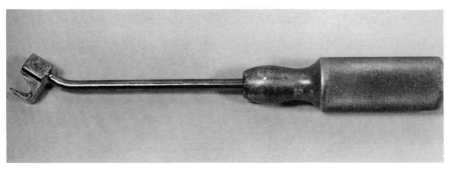

FIG. 10–26. One-piece trial hook.

Corkscrew. The corkscrew device is a modified hook holder with a threaded pusher (Fig. 10-27). It is used to push the rod and eye-bolt into the hook. (Often the spine is actually being pulled up to the rod during this maneuver.) The endplate of the pusher must be placed precisely on the rod and eye-bolt to correctly insert the rod.

Mini-corkscrew. The mini-corkscrew attaches to an ordinary hook holder (Fig. 10-28). When placed in the neck of the hook holder and twisted, it pushes the rod a short distance into the hook.

Eye-Bolt Spreader. The eye-bolt spreader pushes the rod into the hook over a short distance (Fig. 10-29). It fits between the hook holder and the rod and is spread open.

Wrenches. Several wrenches are available to tighten the nuts on the eye-bolts (see Fig. 10-8B). The final tightening of the nuts should be done with the wrench that most closely fits the nut.

Miscellaneous Instruments. In addition to the above, rod benders, rod holders, rod pushers, in situ benders, plate benders, osteotomes, elevators, and gouges are all necessary for the surgical procedure.

SURGICAL TECHNIQUE

The technique that has proved successful in our hands follows a set sequence, which other surgeons may or may not find useful. The sequence we use is as follows: (1) exposure, (2) level identification (radiographically), (3) hook placement, (4) bilateral facetectomy, (5) rod contouring, (6) decortication on the side of first rod placement (usually concave), (7) placement of the first rod and distraction and compression on it, (8) rotation

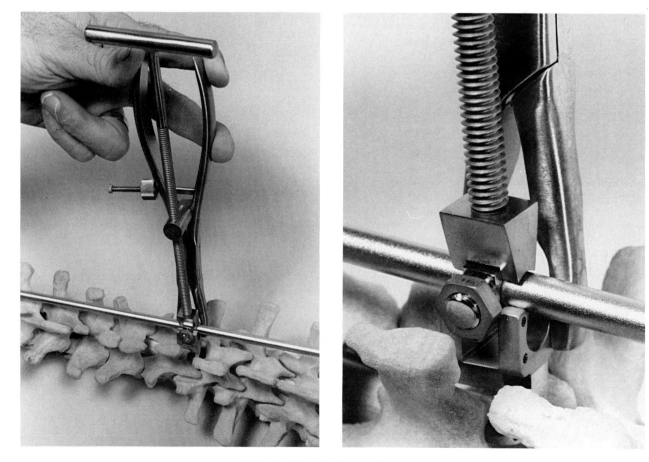

FIG. 10–27. "Corkscrew" in use.

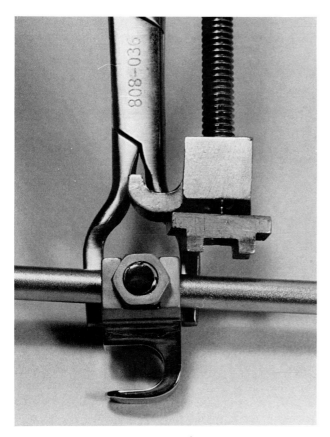

FIG. 10–28. Mini-corkscrew in use.

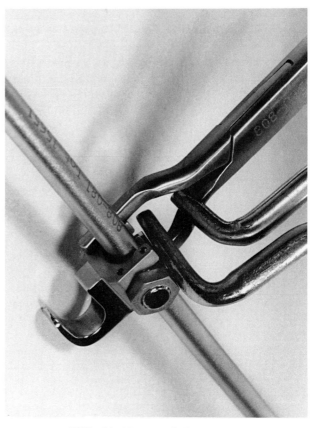

FIG. 10–29. Eye-bolt spreader.

of the first rod, (9) decortication of the second side (usually convex), (10) placement of the second rod and distraction and compression, (11) placement of bone graft, and (12) crosslinking the rods together. The technique described here is that for a single thoracic curve (Fig. 10-30).

The spine is exposed out to the tips of the transverse processes of all the vertebrae to be fused. An additional level often is exposed proximally to facilitate instrumentation. The facet hooks are placed by first excising a portion of the inferior articular process of the vertebra to be instrumented. The pedicle is located at the junction of the transverse process and the lamina. The trial hook can be placed against the lamina to estimate the amount of articular process to remove. Just enough bone should be removed so that when the tines of the hook engage the pedicle, the shoulder of the hook will be in contact with the laminar surface of the articular process (see Fig. 10-18). This provides the

greatest stability of the hook and is quite superior to a hook that impacts the pedicle but does not engage the articular process (see Fig. 10-10D).[4]

The transverse process hook is placed by passing the trial hook just over the transverse process in a subperiosteal plane. The laminar hooks are placed in a caudal-facing position by first removing the adjacent facet joint. The ligamentum flavum is then incised sharply, and the inferior lamina of the adjacent vertebra is removed with a Kerrison rongeur. Considerable space is necessary to allow insertion of the hook over the lamina (see Fig. 10-19).

The buttressed hook best fits the lamina and prevents migration into the canal. Once the trial hook has been placed, it is not necessary to place the final hook until the instrumentation is ready to be inserted.

Cranial-facing laminar hooks are placed by first passing a lamina elevator beneath the lamina, through the ligamentum flavum. Because of the slope of the lamina, it is not necessary to remove any bone to place this hook. The rounded laminar hook best suits this purpose (see Fig. 10-20).

Following hook placement, a bilateral facetectomy is performed. This is done prior to instrumentation in order to increase the flexibility of the spine. The rod is then contoured. The spine is decorticated on the side to be first instrumented. The rod is then placed into the hooks with eye-bolts at each hook site, and two extra eye-bolts are preplaced for Crosslink™ insertion. The Crosslinks™ are placed toward the ends of the rod. The eye-bolt spreader and corkscrew devices are used to seat the rod into the hooks. Once the rod is in the hook, the nut should be tightened enough to prevent the rod from escaping.

The nuts on the hooks are then tightened moderately, and the hooks can be placed in compression and distraction. If a hook slips, the nut needs to be tightened a small amount to maintain position. The rod may then be rotated to correct the curve. During rotation it is essential to watch the alignment of the hooks to avoid rotation of the hooks into the canal. Hook holders placed on the pedicle hooks serve as indicators of hook rotation. After rod rotation, the nuts are fully tightened to prevent derotation.

Next the contralateral side of the spine is decorticated. Hooks are inserted, the contoured rod is placed, and compression or distraction is applied to the hooks. The bone graft is placed over the decorticated surfaces and into the lateral gutters. Finally, the Crosslinks™ are placed. If the rods are not parallel, the plates should be contoured to align the grooves in the Crosslink™ plates with the rods. The nuts are tightened to full tension with the torque wrench. All nuts in the system are then maximally tightened.

USE OF THE SYSTEM

Selection of Levels and Placement of Hooks

Level selection and hook placement will be described for the following curve types:

I. Single thoracic curve, King III type

II. Low single thoracic curve with junctional kyphosis

III. Double thoracic curve

IV. Double curves, right thoracic, left lumbar, King II type
  (A) Instrumentation of the thoracic curve with rotational correction
  (B) Instrumentation of the thoracic curve with translational correction
  (C) Instrumentation of both the thoracic and lumbar curves

V. Thoracolumbar curve
  (A) Posterior instrumentation construct with cantilever correction
  (B) Anterior instrumentation with the TSRH system

VI. Paralytic scoliosis with pelvic obliquity—instrumentation with the TSRH-Galveston construct

Single Thoracic Scoliosis, King III Type[15]

A single thoracic scoliosis is corrected primarily by rotation of a concave rod with a four-hook construct. The surgeon must first decide on the end vertebrae to be instrumented (see Fig. 10-30). From the anterior-posterior radiograph, the cephalad end vertebra, which is in neutral rotation and whose discs are not wedged, is identified. Caudally, the stable vertebra[15]—the vertebra most evenly bisected by a vertical line drawn from the center of the sacrum—is identified. With a King III curve, the upper neutral vertebra, or one level cephalad to neutral, usually is chosen for the most proximal hook. Distally the vertebra next most cephalad to the stable vertebra is tentatively chosen as the end vertebra. The lateral radiograph is then evaluated and the location of any junctional kyphosis noted. (A junctional kyphosis is defined as a mildly kyphotic area around the thoracolumbar junction. The thoracolumbar junction is normally neither kyphotic nor lordotic.) The end vertebra tentatively chosen should not be used if it is close to the apex of a junctional kyphosis. If there is a significant junctional kyphosis, it is usually best to instrument one or two levels below the apex of the kyphotic segment as seen on the lateral radiograph.

Next the concave apical hook sites are selected. Usually two vertebrae proximal and two distal to the apex of the curve are chosen for the concave hooks. The lateral bending radiograph is helpful in making this

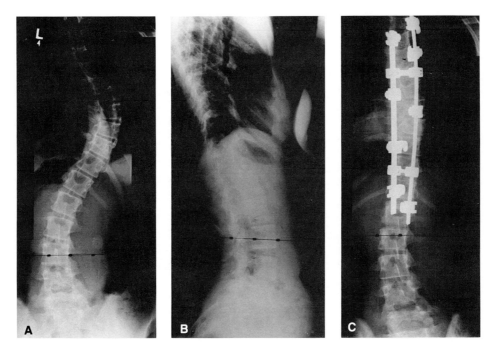

FIG. 10–30. The most common pattern of instrumentation for a single thoracic scoliosis. **A.** Anteroposterior radiograph shows a moderate scoliosis. **B.** Lateral radiograph shows a moderate hypokyphosis. **C.** Postoperative radiograph shows instrumentation from T4 to T12. The hooks on the left rod are pedicle hooks at T4 and T7. There are buttressed laminar hooks at T10 and T12. On the right rod, hooks include a transverse process hook at T4, pedicle hooks at T4 and T8, and a large curved laminar hook at T12.

decision. The vertebrae at the end of the stiff segment (i.e., the first vertebrae in which the disc spaces proximal and distal to the apex open with bending) should be chosen for apical hook placement.

Finally, the placement sites of the convex hooks are chosen. The end vertebrae remain the same, and proximally a standard claw configuration may be used. This construct consists of a transverse process hook and a pedicle hook on the upper vertebrae. The claw may be split with the pedicle hook placed one vertebra lower than the transverse process hook for added strength of fixation.[20] At or just distal to the apex, a pedicle hook is placed. Finally, at the lower end vertebra an upward-facing compression hook is placed.

Low Single Thoracic Curve

The thoracic curve with an apex at or below T9 will require instrumentation of the upper lumbar spine.

The end vertebra should be either the stable vertebra[15] or the one proximal to the stable vertebra at the lower end. It is generally not necessary to go distal to the L2 vertebra unless that vertebra is well out of the midline (Fig. 10-31).

The major conceptual difference in treating this curve is that it is necessary to use compression instrumentation across the thoracolumbar junction to create a neutral or slightly lordotic contour at the T11–L2 area. Thus hooks are placed so that on the concavity there is distraction between the upper thoracic hook and T11, with compression between T11 and L2. The rod is contoured so that when it is rotated, the kyphotic contour ends at T11 and the T11 to L2 segment is lordotic. Because the rod contour does not match the scoliosis, some lateral translation of the rod is necessary to seat it in the hooks. (See the discussion of thoracolumbar curves and cantilever correction.)

The convex rod is applied with compression over

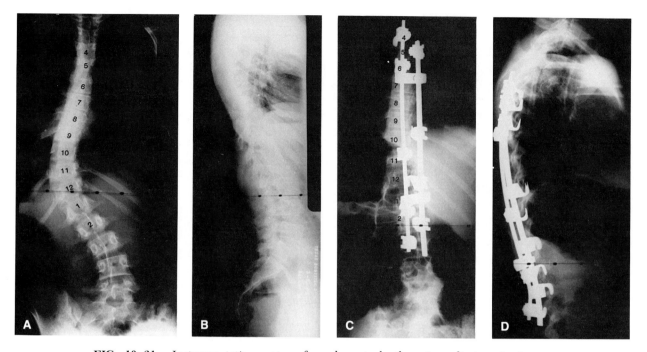

FIG. 10–31. Instrumentation pattern for a low single thoracic scoliosis. **A.** Anteroposterior radiograph of a left thoracic scoliosis with the apex at T10. **B.** Lateral radiograph
showing a normal sagittal contour. **C.** Postoperative anteroposterior radiograph shows
instrumentation from T4 to L2. The right rod is placed first with pedicle hooks at T4 and T9
and buttressed laminar hooks at T12 and L2. This rod is contoured into a kyphosis–lordosis
pattern and is inserted distally first. After placement of the rod into the lower two hooks, the
rod is translated across the midline to the right to place the upper two hooks. This maneuver
produces a cantilever effect that is the major corrective force for the curve. The left rod is then
placed with the claw spaced with the transverse processes hook on T4 and the pedicle hook at
T5. A buttressed laminar hook is placed at T11, and large round laminar hooks are placed at
L1 and L2.

the thoracic curve and distraction across the thoracolumbar junction. The forces applied to the second
rod seat the hooks and stabilize the spine, but do not
change the sagittal contour set by the first rod.

Double Thoracic Curve, King V Type[15]

The double thoracic pattern curve is corrected by a
combination of distraction and cantilever forces (Fig.
10-32). The end vertebrae are usually the stable vertebrae at the upper end of the upper thoracic curve and
the lower end of the lower thoracic curve. The hook
placement of the lower thoracic curve is identical to
that for a single thoracic curve. The upper thoracic

curve is also instrumented as a single curve, but usually it is necessary to place only one hook in the apical
portion, both on the concavity and the convexity of the
curve.

The rod contour is that of a normal kyphosis, and
the rod is placed without any rotation maneuver. The
rod in the kyphotic position is placed in the hooks
beginning at the caudal end of the curve. After passing
the apex of the lower thoracic curve, the rod will tend
to lie to the concave side of the upper portion of the
spine. At each level, the rod is translated to the hooks
and fixed in place. As the rod is translated laterally, the
curves are being gradually corrected. Bringing the rod
to the uppermost hooks may be difficult, since this
represents the final correction of the curve. If it is not

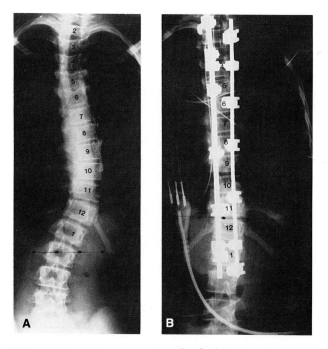

FIG. 10–32. Instrumentation of a double thoracic curve. **A.** Anteroposterior radiograph of a double thoracic curve in a skeletally immature girl. **B.** Posterior radiograph shows instrumentation from T2 to L1. The left rod was placed first from caudal to cephalad. The rod was contoured to a physiologic kyphosis–lordosis pattern and cantilevered across the midline. There is a transverse process hook at T2, pedicle hooks at T3, T5, and T8, and buttressed laminar hooks at T11 and L1. On the right, there is a pedicle hook at T2 and large round laminar hooks at T6, T8, T10, and L1.

possible to bring the rod to the upper hooks, it may have to be contoured in situ to reach them. (This is likely only with stiff curves.)

Double Curves, King II Type[15]

Significant balance problems are associated with the instrumentation of the King II curve.[17, 19] In milder curves and in those with trunk shift to the right, selective fusion of the thoracic curve may be appropriate. There should be no junctional kyphosis present on the lateral radiograph if only the thoracic curve is to be fused. Correction with the standard rotational maneuver may be chosen, or the curve may be corrected with a distraction–transverse loading construct. If the curves are severe, if there is a leftward shift of the trunk, or if there is junctional kyphosis, instrumentation into the lumbar curve may be necessary.

Instrumentation of the Thoracic Curve With Rotational Correction

The levels are selected as in the single thoracic curve. The lower vertebra should be one proximal to the stable vertebra.[17, 19] The remainder of the instrumentation is as described for the single thoracic curve (Fig. 10-33).

Instrumentation of the Thoracic Curve With Transverse Loading

The levels are selected as in a single thoracic curve, instrumenting to the stable vertebra at the caudal end (Fig. 10-34).[15] A distraction construct with one proximal and one distal hook is placed. The rod is contoured into a normal kyphotic curvature. Spinous process wires are placed with button wires as described by Drummond.[9] The wires are drawn to the concave rod and tightened by twisting.

A second rod is placed in a compression construct on the convexity of the curve. Crosslinks™ are then fastened to the rods for final stability.

Instrumentation of Both the Thoracic and Lumbar Curves, Double Major Pattern

The technique for instrumentation of both curves begins with placement of a rod on the left side of the spine (Fig. 10-35). The rod is contoured into a kyphosis–lordosis curvature that approaches the normal sagittal contour for the levels to be instrumented. A four-hook construct is used for the thoracic curve, with the lower thoracic hook also serving as the proximal hook for the lumbar curve, which is instrumented in compression. The lumbar curve will usually also have four hooks, counting the lowest thoracic hook. After compression and distraction, the rod is rotated 90 degrees. Care is necessary to prevent loss of purchase of the lowest lumbar hook during rotation. The right-sided rod is contoured and placed with compression of the thoracic curve and distraction of the lumbar curve. The rods are joined with Crosslinks™.

Thoracolumbar Curve

Posterior Instrumentation

The instrumentation of this curve is quite different from that for the other types of curve (Fig. 10-36). Correction is obtained by using a cantilever force. The concave rod is contoured into a kyphosis–lordosis pattern that approximates normal. It is inserted into the caudal three hooks, which are placed in enough dis-

(text continues on page 247)

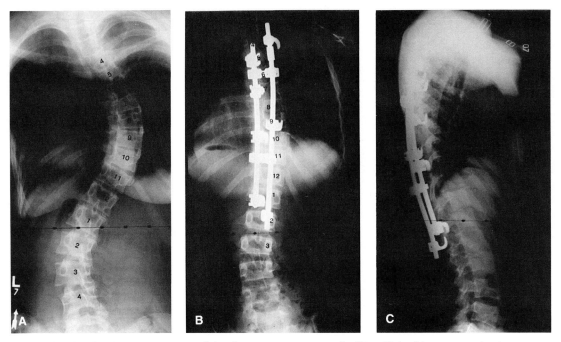

FIG. 10–33. Instrumentation of the thoracic component of a King II double curve. **A.** Anteroposterior radiograph shows a large thoracic curve and a relatively small lumbar curve. There was no junctional kyphosis on the lateral radiograph. **B.** Postoperative anteroposterior radiograph shows instrumentation from T5 to L1. The left rod is placed first and correction obtained by rod rotation. There are pedicle hooks on the left at T5 and T7 and buttressed laminar hooks at T10 and L1. On the right, there is a transverse process hook at T5, pedicle hooks at T5 and T9, and a large round laminar hook at L1. **C.** The lateral postoperative radiograph demonstrates restoration of kyphosis.

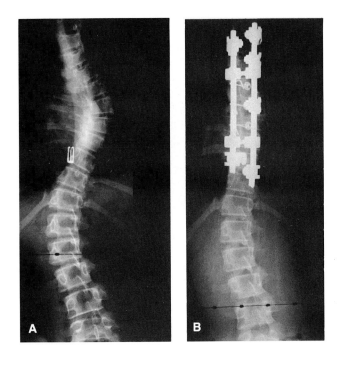

FIG. 10–34. Instrumentation of a King II double curve using transverse loading instead of rod rotation for correction. This patient had trunk shift to the left preoperatively, which would have worsened with rotational correction. **A.** Anteroposterior radiograph shows matched thoracic and lumbar curves. **B.** Posterior anteroposterior radiograph shows dual rods and translational instrumentation. The left rod is placed first with a pedicle hook at T4 and a buttressed laminar hook at T10. Drummond-type spinous process buttons and wires are placed at T6, T7, and T8. The right rod is then placed with a transverse process hook at T4, pedicle hooks at T4 and T7, and a small round laminar hook at T10. The spinal balance was maintained.

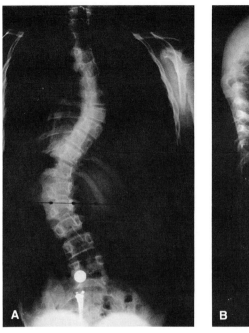

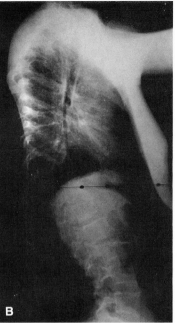

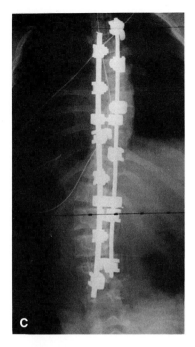

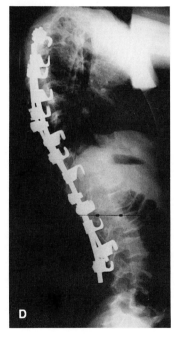

FIG. 10–35. A double major curve with instrumentation of both the thoracic and lumbar curves. **A.** Anteroposterior radiograph shows double curves of equal magnitude. **B.** Lateral radiograph demonstrates a junctional kyphosis at the thoracolumbar junction. **C.** Postoperative anteroposterior radiograph shows instrumentation from T4 to L3. The left rod is inserted first and rotated to achieve correction. There are pedicle hooks at T4 and T6 and buttressed laminar hooks at T10, T12, L2, and L3. On the right rod there is a transverse process hook at T4, a pedicle hook at T5 and T8, large curved laminar hooks at T10 and L1, and a buttressed laminar hook at L3. **D.** Postoperative lateral radiograph shows the contour of the rods into a physiologic kyphosis–lordosis pattern.

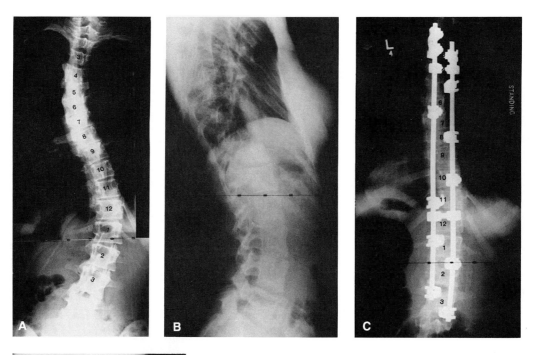

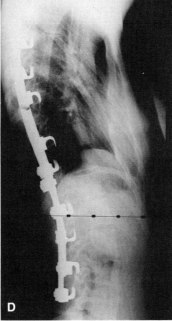

FIG. 10–36. A right thoracolumbar curve with secondary left thoracic curve, instrumented posteriorly. **A.** Anteroposterior radiograph shows the major right thoracolumbar curve and a secondary left thoracic curve. **B.** Preoperative lateral radiograph shows an extended thoracolumbar lordosis. **C.** Postoperative anteroposterior radiograph with instrumentation from T3 to L3. To achieve cantilever correction of the scoliosis, the left rod is contoured into a kyphosis–lordosis pattern and inserted, beginning at the caudal portion. After seating the L3 and L1 hooks, the rod is translated across the midline and the T11 hook is inserted. The remainder of the hooks are then inserted sequentially. When the right rod is placed, the distraction is released from the left rod lumbar hooks. The hooks between T10 and L3 on the right are then compressed to produce lordosis. **D.** Postoperative lateral radiograph shows maintenance of lumbar lordosis and restoration of thoracic kyphosis.

traction to seat them well. The rod is then translated over to the next most proximal hook; this is continued until the rod is in the most proximal hooks. At this point the curve will be corrected to at least its best bend. The hooks are seated with minimal distraction, and if the rod is not in the sagittal plane, it is rotated to that position.

Next the convex rod is placed after contouring it to a kyphosis–lordosis curve. At this point it is necessary to release the distraction on the concave hooks below T10 and compress the hooks on the convex rod, in order to produce normal lordosis of the lumbar segment. Finally the Crosslinks™ are inserted to stabilize the system.

Anterior Instrumentation

In thoracolumbar and lumbar curves, the TSRH system may be used anteriorly much like the Zielke system (see Fig. 10-13). Vertebral screws are inserted through circular collars. After excision of the discs and endplates, a rod is inserted. The rod is contoured into a lordotic posture in its lumbar portion and is straight at the thoracolumbar junction. The rod is rotated to convert the scoliosis to lordosis, and the screws are compressed to the center of the rod. The 4.8-mm ($3/16''$) rod is used for this procedure.

Pelvic Fixation

When fixation to the pelvis is necessary, we prefer to instrument the spine to L5 in the normal manner. We then place rods into the iliac wing by the Galveston technique (Fig. 10-17).[1] It is important to place these rods as close as possible to the hard bone over the acetabulum. They are then contoured so as to lie adjacent to the instrumentation above L5. The main rods are connected to the iliac rods with Crosslinks™. The rods are spread as they are seated on the iliac wings by using a Crosslink™ slightly wider than necessary. If the lumbosacral junction is excessively lordotic, the pelvic obliquity is corrected by distraction against the rod on the higher side. If the junction is kyphotic or flexed, the obliquity is corrected by compression on the low side. The correction is stabilized by firmly tightening the Crosslinks™. It is most important to contour the plates so that the rods fit in the grooves of the plates exactly perpendicularly.

References

1. Allen BL Jr, Ferguson RL: The Galveston technique for L-rod instrumentation of the scoliotic spine. Spine 7:276, 1982
2. Ashman RB, Birch JG, Bone LB, et al: Mechanical testing of spinal instrumentation. Clin Orthop 227:113, 1988
3. Ashman RB, Galpin RD, Corin JD, Johnston CE II: Biomechanical analysis of pedicle screw instrumentation systems in a corpectomy model. Spine 14:1398, 1989
4. Birch JG, Camp JF, Corin J, Ashman RB: Rotational stability of various pedicle hook designs—an in vitro analysis. Presented at the Annual Meeting of the Scoliosis Research Society, Amsterdam, The Netherlands, September 17–22, 1989
5. Boachie-Adjei O, Lonstein JE, Winter RB, et al: Management of neuromuscular spinal deformities with Luque segmental instrumentation. J Bone Joint Surg [Am] 71:548, 1989
6. Broom MJ, Banta JV, Renshaw TS: Spinal fusion augmented by Luque-rod segmental instrumentation for neuromuscular scoliosis. J Bone Joint Surg [Am] 71:32, 1989
7. Camp JF, Candle R, Ashman RB, Roach JW: Immediate complications of C.D. instrumentation to the sacro-pelvis: A clinical and biomechanical study. Spine 15:932, 1990
8. Collins JA: High-cycle fatigue. In Failure of Materials in Mechanical Design: Analysis, Prediction, Prevention. New York, John Wiley, 1981
9. Drummond D, Guadagni J, Keene JS, et al: Interspinous process segmental spinal instrumentation. J Pediatr Orthop 4:397, 1984
10. Gurr KR, McAfee PC, Warden KE, Shih CM: Roentgenographic and biomechanical analysis of lumbar fusions: a canine model. J Orthop Res 7:838, 1989
11. Johnston CE II, Ashman RB, Baird AM, Allard RN: Effect of spinal construct stiffness on early fusion mass incorporation. Spine 15:908, 1990
12. Johnston CE II, Ashman RB, Corin JD: Mechanical effects of cross-linking rods in Cotrel-Dubousset instrumentation. Orthop Trans 11:96, 1987
13. Johnston CE II, Ashman RB, Sherman MC, et al: Mechanical consequences of rod contouring and residual scoliosis in sublaminar segmental instrumentation. J Orthop Res 5:206, 1987
14. Johnston CE II, Haideri N, Ashman RB: Early experience with rigid crosslinking. Presented at the Annual Meeting of the Scoliosis Research Society, Honolulu, Hawaii, September 23–27, 1990
15. King HA, Moe JH, Bradford DS, Winter RB: The selection of fusion levels in thoracic idiopathic scoliosis. J Bone Joint Surg 65A:1302, 1983
16. Luque ER: The anatomic basis and development of segmental spinal instrumentation. Spine 7:256, 1982
17. McAllister JW, Bridwell KH, Betz R, et al: Coronal

decompensation produced by Cotrel–Dubousset de-rotation manuever for idiopathic right thoracic scoliosis. Orthop Trans 13:79, 1989

18. Nasca RJ, Hollis JM, Lemmons JE, Cool TA: Cyclic axial loading of spinal implants. Spine 10:792, 1985

19. Richards BS, Birch JG, Herring JA, et al: Frontal plane and sagittal plane balance following Cotrel–Dubousset instrumentation for idiopathic scoliosis. Spine 14:733, 1989

20. Roach JW, Ashman RB, Allard RN: The strength of a posterior element claw at one versus two spinal levels. J Spinal Disord 3:259, 1990

21. Shufflebarger H: Neurologic injury with Cotrel-Dubousset instrumentation. Report to Scoliosis Research Society, Membership Survey on Morbidity, 1989

22. Weiler PJ: Buckling analysis of spinal implant devices used for the surgical treatment of scoliosis. Thesis, Department of Mechanical Engineering, University of Waterloo, Waterloo, Ontario, 1983

CHAPTER 11

Adult Scoliosis

John Kostuik

■

A dult scoliosis is defined as a presentation of scoliosis after skeletal maturity. Some authors have included in this term all spinal deformities of patients who present for treatment after the age of 20. Scoliosis in adults can be the consequence of a process that began before skeletal maturity, or the scoliosis can arise in adult life secondary to osteoporosis, osteomalacia, or iatrogenic causes, such as multilevel decompressions for spinal stenosis and degenerative changes. This chapter focuses primarily on the resulting adult spinal deformities that began to develop before skeletal maturity, but the principles apply to all scoliosis patients.

Until the late 1960s, surgical treatment of most scoliotic deformities in the adult was not considered possible. The work of Collis, Kostuik, Nilsonne, Ponsetti, Stagnara, and others showed that curves in the adult may progress and that the curves were often painful.[4, 8, 11, 12, 26, 35, 50–53, 56–61, 63, 64, 68, 69] The advent of Harrington instrumentation in the late 1950s and the subsequent improvements in instrumentation by Dwyer in 1970, Luque in 1976, Zielke in 1975, and more recently by Cotrel and Dubousset, combined with improvements in preoperative assessment and postoperative care, markedly improved the surgeon's ability to deal with the complex spinal problems of the adult.[9, 10, 15, 20, 21, 40, 41, 69, 70] There is a greater understanding by family physicians and paramedical personnel that the adult with scoliosis can now safely undergo surgical intervention when required.

CURRENT PROBLEMS

Kostuik and Bentivogilio in 1981 found an incidence of 3.9% of curves involving the thoracolumbar and lumbar spine.[32] They felt that these curves were truly structural in nature and had commenced in adolescence and progressed during adult life. These were not curves generated by osteoporosis or due to local degenerative changes.

In 1968, James stated that 6% of adults over the age of 50 years showed evidence radiographically of scoliosis, but he felt that the majority of these were due to compression fractures, osteoporosis, and osteomalacia.[65]

Illustrations reproduced from Frymoyer JW et al (eds): The Adult Spine: Principles and Practice. New York, Raven Press, 1991, with permission.

Dewar, in the early 1950s (unpublished data), discovered an incidence of structural thoracic scoliosis of 4% on reviewing 10,000 consecutive chest radiographs done for routine hospital admission.

Because many of these curves are mild or moderate in adolescence and do not become apparent until the fourth, fifth, and sixth decades of life, the population with scoliotic curves will continue to grow as the population ages in the industrialized countries, where surgical intervention is warranted.

In 1983, Weinstein and Ponsetti delineated the factors that are responsible for continued curve progression in adults.[67] Thoracic curves between 50 and 75° at skeletal maturity increased an average of 30° during the follow-up period. Thoracolumbar curves between 50 and 75° at skeletal maturity increased 22.3° over 40 years. Lumbar spine curves, where the L5 vertebra was not well seated and where apical rotation was greater than 33%, progressed the most.

In our experience the patient with the worst prognosis in adult life is the young adult or adolescent who presents with an imbalanced lumbar curve or thoracolumbar curve in which the L5 vertebra is not parallel with the sacrum and the curve emanates from the lumbosacral junction (Fig 11-1). This curve presents the greatest technologic difficulties in correction in later adult life, and it is better to treat this condition at an early age if possible.

Other curves with a poor prognosis include those whose apexes fall between L2 and L4 who have a significant Grade 3 rotation, are imbalanced, and have a secondary compensatory curve that is sharp and angular between L4 and S1. In the young adult or adolescent, these curves can often be treated and rebalanced by dealing with the compensatory curve at one or two levels, rather than dealing with the entire proximal curve over five to seven levels.

Reflecting the increasing age of our population, it is not uncommon for the spinal surgeon to be presented with a complex problem of an increasing deformity associated with pain, loss of lumbar lordosis, imbalance, osteoporosis, and spinal stenosis. With a better understanding of spinal mechanics, improved instrumentation, improved postoperative care, and screw fixation in bone, it is possible to treat these patients with little resultant morbidity (Fig. 11-2).

In a review of adult patients with curves in the lumbar and thoracolumbar spine, Kostuik and Bentivoglio found a 60% incidence of back pain.[32] This rate was similar to an unselected, consecutive series of 100 patients without scoliosis of the same age range. These figures are also comparable to those found in local

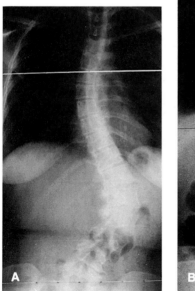
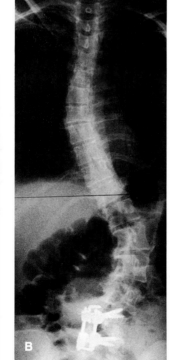

FIG. 11–1. **A.** A 26-year-old woman with a painful scoliosis. Notice the marked imbalance to the left. Pain was reproduced on discography at both L4–L5 and L1–S1 discs. **B.** Rebalanced with relief of pain from the lateral closing wedges. The double Zielke rods control rotational forces.

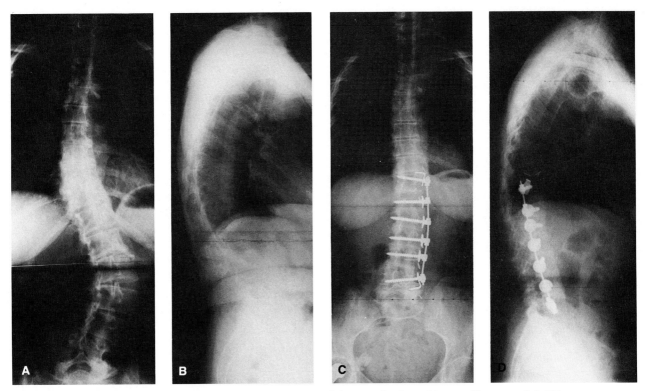

FIG. 11–2. **A.** Documented, progressive, painful curve of 44° in a 45-year-old woman. L4–L5 and L5–S1 discs were not painful during discography. L4–S1 and L5–S1 facet blocks did not relieve pain. Notice previous total hip replacement. **B.** Preoperative lateral radiograph, 66°. **C.** Postoperative Zielke instrumentation corrects to 2°. After 6 years of follow-up, there was no pain. **D.** Lordosis has been fully preserved.

population studies in the industrialized world, in which the incidence of back pain is between 60 and 70% in the general adult population. Results demonstrated that the incidence of pain increased markedly in curves greater than 45°. The pain reached its maximum between the ages of 40 and 60 years, similar to the spondylogenic or discogenic pain patterns in the general population. In 1969, Nachemson found a similar incidence of pain among scoliotics.[44, 45] However, the incidence of severe pain seems to be greater in reports of Kostuik and Bentivoglio than in that of Nachemson, who stated that the pain always seemed to be mild and rarely required treatment.[32, 44, 45]

It is not the degree of deformity that is paramount in determining treatment for adults, as it is in adolescents. The symptoms should be addressed. Most patients should be given a course of nonoperative or conservative treatment first. The exception to this is the patient with significant progression, evidenced radiologically or by loss of height, who is imbalanced and

who has radiologically determined excessive rotation and significant, disabling pain (Fig. 11-3). In my experience, thoracic curves in adults with scoliosis are rarely painful.

Some problems confronting the orthopedic surgeon dealing with adult scoliosis are those related to iatrogenic flat backs caused by correction and fusion with Harrington instrumentation and extending to the distal lumbar spine, usually L5 or S1.[14, 17, 22, 37, 39] This problem may also result from degenerative changes and loss of disc height below a fusion mass ending at L2, L3, L4, or L5 or may occur above a fusion (e.g., L4 to the sacrum) in women with osteopenia and loss of disc height. Precocious degenerative changes can occur below a fusion done in adolescence or young adult life.

After a long-term anatomic and functional review of patients with adolescent idiopathic scoliosis treated by Harrington rod fusion, Cochran and colleagues reported in 1988 that the incidence of degenerative

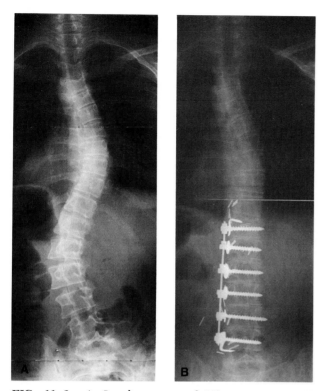

FIG. 11–3. A. Lumbar curve of 60° in a 24-year-old woman. The thoracic curve is 52°. Notice the obliquity of L5. **B.** Postoperative lumbar curve is 15°, and the thoracic curve was reduced to 40°. L5 is more horizontal.

changes increased proportionally with the distal extent of the fusion formed in adolescence. The incidence of degenerative changes with pain was about 20% for fusions ending at L2, 40% for fusions ending at L3, 60% for fusions ending at L4, and 80% for those ending at L5.[6] In 1982, Edgar similarly found an increased incidence of degenerative changes associated with pain at levels of previous fusions below L3 or L4.[16]

When correlating pain with age, the pattern seems to follow a bell curve, with the majority of patients with pain falling in the sixth, seventh, and eighth decades of life. Pain appeared to reach its maximum between the ages of 40 and 60 years, which corresponds to the maximum incidence of pain from a spondylogenic or discogenic causes in the nonscoliotic population.

There appears to be distinct preference for lighter work by scoliotic patients, although only 21% of patients reviewed by Kostuik and Bentivoglio were aware that they had scoliosis.[32] Rogala and Drummond suggested a preference for lighter work by scoliotics as

well.[54] The type of occupation was not a predisposing factor to pain, although those with more labor-intensive jobs seemed to be less able to cope and missed more time from work or were more likely to be incapacitated.

Patients with curves greater than 45° had a statistically significant greater degree of incapacitating pain than those patients with curves less than 45°. The increasing incapacitation due to pain with greater curves, together with an increasing severity of pain with increasing age, suggests that curves 45° or greater at the end of growth tend to become more clinically significant with increasing age. In both the lumbar curves and thoracolumbar curves, pain correlated with the severity of the curves. All patients with radiographic affirmation of degenerative processes at the apex of curves demonstrated similar changes at the lumbosacral junction. Facet sclerosis correlated with a history of pain in 64% of patients.

PATIENT EVALUATION

As with most spinal problems, history is the primary means of evaluating the patient. A relevant family history of deformity may give some indication of prognosis. For example, a close relative who has a progressive, severe deformity and is older than the patient may give some insight into the patient's future.

The date of onset of the deformity is rarely important. A history of curve progression can be obtained from the patient or from relatives. For example, a change in clothes, increasing rib hump, a loss of height, or a loss of waistline is relevant. Ideally, progression is determined through serial radiographs, but these are often not available, particularly in the case of thoracolumbar or lumbar curves, which may not be noticed until adult life. The psychologic aspects of the patient's deformity should be considered. Many adults are reluctant to discuss the esthetics of their deformities unless directly asked. Many of them have learned to live with their deformities without problems, but for about 10% of the patients in our series, deformity continues to play a significant psychological role.[31]

A questionnaire is important to help determine the location of pain. Pain may be apical or below the apex. Patients often indicate the location of pain with the palms of their hands. It is important to know the duration of pain and how it affects activities of daily living, social function, occupation, and family and sexual life. It is important to know what aggravates and what alleviates the pain. If there is radicular pain, which suggests root irritation, it is important to get a history of this as well. Radicular pain may be related to the apex of the curve, and if it is in the thoracic or thoracolumbar curve area, it may be costal in nature. Radicular pain may also arise from the compensatory curve in the case of a thoracolumbar curve.[25] Lumbar pain may be referred into the lower extremities. True sciatica goes below the knee; pain above the knee may simply be referred pain, but it can have a nerve root origin.

A history of bowel and bladder function is important. An associated spinal stenosis may present initially with bladder incontinence, particularly in females. Incontinence in the elderly female is often due to spinal stenosis and not, as commonly assumed, a late effect of childbearing. History frequently reveals a recent onset of bladder incontinence.

Respiratory malfunction may be the presenting symptom in scoliosis, but usually only in the paralytic or in patients with severe congenital curves. The patient may describe respiratory problems, such as shortness of breath while climbing stairs, or may complain about tiredness. A good history of respiratory function is important. My review of 200 consecutive adults with idiopathic scoliosis revealed no cases of severe dysfunction, even in curves of 100° or more. Ventilation was often decreased by as much as 25% of the predicted normal value, but the decrement rarely was functionally significant. Arterial blood gases were usually normal. Presentation of severe problems in perfusion or ventilation in the presence of a scoliosis indicates a congenital scoliosis unless otherwise ruled out. Although there would appear to be a correlation between curve size above 60° and pulmonary insufficiency, I have seen no pulmonary deaths associated with idiopathic scoliosis in over 20 years of experience. All deaths were in congenital or in paralytic curves. The only exception to this rule in cases of idiopathic scoliosis is the patient who has a marked thoracic lordosis.

Current theories about thoracic curves suggest an anterior tether of the thoracic spine, causing lordosis and scoliosis. In patients with a marked thoracic lordosis, pulmonary function may be severely affected. Pulmonary function tests are done only for thoracic curves of greater than 60° or in cases of paralytic or congenital scoliosis.

Physical examination focuses on the spinal deformity, but a complete examination is necessary, including a full neurologic examination and cardiopulmonary evaluation. The three-dimensional nature of the curve should be assessed. A kyphotic or lordotic element should be looked for in patients with scoliosis, and its influence on pulmonary function should be assessed.

The degree of decompensation, the flexibility and the size of the rib hump, and the patient's height should be measured. Signs of subtle neurologic dysfunction should be looked for, particularly in left thoracic idiopathic curves, which are often associated with syringomyelia. Mild clawing of the toes may indicate a tethered cord. Muscle fatigue after exercise in patients with a history of spinal stenosis associated with scoliosis should be looked for.

ROENTGENOLOGY

After clinical determination of scoliosis or kyphosis, initial radiographic analysis should include a posterior-anterior and lateral 3-ft films. These will indicate the degree of the deformity, local abnormalities, and the degree of decompensation. If there is pain, localized x-ray films are used to detect enlarged facets, congenital anomalies, disc narrowing, and other specific findings.

In my experience, bending x-ray films can indicate flexibility of the curve but do not provide any formula for the degree of correction expected after surgical intervention. In mobile thoracolumbar curves treated by anterior Zielke instrumentation, the amount of correction obtained was twice that indicated by bending x-ray films.

Traction films will occasionally indicate whether applying corrective force will overcome decompensation. A supine posterior-anterior film may also help the physician decide the most productive means of treating decompensation.

Hyperextension views of the kyphotic area are useful only if the kyphosis if flexible. Flexion views are used for evaluating excessive lordosis.

Stagnara views can demonstrate the rotational deformity of scoliosis, particularly in kyphoscoliosis. They are essentially oblique views. Special studies include bone scans, myelography, discography, computed tomography (CT), and magnetic resonance imaging (MRI). Bone scans are rarely indicated, but for the young adult with a minor curve, they are sometimes useful in ruling out diseases like tumors as the cause of the scoliosis. Myelography is indicated for patients with neuropathology and congenital curves. For any patient undergoing surgical correction for a painful deformity, preoperative myelography can be used to rule out cauda equina or cord compression before surgery.

CT has not proved to be of great value in assessing the contents of the dural canal in scoliosis, and in our experience it is best combined with myelography using nonionic dyes. The scan is done 3 to 4 hours after the myelogram. In low back problems caused by degenerative disease, 30% of the myelography or CT scans alone can give false-positive results. The combination of myelography and CT scanning, however, can increase accuracy to more than 90%. The role of MRI appears promising, but it is still somewhat experimental in the study of spinal deformity.

Discography and the use of facet blocks are discussed under pain evaluation.

CONSERVATIVE NONSURGICAL CARE

Nonsurgical care is primarily for those patients for whom there are no operative indications or for whom operative intervention is precluded by certain health factors, including serious cardiac or respiratory disease or psychological considerations. The essentials of nonsurgical treatment are drugs, physiotherapy, and orthotic devices.

Excluding cosmetic deformity, significant progression, or neurologic problems, the main indication for operative intervention is pain, but nonsurgical treatment should be tried first. Nonsteroidal anti-inflammatory drugs may relieve pain. Enteric-coated aspirin is often as valuable as more expensive nonsteroidal anti-inflammatory drugs and can be used for a longer period. Muscle relaxants or analgesics with high doses (30 mg or greater) of narcotics like codeine or some of the synthetic narcotic drugs like percodan should be avoided except for very acute phases of severe pain.

Physiotherapy, especially exercise, is rarely successful in controlling pain in adult scoliotics. Instead, motion usually aggravates pain. However, flexibility and stretching exercises may be of value for a short period, but the exercises must be tailored to motions that avoid pain. Low-impact aerobics, cycling exercises, and swimming exercises are useful.

No physiotherapy can prevent the progression of a curve, but tailored exercise may maintain some flexibility and augment subsequent surgical treatment.

For patients with scoliosis who are over the age of

50, especially women, orthoses can have great value. These need to be rigid and formed to the patient's deformities. They should be worn while the patient is ambulatory and may sustain the patient for many months or years. However, in my experience, most of these patients eventually require surgery. If an orthosis is provided, the patient should also be involved in an exercise program to maintain mobility of the deformity and general muscle tone.

Other factors influencing nonsurgical treatment are diet, a general understanding of the cause of scoliosis, and a prognosis for the patient's individual deformity. A normal diet is advised.

Because osteoporosis plays a major role in the progression of deformity in postmenopausal women, it is important that premenopausal women with scoliosis exercise. Twenty minutes of low-impact aerobics four times a week for 10 years before menopause can prevent postmenopausal osteoporosis in most women. For postmenopausal women, exercise combined with hormonal therapy and calcium taken under the supervision of a physician may retard osteoporosis during the first 10 years after menopause.

SURGICAL INDICATIONS

The indications for surgery, in order of their importance, are pain, progression of deformity, neurologic disability, cosmesis, structural imbalance in paralytic or neuromuscular disease, curve progression associated with pain below previous fusions for spinal deformity, and iatrogenic flat back (kyphosis).

The adult younger than 35 years of age, without pain but with documented increasing curvature, whose lumbar or thoracolumbar curve measures aproximately 45° and who is unbalanced, is best treated surgically, because he or she will inevitably go on to develop a painful low back. This is particularly true of a female patient with significant lumbar or thoracolumbar curve who, because of degenerative changes, may later convert from scoliosis with retention of lumbar lordosis to kyphoscoliosis, which becomes rigid and may require two-stage surgery to correct.

The younger adult can be readily treated anteriorly with good correction of the deformity using Zielke instrumentation with minimal morbidity (see Fig. 11-3). The unanswered question is what may happen to the levels below the fusion. In separate studies, Edgar and Cochran pointed out the increased incidence of pain and degenerative changes below the level of previous fusion with posterior instrumentation, which has been extended to the L3, L4, or L5 level.[6, 16] My advice to these and all patients after surgery is that they must become involved in athletic endeavors and maintain a satisfactory level of physical fitness. They must practice good back hygiene routinely and do low-back exercises on a daily basis. Physical fitness must also be attempted by the older patient, but because of age and a previous sedentary lifestyle, this is not often as practical as it is for the younger adult.

The unbalanced younger patient whose major curve may measure 40° or more and extend to L3 or L4, but who has a compensatory curve at L4 or L5 to L5 or S1 and who is imbalanced, may often have the primary curve significantly reduced by rebalancing through the lower curve. This should only be done if the lower curve is painful. Pain patterns must be proved preoperatively by discography and facet blocks. These patients may run the risk of upper curve progression later in life, and it should be explained that they may then require proximal extensions of their fusions. The technique has worked satisfactorily in 6

patients, and although the follow-up is short, the average degree of correction of the major curve has been more than 40% (see Fig. 11-1).

Curve progression is best documented by a careful history taken from both the patient and the relatives, with particular reference to current height and the height at completion of growth. A loss of height indicates progression of the spine deformity. Radiologic documentation is ideal but rarely available for adults. In 1983, Ponsetti and Weinstein showed that curves in the thoracolumbar spine and lumber spine are more likely to progress if the L5 vertebra is not well seated (oblique) and apical rotation is greater than 33%.[67] In my estimation, imbalance seems to play a major role in progression of the curve in conjunction with a significant degree of rotation.

Neurologic deficit in a series of more than 1000 adults with scoliosis treated surgically was rarely an indication for surgical intervention. However, in an increasingly aging population, more patients are seen with an associated spinal stenosis (Fig. 11-4). Surgical decompression by laminectomy is rarely indicated,

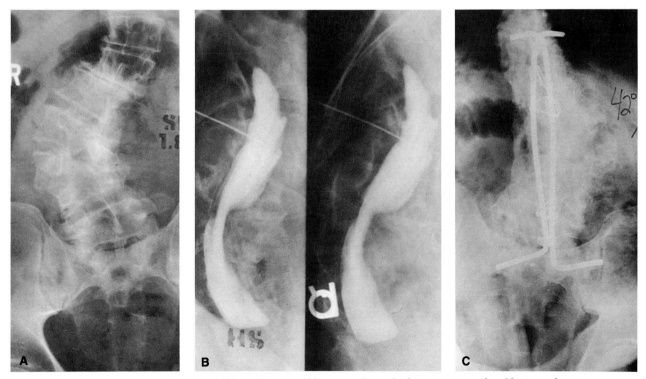

FIG. 11–4. **A.** Curve of 68° in a 56-year-old man with marked symptoms and mild signs of spinal stenosis. **B.** Preoperative myelogram indicates severe compromise of the canal at the apex of the curve. **C.** Postoperative anterior-posterior view shows a curve of 42°. Five years later, the patient was pain-free and working.

and in a 1978 review, only 5 of 227 patients treated surgically for a painful scoliosis required associated decompression.

In 1983, Simmons reported that patients with radicular symptoms arising from the compensatory curve frequently had marked improvement after correction of the major curve with an anterior procedure.[25] In my experience, this has been less successful.

All patients who complain of significant pain should undergo preoperative myelography to rule out causes such as intradural or extrdural tumors. Older adults with lumbar and thoracolumbar curves greater than 45° and pain should also have preoperative myelography. Spinal stenosis may be the cause of pain, especially patients over the age of 60.

The problem of cosmesis in the lumbar and thoracolumbar spine is rare in adults, with the exception of the young adult who is imbalanced. Some adults (10%) with scoliosis present with thoracic curves, which are not painful, requiring surgical correction for cosmetic reasons. Surgical intervention is warranted after repeated discussions with the patient and close relatives about the complexities and risks of the surgery if the patient has a strong desire for improvement of the deformity, even though the spinal deformity unlikely to progress or lead to pain later in life.

With the advent of Cotrel–Dubousset instrumentation, excellent cosmetic correction can safely be obtained in adults, especially for hypokyphosis of the thoracic spine. Thoracoplasty involving partial rib excision (usually four to six ribs) enhances the postoperative cosmetic appearance.

A functional analysis of 100 patients followed for more than 10 years postoperatively found that body image and cosmesis played a much greater role in adults' decisions to have surgery than was previously suspected.[38]

POSTOPERATIVE CARE

In postoperative care of the adult today, recumbency is not permitted. Patients usually become ambulatory by the third or fourth postoperative day. A thoracolumbar curve in the postoperative phase is usually fitted with orthosis, the modular Boston overlap-type brace or a molded plastic corset. Thoracic curves require no exterior support.

PAIN ASSESSMENT

Early attempts in the 1960s and 1970s at treating painful lumbar and thoracolumbar curves with Harrington instrumentation and fusion without preoperative pain assessment by discography and facet blocks left a significant number of patients complaining of pain.[35] Pain management helped 65 to 70% of these patients. Subsequent evaluation of pain using discography and facet blocks has increased the number obtaining good pain relief to between 80 and 90% of patients.[31]

It is important to have a thorough understanding of the patient's physical pain, which should not be clouded by psychological difficulties. Careful assessment of the patient requires a careful history. Patients may localize their pain to their low back or the apex of their curvature or both, but their symptoms may be vague. In 1977, Macnab showed that a hypertonic saline injection into the supraspinous ligament at the thoracolumbar junction reproduced pain at the lumbosacral junction.[42] With this in mind, I did a prospective study using discography to help differentiate sources of pain.[31] Today the use of discography is limited to an assessment of the lower levels of the lumbar spine (i.e., L3 to L4, L4 to L5, and the lumbosacral junction); rarely are discograms performed at the apex of the curve.

Discography is used to assess degeneration or pain. Facet blocks are similarly used. Discography is usually done from a posterolateral approach, although it may be necessary to trangress the dura because of deformity. Facet blocks are done using Marcaine with infiltration of the posterior ramus. Levels other than the L5 to S1 articulation have multiple innervation, and if the L4 to L5 level is to be assessed, the L3 to L4 level must be infiltrated as well. It is current practice in painful lumbar and thoracolumbar curves to do discography at the lower levels of the lumbar spine and facet blocks at the lowest level, L5 to S1, which has a single innervation.

If facet blocks relieve pain and discography reproduced pain at the lumbosacral junction, I believe the fusion must be extended to the sacrum. Before discography was used for cases in which the fusion was not extended to the sacrum, many patients continued to complain of pain despite correction of the deformity by a posterior or anterior approach.[35] Extension of fusion to the sacrum with preservation of lumbar lordosis and the ability to obtain a solid arthrodesis yielded good results in 90% of such cases.

If the discograms do not reproduce the patient's pain and facet blocks at the lumbosacral junction do not relieve the pain, it can be assumed that the pain arises in the curve itself. If the L5 to S1 area is not part of the curve, the curve alone is corrected and the lumbosacral junction is not fused.

SURGICAL TECHNIQUES

For adults, Harrington posterior instrumentation is rarely indicated for treatment of scoliotic deformities, especially in the lumbar and thoracolumbar spine, because loss of lumbar lordosis inevitably occurs with any form of this technique. Most lumbar and thoracolumbar curves today are being treated with anterior instrumentation using the Zielke technique.

Zielke instrumentation, however, is not useful if there is a true kyphosis, because it may exacerbate the condition. This can be evaluated only by oblique Stagnara views. In a kyphoscoliosis in the lumbar spine, which is a common problem encountered in patients over the age of 50, it is necessary to restore lumbar lordosis to restore balance and relieve pain. This can only be achieved by a two-stage procedure, an anterior approach done with multiple-level discotomies and fusions followed 2 weeks later by Cotrel–Dubousset instrumentation (Figs. 11-5 and 11-6). If the kyphoscoliosis is mobile, good results may be achieved by a single-stage posterior Cotrel–Dubousset instrumentation. The use of Cotrel–Dubousset instrumentation serves to derotate the spine, restore lordosis, and increase spinal rigidity.[9, 10, 13]

With the advent of Luque instrumentation in 1976, posterior segmental fixation gained great popularity.[10, 41] I do not feel that Harrington instrumentation with segmental wiring suffices for lumbar or thoracolumbar curves. The use of double-L rods or rectangular rods may be indicated. Initially, fixation to the pelvis with Luque rods contoured using the Galveston technique showed great promise.[1] However, many of these patients developed pain related to the sacroiliac joint after a solid fusion of the lumbar spine. We have abandoned the use of sublaminar wiring, except in cases of tumors and some cases of paralytic scoliosis.[7, 19, 23, 24, 27, 36, 48, 55, 62, 66] The advent of Cotrel–

Dubousset instrumentation has obviated the need for sublaminar wiring.

Zielke Instrumentation

The primary indication for Zielke instrumentation is a thoracolumbar or lumbar curve that does not require extension of the fusion to the sacrum, is mobile on bending x-ray films, and has preserved lordosis. In these cases associated with pain, if accurately assessed preoperatively with discography and facet blocks, correction of the deformity should be obtained with the use of Zielke instrumentation. In the older adult, the entire curve should be incorporated in the instrumentation. In the younger adult, levels comparable to those instrumented in adolescents will suffice.

From a technical viewpoint, the major problem in many adults is osteoporosis. This can be overcome with the injection of methylmethacrylate into predrilled screw holes in the vertebral bodies. If possible, the screw should be angled toward the contralateral junction of the pedicle with the vertebral body. This necessitates very careful cleaning of the disc space, including the end plates, to the posterior longitudinal ligament so that an accurate line can be obtained for insertion of the screws. To ensure that the opposite cortex is penetrated, a depth gauge is used to measure to the line in the interspace that the screw will follow. After measurement, 2 mm can be added to the depth of the screw, although frequently this is unnecessary if there is lipping of the vertebral body, particularly in cases associated with marked degeneration. Cooling the methylmethacrylate or using a low-viscosity methylmethacrylate increases the time available for its injection into enlarged screw holes. Frequently the use of a curette inside the screw hole can enlarge the space within the vertebral body for retention of the cement, enhancing fixation of the screws (Fig. 11-7).

The most significant technical difficulty has been withdrawal of the most proximal screw. I do not believe that an extra level should be incorporated across a nonfused space to prevent this problem (Fig. 11-8). In postmenopausal women, I routinely add cement to the upper level at the time of screw insertion.
tion.

There has been no difficulty with fusions extending proximally from L5. It is important to ligate the iliolumbar veins at the L5 level to allow mobilization of the common iliac system.

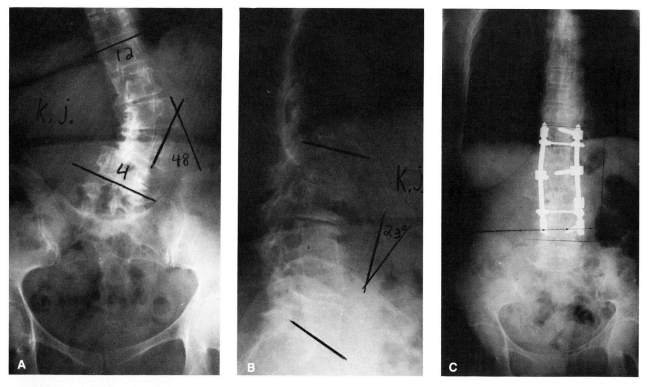

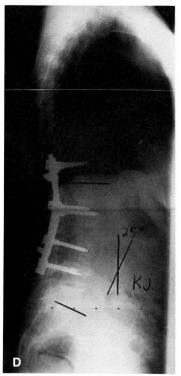

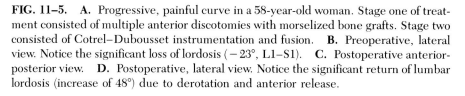

FIG. 11–5. **A.** Progressive, painful curve in a 58-year-old woman. Stage one of treatment consisted of multiple anterior discotomies with morselized bone grafts. Stage two consisted of Cotrel–Dubousset instrumentation and fusion. **B.** Preoperative, lateral view. Notice the significant loss of lordosis (−23°, L1–S1). **C.** Postoperative anterior-posterior view. **D.** Postoperative, lateral view. Notice the significant return of lumbar lordosis (increase of 48°) due to derotation and anterior release.

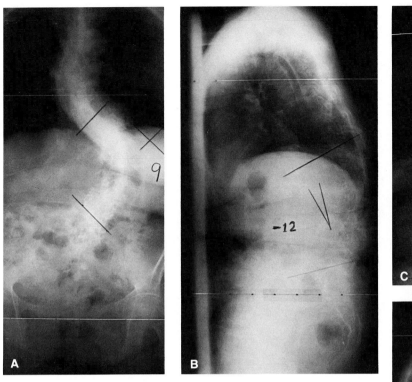

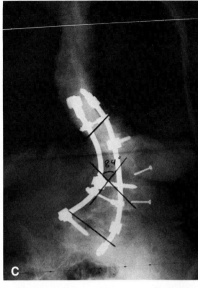

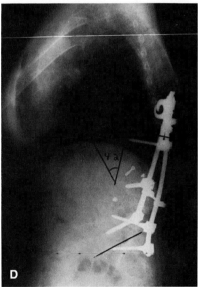

FIG. 11–6. **A.** Progressive kyphoscoliosis, with a curve of 92°, in a 63-year-old woman. Stage one of treatment consisted of multiple anterior discotomies and morselization of L2–L3. In stage two, Cotrel–Dubousset instrumentation and fusion were done. **B.** Preoperative lateral view of − 12° lordosis. **C.** Postoperative anterior-posterior view showing minimal correction. **D.** Postoperative lateral view showing marked restoration of lordosis to 42° (gain of 54°).

Extension with Zielke instrumentation to the sacrum is based on preoperative assessment and combined with a posterior fusion. Extension of Zielke instrumentation beyond T9 or T10 is rarely of value because the disc spaces are so narrow that little correction can be obtained. Routine use of the derotator reproduces lordosis or reduces kyphosis of the thoracolumbar spine. This provides a marked advantage over the previously used Dwyer instrumentation, which tended to produce a kyphosis despite accurate screw placement.

Autogenous bone graft consists of the excised rib cut up into very small fragments. I do not use iliac crest bone. Bits of block graft or placement of minced graft anteriorly in the disc space helps to maintain or increase lordosis with the use of Zielke instrumentation.

With the use of hypotensive anesthesia and cell

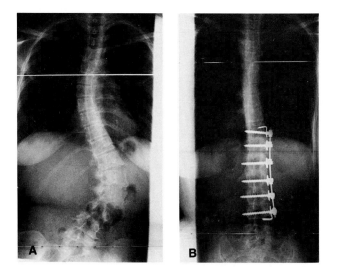

FIG. 11–7. **A.** A 77-year-old woman with severe, incapacitating, painful curve of 75°. **B.** Postoperative curve of 15°. Methylmethacrylate was used to hold the screws. The patient was free of pain 1 year later.

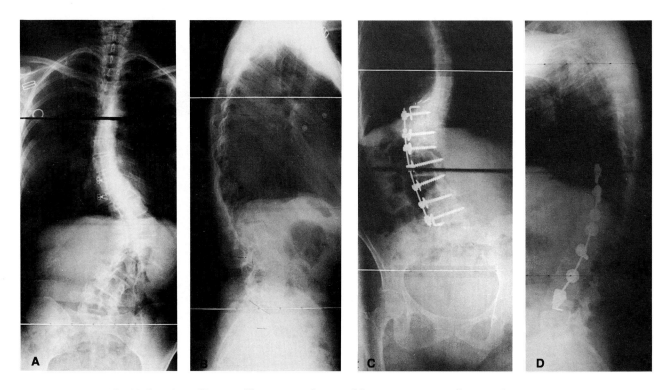

FIG. 11–8. **A.** A 52-year-old woman with a painful, progressive, rigid curve of 68°. **B.** Preoperative view of lordosis of 50°, L1–S1. **C.** Postoperative curve of 34°; notice the proximal hook pullout. **D.** Postoperative lateral view of curve of 38°, showing a good, long-term result.

savers, the average blood loss during Zielke instrumentation procedures has been 1750 ml. Transfusions using bank blood have been kept to a minimum. Hypotensive anesthesia is not used for patients over 50 years of age.

Zielke instrumentation can be used safely for patients over 70, although it is usually necessary to incorporate methylmethacrylate with the screws (see Fig. 11-7).

Correction using Zielke instrumentation has markedly improved on the results obtained with Dwyer instrumentation and posterior segmental instrumentation. A long-term follow-up of my first 57 patients treated with Zielke instrumentation revealed the average correction was 70% with no pseudoarthrosis, compared with an improvement of 45% with Dwyer instrumentation.[15, 20, 28, 33, 43, 51, 69, 70]

The use of the derotational device improved correction of the curve in the sagittal and anterior-posterior planes. Rotation improved by approximately one grade using the Nash-Moe classification.[46] Intraoperative complications included five fractured vertebral bodies, which were repaired with the use of methylmethacrylate. Postoperative complications included three lateral femoral cutaneous nerve entrapments, one of which required surgical decompression. Two post-thoracotomy syndromes were resolved with time. There were 10 cases of atelectasis and pleural effusions that did not require major treatment. One case of instrumentation failure was caused by staples pulling out at two levels, which required posterior surgery. Five other patients had partial staple disengagement. Nuts backed out of the screw heads in 10 cases without any curve deterioration or rod displacement. Rod disengagement from the screw heads occurred in 6 cases without short-term loss of correction. After an average follow-up of 2 years, the average loss of correction was less than 1°.

In double idiopathic curves, the average correction was 62%. At 24 months, the mean loss was 3.4° (4%). The noninstrumented proximal thoracic curve improved 38% after correction of the distal lumbar curve without deterioration during follow-up.

Cumulative surgical results revealed an improvement of 50% correction over that anticipated from the preoperative bending anterior-posterior radiographs.

An analysis of Zielke instrumentation, designed for anterior derotation in cases of scoliosis and used posteriorly as pedicle fixation for degenerative disease, revealed a high incidence of rod breakage. As a result, we no longer use Zielke instrumentation posteriorly. It has been surpassed by Cotrel–Dubousset instrumentation.

Zielke instrumentation has also been used for the distal convex side of fractional lumbosacral curves for 6 patients with imbalance and pain (see Fig. 11-1). This produced a slightly greater than 40% correction of the proximal major curve. The follow-up period is only 4 years for these patients, and they may require further treatment of their major curves at a later date. I feel this technique should be reserved only for those fractional curves in the lower lumbar and lumbosacral spine that are the source of pain, as shown by discography and facet blocks, and if the patient is imbalanced.

Cotrel–Dubousset Instrumentation

The Universal Instrumentation System of Cotrel and Dubousset became available in the 1980s.[9, 10, 13] The Cotrel–Dubousset instrumentation system attempts to combine the rigidity of segmental fixation and the concept of curve derotation to obtain correction. This report details our initial experience with Cotrel–Dubousset instrumentation in the treatment of adult idiopathic scoliosis (Fig. 11-9).

Between August 1985 and June 1988, 49 patients (43 women and 6 men) who had developed their deformities because of idiopathic scoliosis were operated. The average age of the patients was 43 years (range, 21–75 years). There were 19 patients older than 50 years at the time of surgery.

There were 16 primary thoracic, 15 primary lumbar, 14 double-major, and 4 thoracolumbar curves. Twelve patients had previous spinal fusions. (Another 45 patients underwent Cotrel–Dubousset instrumentation for other causes.)

For the entire series, the curves that were instrumented averaged 60° preoperatively in the frontal plane, with a range between 13° to 115°. Preoperatively, the primary thoracic curves averaged 58°, the primary lumbar curves averaged 48°, the thoracolumbar curves averaged 55°, and in the double-major curves, the thoracic curve averaged 76° and the lumbar curve averaged 66°.

The surgical indications were disabling back pain with or without neurologic symptoms in 44 patients. In 5 patients, the indication for surgery was curve progression.

The technical details regarding the use of Cotrel–Dubousset instrumentation are extensively described

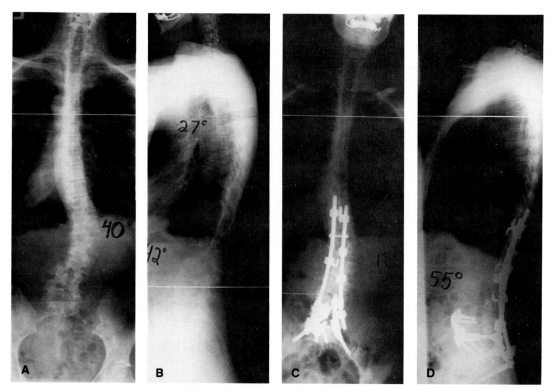

FIG. 11–9. **A.** A 53-year-old woman with progressive, painful scoliosis with a curve of 40°. **B.** The curve was flexible. Preoperative discography revealed painful, degenerative L4–L5 and L5–S1 discs. **C, D.** To achieve solid fusion, two-stage surgery was performed. The first stage consisted of anterior L4–L5 and L5–S1 discectomies, interbody iliac crest grafts, and internal fixation with an "I" beam Yuan plate at L4–S1 and two A-O 6.5-mm screws at L5–S1. The second-stage Cotrel–Dubousset instrumentation and fusion derotated the spine and increased lordosis. Pain was relieved.

elsewhere.[9, 10] In general, for previously unoperated thoracic curves, the selection of fusion levels was that advocated by King and colleagues, and the hook and rod placement was that described by Cotrel and Dubousset.[9, 10, 29]

For patients with severe, rigid thoracic curves greater than 90° or for previously fused patients, anterior or posterior release, as appropriate, was performed before the Cotrel–Dubousset instrumentation. In the interval between the two stages, halo-dependent traction was used to improve curve flexibility and correction. This was done in 4 patients.

Treatment of thoracolumbar and lumbar curves often involved staged surgery. This was to reduce the high rate of complications, including pseudarthrosis, poor curve correction, residual truncal imbalance, and loss of or failure to improve lumbar lordosis associated with single-stage posterior surgery (see Figs. 11-5 and 11-6). The flexible thoracolumbar or lumbar curve with reasonable preservation of lumbar lordosis, in which the fusion need not be extended to the sacrum, may be treated with a single-stage anterior Zielke procedure or a single-stage posterior Cotrel–Dubousset instrumentation.

For the rigid lumbar kyphoscoliosis, an initial anterior lumbar release with morselized bone grafting of the interspaces is followed by a second-stage Cotrel–Dubousset instrumentation to derotate the curve and restore lumbar lordosis (see Figs. 11-5 and 11-6). If the fusion had to be extended to the sacrum because of painful disc degeneration, an anterior release extending the length of the curve, including the L4–S1 and L5–S1 interspaces, and wedged-shaped bone blocks for fusion and to improve lumbosacral lordosis were used. This is supplemented by anterior internal fixation at these two levels (Fig. 11-10). The remaining levels were grafted anteriorly with morselized bone. A second-stage Cotrel–Dubousset instrumentation extending posteriorly to the sacrum was performed 7 to 10 days later. Fusions extended to the sacrum in 4 patients.

Nineteen patients had staged or associated surgery, including 2 anterior thoracic releases, 2 posterior thoracic releases, 10 anterior thoracolumbar or lumbar releases, 4 nerve root decompressions, and 1 thoracoplasty.

Braces or casts are not routinely used, except in the elderly osteoporotic patient in whom fixation of the instrumentation is felt to be at risk. In these cases, a custom-molded polypropylene thoracolumbar orthosis is provided. This was deemed necessary for 14 patients.

Follow-up averaged 28 months (range, 15–49 months). For the entire series, the average preoperative scoliosis was 60°, with a range of 13° to 115°. At

final follow-up, the curves were reduced to an average of 35° (42% correction). For the subset of previously unoperated patients, curve correction averaged 50%. For those patients having an associated anterior release, curve correction averaged 63%. Correction in those patients previously fused averaged 35%.

There was significantly greater correction for the primary lumbar and thoracolumbar curves. This reflected the influence of associated anterior release, which was performed more commonly in this group. For the thoracic curves, correction at final follow-up averaged 45%. For the lumbar curves, correction averaged 58%. For the thoracolumbar curves, correction averaged 60%. For the double-major curves, correction for both the lumbar and thoracic components averaged 41%.

Loss of correction for the entire series was negligible. There was a significant loss of correction (i.e., greater than 5°) in 7 patients. This averaged 13° (range, 6–28°) or 49% (range, 19–93%) of initial correction.

Changes in the sagittal plane were a function of the preoperative size of the curves. In the relatively kyphotic lumbar spine (less than 20°), lordosis improved an average of 133%, from a preoperative average of 15° to 35° after the operation (Figs. 11-5 and 11-6). In the 20° to 50° range (average, 38°), lordosis improved only 32% (average, 47°). In the relatively hyperlordotic lumbar spine (greater than 50°; average, 66°), the postoperative lumbar lordosis declined an average of 11% to 59°.

Similarly, in the hypokyphotic thoracic spine (less than 20°; average, 11°), the thoracic kyphosis improved an average of 173% to 30°. In the 20° to 60° range, the change was insignificant. In the excessively kyphotic spine (average, 73°), the thoracic kyphosis decreased by an average of 11°.

Apical vertebral rotation, determined by the method of Nash and Moe, improved an average of one half grade, from 2.5 before the operation to 2.0 after the operation.[46] Preoperatively, 30 patients were imbalanced; postoperatively, 36 were balanced. Significant imbalance postoperatively (greater than 2 cm) remained in 5 patients.

Fourteen patients, usually the more elderly and osteoporotic, wore orthoses postoperatively, usually for 4 to 6 months. Blood loss for the Cotrel–Dubousset procedure averaged 1400 ml.

Significant or disabling pain in 44 patients before surgery was eliminated in 30, was significantly improved in 6, and was the same or worse in 8.

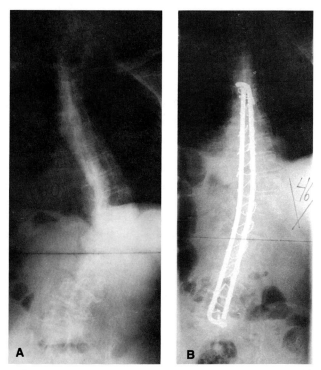

FIG. 11–10. **A, B.** Luque instrumentation in a 58-year-old woman with a progressive, painful thoracolumbar kyphoscoliosis. The kyphosis precluded the use of Zielke instrumentation. Today, Cotrel–Dubousset instrumentation with derotation would be used.

Twenty-eight complications occurred in 20 patients: 2 pneumothoraces, 1 pancreatitis, 3 urinary tract infections, 1 dural tear closed primarily, and 1 superficial wound infection that responded to dressing changes. One 66-year-old patient developed a hemothorax after a thoracoabdominal approach for an anterior release that required repeat thoracotomy for control of bleeding. This same patient developed chronic post-thoracotomy incisional pain.

Eight patients complained about prominent rods, 5 of whom underwent partial removal owing to persistent irritation. Neurologic complications were fortunately transient and consisted of neuropraxias. Two followed anterior approaches. The first was a L4 nerve root neuropraxia with associated quadriceps weakness that resolved. The second was a persistent pain in the distribution of the genitofemoral nerve that resolved after resection. The only injury directly attributable to the Cotrel–Dubousset instrumentation procedure was the L4 nerve root neuropraxia, which resolved.

The most frequent complication readily attributable to the instrumentation system was hook disengagement due to bone failure (i.e., lamina fractures). Four of the 5 failures occurred in the lumbar region at the distal fixation site. They occurred in patients over 50 years of age who had undergone a preliminary anterior lumbar release before the Cotrel–Dubousset instrumentation. Six other cases of anterior lumbar releases were unaffected. It seems prudent to supplement the distal lumbar fixation with pedicle screws when possible, instead of relying on laminar hooks. In a subsequent 10 similar cases in which lumbar pedicle screw fixation was used, instrumentation failure did not occur. The remaining fixation failure occurred in the thoracic region in a previously multiply-operated patient who had also undergone a first-stage anterior thoracic release.

Four of the 5 failures were reinstrumented in the immediate perioperative period, and 2 of these had good results. One of the 5 had a delayed revision 10 months later. She had fused, but with loss of lumbar lordosis and the development of a flat back. This was corrected with a lumbar extension osteotomy. Thus, 3 of 5 instrumentation failures were ultimately salvageable. The remaining 2 patients have both fused with loss of lumbar lordosis. Both have pain and fatigue with ambulation. One patient is scheduled for an extension osteotomy.

One patient required extension of her fusion to the sacrum 18 months after her Cotrel–Dubousset instrumentation. At age 16, she had undergone a Harrington instrumentation but developed multiple pseudarthroses in the lumbar region with progressively debilitating pain. Her pain was attributed to the pseudarthroses, and discography at the L5–S1 level was not performed before the Cotrel–Dubousset instrumentation. Because of persistent pain after the surgery, discography was performed, demonstrating a painful lumbosacral disc. She improved after extension of the fusion to the sacrum.

The pseudarthrosis rate appears low. One patient has an obvious pseudarthosis at L4–L5, despite having a circumferential fusion attempt at that level. She has persistent pain but does not want further surgery currently. A 54-year-old woman was recently found to have three pseudarthroses in the lumbar region after instrumentation of a double-major curve. Tomograms were not helpful in confirming the pseudarthroses, but she had persistent pain and lost some correction, prompting exploration and pseudarthrosis repair.

Another patient had a pseudarthosis in the thoracic region, with persistent pain and loss of correction. A bone scan demonstrated uptake in the midthoracic region. Surgical exploration revealed two pseudarthroses, which were corrected and refused.

Cotrel–Dubousset instrumentation seems to have its greatest benefit in maintaining improvement of the sagittal plane curves in the thoracic and lumbar regions. In the initial enthusiasm for frontal plane curve correction with Harrington instrumentation, the sagittal plane curves were often ignored.

The results from this series indicate that Cotrel–Dubousset instrumentation is able to effect beneficial changes in lumbar lordosis and thoracic kyphosis. This success was influenced by the use of a staged anterior release in many cases, but it also appears that Cotrel–Dubousset instrumentation allows the surgeon to take full advantage of the benefits available from staged anterior surgery.

There were several complications in the series, but several of these patients had complex deformities, and 12 patients had undergone previous fusions. Also, 19 patients had staged surgery in the course of their treatment with Cotrel–Dubousset instrumentation. Neurologic injuries were all neuropraxias and all resolved. Two of these occurred in multiply-operated patients, and only one could be attributed to the Cotrel–Dubousset instrumentation procedure. The wound infection rate was very low, despite multiple procedures that were often long and complex.

The 16% incidence of rod irritation is somewhat high. Cotrel–Dubousset instrumentation is bulky compared with Harrington instrumentation. However, instrument removal is commonly performed after other orthopedic procedures (e.g., fracture fixation), and instrument removal after scoliosis surgery may be a reasonable trade-off if the initial fixation is enhanced by a somewhat bulkier segmental system like the Cotrel–Dubousset instrumentation.

Ultimate satisfaction with the procedure must be judged in terms of pain relief, because this was the primary indication for surgery in 85% of the patients. In 30 patients preoperative pain was relieved, and in 6 it was reduced to a level that required only occasional non-narcotic analgesics. Eight patients continued to complain of pain postoperatively that was the same or worse than that before surgery. Three of these patients appear to have pseudarthroses. Ultimately, 86% of the patients had improvement in their preoperative pain.

Cotrel–Dubousset instrumentation is a complex system, but it is this complexity that provides the surgeon with the versatility necessary to tackle difficult surgical problems. With experience, operative time approaches that needed for other scoliosis systems.

COSMESIS

The correction of thoracic deformities for cosmetic reasons in the adult should be given serious consideration. In a review of the first 1000 patients with scoliosis treated by me, approximately 10% were treated for cosmetic reasons. These were primarily thoracic curves with a range from 45° to 75°. The age range of the patients was from 20 to 42 years; 90% of the patients were women. Some were single, but many had happy marriages.

The operation should not be denied to the adult who wants it only for cosmetic reasons, provided that the surgeon is experienced, has the backing of good institutional facilities and care, and has explained the course and complications of the procedure.

The past few years have seen a return to excision of the rib hump. This is particularly valuable in rigid curves in the thoracic spine, especially for sagittal-plane hypokyphosis. In more mobile curves, using Cotrel–Dubousset instrumentation to derotate the spine helps to decrease the rib hump. An associated rib excision can be done at the same time. Because of its enhanced stability, Cotrel–Dubousset instrumenta-

tion is also used for rigid curves. No postoperative orthoses are necessary.

A review of 20 patients with rigid deformities of 90° or greater who underwent rib excision consisting of five to six ribs on the convexity in patients revealed no serious morbidity. There were no changes between the preoperative and postoperative ventilation studies. Rib hump excision for patients with severe, rigid thoracic scoliosis can markedly improve the cosmetic result.

At the time of rib excision, bone may be cut into small fragments to be used as graft. The ribs are excised subperiosteally through an incision created at right angle to the longitudinal spinal excision. Two myocutaneous flaps are created to expose the ribs.

TREATMENT OF SEVERE RIGID SCOLIOTIC DEFORMITIES

In 1979, I reported on 85 patients with large deformities whose curves on bending x-ray films failed to change.[31] The age range of the patients was from 20 to 55, and the magnitude of the curves was between 75° and 180°. Fifteen of these patients were primarily kyphotic, 42 had idiopathic curves, and 28 had congenital curves. The majority were thoracic and thoracolumbar curves. Included were 28 patients who had fusions because of congenital failures of segmentation and 4 patients with spontaneous fusions. Thirty-three previously untreated patients were rigid on bending x-ray films but were found at the time of surgery to have no spontaneous fusion. Twenty patients had had previous fusions and presented with curve progression and pain. All patients underwent posterior releases, including, when necessary, osteotomies of previous fusions or congenitally fused spines. Posterior osteotomies were done at multiple levels, usually averaging four. These were associated with rib releases over three to four levels on the concavity, transverse process osteotomies, and rib resections of five to six ribs on the convexity. Forty patients had associated anterior osteotomies as well.

At the time of primary release surgery, traction was applied in the form of halo femoral traction for 32 patients or halo pelvic corrective force for 53 patients. The latter form of traction is still used in treating very severe curves, but it has been replaced to some degree from by halo-dependent traction in the circo-electric bed at 30° of dependency or associated with halo wheel-chair traction. Second-stage procedures done 2 weeks later consisted of posterior instrumentation, originally with Harrington instrumentation, but superseded first by sublaminar wiring techniques and more recently by Cotrel–Dubousset instrumentation.

The degree of correction averaged 40% with halo pelvic traction and 32% with halo femoral traction. Subsequent Harrington instrumentation added a further 8% to correction. Overall correction in the rigid group of curves was 40%. This was comparable to a series previously reported of mobile curves. The average correction was 48% for idiopathic curves and 33% for congenital curves.

Sublaminar wiring described by Luque is no longer used in the treatment of scoliosis, with the exception of some cases of paralytic scoliosis.[40, 41] Before it was supplanted, it was used in more than 200 cases of adult spinal deformity. Cotrel–Dubousset instrumentation and pedicle fixation allow more rigid fixation and provide a true means of deformity correction, particularly derotation. For some mobile curves, as in cases of significant arteriosclerosis with anterior calcification of the aorta or cases of marked anterior osteopenia in which the curve is still mobile, Cotrel–Dubousset instrumentation can serve to derotate the spine and restore lordosis.

In cases of significant, rigid kyphoscoliosis, Cotrel–Dubousset instrumentation has proved to be invaluable for restoring lordosis and relieving pain after anterior multiple discectomies with the use of minced bone graft in the interbody spaces. The instrumentation is carried about 2 weeks after anterior surgery and can be used even in cases of extensive laminectomies for spinal stenosis (Figs. 11-5 and 11-6). My experience has demonstrated a means of dealing with rigid, painful kyphoscoliosis, especially in the elderly person, with excellent correction and no neurologic or vascular complications related to instrumentation.

Structural Disabilities

Patients who have a paralytic scoliosis may find sitting at a desk or in a wheelchair difficult because of marked pelvic obliquity or kyphosis associated with a collapsing spine or a hyperlordosis (Fig. 11-11). The latter is encountered particularly in patients who have had peritoneal shunts in childhood. Patients with paralytic scoliosis are best treated by a combined anterior and posterior approach, which eliminates the need for heavy postoperative immobilization and allows early ambulation in a wheel chair.

Certain collapsing, paralytic curves that limit respiratory function can be significantly corrected, improving diaphragmatic breathing. A preoperative trial of

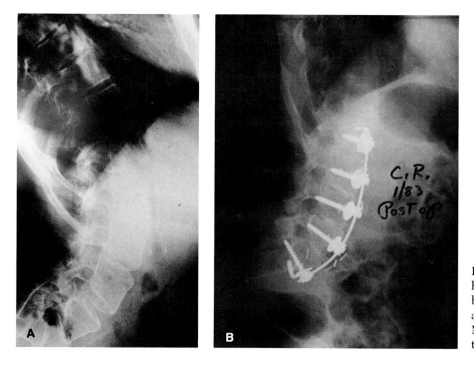

FIG. 11–11. **A.** Marked paralytic hyperlordosis. **B.** Lordosis has been reduced to 60° at L1–S1 by anterior Zielke instrumentation. Notice the anterior-posterior orientation of the screws.

halo-dependent traction may demonstrate an improvement in respiratory function by lifting the diaphragm out of the abdomen, depicting the advantages of surgical correction of the deformity

The use of Cotrel–Dubousset instrumentation has not yet proven itself in the treatment of paralytic deformities that extend into the distal lumbar spine, and I advocate an anterior and posterior approach. In children, the use of Luque instrumentation to the pelvis, using L rods or the Galveston or other modifications, has proven useful, but in my experience with adults these were insufficient, and a two-stage anterior and posterior procedure was necessary.

Spinal Deformities in Patients Over the Age of Fifty

The adult over 50 often presents with a rigid, painful deformity that is associated with significant imbalance and loss of normal lordosis of the lumbar spine. The bone is frequently osteopenic, and there may be associated neurologic problems related to spinal stenosis. My early experience was that major spinal deformities in patients over the age of 50 could be corrected only with great risk to neurologic structures, because most of these curves are rigid. As a result, most of these deformities were stabilized with Harrington instrumentation with little attempt at correction. This often meant continuing kyphosis, which was in itself a problem.

With the addition of improved techniques of anterior fixation like Zielke instrumentation and posterior fixation techniques like Cotrel–Dubousset instrumentation, correction can now be safely achieved.[9, 70] For a thoracolumbar or lumbar deformity with good preservation of lordosis, an anterior Zielke instrumentation can be safely used. The use of methylmethacrylate has greatly enhanced the holding power of screws in the vertebral bodies. Methylmethacrylate should not be used posteriorly in the pedicles, with the exception of the first sacral pedicle, because the cement may exude from the osteopenic pedicle in elderly adults and compromise the canal.

In the case of a rigid kyphoscoliosis or if there is minimal lumbar lordosis, a two-stage procedure is preferable. The first stage consists of multiple-disc excisions and interbody grafts using small bone fragments. This is followed 10 days later by posterior derotation using Cotrel–Dubousset instrumentation to correct the curve and restore lumbar lordosis. This has proven to be a valuable technique over the last few years.

I followed 80 patients over the age of 50. Fifty of them had idiopathic curves, and the remainder had congenital curves, paralytic curves, or a pure kyphotic deformity. Twelve of the idiopathic curves were thoracic, 9 were thoracolumbar, 17 were lumbar, and 12 were double curves. All patients presented with back pain. Eight patients had a progressive pulmonary dysfunction, usually related to an increasing kyphosis. Fifty-seven percent of the patients had documented evidence of progression of greater than 10° in 3 years preoperatively. Sixteen patients had associated root pain. The 80 patients underwent 100 procedures. Twenty patients had a second-stage procedure, either anterior or posterior, for increased stabilization. Twelve patients had concurrent anterior and posterior procedures to correct flat-back syndromes; these were performed through a single-stage combined posterior and anterior osteotomy with anterior and posterior fixation. Although 20 patients underwent a second-stage procedure for stabilization, most patients had rigid kyphoscoliosis. Fourteen had second-stage anterior procedures because fusion was carried to the sacrum posteriorly. To ensure a solid fusion, anterior fixation and fusion was carried out as described in the next section. In a review of all cases, good results were achieved in 56.5% of the patients, and excellent results were achieved in 12.5%. Fair or poor results occurred in 6% and 25% of the patients, respectively. No pain was reported in 27 (34%) postoperatively, and root pain was relieved in all patients.

It is absolutely contraindicated in cases of scoliosis with spinal stenosis or other causes of root pain to perform a posterior decompression alone, particularly if more than one side at one level is decompressed. An associated stabilization procedure should always be performed. I have encountered many patients with scoliosis who have undergone posterior decompression for spinal stenosis and who, within months or years, presented with collapsing, progressive, painful scoliosis (Fig. 11-12). These patients present marked difficulties in obtaining stable, fused spines because they lack bone stock as a result of the decompression and subsequent scarring.

In the group of 80 patients over the age of 50, curve correction averaged 22% with Harrington instrumentation and 22% using Harrington rods with sublaminar wires. Twenty-one percent correction was achieved with Harrington rods combined with L-rods, and 33%

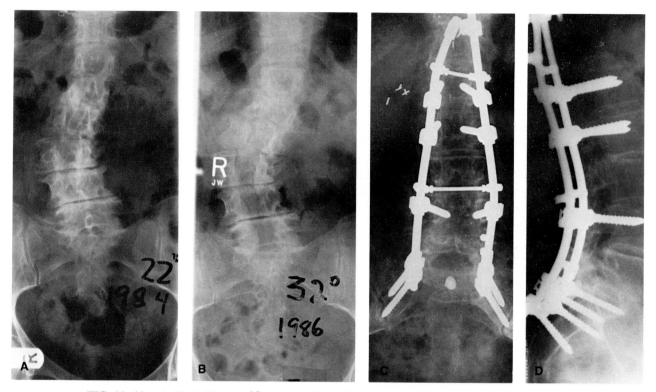

FIG. 11–12.   A, B. A 68-year-old woman with a prelaminectomy scoliosis measuring 22°. After decompression, the deformity increased to 32° with totally disabling back pain and subsequently to 50°. Notice the loss of lumbar lordosis after decompression.   **C, D.** Two-stage surgery restored lordosis and relieved the pain. The first stage consisted of multiple anterior discectomies and bone grafts. The second-stage Cotrel–Dubousset instrumentation and fusion corrected the deformity and restored lordosis.

was achieved with double L-rods. Curve correction with Dwyer instrumentation was 42% and 67% with Zielke instrumentation (Figs. 11-2 through 11-7). This compares favorably with the 70% of all adults over the age of 20 corrected by Zielke instrumentation.[33] The average correction obtained with Cotrel–Dubousset instrumentation was 50% (Figs. 11-5 and 11-6). Thirteen of the patients treated with Harrington instrumentation alone developed flat backs. Four of these subsequently underwent restoration of lordosis by single-stage anterior and posterior osteotomies. One patient who became paraparetic as a result of surgery had partial improvement. Applying posterior corrective force in the lumbar spine at any age should be avoided, except for anterior corrective force for kyphotic deformities. Pure kyphotic deformities are best treated by anterior instrumentation.

Instrumentation failure (14%) in this group of elderly adults occurred in 11 patients: 6 had Harrington rod fractures, 1 had a dislodged rod, 2 had L-rod migration, 1 had anterior screw breakage, and 1 had posterior Zielke rod breakage. The intraoperative bone fracture of lamina or vertebral bodies that occurred in 7 patients was overcome with methylmethacralate and internal fixation devices.

The infection rate was 1%. Pulmonary complications, including atelectasis, pneumonia, and adult respiratory distress syndrome, occurred in 24%.

Pseudarthrosis occurred in 21%, primarily in the Harrington series. There were no pseudarthroses with the use of Zielke instrumentation or Cotrel–Dubousset instrumentation. Twenty-five percent of pseudarthroses occurred in fusions carried to L5, and 24% occurred in fusions carried to the sacrum, which were done before the development of two-stage surgery. Nine patients developed kyphosis secondary to osteopenic fractures proximal to their instrumentation. Because of improved diagnostic capabilities, postoperative care, and fixation procedures, morbidity has decreased significantly in the last 5 years. Restoration of lordosis cannot be overemphasized, particularly in cases of kyphoscoliosis. The use of multiple-level releases anteriorly followed by posterior derotation with Cotrel–Dubousset instrumentation and, if necessary, posterior osteotomy through the pars interarticularis to increase lordosis has appreciably improved the quality of life for these senior patients.

Fusions to the Sacrum

In 1978, as Chairman of the Morbidity Committee of the Scoliosis Research Society, I noticed that 4% of all scoliosis fusions resulted in a clinically significant loss of lumbar lordosis (unpublished data). This included all forms of posterior instrumentation in all areas of the spine. A review of fusions to the sacrum revealed that clinically significant loss of lumbar lordosis occurred in approximately 50% of adult cases, requiring revision surgery in half of these patients.[34] Balderson and colleagues had similar experiences.[2] It was not recognized until the late 1970s that correction of the thoracolumbar and lumbar spine could cause the loss of lordosis, even with contouring of the Harrington rod and the use of square-ended Moe rods and sacral-alar hooks.[5] The advent of Luque L-rods across the sacroiliac joint and its subsequent refinement with the Galveston technique were thought to improve maintenance of lordosis and enhance the rate of fusion for posterior instrumentation to the sacrum.[41]

The initial incidence of pseudarthrosis to the sacrum using Harrington rods with a sacral bar or alar hooks was 40%.[34] A review of Luque instrumentation to the sacrum revealed that the incidence of pseudarthrosis had been decreased to 15%.[36] The incidence of flat back in fusions to the sacrum was reduced to 20% and was significant in only a fifth of those patients. Flat backs occurred despite marked contouring of the rods into lordosis and occurred only in kyphoscoliotic cases. The use of Cotrel–Dubousset instrumentation has not generated this problem owing to the introduction of increased lordosis. Fusion to the sacrum in idiopathic scoliosis is indicated only if the last motion segment is a source of the pain.

Since 1981, if fusion to the sacrum is indicated, a two-stage procedure is carried out.[30] If the patient is scoliotic with reasonable lordosis, an initial anterior procedure using Zielke instrumentation is done. The use of Zielke instrumentation anterior to the sacrum, although technically demanding, has not caused any problems related to the common iliac vessels. Careful technique, avoiding any impingement of screw heads against the vessels, has resulted in no vascular complications. The rod can safely pass beneath the common iliac vessels because it is small and lies close to the vertebral body. Occasionally, two rods are used at the distal two or three levels to help control rotation at the lumbosacral junction. A second-stage posterior fusion using segmental wiring was initially done, but this was replaced by pedicle fixation (Cotrel–Dubousset or plate instrumentation).

If the patient has a rigid kyphoscoliosis and requires fusion to the sacrum, the first stage consists of multiple anterior discotomies. The interbody spaces are filled with bone chips, except for the L4–L5 interspace and the L5–S1 interspace. At those levels, interbody bicortical or tricortical grafts are used to fill the disc spaces and increase lordosis. Internal fixation is performed to enhance stability over these two levels. This is followed about 2 weeks later by posterior Cotrel–Dubousset instrumentation, which derotates the lumbar spine and restores lordosis.

If the kyphoscoliosis is mobile, the scoliosis is corrected and the lordosis restored by a first-stage posterior Cotrel–Dubousset instrumentation and fusion, followed by a second-stage anterior fusion from L4 to the sacrum with solid interbody grafts and instrumentation. For instrumentation from L4 to the sacrum, a rigid, contoured I-plate designed by Yuan or two 6.5-mm AO cancellous screws have replaced Zielke instrumentation (see Fig. 11-9).

In over 450 cases of of anterior instrumentation of the thoracic and lumbar spine, I have not encountered any late vascular problems. During an anterior instrumentation, ligation of the segmental vessels, particularly in a left retroperitoneal approach, allows the aorta and common iliac vessels to fall away from the vertebral bodies, providing more room for placement of the internal fixation devices. Because lumbar and thoracolumbar curves are usually left-sided, this approach is most commonly used.

Bicortical grafts from the iliac crest in younger people or tricortical grafts in more osteoporotic people are used to maintain disc height at L4–L5 and L5–S1 and to enhance lordosis anteriorly. Internal fixation is used because iliac crest bone is unable to support loads much greater than the body weight in the erect position. With combined anterior and posterior approaches, the incidence of pseudarthrosis has been reduced to 5% in the last 30 cases.

Extensions of Fusions in the Lumbar Spine

Recent reports and a review of my own statistics show that patients who have had previous fusions to L2, L3, L4, or L5 are at increased risk of developing degenerative changes below their fusions (Fig. 11-13).[6, 16] These patients require extension of their fusions if nonsurgical means fail to control pain and their problems progress. If after myelography, CT scanning, and discography and facet blocks, a fusion does not require extension to the sacrum, posterior instrumentation or anterior instrumentation can be used alone. If, however, extension of the fusion to the sacrum is required, a combined approach is necessary.

Extension of fusion to the sacrum is usually done in a single stage (Fig. 11-14).[3] This is done with posterior pedicle fixation and anterior instrumentation. In order to improve lordosis some of the posterior lamina at L4–L5, L3–L4, and L5–S1, instrumentation can be removed and compression applied to the pedicles to increase lordosis. Interbody grafts are done anteriorly after opening the disc space as widely as possible. Anterior instrumentation using Zielke rods or a plate enhances the fusion. The best results have been obtained with removal of posterior bone to increase lordosis, rather than simply fusing the spine in situ posteriorly with instrumentation and then anteriorly with interbody graft and instrumentation. Review of 24 cases (unpublished data) of extension fusion to the sacrum revealed that of 6 fused posteriorly with Harrington rods only, 5 failed due to the development of pseudarthrosis and a flat back. Nine were fused in situ anteriorly with interbody grafts used to maintain lordosis and supplemented at the same stage or at a second stage with posterior instrumentation and fusion; 3 of these were failures with pseudarthrosis and flat back.

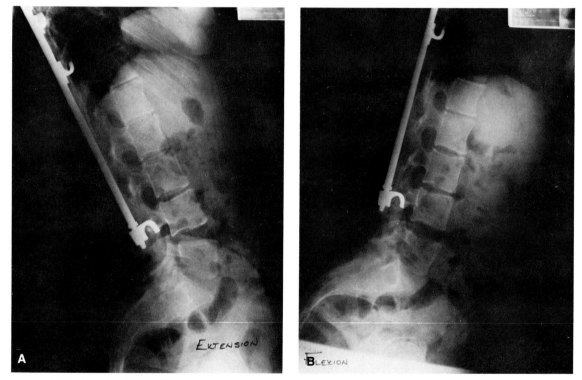

FIG. 11–13.   A, B. Flexion-extension view demonstrates marked instability at the L4–L5 disc space. The patient had undergone Harrington instrumentation 12 years earlier.

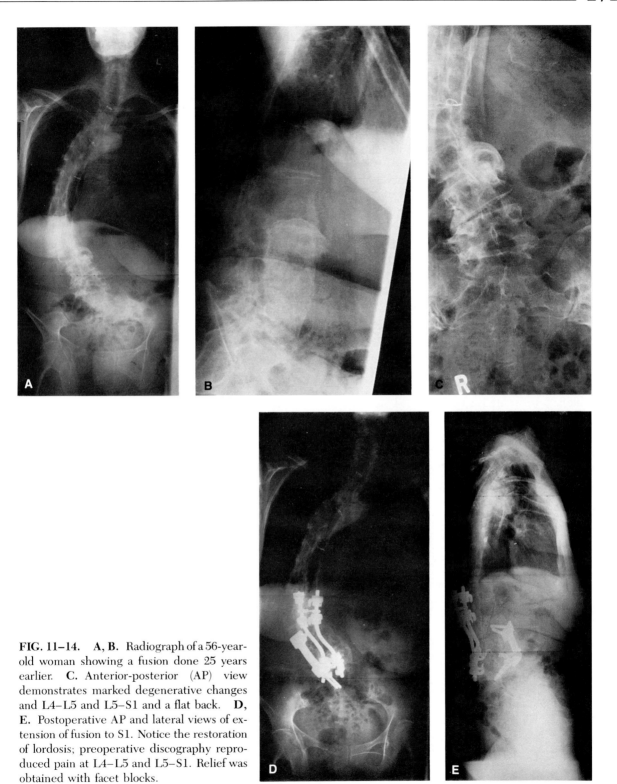

FIG. 11–14. A, B. Radiograph of a 56-year-old woman showing a fusion done 25 years earlier. **C.** Anterior-posterior (AP) view demonstrates marked degenerative changes and L4–L5 and L5–S1 and a flat back. **D, E.** Postoperative AP and lateral views of extension of fusion to S1. Notice the restoration of lordosis; preoperative discography reproduced pain at L4–L5 and L5–S1. Relief was obtained with facet blocks.

However 10 fusions done in a single stage with associated removal of bone posteriorly had good results, with only 1 case of pseudarthrosis.

Restoration of Iatrogenic Lumbar Lordosis

Fusions to the sacrum with posterior instrumentation, particularly Harrington instrumentation, produce a loss of lumbar lordosis in 50% of the patients, many of whom with require restoration surgery.[14, 17, 34, 39] Although adolescents compensate well, it is not unusual for those who had fusions to the sacrum to complain about fatigue and pain in their low backs during the third, fourth, or fifth decades of their lives. Care must be taken to ascertain that pain does not arise from the sacroiliac joint. Loss of lumbar lordosis causes an increasingly forward-flexed attitude as the day progresses, and the patients walk with their knees flexed and hips flexed. This is an unsightly deformity (Fig. 11-15). Despite a solid fusion, these patients complain of increasing pain and fatigue. This problem was not recognized until the late 1970s.

In 1988, I presented a review of 54 patients for whom combined anterior and posterior osteotomies were used for restoration of lordosis.[37] A combined approach offers more than a posterior osteotomy of an old fusion mass. Greater correction can be obtained,

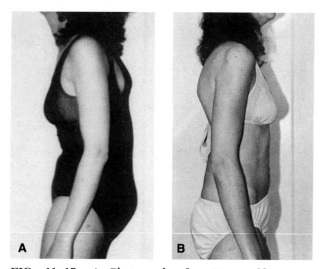

FIG. 11–15. **A.** Photograph of a 24-year-old woman showing the results of a previous lumbar fusion. Notice the marked kyphosis (flat back) caused by the applied corrective forces. **B.** Postoperative photograph demonstrating the restoration of lordosis.

and is not necessary to immobilize the patient in a hip spica postoperatively. Moreover, the use of posterior osteotomy alone has led to late recurrences of deformity. In 1987, Lagrone and colleagues also indicated that the best results can be obtained with anterior and posterior procedures.[37] A combined anterior-posterior approach, with internal fixation and postoperative use of a simple lumbar orthosis, allows early ambulation.

Etiologic factors that influence the loss of lumbar lordosis are, in descending order of frequency, corrective instrumentation of the lumbar spine that ends caudally at L5 or S1; a thoracolumbar junction kyphosis greater than 15°, especially if associated with hypokyphotic thoracic spine; and degenerative changes above or below a previous fusion because of the loss of disc height.

If loss of lumbar lordosis is associated with pseudarthrosis, repair of the pseudarthrosis alone will not relieve the patient's symptoms. If the patient is imbalanced in the anterior-posterior plane, a quadralateral wedge osteotomy done anteriorly and posteriorly can restore balance in the frontal plane and restore lumbar lordosis in the sagittal plane. If the fusion is solid, the osteotomy is carried out usually at the L3 to L4 level, or it may be carried out through the posterior pseudarthrosis, which is enlarged. The nerve roots at the level of the posterior osteotomy must be clearly, identified and an osteotomy analogous to that described by Smith Peterson is used. I have found the use of 8 Dwyer screws posteriorly in the lateral fusion mass to be ideal, using cables to close the osteotomy site. Four screws are proximal and four screws are distal to the osteotomy site on either side of the midline (Fig. 11-16A). This is easier to use than other forms of fixation. A midline contoured AO plate is used to help control rotation with at least two screws proximal and distal to the osteotomy site.

The anterior approach is carried out at the L3 or L4 level or at the apex of the frontal curve, corresponding to the posterior osteotomy (Fig. 11-17). An opening wedge osteotomy is done through the disc, or if there has been a previous anterior fusion, through the anterior fusion mass. The opening of the osteotomy anteriorly is carried out simultaneously with Kostuik-Harrington instrumentation while closing the posterior osteotomy with a Dwyer instrumentation. A tricortical or bicortical iliac crest graft is used anteriorly (Fig. 11-16B).

A review of 54 patients treated in this fashion revealed excellent results with pain relief in 48 (90%).[37] Nonunion occurred in 3 patients owing to anterior graft

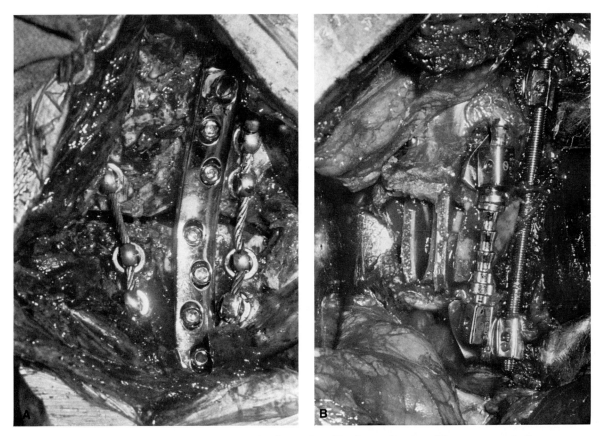

FIG. 11–16. **A.** Posterior osteotomy has been closed by the application of Dwyer screws in the lateral fusion mass. An AO plate has been added in the midline to help control rotation. **B.** Simultaneous to posterior closure, the anterior osteotomy site is opened with Kostuik-Harrington instrumentation. Iliac crest grafts are added, and a second Kostuik-Harrington compression rod is added to enhance stability.

collapse; 1 patient requested another operation. Neurologic complications occurred in 2 patients, 1 with a permanent weakness of the dorsal extensors and plantar flexors of her feet and inconsistent bladder control. Minimum follow-up was 4 years. The average pre-osteotomy lordosis, L1 to S1, of 21.5° was restored to 49°, which was equal to lordosis before initial posterior scoliosis surgery. This is an average of 29° of correction, with a range from 24° to 63°. Although correction is possible, prevention is paramount.

DEGENERATIVE ADULT SCOLIOSIS

Considerable controversy has existed about the definition of adult scoliosis and the differentiation between adolescent-onset scoliosis and the subsequent development of scoliosis and preexisting straight spine in the frontal plane.

James and co-workers performed a study in Edinburgh, where the incidence of osteoporosis and osteomalacia is high, and found an incidence of scoliosis to be approximately 6% of the adult group.[65] Many of these patients presented with evidence of osteoporosis and osteomalacia, and James felt that many of the cases of scoliosis were results of these diseases.

My colleagues and I, in a review of 5000 intravenous pyelograms, found an incidence of 3.9% of thoracolumbar lumbar curves.[32] These were all cases of adolescent onset.

The difficulty in differentiating between the two groups lies in the fact that lumbar and thoracolumbar curves in the frontal plane are frequently not noticed until the onset of back pain or until progression occurs

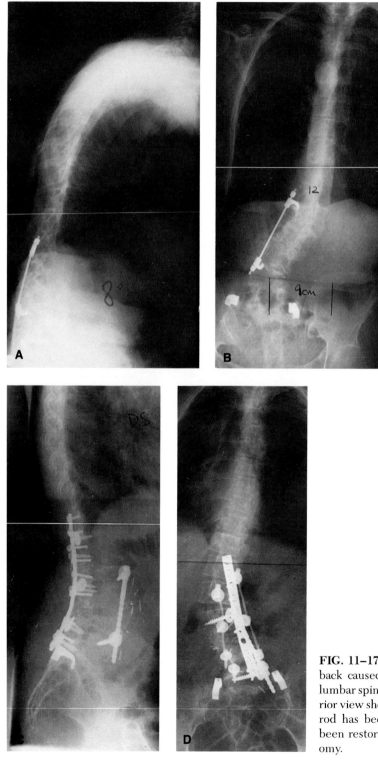

FIG. 11–17.   A. Notice the loss of lordosis and a marked flat back caused by a previous corrective attempt and fusion of lumbar spine in a 45-year-old woman.   **B.** The anterior-posterior view shows an imbalance 9 cm to the right. The Harrington rod has been removed.   **C, D.** Lordosis and balance have been restored by a single-stage anterior and posterior osteotomy.

as a result of degenerative changes in a preexisting adolescent curve.

Grubb compared two groups, one with onset in adolescent life and one with later onset in which the deformity was felt to occur as a result of degenerative changes.[18] He found significant differences in densitometric measurements between the idiopathic and adult degenerative curves when measurements were made for age-matched controls. Pain patterns in both groups predominantly involved the low back, buttocks, and legs, but the adult degenerative patients had a much higher incidence of stenotic symptoms and up to 90% were aggravated by activity, compared with 31% in the idiopathic group. Activities that provoked stenotic symptoms were primarily those involving extension of the lumbar spine. The curve magnitude was significantly different with idiopathic patients, ranging from 34° to 78°, with a mean of 52°. The degenerative group ranged from 15° to 53°, with a mean of 28°. Although the curvature in the idiopathic group was significantly greater, the mean degree per segment measurement was the same (9°) in both groups. All the idiopathic scoliotic group in Grubb's series were women, with a mean age of 42, but in the degenerative group, men and women were equally represented, and the mean age was 60 years.

In radiologic studies, the idiopathic group showed myelographic defects primarily in the compensatory lumbosacral curve; in the degenerative group, the myelographic defects were seen most frequently within the curve. In Grubb's analysis of the discography, there was grossly degenerative discs throughout the lumbar spine in the adult onset group. Pain was frequently not reproduced on distension of the disc. One explanation is that, in markedly degenerative discs, it is impossible to distend the disc quickly enough to reproduce pain, which makes the study invalid. In idiopathic patients with mechanical back pain, discography revealed abnormal, painful discs with reproduction of symptoms within the curve. In the untreated group, pain was often reproduced on discography at the lower end of the curve in the lumbar spine or in compensatory lumbosacral curve.[18, 31] Grubb and I also concluded that no assumption could be made that only a structural problem caused the pain. The pain may arise below the curve in a compensatory part of the lumbosacral curve. The structural problem may contribute to development of pain by producing abnormalities within and below the curve.

The reason for adult progression of an adolescent

curve is degenerative change. In the lumbar and thoracolumbar spine lordosis, is initially well preserved, but with progressive degeneration of discs in the fifth and sixth decades of life, the patient may develop a lumbar kyphosis. The management of these curves is discussed elsewhere in this chapter.

Because most of the adult-onset deformities developed spinal stenosis, decompression alone should be avoided unless it can be limited to one nerve root with preservation of the facet joints. Any more than this should be accompanied by fusion in situ or by correcting the deformity (see Fig. 11-17).

Nash and colleagues analyzed fusion done in the lumbar spine to see whether the criteria used for adolescents were valid in adults.[47] Criteria included the stable zone, central sacral line, neutrally rotated vertebra, degenerative arthritis, displaced wedging, rotatory subluxation, vertebral body wedging, lumbosacral take-off, and hemisacralization. They concluded that multiple anatomic factors needed to be considered in selecting lumbar vertebrae for fusion in adult scoliosis patients. They felt that the stable zone, although helpful in younger patients for correcting the upper lumbar, was not valid in the older patients. Degenerative and deforming factors play a role in older patients who have increased disease in the lower lumbar spine and necessitate fusions to lower levels, as I pointed out in a previous publication.[31] This substantiates the value of using facet blocks and discography at these lower levels to determine all painful levels.

Nash and co-workers concluded that patients undergoing fusion into the lumbar area appear to have a significant improvement of the pain and were satisfied with their surgery in 89% of the cases when the selection criteria were applied.[47] Nash felt that the central sacral line determination did not help in selecting the lumbar fusion vertebra in adult scoliosis patients.

Many criteria proved to be of little value; one factor was of value in only 16 of 53 cases, two factors were useful in 20 of 53 cases, three factors in 11 of 53 cases, four factors in 3 of 53 cases, and five factors in 2 of 53 cases in Nash's series. Degenerative changes, including rotatory subluxation, disc narrowing, and disc-space wedging, must be included in the determining the fusion level. In fusion to L2, most patients had only two or fewer criteria for selection. The stable zone was a factor in the majority of cases fused to L2, L3, or L4. Displaced wedging was a factor in only 53% of cases fused between L2 and L5, and rotatory subluxation was a factor in only about 50% of the cases fused to L4 or L5. This was similarly true for obique take-off in patients fused to L5 or S1, and hemisacralization affected only 25% of patients fused to S1. The most important thing learned from this review is that degenerative changes must be included in determining the fusion mass, and these are best evaluated with discography and facet blocks.

References

1. Allen BL Jr, Ferguson RL: The Galvestion technique for L-rod instrumentation of the scoliotic spine. Spine 7:276, 1982
2. Balderston RA, Winter RB, Moe JH, et al: Fusion to the sacrum for nonparalytic scoliosis in the adult. Spine 11:824, 1986
3. Byrd JA III, Scoles PV, Winter RB, et al: Adult idiopathic scoliosis treated by anterior and posterior spinal fusion. J Bone Joint Surg [Am] 69:843 1987
4. Bradford DS: Adult scoliosis: current concepts of treatment. Clin Orthop 229:70, 1988
5. Casey MP, Asher MA, Jacobs RR, Orrick JM: The effect of Harrington rod contouring on lumbar lordosis. Spine 12:750, 1987
6. Cochran T, Irstam L, Nachemson A: Long-term anatomic and functional changes in patients with adolescent idiopathic scoliosis treated by Harrington rod fusion. Spine 8:576, 1983
7. Coe JD, Becker PS, McAfee PC, Burr KR: Neuropathology with spinal instrumentation. J Orthop Res 7:359, 1989
8. Collis DK, Ponsetti IV: Long-term follow-up of patients with idiopathic scoliosis not treated surgically. J Bone Joint Surg [Am] 51:425, 1969
9. Cotrel Y: New Instrumentation for Surgery of the Spine. London, Freud Publishing House, 1986
10. Cotrel Y, Dubousset J, Guillaumat M: New universal instrumentation in spinal surgery. Clin Orthop 227:10, 1988
11. Cummine JL, Lonstein JE, Moe JH, et al: Reconstructive surgery in the adult for failed scoliosis fusion. J Bone Joint Surg [Am] 61:1151, 1979
12. Dawson EG, Caron A, Moe JH: Surgical management of scoliosis in the adult. J Bone Joint Surg [Am] 61:1151, 1973
13. Denis F: Cotrel–Dubousset instrumentation in the treatment of idiopathic scoliosis. Orthop Clin North Am 19:291, 1988
14. Doherty JH: Complications of fusion in lumbar scoliosis. J Bone Joint Surg [Am] 55:438, 1973
15. Dwyer AF: Experience of anterior correction of scoliosis. Clin Orthop 93:191, 1973
16. Edgar MA, Mehta MH: A long-term review of adults with fused and unfused idiopathic scoliosis. Orthop Trans 6:462, 1982
17. Grobler LJ, Moe JH, Winter RB, et al: Loss of lumbar lordosis following surgical correction of thoracolumbar deformities. Orthop Trans 2:239, 1978
18. Grubb SA, Lipscomb HS, Conrad RW: Diagnostic findings in painful adult scoliosis. Presented at the Meeting of the Scoliosis Research Society, Amsterdam, The Netherlands, September 1989
19. Haher JE, Devlin V, Freeman B, Rondon B: Long-term effects of sublaminar wires on the neural canal. Orthop Trans 11:106, 1987
20. Hall JD: Dwyer instrumentation in anterior fusion of the spine. J Bone Joint Surg [Am] 63:1188, 1981
21. Harrington PR, Dickson JH: An eleven-year clinical investigation of Harrington instrumentation. A. Preliminary report on 578 cases. Clin Orthop 93:113, 1973
22. Hasday CA, Passoff TL, Perry J: Gait abnormalities arising from iatrogenic loss of lumbar lordosis secondary to Harrington instrumentation in lumbar fractures. Spine 8:501, 1983
23. Herndon WQ, Sullivan JA, Yngve DA, et al: Segmental spinal instrumentation with sublaminar wires. J Bone Joint Surg [Am] 69:851, 1987
24. Herring JA, Wenger DR: Segmental spinal instrumentation. A preliminary report of 40 consecutive cases. Spine 7:285, 1982
25. Jackson RP, Simmons EH, Stripinus D: Incidence and severity of back pain in adult idiopathic scoliosis. Spine 8:749, 1983
26. Johnson JR, Holt RT: Combined use of anterior and posterior surgery for adult scoliosis. Orthop Clin North Am 19:361, 1988
27. Johnston CE II, Happel LT Jr, Norris R, et al: Delayed paraplegia complicating sublaminar segmental spinal instrumentation. J Bone Joint Surg [Am] 68:556, 1986
28. Kaneda K, Fujiya N, Satoh S: Results with Zielke instrumentation for idiopathic thoracolumbar and lumbar scoliosis. Clin Orthop 205:195, 1986
29. King HA, Moe JH, Bradford DS, Winter RB: The selection of fusion levels in thoracic idiopathic scoliosis. J Bone Joint Surg [Am] 65:1302, 1983
30. Kostuik JP: Treatment of scoliosis in the adult thoracolumbar spine with special reference of fusion to the sacrum. Orthop Clin North Am 19:371, 1988
31. Kostuik JP: Decision making in adult scoliosis. Spine 4:521, 1979
32. Kostuik JP, Bentivoglio J: The incidence of low back pain in adult scoliosis. Spine 6:268, 1981
33. Kostuik JP, Carl A, Ferron S: Anterior Zielke instrumentation for adult spinal deformity. J Bone Joint Surg [Am] 71:898, 1989
34. Kostuik JP, Hall BB: Spinal fusions to the sacrum in adults with scoliosis. Spine 8:489, 1983
35. Kostuik JP, Israel J, Hall JE: Scoliosis surgery in adults. Clin Orthop 93:225, 1973
36. Kostuik JP, Maurais GR, Richardson WJ: Primary fusion to the sacrum using Luque instrumentation. Presented at the Meeting of the North American Spine Association, Colorado Springs, CO, June 1988
37. Kostuik JP, Maurais GR, Richardson WJ, Okajima Y: Combined single-stage anterior-posterior osteotomy for

correction of iatrogenic lumbar kyphosis. Spine 13:257, 1988

38. Kostuik JP, Worden Hawker R, Salo P: Long-term functional outcome following surgery for adult scoliosis. Presented at the Meeting of A.O.A., Boston, MA, June 1990

39. Lagrone MO, Bradford DS, Moe JH, et al: Treatment of symptomatic flat back after spinal fusion. J Bone Joint Surg [Am] 70:569, 1988

40. Luque ER: The anatomic basis and development of segmental spinal instrumentation. Spine 7:256, 1982

41. Luque ER: Segmental spinal instrumentation for correction of scoliosis. Clin Orthop 163:192, 1982

42. Macnab I: Backache. Baltimore, Williams & Wilkins, 1977

43. Moe JH, Purcell GA, Bradford DS: Zielke instrumentation (VDS) for the correction of spinal curvature. Analysis of results in 66 patients. Clin Orthop 180:133, 1983

44. Nachemson A: A long-term follow-up study of nontreated scoliosis. Acta Orthop Scand 39:489, 1983

45. Nachemson A: A long-term follow-up study of nontreated scoliosis. J Bone Joint Surg [Am] 50:203, 1969

46. Nash CL Jr, Moe JH: A Study of vertebral rotation. J Bone Joint Surg [Am] 51:223, 1969

47. Nash CL, Goldstein JM, Wilham MR: Selection of lumbar fusion levels in adult idiopathic scoliosis patients. Presented at the Meeting of the Scoliosis Research Society, Amsterdam, The Netherlands, September 1989

48. Nicastro JF, Hartjen CA, Traina J, Lancaster JM: Intraspinal pathways taken by sublaminar wires during removal. An experimental study. J Bone Joint Surg [Am] 68:1206, 1986

49. Nilsonne U, Lundgren DD: Long-term prognosis in idiopathic scoliosis. Acta Orthop Scand 39:455, 1968

50. Nuber GW, Schafer MF: Surgical management of adult scoliosis. Clin Orthop 208:228, 1986

51. Ogiela DM, Chan DPK: Ventral derotation spondylodesis. A review of 22 cases. Spine 11:18, 1986

52. Ponder RC, Dickson JH, Harrington PR, Erwin WD: Results of Harrington instrumentation and fusion in the adult idiopathic scoliosis patient. J Bone Joint Surg [Am] 57:797, 1975

53. Ponsetti IV: The pathogenesis of adult scoliosis. In Zorab PA (ed): Proceedings of Second Symposium on Scoliosis. Cansation, Edinburgh, E & S Livingstone, 1968

54. Rogala EJ, Drummond DS, Gurr J: Scoliosis: incidence and natural history. A prospective epidemiological study. J Bone Joint Surg [Am] 60:173, 1978

55. Schrader WC, Betham D, Scherbin V: The chronic local effects of sublaminar wires—an animal model. Orthop Trans 11:106, 1987

56. Sponseller PD, Cohen MS, Nachemson AL, et al: Results of surgical treatment of adults with idiopathic scoliosis. J Bone Joint Surg [Am] 69:667, 1987

57. Stagnara P: Scoliosis in adults. Surgical treatment of severe forms. Excerpta Med Found Int Cong 192:1969.

58. Stagnara P, Jouvinoux P, Peloux J, et al: Cyphoscoliosis essentielles de l'adulte. Formes severe de plus de 100. Redressment partial et arthrodese. Presented at the XI SICOT Congress, Mexico City, Mexico, 1969

59. Stagnara P: Utilization of Harrington's device in the treatment of adult kyphoscoliosis above 100°. Presented at the Fourth International Scoliosis Symposium, 1971. Stuttgart, George Thieme Verlag, 1973

60. Stagnara P, Fleury D, Faucher R, et al: Scoliosis majeures de l'adultes superieures a 100–183 cas traites chirurgicalement. Rev Chir Orthop 61:101, 1975

61. Swank S, Lonstein JE, Moe JH, et al: Surgical treatment of adult scoliosis. A review of two hundred and twenty-two cases. J Bone Joint Surg [Am] 63:268, 1981

62. Thompson GH, Wilber RG, Shaffer JW, et al: Segmental spinal instrumentation in idiopathic scoliosis. A preliminary report. Spine 10:623, 1985

63. van Dam BE: Nonoperative treatment of adult scoliosis. Orthop Clin North Am 19:347, 1988

64. van Dam BE, Bradford DS, Lonstein JE, et al: Adult idiopathic scoliosis treated by posterior spinal fusion and Harrington instrumentation. Spine 12:32, 1987

65. Vanderpool DW, James JIP, Wynne-Davies R: Scoliosis in the elderly. J Bone Joint Surg [Am] 51:446, 1969

66. Wilber RG, Thompson GH, Shaffer JW, et al: Postoperative neurologic deficits in segmental spinal instrumentation. A study using spinal cord monitoring. J Bone Joint Surg [Am] 66:1178, 1984

67. Weinstein SL, Ponseti IV: Curve progression in idiopathic scoliosis. J Bone Joint Surg [Am] 65:447, 1983

68. Winter RB, Lonstein JE, Denis F: Pain patterns in adult scoliosis. Orthop Clin North Am 19:339, 1988

69. Winter RB: Combined Dwyer and Harrington instrumentation and fusion in the treatment of selected patients with painful adult idiopathic scoliosis. Spine 3:135, 1978

70. Zielke K, Stunkat R, Beaujean F: Ventrale Derotationsspondylodese. Arch Orthop Unfallchir 85:257, 1976

CHAPTER
12

■ ■ ■

Paralytic Spinal Deformity

James E. Shook
John P. Lubicky

■

Paralytic spinal deformities caused by polio motivated Dr. Paul Harrington to develop a better way of treating these unfortunate patients. Through trial and error, he came to realize that, although instrumentation greatly improved correction, a solid arthrodesis was still essential. The instrumentation has evolved significantly since Harrington fabricated each implant himself, but his idea revolutionized the care of patients with spinal deformities.

Probably no other group of patients with spinal deformities benefits from corrective surgery as much as the paralytics. An adolescent girl with a 45° idiopathic curve benefits from surgery because her cosmesis is better and further curve progression is arrested. However, other than her rib hump and perhaps ill-fitting clothes, this girl has very few symptoms from her curve. Contrast this with the child with myelomeningocele with a severe curve and associated pelvic obliquity, who cannot sit well or comfortably and may have recurrent problems with pressure sores beneath the low ischium. For children like this, corrective spinal surgery has made a big difference in their quality of life.

Those with paralytic scoliosis consitute a varied group, and each subset has its special problems. However, the goals of surgical treatment are basically the same for all—a spine as straight as possible over a pelvis that is as level as possible with the achievement of a solid arthrodesis. These goals are met by selecting the appropriate procedure(s) combined with appropriate instrumentation and an adequate amount of bone graft to insure a stable construct and a solid arthrodesis. Instrumentation without fusion as the definitive procedure is inappropriate in the neuromuscular patients. Except for those with muscular dystrophy or spinal muscular atrophies, most of these patients have a relatively normal life expectancy, and achieving a solid arthrodesis is essential.

As in other areas of spinal surgery, it is important not to "reinvent the wheel." We should avoid making the same mistakes made by the pioneers of spinal surgery in their early efforts to improve the procedures. For example, there is no reason to end the posterior instrumentation in a paralytic curve at T4 or T5 and suffer the consequences of "fall off" over the top of the instrumentation (particularly with Luque instrumentation). The instrumentation should cross over the apex of any upper thoracic kyphosis to prevent iatrogenic problems. There is no functional disadvantage in extending the fusion to T1 or T2 in these patients.

Although more stable, complicated, and powerful instrumentation systems have been produced, the principles of spinal surgery remain constant. If large paralytic curves are demonstrated to be stiff on side bending, anterior release by discectomy and bone graft should be used to improve the curve correction and pelvic obliquity and to decrease the force needed to achieve that correction by the posterior instrumentation. This surgical plan also provides circumferential arthrodesis to insure a solid bony construct after healing. Efforts to achieve these goals by powerful posterior instrumentation and fusion alone will often fail. Similarly, there are very few curves associated with myelomeningocele that can be handled adequately by posterior instrumentation and fusion alone.

Broad knowledge and experience is needed to care properly for these patients, because many of them are debilitated and have multisystem involvement. Maintaining good nutrition is very important, especially for those undergoing two-stage procedures or those with total-body involvement by cerebral palsy. The use of small-caliber feeding tubes with supplemental enteral feedings helps maintain caloric intake without the high cost and potential problems of parenteral administration of hyperalimentation. An alternative is to do both stages of two-stage reconstruction during the same anesthesia. For many of these patients, respiratory care before and after surgery is especially critical and often difficult. Although the routine use of preoperative tracheostomy is probably not indicated, ventilatory support through an endotracheal tube for several days after surgery may be necessary.

The surgeon must be open and truthful in dealing with the families of these patients. They need to know all the advantages and disadvantages of the surgery. They must understand—particularly patients who are debilitated—that although the vast majority of patients do very well, some of them have a difficult course until their surgical treatment has been completed. The parents also need to know that the goal of surgery is limited to correcting spinal deformity in an effort to improve the quality of life. They must understand that the underlying disease process will most likely not be changed by the spinal surgery.

With this background, this chapter discusses paralytic deformities in general and addresses specific groups of neuromuscular diseases in particular.

NEUROMUSCULAR SCOLIOSIS

Neuromuscular diseases are a group of disorders characterized by a compromise in the normal, integrated function of the brain, spinal cord, peripheral nerves, neuromuscular junctions, and muscles.[143] The final functional unit in this integrated sequence is the muscle.[18] Muscle dysfunction manifests as not enough motion (flaccidity), too much motion (spasticity), or out-of-sequence (dyskinetic) motion.

Scoliosis is frequently encountered in these neuromuscular dysfunctional states. A classification system has been established for neuromuscular scoliosis by the Scoliosis Research Society:[16]

A. Neuropathic
  1. Upper motor neuron
    a. Cerebral palsy
    b. Spinocerebellar degeneration
      i. Friedreich's ataxia
      ii. Charcot-Marie-Tooth
      iii. Roussy-Levy
    c. Syringomyelia
    d. Spinal cord tumor
    e. Spinal cord trauma
  2. Lower motor neuron
    a. Poliomyelitis
    b. Other viral myelitides
    c. Traumatic
    d. Spinal muscular atrophy
      i. Werding-Hoffman
      ii. Kugelberg-Welander
    e. Dysautonomia (Riley-Day)

B. Myopathic
  1. Arthrogryposis
  2. Muscular dystrophy
    a. Duchenne (pseudohypertrophic)
    b. Limb-girdle
    c. Facioscapulohumeral
  3. Fiber-type disproportion
  4. Congenital hypotonia
  5. Myotonia dystrophica

Causes of Neuromuscular Scoliosis

A spine that is straight in the anterior-posterior plane in the upright position and has sagittal cervical and lumbar lordotic and balancing thoracic kyphotic curves requires a precise interplay between the intrinsic mechanical stability of the bony vertebral column and its supporting ligaments and muscles.

Although the precise cause of any case of scoliosis is unknown, what is known about scoliosis can be applied to neuromuscular diseases, and, by identifying contributing factors, possible solutions can be examined.

The vertebral column can be viewed as a long, flexible rod. In bending, it can be deformed by a vertical force that is known as buckling. The vertical force that initiates buckling is called the critical load.[133] The Swiss mathematician Leonhard Euler (1707–1783) derived the formula to calculate the critical load (Per) for a certain column length (L), elasticity (E), and area moment of inertia (I), with both ends of the column clamped:

$$Per = \frac{4K\ EI}{L^2}$$

If one end is unclamped and left free while the other end remains fixed, the solution for the Per is:

$$Per = \frac{K\ EI}{4L^2}$$

By allowing one free end, the column's weight-bearing ability is decreased by a factor of 16. A child with weakness in the shoulders can be considered to have unclamping of the upper end of the spinal column.[25]

The length (L) of the spinal column affects the critical load. With growth, the trunk length increases, and the load that the spine can support decreases rapidly.

Extrinsic muscles contribute significantly to the dynamic stability of the spine. The resistance of the spinal column, the vertebrae, discs, and ligaments to buckling is small. It requires only about 20 N to buckle a thoracolumbar spine that has been dissected out of a human cadaver.[133] Neuromuscular diseases all produce a compromise in muscular function and thus a compromise in the dynamic support for vertebral column stability.

The biomechanically compromised spine is initially straight in the recumbent position but buckles or deforms in the upright position. However, these postural curves become structural with time owing to biologic factors, especially in the growing spine. "As soon as a small curve develops, forces on the vertebral end plates become asymmetrical, paving the way for the relentless development of a progressive curve with permanent disc, vertebral, and facet joint alterations."[19] The explanation of the permanent deformation of the vertebral column is based on the Heuter Volkmann Law. This theory suggests that increased loading across an epiphyseal growth plate inhibits growth and that decreased pressure tends to accelerate growth. In the deformed, growing spine, the vertebral end plate on the concave side of the curve is subject to increased compression loading, causing decreased growth, and on the convex side is subject to relatively decreased loading, causing increased growth. The result of these forces is a wedge-shaped, deformed vertebral body.[160] In many neuromuscular disorders, scoliosis starts when the patient is very young and the spine is abnormally loaded; thus, the potential for vertebral body deformity is great.

The vertebrae may be structurally compromised as a result of metabolic bone disease secondary to nutritionally or anticonvulsant-induced rickets.[72, 107, 156] Disuse osteopenia is also a significant factor in neuromuscular patients. These structurally compromised vertebrae may become permanently deformed when subjected to adverse biomechanical forces.

The cause of spinal deformity in neuromuscular scoliosis is a complex interaction between adverse biomechanical conditions superimposed on biologic factors. The earlier and greater the disease process is incurred, the greater the potential for spinal deformity.[63, 88]

Characteristics of Neuromuscular Scoliosis

Although neuromuscular diseases are a diverse group of disorders having primary abnormalities at different sites in the brain, spinal cord, peripheral nerves, and muscle axis, they share many characteristics. The final common pathway of dysfunction is the muscle cell. Common characteristics of neuromuscular scoliosis include:

Early onset
Rapid progression
Progression after skeletal maturity
Compromised functional abilities
Long curves, which may include the sacrum
Pelvic obliquity

Many of the neuromuscular disorders exist at birth because of hereditary (e.g., spinal muscular atrophy) or acquired (e.g., cerebral palsy) abnormalities. Disorders that appear later are acquired (e.g., spinal cord injury) or genetic defects that manifest themselves during childhood (e.g., Duchenne's muscular dystrophy). The earlier the neuromuscular disorder is evident and the more severe the disorder, the greater the likelihood of scoliosis. The average age of onset of scoliosis in patients with infantile spinal muscular atrophy of the acute variety is less than 2 years, and for those with the chronic variety, 3 years. Children who become quadriplegic show a spinal deformity an average of 2.3 years after skeletal injury.[19] In Duchenne's muscular dystrophy, the patients are ambulatory until an average age of 10; they become wheelchair bound, and scoliosis is detected at an average age of 12 years.[152] Patients who sustain a spinal cord injury after the adolescent growth spurt have only a small chance of developing a scoliosis.[110]

Neuromuscular scoliosis is progressive even after skeletal maturity. Thometz and Simon, in a study of 51 adult patients with cerebral palsy followed for at least 4 years after they reached skeletal maturity, found scoliosis progressed even in adults, with the greatest progression in the patients with the largest curves at the time of skeletal maturity.[155] The rate of progression was 0.8° each year for those with curves less than 50° and 1.4° per year for those with curves greater than 50°. Cady and Bobechko, in a review of 42 patients with Friedreich's ataxia, confirmed that curves tend to progress with the severity of the disease and often tend to progress after skeletal maturity.[28]

The functional independence of patients already compromised by flaccid, spastic, or dyskinetic states may be further impaired by progressive scoliosis.[100, 149] Hensinger and MacEwen, after reviewing patients with spinal muscular atrophy, felt the loss of ambulatory ability was due, in some patients, to the development of scoliosis.[76] In a study of arthrogrypotic patients, Hoffer reported that a progressive spinal deformity with extremity deformities resulted in loss of ambulation.[81] A study of patients with Duchenne's muscular dystrophy showed that, when the scoliosis was in excess of 40°, patients had to use their upper extremities to support their trunk and became functional quadriplegics.[83] Bonnet and associates, in a study of patients with paralytic scoliosis, revealed that a progressive scoliosis can reduce a patient from household-ambulatory to wheelchair-bound status.[14]

Neuromuscular scoliotic curves are frequently long curves that extend to and may include the sacrum and pelvis, resulting in pelvic obliquity.[59, 127] Pelvic obliquity is the failure of the pelvis to be in a perfectly horizontal position and perpendicular to the spine in the frontal plane.[167] The functional problems, evaluation, and management of pelvic obliquity in the neuromuscular patient offer some of the most challenging aspects of these disorders and deserve special attention.

Pelvic obliquity is associated with uneven weight-bearing in the sitting position, causing decreased surface area for weight bearing and increased contact-surface pressures.[99] This leads to painful sitting for the patient with intact sensation and to pressure sores for patients who are without protective sensation. In patients with sensation, the pain may limit sitting tolerance. In patients with pressure sores, osteomyelitis of the ischium or trochanter may result.[139] An uneven pelvis also leads to an unstable base for the spine in the upright position and requires the use of the patient's hands or elbows to support the spine. The patient becomes a functional quadriplegic. Pelvic obliquity

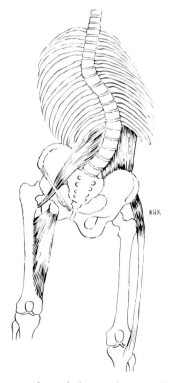

FIG. 12–1. Muscular imbalance of spinopelvic, spinofemoral, or pelvofemoral muscles may cause pelvic obliquity.

may lead to subluxation or dislocation of the hip on the high side of the pelvis, and hip dislocation may become painful.[100]

The cause of pelvic obliquity is contracture of muscles spanning from the pelvis to the femur, from the spine to the femur, from the spine to the pelvis, or a combination of these (Fig. 12-1).[71] Among patients with polio or Duchenne's muscular dystrophy, a contracture of the iliotibial band may cause pelvic obliquity.[29, 87] Tight iliopsoas and adductor muscles can cause progressive subluxation and dislocation of the affected hip in patients with cerebral palsy.[100] The dislocated hip was followed by pelvic obliquity and scoliosis. Letts noticed that in children with spasticity the pelvis functions as part of the spine and participates in the severe rotation that accompanies the scoliosis.[100] Mayer incriminated unilateral contracture of spinal pelvic musculature (i.e., quadratus lumborum, external oblique, and internal oblique muscles) as a cause of pelvic obliquity in patients with polio.[108]

To determine whether the pelvic obliquity is caused by contracted spinal femoral, pelvic femoral, or spinal pelvic muscles, the patient should be prone on the examining table with his or her hips flexed over the end of the table. On adduction or abduction of the hips, if scoliosis is alleviated, fixed spinal pelvic deformity is exonerated, and release of the contracted muscles will alleviate the pelvic obliquity (Fig. 12-2). If pelvic obliquity persists on this maneuver, a fixed spinal pelvic deformity exists, which can be overcome only by surgical release of the contracted muscles, traction, or relative lengthening of these muscles by a spine-shortening procedure (i.e., anterior spinal discectomy and fusion).[126]

TREATMENT OF NEUROMUSCULAR SCOLIOSIS

The goal of treatment in neuromuscular scoliosis is to maintain a spine balanced in the coronal and sagittal planes over a level pelvis.[18, 102, 119] In achieving this goal, respiratory compromise is minimized and functional ability is optimized.

After a child is diagnosed as having a neuromuscular disorder, the spine should be carefully followed for the development of the deformity. Yearly checks for scoliosis and kyphosis should be instituted, and at the first sign of deformity, appropriate x-ray films taken. Thereafter, visits every 3 to 6 months are warranted. After the curve exceeds 20°, orthotic management should be considered. Observation is also appropriate for severely mentally retarded patients with large curves to ascertain that the spinal deformity has not caused a functional loss. If the deformity increases or if functional ability is compromised because of an increasing curve, treatment should be instituted.

Orthotic Management

Spinal orthotics have been used in neuromuscular spinal deformities with varying degrees of success. The goals of orthotic management include:

1. Correction of spinal deformity
2. Control of curve progression
3. Stabilization of the spine and pelvis to allow the patient to be in an upright posture without hand support
4. Control of abnormal reflexes

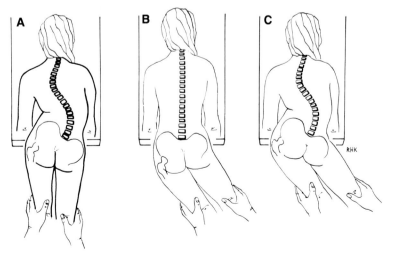

FIG. 12–2. A. Pelvic obliquity. **B.** If the pelvic obliquity is eliminated by abduction or adduction of the hips, a pelvofemoral muscle contracture is the cause. **C.** If pelvic obliquity persists despite abduction or adduction of the hips, a fixed spinopelvic obliquity exists.

Spinal orthotics function in active and passive ways. The Milwaukee brace, which is the classic active spinal orthosis,[22, 24, 122] furnishes pelvic fixation, a thoracic pad that provides a lateral irritant over the apical ribs of the spinal deformity. The patient relies on an intact "righting reflex" to pull away from the thoracic pad on the convexity of the spinal curve, actively correcting the spinal deformity. The anterior-posterior shell Kidex jacket is an example of a passive device.[166] After the spine is passively straightened to a maximal degree, a plaster cast is applied. The cast is removed, and from this a positive impression of the patient's pelvis and trunk is fabricated. From this positive mold, a plastic jacket is fabricated that conforms to the spine in the corrected position. When placed on the patient, it holds the spine in its corrected position.

Active devices in the management of neuromuscular spinal deformities have been largely unsuccessful. Most patients with neuromuscular scoliosis lack voluntary control, normal righting reflexes, or the ability to cooperate with an active orthotic program. Two groups of patients who seem to benefit from active spinal orthosis are those with minimal cerebral palsy who are capable of cooperating with an active exercise program and patients with Charcot-Marie-Tooth disease, especially with kyphoscoliosis, who seem to benefit from using Milwaukee braces.[40, 76]

Passive orthotic devices have met with considerably greater success in the management of neuromuscular scoliosis than active devices. Passive devices applied to a child with a flexible neuromuscular scoliosis initially substantially improve the spinal deformity. This should be confirmed with a spinal x-ray film taken in the orthosis. Eventually, with growth and weight gain, especially as the child enters the pubertal growth spurt, the device begins to fail, and curves invariably progress. In neuromuscular spinal deformities, passive devices should be viewed as slowing the inevitable progression until the child has completed most of his or her spinal growth and can undergo surgery.[23, 24] The spinal deformity should be monitored with periodic x-ray films in the orthosis, and curve progression should not be allowed beyond 50° before other measures are instituted.

Wheelchair seating orthoses have found great application in the management of neuromuscular spinal deformities. They allow an upright position of the child without trunk support, a method for controlling abnormal pathologic reflexes, and a method of safe transport of patients in the upright posture. They permit mobilization of the patient with a severe spinal deformity, allowing him or her to be in the upright posture while accommodating the deformity.[31] Three basic seating systems are available for use in patients with neuromuscular disease (Fig. 12-3):

1. Modular seating systems that provide for control of the pelvis and trunk and have attachments for control of the head have found particular application among small children with spastic neuromuscular diseases.
2. Commercially available wheelchairs with attachments to provide an abduction pad to control the pelvis, lateral trunk supports to prop up the spine, and mobile arm supports provide increased independence in seating skills. These systems have found particular application among older children and adolescents with moderate trunk control and the cognitive ability to use arm supports and electric-powered controls to drive the wheelchairs.
3. Custom-molded seating-support orthoses are made from a mold of the patient. They extend from the distal thighs to the upper back, with side extensions on the pelvis and trunk. An anterior thoracic vest holds the patient back into the orthosis, and a head support can be added if the patient lacks head control. Custom-molded seating-support orthoses have found particular application among patients who are quite flaccid, with little or no trunk and head control, and among those with severe spinal deformities who are not candidates for reconstructive spinal surgery.

Surgery

Garrett has enumerated the benefits of surgical stabilization of a paralytic collapsing spine:[62]

1. The upright posture is maintained with greater ease.
2. Trunk movement is accomplished with less fatigue.
3. There is a conspicuous relief from fatigue and an unmistakable improvement in general physical well-being.

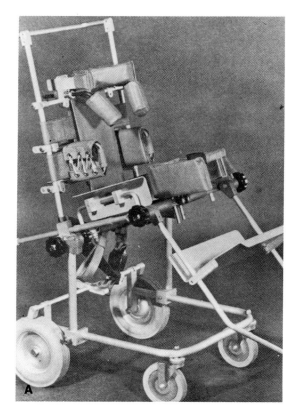

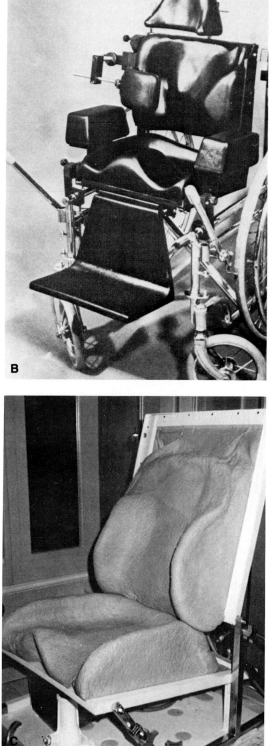

FIG. 12–3. **A.** Mullholland child traveler (Mulholland Corporation, Santa Paula, CA). **B.** Contour U-shaped custom-molded seating system (Pin.dot Products, Northbrook, IL) **C.** Custom-molding technique.

Other important factors are relevant to stabilization of a progressive neuromuscular deformity:

4. For patients who preoperatively require the use of their upper extremities for trunk support, the arms are freed for more useful activities.
5. For patients with static neuromuscular disease, pulmonary function is stabilized and further compromise that would result from a progressive spine deformity is averted.
6. By correcting the scoliosis and pelvic obliquity, pain from a decreased surface area for seating and pain from rib-pelvis impingement is alleviated.

Preoperative Considerations

The physiologic stress to a patient undergoing reconstructive spine surgery can be extreme. This patient is already debilitated because of neuromuscular disease. To ensure that he or she can tolerate reconstructive spinal surgery, a detailed preoperative assessment must include an evaluation of respiratory competency, cardiac status, nutrition, possible feeding difficulties, seizure disorders, and metabolic bone disease.

The clinical assessment of a patient's breathing ability begins with a detailed history. Questions concerning whether the patient has dyspnea with exertion, at rest, or at night and if there is a history of frequent upper respiratory infections or recurrent pneumonia should be answered.

A detailed physical examination should be performed, noting the patient's breathing pattern and measuring the strength of the diaphragm, intercostals, neck flexors, and abdominals. The diaphragm normally accounts for 60% of the vital capacity during maximal deep breathing and for nearly 100% during quiet breathing. The intercostal muscles increase the anterior-posterior diameter of the upper part of the thorax and the transverse diameter of the lower part. Normally, the upper part of the chest expands as the diaphragm descends. However, with intercostal muscle paralysis, as the diaphragm descends, there is a retraction of the soft tissues in the intercostal spaces and distention of the abdomen. The neck flexors are normally considered accessory muscles of respiration. With paralysis or weakness of both the diaphragm and intercostals, the cervical accessory muscles attempt to elevate the thorax during inspiration and contraction becomes conspicuous.[14]

An efficient cough is essential for successful respiration and should be carefully evaluated.[59, 123] Coughing requires the use of all muscles of respiration. The patient with poor strength or difficulty in controlling muscles of respiration will have a poor cough and may have difficulty clearing pulmonary secretions postoperatively.

All patients with neuromuscular diseases who are capable of cooperating should attempt an evaluation of pulmonary function with a spirogram (Fig. 12-4). The patient is asked to inhale to total lung capacity and exhale as forcefully and rapidly as possible to empty the lungs. The amount of air that is forcefully exhaled is the forced vital capacity (FVC), the volume of air exhaled during the first second is the forced expiratory volume (FEV_1), and the remaining air in the lungs after maximal exhalation is the residual volume (RV).

Patients with vital capacities less than 30% of the predicted normal value require postoperative respiratory aid. In patients with progressive terminal neuromuscular disease (Duchenne's muscular dystrophy and Friedreich's ataxia), a FVC of less than 30% of predicted normal value should be considered a relative contraindication to surgery. Patients with a vital capacity above 70% can be expected to tolerate surgery without postoperative respiratory support. Patients with a vital capacity between 35 and 70% occasionally require postoperative respiratory support, depending on the amount of postoperative narcotic that is required for pain relief and whether an anterior or posterior spinal surgery is performed.[106, 123]

An arterial blood gas test should be performed. This is especially important for patients with neuro-

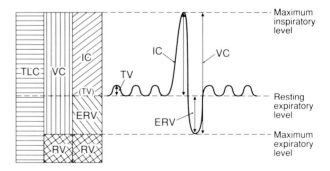

FIG. 12–4. Pulmonary function tests. RV, residual volume; ERV, expiratory reserve volume; VC, vital capacity; TV, tidal volume; IRV, inspiratory reserve volume; TLC, total lung capacity. (Adapted with permission from Comroe JH et al (eds): The Lung, Clinical Physiology, and Pulmonary Function Tests, p 8. Chicago, Year Book Medical Publishers, 1962)

muscular disease who are unwilling or unable to cooperate with a spirogram. Hypercarbia with a $PaCO_2$ greater than 50 and hypoxemia with a PaO_2 less than 50 should be considered contraindications to surgery.[62, 73]

Several neuromuscular diseases are complicated by progressive cardiac impairment, mandating preoperative cardiac assessment that includes an electrocardiogram (ECG) and echocardiogram.

In Duchenne's muscular dystrophy, myocardial involvement is common.[6] The cardiac dysfunction is progressive and often parallels skeletal muscle dysfunction.[85] Electrocardiographic abnormalities are seen in 50 to 90% of cases. These include tall R waves on the right precordial leads and increased R/S amplitude ratios with narrow and deep Q waves. Cardiac conduction abnormalities are frequent and include a prolonged intra-atrial conduction and right bundle branch block. The echocardiogram shows impairment of both systolic and diastolic function. Left ventricular wall thickness and left ventricular size may be reduced. Generally, the pulmonary functional impairment is greater than cardiac impairment, and pulmonary disease is the limiting factor when considering reconstructive spinal surgery in the patient with Duchenne's muscular dystrophy.

Friedreich's ataxia is complicated by a progressive cardiomyopathy with cardiac failure, a frequent cause of the patient's ultimate demise.[1] The ECG shows T-wave abnormalities, sinus tachycardia, atrial flutter, atrial fibrillation, premature ventricular beats, and left and right ventricular hypertrophy.

Patients with myotonic dystrophy frequently have cardiac abnormalities.[6] Although most patients will have a normal cardiac examination, 29% reveal mitral valve prolapse. ECG abnormalities are seen in up to 90% of the patients. First-degree heart block and intraventricular conduction disturbances have been the most common findings, but atrial or ventricular tachyarrhythmias do occur. These cardiac conduction defects can lead to sudden death. In view of the frequency of conduction abnormalities, patients with symptoms or ECG evidence of dysrhythmias should be investigated.

The relationship between poor nutrition and perioperative complications in patients undergoing orthopedic procedures is well documented.[89] Protein depletion correlates with increased mortality rates, impaired wound healing, and impaired humoral and cell-mediated immunity that lowers host resistance and leads to an increased rate of wound infections and sepsis.[97]

Patients with neuromuscular scoliosis may have suboptimal nutrition for many reasons, including incoordination of the muscles of the lips, tongue, palate, and pharynx, leading to difficulties in mastication and swallowing.[27, 92, 129, 146] In addition, gastroesophageal reflux is a frequent problem encountered in children with cerebral palsy with spastic, total body involvement and scoliosis. Gastroesophageal reflux leads to recurrent vomiting, esophagitis, and aspiration pneumonia.[13, 41, 90, 146] Major surgical procedures intensify the preexisting state by raising the metabolic requirements, altering nutrient ingestion and absorption, and consuming endogenous energy stores.[89] Fortunately, appropriate nutritional therapy can restore the patient's cell mass and immunocompetency.[120] This improves the patient's prognosis for wound healing and decreases the rate of infections.

Patients with histories of feeding difficulties should have a preoperative nutritional assessment consisting of body weight, total lymphocyte count (N > 1550 cells/mm^3), total protein (N = 6.0–8.0 g/dL), and albumin (N = 3.8–4.8 g/dL).[47, 89] Patients identified as being malnourished preoperatively should have these abnormalities corrected before elective spinal surgery.

Children with neuromuscular diseases and a history of feeding difficulties, recurrent vomiting, or recurrent pneumonia should have a gastrointestinal evaluation of the swallowing mechanism, looking for discoordination in swallowing, trachial aspiration, gastroesophageal reflux, and hiatal hernias. These abnormalities should be corrected before reconstructive spinal surgery by medical means or surgery (i.e., Nissen fundoplication, gastrostomy, or both).[47]

Seizure disorders are not uncommon in neuromuscular diseases and present the dual problem of perioperative seizure control and metabolic bone disease. For patients taking seizure medications, preoperative anticonvulsant levels should be obtained, and their levels should be optimized within a therapeutic range. Perioperative parenteral administration of anticonvulsant medications may be necessary to keep these levels in a therapeutic range.

Metabolic bone disease is seen in patients with neuromuscular disease and may have an adverse affect on spinal fixation, rates of spinal fusion, and perioperative pathologic fractures of long bones. The bone disease may be secondary to disuse osteopenia, nutritional rickets, and anticonvulsant-induced rickets. Active metabolic bone disease should be corrected, if possible, before elective reconstructive spinal surgery. If, despite nutritional supplementation, metabolic bone disease persists, surgical fixation systems that entail the use of segmental fixation should be used.[44, 103, 147]

Operative Considerations

General Considerations. The operative treatment of spinal deformities in patients with neuromuscular disease is more complicated than is implied by the technical management of the deformities. Surgical success depends on having a stable operating room environment and keeping tight physiologic control of the patient.

Intraoperative hypothermia can have an adverse effect on patient physiology. It can cause myocardial depression and arrythmias, and these problems—superimposed on a heart already compromised by neuromuscular cardiomyopathy—may be especially severe. Hypothermia may diminish ventilatory response to hypoxemia and hypercarbia, or it may delay emergence from anesthesia and cause a relative hyperglycemia. Controlling the patient's temperature makes anesthesia, surgery, and emergence from anesthesia safer. Preventing inadvertent hypothermia includes controlling room temperature, covering all areas of the patient's body that do not need to be exposed, warming skin preparations, irrigation fluids, and infusions, and using heated, humidified anesthesia gas and a heating mattress.[144]

Reconstructive spinal surgery for the patient with neuromuscular disease is associated with greater blood loss than for patients with scoliosis associated with other causes. The amount of blood loss that necessitates intraoperative replacement should be established preoperatively. The estimated blood volume (EBV) in most children is approximately 70 ml/kg. Factors like obesity can reduce the EBV to 60 to 65 ml/kg. The preoperative hematocrit, coupled with the preoperative EBV, allows the calculation of a maximal allowable blood loss (MABL) before initiating erythrocyte transfusion. Adverse anesthetic and surgical effects from anemia are rarely seen with hematocrits above 10. A sample calculation of MABL is given:[35]

$$\frac{\text{estimated blood volume (EBV)} \times (\text{patient hematocrit} - 30)}{\text{patient hematocrit}} = \text{MABL}$$

For example, a 30-kg patient has an EBV of 30 kg times 70 ml/kg or 2100 ml, and his hematocrit is 45. The patient's MABL is calulated below:

$$\frac{2100 \times (45 - 30)}{45} = 700 \text{ cc}$$

These estimates of MABL are rough and serve only as guidelines for erythrocyte replacement.

Control of blood loss is a significant operative consideration. Hemodilution, controlled hypotension, use of a cell saver, and meticulous surgical technique are all effective means of reducing intraoperative need for blood replacement.

Neurologic complications in reconstructive spinal surgery occur with a frequency of 0.5 to 17%, depending on the type of spinal surgery (i.e., anterior or posterior), the type of spinal instrumentation, the degree of preoperative spinal deformity, and the amount of correction obtained.[4, 77, 163] An intraoperative wake-up test has been used quite successfully for ensuring the safety of spinal cord function.[12] The intraoperative wake-up test requires a patient who is able and willing to respond to verbal commands. After spinal instrumentation, the level of anesthesia is decreased to the point that the patient is awake enough to respond to verbal commands. The patient is asked to squeeze the anesthesiologist's hands, demonstrating intact cord function cranial to the level of spinal instrumentation. The patient is then asked to move his or her feet, demonstrating intact cortical control of cord function caudal to the level of spinal instrumentation. If the patient is able to demonstrate cord function cranial but not caudal to the level of spinal instrumentation, spinal cord compromise has occurred and immediate removal of the spinal instrumentation is imperative. This method has proved effective in reversing spinal cord compromise caused by the instrumentation.

Many patients with neuromuscular scoliosis are either unable or unwilling to cooperate with an intraoperative wake-up test. The electrophysiologic monitoring of spinal cord function has proved to be an effective alternative. The principal of spinal cord monitoring is stimulation of a peripheral nerve caudal to the level of spinal instrumentation and recording of cortical evoked response cranial to the level of spinal instrumentation. A preoperative baseline recording is obtained, and a stable intraoperative recording is established before spinal instrumentation. After spinal instrumentation, a sudden change in latencies or reduction in wave amplitude can indicate an alteration in spinal cord function. Early removal of spinal instrumentation is usually followed by a return to baseline evoked potentials and preservation of cord function.[12]

Technical Considerations. Surgical treatment of neuromuscular deformities involves the ability to correct the spinal deformity in coronal and sagittal planes, the ability to hold the correction without instrumentation failure, and the ability to obtain a solid fusion without pseudarthroses.

In 1956, Gucker reported the treatment of 78 patients with spinal deformities caused by poliomyelitis.[69] The surgical technique used was a posterior spinal fusion and postoperative recumbency in a plaster jacket for 4 months followed by ambulatory jacket management. In the follow-up of these patients, 9% had worse postoperative deformities than before surgery, 47% remained the same, and 44% were improved. Pseudarthroses were identified as significant factors in poor results. The overall pseudarthrosis rate was 56%, and the rate was 71% in those patients who had worse curves postoperatively than preoperatively and 44% in patients with improved postoperative curves. In 1970, Pavon reported on the treatment of 118 patients with polio and spinal deformity.[130] These patients were managed with cast correction, posterior fusion without instrumentation, recumbency for 6 months, and ambulatory treatment with a Milwaukee brace for 6 months. Curve correction was poor, averaging 7.7% for preoperative curves between 50 and 75°, 14.8% for preoperative curves between 76 and 100°, and 22% for preoperative curves greater than 100°. Bonnet was able to reduce the pseudarthrosis rate from 38% to 28% in patients treated with posterior fusion without instrumentation by adding a facet fusion to the posterior spine fusion.[14] In Bonnet's patients, curve correction was still poor, averaging only 20%.

In an effort to improve curve correction, Harrington introduced spinal instrumentation with posterior rod fixation of the corrected spine. Bonnet applied Harrington's instrumentation system to patients with neuromuscular scoliosis.[14] Curve correction in 113 patients treated with posterior instrumentation and spinal fusion increased to 34%, compared with an average 20% curve correction for the 155 patients treated with fusion without instrumentation.

Anterior surgical exposure of the spine for treatment of tubercular spine infections introduced a new option for treating spinal deformities.[80] In 1976, Bonnet reported on a series of 10 patients with cerebral palsy treated with posterior instrumentation and spinal fusion using a Harrington rod, producing a disappointing curve correction rate of only 30% and a 40% incidence of pseudarthrosis.[15] Bonnet and associates then adopted an anterior spinal instrumentation and fusion using a Dwyer apparatus.[53] Curve correction in this series increased to 48%, but the pseudarthrosis rate was 72%.

To preserve the correction obtainable with an anterior procedure by limiting instrumentation failure and pseudarthroses, several physicians have used a first-stage anterior discectomy, instrumentation, and fusion, followed by posterior instrumentation and spinal fusion. In 1975, DeWald reported the results of 23 patients treated with anterior and posterior instrumentation and spinal fusion using a Dwyer apparatus anteriorly and a posterior Harrington rod.[42] In this series curve correction averaged 63%; there were no pseudarthroses but 5 patients (22%) had superior hook dislocation. In the same year, O'Brien reported the results of patients managed with a circumferential spinal instrumentation and fusion using an anterior Dwyer apparatus and, posteriorly, a Harrington rod.[128] Curve correction in these patients averaged 75%, and there were no pseudarthroses.

As the ability to obtain and maintain excellent curve correction and limit pseudarthroses was achieved, techniques that would preserve sagittal contours of the spine, that would allow for segmental fixation and curve control, and that would possibly eliminate postoperative external support of the spine were all explored.[158]

Moe introduced a square-ended Harrington rod that couples to a square-holed hook and allows for contouring lumbar lordosis and thoracic kyphosis (Fig. 12-5). This rod has been employed in neuromuscular curves, especially those that required fusion to the lumbar spine and pelvis. The reported attributes of this rod include the ability to maintain lumbar lordosis and decrease the incidence of hook dislodgment from the sacrum. In 1987, Casey reported on a series of 36 patients in whom rod contouring was used to preserve lumbar lordosis.[32] He concluded that additional steps beyond concave rod contouring appeared to be necessary to preserve lumbar lordosis.

Eduardo Luque and colleagues developed a segmental spinal instrumentation system that provided for the maintenance of normal sagittal spine contours.[103] It was thought that postoperative immobilization would not be necessary with a more stable spinal fixation.

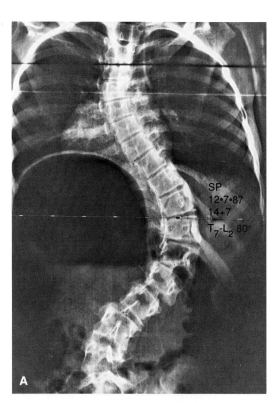

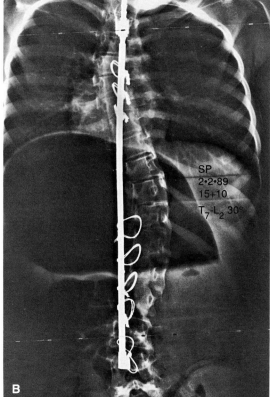

SP
12·7·87
14+7
T₇-L₂ 80°

SP
2·2·89
15+10
T₇-L₂ 30°

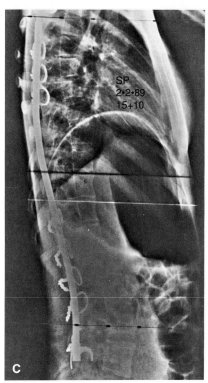

SP
2·2·89
15+10

FIG. 12–5. **A.** 14 + 7-year-old ambulatory patient with cerebral palsy and an 80° scoliosis without pelvic obliquity. **B.** Postoperative curve reduced to 30°. Instrumentation with a Moe rod to L4. **C.** Sagittal lumbar and thoracic curves maintained by contouring of the square ended rod.

The use of posterior spinal instrumentation and fusion using Luque rods without the use of antecedent anterior spinal procedures has been reported. In 1989, the results of 10 patients treated with a single-stage posterior procedure using 3/16-in dual-contoured Luque rods were reported by Swank.[153] Curve correction averaged 53%, but the pseudarthrosis rate was high at 40%, and there was a 10% rate of instrumentation failure. In the same year, Gersoff reported the results of 33 patients managed with a single-stage posterior procedure using Luque instrumentation.[65] Curve correction was 52%, there were no pseudarthroses, and the only instrumentation failures were in cases where 3/16-in rods were used instead of 1/4-in rods.

Allen and Ferguson have reported extensively on the use of Luque rod instrumentation for the treatment of neuromuscular curves.[5, 58] In most patients a two-stage procedure is recommended. After reviewing patients treated with a first-stage anterior instrumentation and fusion followed by posterior instrumentation and fusion, they questioned whether anterior instrumentation was really necessary. They recommended an anterior release and fusion, followed by tong gravity traction and posterior instrumentation and spinal fusion using Luque rod instrumentation. Using this technique for 10 patients with neuromuscular scoliosis, curve correction averaged 63.8%, and although no pseudarthroses were identified, poor fusion occurred in 20% of patients.[57] They believed that their results were comparable with those in which anterior and posterior instrumentation were used, and complications associated with anterior instrumentation were avoided.

The problems of fixed pelvic obliquity in patients with neuromuscular scoliosis include pressure sores; loss of sitting balance, necessitating the use of upper extremities for trunk support; and paralytic hip dislocation. The causes of pelvic obliquity include a fixed lumbar curve in which the sacrum and pelvis are structurally the last vertebrae in the curve, fixed spinal pelvic or pelvofemoral muscle contractures, and paralytic hip dislocation. If muscle contracture is the cause of pelvic obliquity, release should rectify the problem.[71, 100, 109] If a fixed lumbar scoliosis is the cause of pelvic obliquity, surgical treatment of the scoliosis is usually required with an anterior discectomy and fusion. O'Brien has made the observation that the L5 vertebra is usually parallel with the intercrest line and that inclusion of L5 in an anterior procedure usually

corrects pelvic obliquity (Fig. 12-6).[126] If the top of the L4 vertebra is parallel to the intercrest line, anterior instrumentation to L4 is all that is required to correct pelvic obliquity.

For 17 patients treated with halo-femoral or halo-pelvic traction followed by a two-stage surgery consisting of anterior discectomy, Dwyer instrumentation, and fusion followed by posterior Harrington rod instrumentation and fusion, pelvic obliquity was corrected in 66%.[128] DeWald reported another group of 23 patients for whom a similar technique yielded an average correction of 68.4%. Swank, using a first-stage anterior instrumentation and spinal fusion with a Zielke apparatus followed by posterior instrumentation and spinal fusion using Luque rod instrumentation, reported an average of 54% correction of pelvic obliquity.[42, 153]

Allen and Ferguson developed a method of pelvic fixation using Luque rod instrumentation called the "Galveston technique" (Fig. 12-7).[3] The rods are contoured to fit along the spine and transversely on the flat of the sacrum. They are then impacted longitudinally between the cortices of the ilium for a distance of greater than 6 cm, just superior to the greater sciatic notch (within 1.5 cm of the notch). Pelvic fixation is excellent, and lumbosacral fusion rates are high. Allen and Ferguson, using this technique, did not feel that anterior instrumentation was necessary to correct pelvic obliquity or obtain a solid circumferential fusion. Pelvic obliquity correction in their series averaged 67.4%.

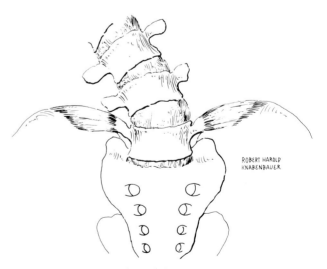

FIG. 12–6. L5 vertebra held parallel to the intercrest line by strong iliolumbar ligaments.

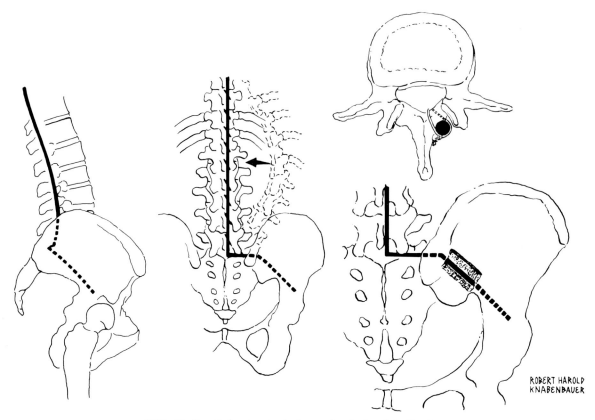

ROBERT HAROLD
KNABENBAUER

FIG. 12–7. Galveston technique of spinal pelvic fixation.

Many authors have questioned whether surgical fusion should include the sacrum or pelvis. All patients with a fixed spinopelvic obliquity should have a fusion to the sacrum to prevent recurrent pelvic obliquity after surgical correction. Patients with collapsing neuromuscular scoliosis should also have instrumentation to the sacrum and pelvis to prevent progressive trunk decompensation and pelvic obliquity. Spinal fusion to the sacrum and pelvis is not necessary if there is no pelvic obliquity. It should also be avoided in patients who are still ambulatory for fear of compromising their precarious mobility (Fig. 12-8).

The issue of whether or not an anterior spinal surgery is necessary can be addressed by reviewing the previously stated studies. Patients with a large fixed spinal pelvic obliquity require an anterior release to overcome the pelvic obliquity. If the lumbar curve is flexible and the pelvic obliquity can be overcome on side-bending x-ray films, an anterior release is not necessary. Patients with large, rigid curves that on bending films do not correct to less than 30° should have a first-stage anterior release and fusion, followed by posterior segmental fixation. When curves are flexible and correctable to less than 30° on bending x-ray films, posterior instrumentation with segmental fixation and fusion is all that is usually required. Patients with severely deficient posterior elements usually require anterior fusion to decrease the possibility of pseudarthrosis. Patients with severe spasticity usually require a circumferential fusion to limit the incidence of failure of instrumentation and failure of fusion.

There is a high incidence of osteopenia in patients

FIG. 12–8. **A.** Ambulatory cerebral palsy patient with a 50° lumbar curve and a small pelvic obliquity. **B.** The curve is supple on side bending, and the pelvic obliquity is flexible. **C.** Scoliosis is reduced to 3° by circumferential instrumentation and fusion to L5 (patient has 6 lumbar vertebrae) in this standing anterior-posterior x-ray film. **D.** Postoperative standing lateral x-ray film.

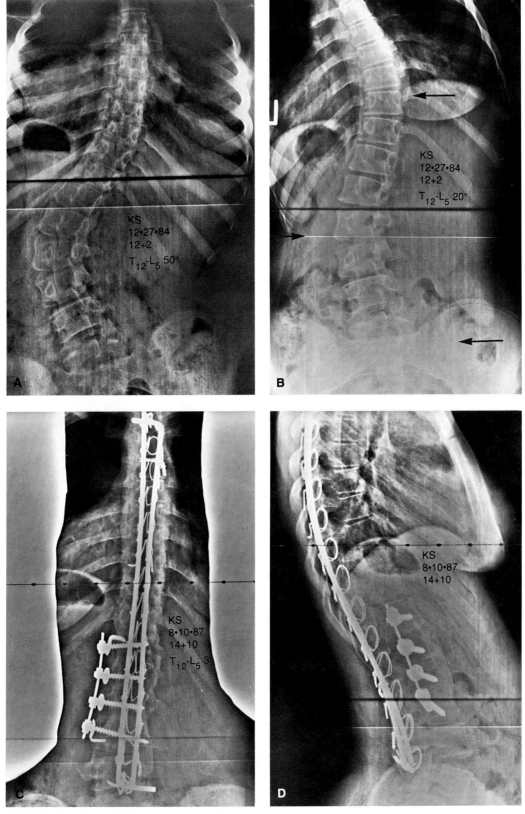

KS
12•27•84
12+2
T₁₂-L₅ 50°

KS
12•27•84
12+2
T₁₂-L₅ 20°

KS
8•10•87
14+10
T₁₂-L₅ 3°

KS
8•10•87
14+10

FIG. 12–8. (*continued*)

with neuromuscular disease. In systems that rely on two or four points of fixation between the spine and instrumentation, there is a significant risk of hook cut-out. Systems that use segmental spinal instrumentation markedly decrease postoperative loss of correction.

Anterior Spinal Instrumentation

The issue of anterior spinal instrumentation in neuromuscular scoliosis remains a controversial one. If a posterior spinal fixation system using only two points of fixation is to be used after an anterior spinal fusion, anterior spinal instrumentation is warranted to create a segmental, more stable spinal construct. Anterior spinal instrumentation does entail significant risk, including increased operative time and blood loss and the chance of instrumentation erosion into the aorta.[60, 74] Therefore, in many patients in whom a second-stage posterior segmental instrumentation system is to be used after an anterior spinal fusion, anterior instrumentation may not be necessary (Fig. 12-9).

Bank Bone

Many patients with neuromuscular scolioses have deficient bone stock to harvest for a spinal fusion. This deficiency is usually associated with metabolic disease or with the underdevelopment of the pelvis because of decreased muscle tone. Banked bone has been used extensively in reconstructive spinal surgery, especially for patients with neuromuscular scoliosis.[61, 112] The results with banked allograft bone have been excellent, with low rates of infection and high rates of solid arthrodeses. Allograft banked bone should be readily available for use in patients with neuromuscular scoliosis because there is not enough iliac crest bone to forge a solid spinal arthrodesis.

Traction

Traction has been used extensively in patients with neuromuscular scoliosis. Most series have used halo-pelvic, halo-femoral, or halo-gravity traction (Fig. 12-10). Traction offers greater correction of deformity, safer correction of deformity, the ability to assess

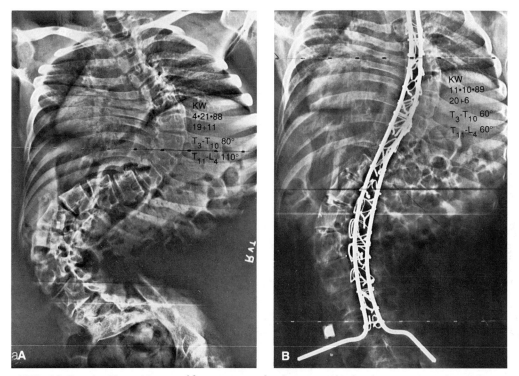

FIG. 12–9. **A.** 19 + 11-year-old spastic, quadriplegic, cerebral palsy patient with a pelvic obliquity, thoracic scoliosis of 80°, and lumbar scoliosis of 110°. **B.** Postoperative correction of pelvic obliquity and residual balanced thoracic and lumbar curves obtained with a first-stage anterior release followed by Luque rods to the pelvis.

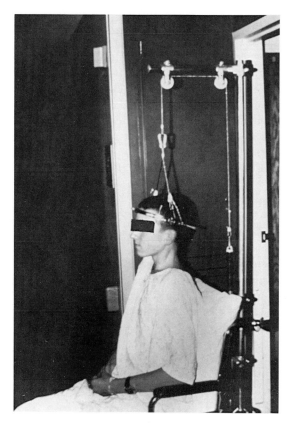

FIG. 12–10. Halo gravity traction.

whether surgery will improve cor pulmonale or the patient will tolerate reconstructive spinal surgery, and ease in managing the patient between first-stage anterior and second-stage posterior spinal surgery.[101, 151]

Complications of traction are frequently seen, and in some cases they can be severe. They include pain and weakness of neck muscles, avascular necrosis of the dens, cranial nerve damage, paraplegia, and pin tract infections.

O'Brien stated that cranial pelvic or cranial femoral traction was especially useful for correcting pelvic obliquity, and Leong, despite a rather high rate of complications, believed that traction played a role in the management of neuromuscular curves of greater than 80°.[99]

After reviewing patients treated with circumferential spinal instrumentation and fusion for spinal deformities and pelvic obliquity secondary to polio, Mayer felt that Dwyer instrumentation provided most of the correction for both the spinal deformity and pelvic obliquity and that 2 weeks of halo-femoral traction did not achieve significantly greater curve correction.[109] In

a study of patients with cerebral palsy treated with a two-stage procedure for scoliosis, Lonstein stated that traction was not useful for curve correction but was of great use in controlling the uncooperative patient and facilitating nursing care.[101]

Currently it seems that cranial-gravity or cranial-femoral traction is most useful for patients with cor pulmonale to discern the possibility of partial reduction before spinal instrumentation and to control the uncooperative, retarded patient between anterior and posterior spinal surgeries.[151] The patient's neurologic status must be monitored closely, watching for cranial nerve damage, and traction should not be used for longer than 2 to 3 weeks.

UNCONTROLLED SPINAL DEFORMITIES IN THE CHILD

A child with a rapidly progressive spinal deformity that remains uncontrolled despite orthotic management presents a challenge. In 1984, Moe suggested the use of a subcutaneous Harrington rod without spinal fusion and with a postoperative Milwaukee brace as an alternative to definitive spinal instrumentation and fusion.[118] Moe suggested elongation of the instrumentation every 6 months until full growth potential was attained; at that time, definitive fusion would be performed. In the same year, Winter reported the use of this technique in 30 children.[168] Fourteen of Winter's patients had paralytic neuromuscular scoliosis. The complication rate in the paralytic patients was 78%, with 11 hook dislocations, 2 rod fractures, 5 severe infections, 8 bone erosions of sacral hooks, and 2 progressive kyphoses. Winter's conclusion was that spinal instrumentation without fusion in neuromuscular conditions has a high complication rate and that expectations for growth may not be met.

Work done in dogs supported the theoretical benefit of using Luque rods with sublaminar wires and without fusion for correcting a spinal deformity and allowing continued spinal growth.[111] In 1985, Rinsky reported the results of the use of Luque rods without arthrodesis in 9 children with neuromuscular scoliosis.[136] Postoperative spinal orthotics were not used in this group of patients. Follow-up averaged 28 months. Only 4 of 11 patients maintained their original corrections, with a mean loss of correction of 32%. All patients demonstrated some continued spinal growth, but the growth was only 38% of the predicted normal value. Much of the growth was stunted from the procedure or lost in the increase of the curvature. Significant technical difficulties were encountered in converting the cases to a fusion. The authors abandoned the procedure.

In 1988, Eberle reported the results of using segmental spinal instrumentation without arthrodesis in 16 patients with spinal deformity secondary to poliomyelitis.[54] In 15 patients, the implant system failed to control the deformity. Rod fracture occurred in 6 patients, longitudinal rod shift allowed recurrence of deformity in 5 patients, and rod rotation caused skin perforation and infection in 4 patients, necessitating rod removal. Eberle's conclusion was that segmental instrumentation of the spine without arthrodesis does not effectively control paralytic scoliosis in a growing child.

Currently, we recommend definitive spinal instrumentation and fusion on any child over the age of 8 with a progressive, rigid scoliosis greater than 60°. If the child is less than 8, a trial of subcutaneous Moe rod instrumentation without fusion is implemented for curves greater than 50 to 60°, and every 6 months further corrective force is applied. If this system fails, definitive spinal instrumentation and fusion are performed.

Postoperative Considerations

The postoperative care can be complicated for patients who are weak with respiratory and cardiac impairment, who have undergone a major surgical assault, and who may be unable or unwilling to cooperate with their postoperative recovery.

The postoperative pulmonary problems in these patients may be critical, and the assistance of a pulmonologist is invaluable. Postoperative ventilatory support may be warranted. The use of Triflows in cooperative patients and Med-neb or IPPB in uncooperative patients helps prevent atelectasis. Perhaps the best measure taken to prevent postoperative pulmonary problems is an intraoperative spinal construct that allows early mobilization of the patient after surgery without an external orthosis.

Fluid balance requires careful monitoring postoperatively to prevent congestive heart failure and pulmonary edema. After prolonged spinal surgery, especially when hypotensive anesthesia has been used, antidiuretic hormone levels may be quite high for 24 to 48 hours, with oliguria resulting.[10] Pushing fluids to overcome the oliguria will lead to fluid overload and should be avoided.

The nutritional status of these patients should be closely monitored in the first 2 weeks postoperatively. If there is inadequate nutritional intake to meet the perioperative metabolic demands, supplemental enteral or parenteral nutrition should be implemented.

Every effort should be made to mobilize the patient as soon as possible after surgery. Early mobilization to the upright posture optimizes the patient's pulmonary status, minimizes further muscle weakness, and decreases the chance of further osteopenia.[154]

Postoperative orthotic management has been in most cases obviated by the advent of circumferential spinal surgery in neuromuscular scoliosis, especially if segmental spinal instrumentation has been used. However, if bone is extremely osteoporotic or if the patient is unusually large, spastic, or dyskinetic so that the spine and spinal instrumentation are excessively stressed, postoperative orthotic management is still warranted.

CEREBRAL PALSY

Incidence and Natural History

Cerebral palsy is a static encephalopathy caused by a nonprogressive brain dysfunction arising from prenatal, perinatal, or postnatal causes. It is characterized by problems of muscle tone and muscle control, mental retardation, and seizure disorders. The prevalence of cerebral palsy is between 1 and 5 children per 1000 live births. Although the field of neonatology has markedly improved the care of premature or seriously ill newborn children, the incidence of cerebral palsy has changed very little.[134]

Cerebral palsy can be classified by motor or geographic categories. Motor classifications include "spastic" (children with increased tone), "hypotonic" (those with decreased tone), and those with "motion disorders," including athetosis and ataxia. Geographic classification includes hemiplegia (one-sided involvement), diplegia (legs that are affected more than hands), quadriplegia (all four extremities involved but fair cognitive function), and total body involvement (profound four-extremity motor involvement and cognitive functional impairment).

The overall incidence of scolosis in patients with cerebral palsy is substantially higher than in the general population. Shands, in a review of 50,000 chest x-ray films of otherwise normal individuals, identified an incidence of scoliosis of 1.9%. Of these, 0.2% had curves greater than 35°.[142] Balmer and MacEwen, in a review of 100 patients with cerebral palsy from the outpatient clinics at the Alfred I. duPont Institute, found that 21% of patients had curves greater than 10° and 6% had curves in excess of 30°.[9]

The severity of scoliosis is adversely influenced by the degree of neurologic impairment. Rosenthal, in a review of 50 ambulatory children with cerebral palsy, found a 38% (19 of 50) incidence of scoliosis, but only 2% had curves greater than 40°.[138] Madigan, in a review of 272 institutionalized patients with cerebral palsy, identified a 76% incidence of scoliosis curves greater than 10° in bedridden patients.[105]

Scoliosis continues to progress after skeletal maturity in patients with cerebral palsy. In a review of 180 institutionalized adult patients with cerebral palsy followed for at least 4 years, Thomez documented progression of curves, sometimes extreme, into the third decade of life.[155] The greatest progression was seen in spastic, quadriplegic patients who were unable to walk and who had thoracolumbar or lumbar curves. Curve progression averaged 0.8° per year for curves less than 50° and 1.4° per year for curves greater than 50°.

Curve progression in patients with cerebral palsy can cause significant functional impairment.[2] It can decrease walking ability, necessitate the use of upper extremities to support the trunk in the upright, sitting posture, and lead to severe discomfort and limited sitting tolerance from a rib-pelvis impingement or pressure sores from a pelvic obliquity.[15, 139]

Two basic scoliotic deformities have been identified in patients with cerebral palsy: Group 1 curves with a thoracic and lumbar component (Fig. 12-11) and Group 2 curves with a large lumbar or thoracolumbar curve and marked pelvic obliquity (Fig. 12-12).[101] Sagittal-plane deformities are also seen. Postural kyphotic deformity is identified in the patient with poor trunk control and hypotonicity, and a long, rigid thoracolumbar kyphosis is identified in the child with tight hamstrings, weak trunk extensors, and tight abdominal muscles. The most complex deformity is a kyphotic deformity caused by spinal rotation—the Stagnara rotational kyphosis.[148]

Treatment

There is great controversy about the fundamental issue of treating the deformity of the patient with cerebral palsy. What to do with the child with spastic, total body

involvement who has major nutritional problems, a severe seizure disorder, no head or trunk control, and minimal cognitive function is a difficult question. The functional gains in treating a scoliosis in such a patient would be difficult to gauge. Fortunately, the number of patients with this severe involvement is limited. The largest group of patients with cerebral palsy do have some cognitive or functional capabilities that should be preserved, and if progression of a spinal deformity compromises these capabilities, causes pain, or increases nursing care of the patient, the deformity should be treated.[2, 15, 101]

Nonoperative Treatment

Observation is warranted in two groups of patients: those with curves less than 20° and those with large, rigid curves that are not causing pain or functional disability.

Most nonambulatory patients with cerebral palsy lack head and neck control during the first decade of life. This results in a buckling paralytic kyphosis or kyphoscoliosis when the patient is in the upright posture. Custom or modular seating systems may be quite effective in providing these patients with a straight spine and level pelvis, reducing the strength of spastic reflexes and controlling pressure distribution. Custom seating systems have also been effective in accommodating severe spinal deformities and allowing these patients to be positioned in an upright posture.

Spinal orthotics have been used in cerebral palsy. The Milwaukee brace has been tried and found impractical. Balmer and MacEwen reported that the Milwaukee brace failed in these patients because of their inability or unwillingness to cooperate with the required exercise program or because of skin intolerance, especially in patients with dyskinetic movements.[9] Bunnell and MacEwen, in a short-term study of 48 patients, demonstrated curve control in 35 patients treated with a removable plastic jacket.[26] The patient with a progressive curve between 25 and 45° who is still growing should try a thoracolumbosacral orthosis. A spinal orthosis can slow curve progression and allow definitive surgical correction when the child is older, larger, and near the end of spinal growth. In those with flexible curves, the orthosis improves spinal alignment, increases trunk height, and makes sitting better without elaborate seating systems.

Surgical Treatment

Surgery has been used in the treatment of spinal deformity in cerebral palsy. Surgical indications include

(text continues on page 300)

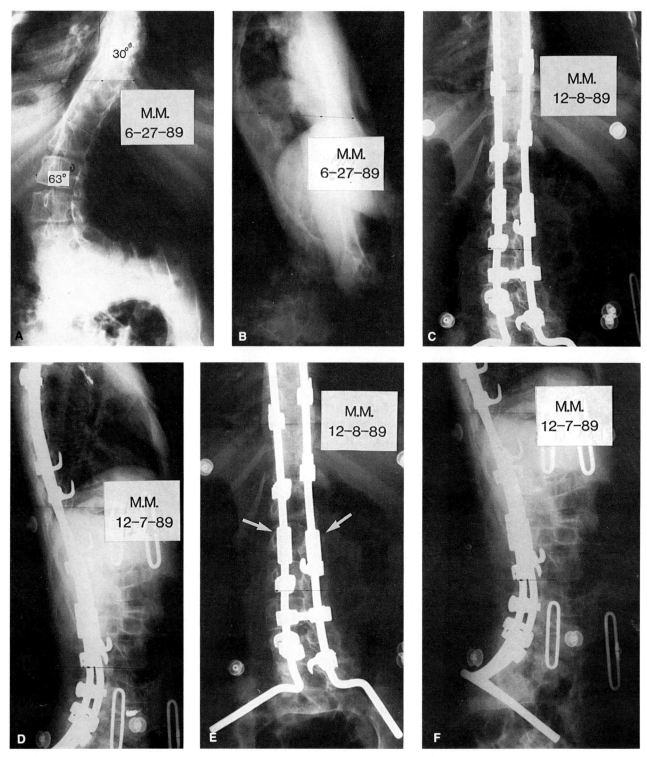

FIG. 12–11. A 13-year-old girl with cerebral palsy with a progressive scoliosis and painful dislocated left hip. **A, B.** posterior-anterior and lateral spine radiographs showing deformity and pelvic obliquity. **C, D.** Postoperative sitting posterior-anterior and lateral spine radiographs showing excellent correction alignment. **E, F.** Fixation into pelvis using the Galveston method and four-rod Cotrel–Dubousset construct, in this case joining the two rods on each side with axial connectors (*white arrows*). The construct was then coupled with TSRH Crosslinks™

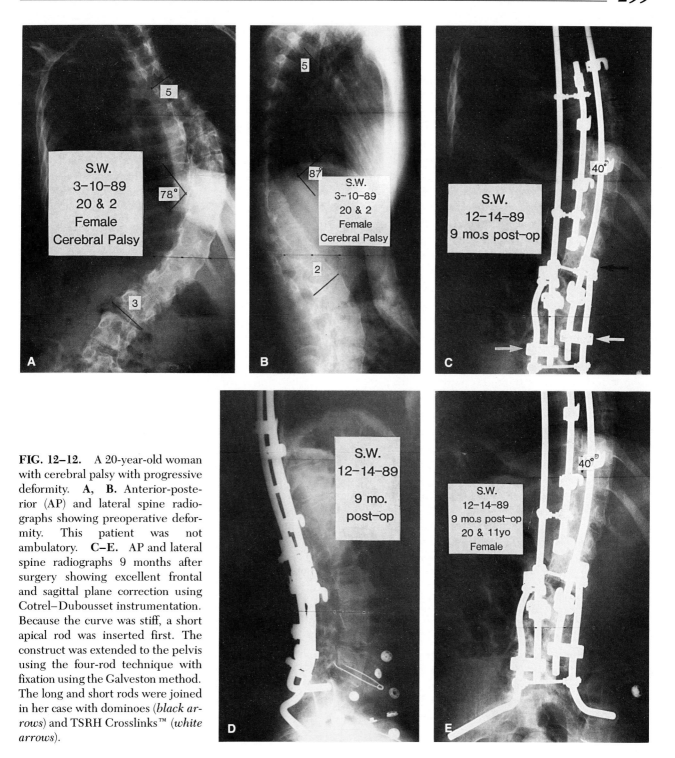

FIG. 12–12. A 20-year-old woman with cerebral palsy with progressive deformity. **A, B.** Anterior-posterior (AP) and lateral spine radiographs showing preoperative deformity. This patient was not ambulatory. **C–E.** AP and lateral spine radiographs 9 months after surgery showing excellent frontal and sagittal plane correction using Cotrel–Dubousset instrumentation. Because the curve was stiff, a short apical rod was inserted first. The construct was extended to the pelvis using the four-rod technique with fixation using the Galveston method. The long and short rods were joined in her case with dominoes (*black arrows*) and TSRH Crosslinks™ (*white arrows*).

curve progression in excess of 40°, curves that cause loss of function, and curves that cause pain. The surgical treatment of scoliosis in patients with cerebral palsy has paralleled the advancement and improvements in techniques in spinal surgery in general. MacEwen, in 1972, reported 15 patients treated with a posterior Harrington rod, and although initial correction averaged 50%, there was a 20% pseudarthrosis rate and a 6% incidence of failure of instrumentation.[104] Bonnet, in 1976, in a similar series of 10 patients treated with a posterior Harrington rod, demonstrated curve correction averaging 30%, a pseudarthrosis rate of 40%, and a 30% rate of failure of instrumentation.[15] To improve curve correction, Bonnet and associates treated a group of these patients with a single-stage anterior discectomy, interbody fusion, and instrumentation using a Dwyer apparatus. In this series, curve correction was increased to 48%, but there was a 72% incidence of pseudarthrosis, a 17% incidence of failure of instrumentation, and a 6% incidence of infection. To maintain the correction obtained with the anterior procedure by limiting the incidence of pseudarthrosis, Bonnet and associates treated 5 patients with a first-stage anterior discectomy, fusion, and instrumentation using a Dwyer apparatus, followed by posterior instrumentation and fusion using the Harrington rod. In this series, the curve correction was 62%, no pseudarthroses, and no instrumentation failures. In 1982, Brown reported results of 17 patients managed with a first-stage anterior instrumentation and fusion using a Dwyer apparatus, followed by a second-stage posterior Harrington rod to the sacrum.[17] Curve correction was 60%, and correction of pelvic obliquity was 75%. However, instrumentation problems still occurred in 35% of the patients.

As the ability to obtain and maintain curve correction was achieved and the ability to control pelvic obliquity accomplished, the remaining problems of maintenance of sagittal-plane alignment and the possibility of eliminating postoperative orthotic support was addressed. During the 1970s, Dr. Eduardo Luque and colleagues developed a segmental spinal instrumentation system that coupled the spine at each lamina to a contoured rod.[103] This system provided a means of increased stability of the corrected spine and a way to stabilize the spine to the pelvis, further correcting pelvic obliquity. Because of the increased stability of this spinal construct, it was felt that postoperative orthotic management could be avoided.

Gersoff reported a series of 33 patients with curves less than 110° treated with a single-stage posterior spinal fusion using Luque instrumentation.[65] Curve correction was 52%, there were no pseudarthroses, and the two instrumentation failures were caused by the use of 3/16-in rods rather than 1/4-in rods. Swank and associates reported on 10 patients treated with the single-stage posterior technique using 3/16-in dual-contoured Luque rods.[153] This series showed a postoperative curve correction of 53% and 52% correction of pelvic obliquity. There was, however, a 40% pseudarthrosis rate, a 10% rate of instrumentation failure, and a loss of greater than 10° of correction in 6 of 10 patients. In the same study, Swank and associates also reported 21 patients treated with a first-stage anterior spinal instrumentation and fusion using a Zielke apparatus, followed by a posterior Luque procedure to the pelvis. The postoperative curve correction was 63%, correction of pelvic obliquity 54%, there was only a 9.5% incidence of pseudarthroses, and there were no failures of instrumentation. The authors thought that a failure to extend the fusion to the sacrum caused a much greater postoperative loss of sitting balance and an increase in torso decompensation.

Allen and associates have questioned the need for anterior instrumentation.[2] They believe that the instrumentation decreases the overall correction and prefer instead to do an anterior release and fusion followed by a second-stage Luque procedure to the pelvis.

A few technical points are important for using Luque instrumentation. The instrumentation should extend above the apex of any thoracic kyphosis, and probably should end no lower than T2 in most instances. This is particularly important in preventing "fall off" over the end of the rods, with the creation of a high thoracic kyphosis. Extending to T1 or T2 has no functional disadvantages for the patient. To make the exposure and the instrumentation easier, the use of skull tongs to position the head and neck during surgery is helpful. The tongs are connected to a head-holding clamp or to the ether screen with the patient's neck slightly extended to avoid stretch of the spinal cord. Longitudinal traction on the spine is not needed. An effort should be made to remove only a small portion of the ligamentum flavum on either side of the superior interspinous space to be instrumented. Also, the supraspinous and intraspinous ligaments should be preserved as much as possible. An alternative or additional maneuver is to wire the last instrumented spinous process to the one above to close the intraspinous space and to add bone graft to that level as well. The rods should be joined to prevent shifting. This is most likely to occur in a situation with a large preoperative curve with a significant pelvic obliquity. Joining the rods with a Texas Scottish Rite Crosslink™ System (Danek, Memphis, TN) is very helpful in accomplishing this.

During the last 2 years, one of us (J.P.L.) has gained increasing experience with the use of Cotrel–Dubousset instrumentation (Stuart, Greensburg, PA) in paralytic scoliosis. This system offers the advantage of being able to use distraction and compression along the rods in addition to bending and rotation forces to obtain correction. The principles remain the same: If the curve is large and stiff before surgery, anterior release by discectomy and anterior bone grafting are done first. Pelvic fixation has been accomplished by using the Galveston technique, using either one or two rods on each side to accomplish it. When the curve is very flexible, one long rod on each side can be used. However, in larger curves that are not readily correctable, a shorter rod is contoured in the Galveston configuration and inserted into the pelvis. The second rod is contoured to the scoliosis and kyphosis of the thoracolumbar spine. Hooks are placed in the appropriate configurations, and the rods are inserted into them. Correction can be obtained with the derotation maneuver or with simple distraction force or compression along the rod. The two rods are then joined with axial connectors or dominoes (Figs. 12-11 and 12-12). Two more rods are then inserted in the other side in a similar fashion. The construct is completed by using a Texas Scottish Rite Crosslink™ System or the Cotrel–Dubousset DTTs. Sublaminar wires have also been used to supplement hook fixation.

The versatility of the Cotrel–Dubousset system has made it well-suited to treating these patients. Although sacral fixation by pedicle screws is possible, it has been shown to be problematic in osteopenic small patients,[29a] and for this reason, the Galveston technique has been used. The same cautions about the Luque instrumentation regarding the superior extent of the instrumentation apply to the Cotrel–Dubousset instrumentation as well. However, hooks over the superior end vertebrae suffice to prevent fall-off. Special cervical hooks placed in the canal over the top of the most superior lamina are very helpful.

Authors' Preferred Treatment

Children with cerebral palsy are managed expectantly. If, when young, they have poor trunk and head control and collapse into a postural kyphosis or kyphoscoliosis while in the upright posture, they are treated with a seating system. When curves become structural, are in excess of 20 to 25°, and interfere with proper sitting, the patients are fitted with plastic removable thoracolumbosacral orthosis. Curves that progress to 45 or 50° are treated surgically. If on preoperative bending films the spine can be balanced and the curve is corrected to less than 30°, a posterior segmental instrumentation system is used. If the patient is ambulatory, an effort should be made to end the instrumentation above the pelvis. This decreases the problems associated with fusion across the lumbosacral junction and also interferes less with walking ability. However, preoperative evaluation with bending films should show that adequate correction, balance, and improvement in pelvic obliquity will occur without extension of the instrumentation to the pelvis. It is especially important in this group to recreate the normal sagittal contour (Fig. 12-13). In patients whose curves are not correctable on bend films to less than 30°, an anterior release and fusion is followed by posterior segmental instrumentation and fusion.

In patients with a pelvic obliquity or lack of sitting ability, the posterior instrumentation and fusion are carried to the pelvis. If the pelvic obliquity is correctable on preoperative bend films, a single-stage posterior segmental fixation and fusion is all that is required (Fig. 12-14). If the pelvic obliquity is not correctable on preoperative bend films, a first-stage anterior release and fusion are required, followed by a second-stage posterior segmental instrumentation and fusion. Anterior instrumentation with the Dwyer or Zielke apparatus is considered only as the first of two stages and only when there is a major rigid pelvic obliquity or a curve in excess of 75° that is rigid. All patients are maintained in postoperative removable thoracolumbosacral orthoses until x-ray films reveal a solid fusion.

FRIEDREICH'S ATAXIA

Friedreich's ataxia is a spinal cerebellar degenerative disorder. It is an autosomal recessive genetic disease, and although there are autosomal dominant varieties, they are one-tenth as common as the recessive type.[143] Clinical onset occurs between the age of 6 and 20. According to the criteria of Geoffrey, primary symptoms and signs include an onset before the age of 20, progressive ataxic gait, dysarthria, decreased proprioception or vibratory sense, muscle weakness, and a lack of deep tendon reflexes. Secondary symptoms and

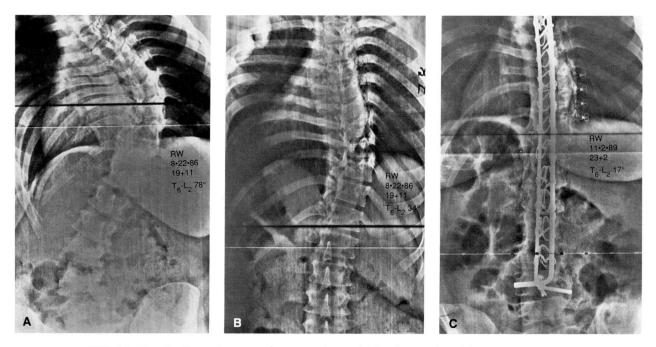

FIG. 12–13. **A.** Group I curve: a thoracic scoliosis of 78° without pelvic obliquity. **B.** Curve is supple and reduces to 34° as shown on a recumbent x-ray film. **C.** Curve reduced to 17° by circumferential fusion and posterior instrumentation to L4.

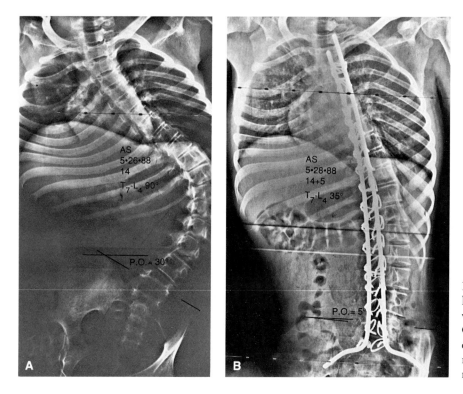

FIG. 12–14. **A.** Group II curve: large thoracolumbar curves of 90° with a 30° pelvic obliquity. **B.** Curve reduced to 35° and pelvic obliquity to 5° by posterior instrumentation and fusion with Luque rod instrumentation to the pelvis.

signs are pes cavus, scoliosis, a Babinski sign, and cardiomyopathy.[64] Affected individuals frequently become wheelchair bound in the second and third decades of life. Affected individuals develop a progressive cardiomyopathy and usually die in the third or fourth decade of life. The average age at death is 36 years.[79]

Scoliosis occurs in 75 to 100% of these patients. The scoliosis is generally not the classic neuromuscular variety. In Daher's series of 19 patients, there were no long C-shaped curves with pelvic obliquity. In Cady's study of 42 patients, only 3 (7%) were C-shaped curves with pelvic obliquity, and in Labelle's series of 56 patients, only 8 (14%) had a typical neuromuscular curve.[28, 38, 95] Like Charcot-Marie-Tooth disease, with which it is frequently confused, kyphosis frequently accompanies the scoliosis, with 8 (42%) of 19 patients in Daher's series and 66% of the patients in Labelle's series having hyperkyphosis.[38, 95]

Scoliosis can be progressive in Friedreich's ataxia, but not inevitably so. In Labelle's study of 36 patients followed for at least 10 years, there were 20 patients whose curves were greater than 60° and progressed and 16 whose curves were 40° or less and did not progress.[95] There was a statistically significant difference between patients whose scoliosis progressed and those that did not, with children whose disease started before the age of 10 and in whom scoliosis was detected before the age of 15 having the greatest likelihood of progression. Based on this, Labelle recommended observation for curves less than 40°, surgery for those greater than 60°, and treatment for curves between 40 and 60° based on the patient's age, the age at which scoliosis was first detected, and evidence of progression of the curve.

Treatment

Orthotics tried in the management of scoliosis for patients with Friedreich's ataxia have generally failed. Hensinger reported on a single patient tried in a Milwaukee brace for whom orthotic management was abandoned because of a loss of walking balance.[76] Daher reported on 6 patients who tried an orthosis; 3 of these patients went on to surgery, 1 was still under treatment, and 2 patients who were started on orthotic management and close to skeletal maturity were felt to be inappropriate choices for orthotic management.[38] Cady and Bobechko managed 5 patients with spinal orthosis for 2 years, during which the average degree of progression was 10.9° per year.[28] Orthotic management seems impractical for two reasons: An orthosis simply fails to control the curve, and by the time patients develop scoliosis, they have a significant degree of ataxia and a very precarious gait, and the restriction a spinal orthosis imposes on them may further compromise their ambulation.

Surgery has been implemented in the treatment of spinal deformity in patients with Friedreich's ataxia. Hensinger reported on 2 patients managed with posterior instrumentation and spinal fusion using Harrington rods.[76] Curve correction averaged 33%. Recommendations were for rapid postoperative mobilization in a cast. Cady reported on 11 patients treated surgically with posterior instrumentation and spinal fusion using Harrington rods; curve correction averaged 41%.[28] There was one early postoperative death from cardiac causes. Daher reported on 12 patients treated surgically with posterior instrumentation and spinal fusion using a Harrington rod in 10 patients and Luque rods in 2 patients.[38] Two patients lost general function because of prolonged postoperative recumbency or the weight of the postoperative cast, 1 patient had cardiac failure due to cardiomyopathy, and 1 patient's thoracic kyphosis progressed because of a fusion that was too short. Recommendations were for fusion levels from T2 to L3 or L4, and extension to the cervical spine or pelvis was not considered necessary.

Authors' Preferred Treatment

We are in general agreement with the recommendations of Labelle.[95] Patients with Friedreich's ataxia should be managed expectantly. If a curve develops before the adolescent growth spurt, it will probably progress. When the curve gets to 40°, it should be treated surgically. Patients with curves greater than 60° at presentation should be considered for surgical care. Before surgery, a detailed cardiac evaluation is mandatory, and surgery should be avoided for patients with significant cardiomyopathy. Patients with curves between 40 and 60° at presentation should be assessed for age and evidence of progression. Young adolescents and those with documented evidence of progression should have surgery. Adults or younger patients without evidence of progression should be examined at 6-month intervals. Documented progression mandates surgery. The surgery of choice is a long posterior instrumentation using a rigid segmental fixation (1/4-in Luque rods with sublaminar wires or the Cotrel–Dubousset system), taking care to preserve sagittal contours. The posterior fusion should be from T2 to L3 or L4. There is no need to go to the pelvis unless a pelvic obliquity exists, which is unusual for this class of patients. Careful perioperative monitoring of cardiac function is mandatory. An early postoperative return to preoperative levels of mobility should be the goal.

CHARCOT-MARIE-TOOTH DISEASE

Charcot-Marie-Tooth disease is a genetically determined demyelinating neuropathy. The disease is autosomal dominant, with considerable variation in its severity. Patients are areflexic and have symmetric distal muscle weakness that is usually worse in the lower extremities. Nerve conduction velocities are quite slow, and nerve biopsy specimens show demyelination and increased fibrosis.[143]

Scoliosis occurs in approximately 10% of patients with Charcot-Marie-Tooth disease.[76] The curves are not the classic neuromuscular variety in that they rarely include the sacrum, and the incidence of pelvic obliquity does not increase with the curve. Kyphosis frequently accompanies the scoliosis. In Hensinger's series, 3 (43%) of 7 patients had kyphosis, and in Daher's series, 6 (50%) of 12 patients had kyphosis.[40, 76]

Treatment

Observation is warranted in patients with Charcot-Marie-Tooth disease who have curves less than 20°. In Hensinger's series, 2 of 7 patients with scoliosis had mild to moderate degrees of curvature and did not require treatment. In Daher's series, 2 of 5 patients with scoliosis had small curves (less than 15°) and were under observation; 1 patient had a thoracic curve (38°) and lumbar curve (45°) that did not progress; and 2 patients had curves that averaged 31° of progression and required surgical intervention.[40, 76]

Orthotics have successfully been used in the management of scoliosis in these patients. In Hensinger's series, 2 of 4 patients managed with a Milwaukee brace curves were controlled.[76] In Daher's series, 3 patients were managed with a spinal orthosis.[39] In 1 patient treated with a Milwaukee brace, the curve was successfully controlled; 1 patient was still under observation; and in 1 patient, the curve progressed and required surgical intervention.

Surgical treatment is occasionally necessary. In Hensinger's series, 3 of 7 patients with scoliosis required surgery.[76] In each of these patients, posterior fusion was from the upper thoracic spine to the upper or mid-lumbar spine, and Harrington instrumentation was used in 2 of 3 patients. In Daher's series, 5 patients were managed with surgery. There were 2 pseudarthroses.[40] The only patient treated with fusion to the sacrum developed a pseudarthrosis, and in review, this patient did not need the fusion to the sacrum.

Spinal deformities in patients with Charcot-Marie-Tooth disease can be managed with the same techniques used for idiopathic scoliosis. The sagittal-plane deformity accompanying the scoliosis is most frequently a kyphosis. The fusion need not be taken to the pelvis unless a pelvic obliquity exists (Fig. 12-15).

SYRINGOMYELIA

Syringomyelia is a chronic, slowly progressive degeneration of the spinal cord and medulla.[84] There is spinal cord cavitation and gliosis. The spectrum of presenting complaints in patients with syringomyelia includes several orthopedic features:[162]

1. Pain affecting the head, neck, trunk, or limbs
2. Bony deformities with scoliosis, deformity of the hands and feet, and Charcot changes of joints
3. Muscle wasting and fasciculations
4. Sympathetic disturbances, including Horner's syndrome, sweating disorders, and temperature changes

Scoliosis is a common feature in patients with syringomyelia. MacIlroy and Richardson found scoliosis in 33 (44%) of 75 cases of syringomyelia.[113] McRae and Standen identified 17 (85%) of their 20 cases as having scoliosis associated with syringomyelia.[114] Huebert identified scoliosis in 27 (63%) of 43 patients.[84] Williams identified scoliosis in 108 (73%) of 148 of their patients with syringomyelia.[162]

Scoliosis may be the presenting complaint in patients with syringomyelia.[8] The diagnosis of syringomyelia in patients presenting with scoliosis depends on an accurate history, probing for symptoms of pain and physical findings suggesting a neurologic disorder, such as deformities of the hands with intrinsic muscle wasting, dissociated disturbance of pain and temperature, loss of superficial abdominal reflexes, cavus deformities of the feet, and possible Charcot changes in joints, and associated x-ray film findings, such as bony anomalies of the cervical spine, including basilar impression, cervical vertebral synostoses, cer-

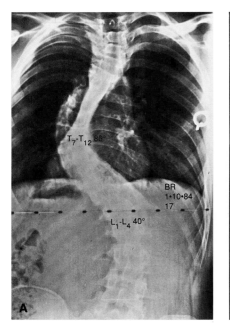
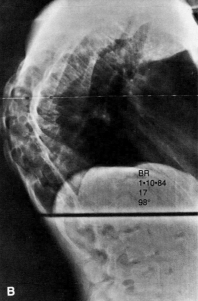
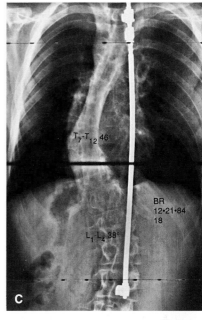

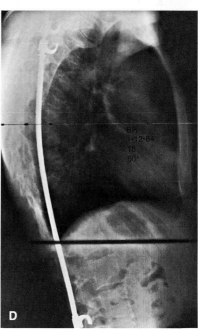

FIG. 12–15. **A.** A 17-year-old patient with Charcot-Marie-Tooth disease and a preoperative T7–T12 curve of 86°. **B.** Thoracic kyphosis is 98°. **C.** Scoliosis reduced to 46° with single-stage procedure using Harrington rod intrathoracic and extrapleural placement. **D.** Kyphosis reduced to 50° after surgery. (Courtesy of Dr. Kenneth Roth)

vical-thoracic spina bifida, and enlargement of the cervical spinal canal.[114, 132, 162]

As the cystic cavitation in syringomyelia enlarges, pressure erosion of the cervical vertebrae occurs. This is seen radiographically as erosion of the bodies of the cervical vertebrae and widening of the canal. If the size of the canal at C5 exceeds that of the vertebral body by 6 mm in the adult, pathologic dilation is confirmed.[162]

Scoliosis in patients with syringomyelia may have some unusual features. The scoliosis may be of the high left thoracic variety, a high double curve, or a painful curve.[34] In the growing child or adolescent, the curves tend to progress rapidly, even if a spinal orthosis is used.[124]

If a syrinx is suspected, cord imaging is warranted. In the past, metrizamide myelography with CT scanning was used, but MRI is currently recommended for cord imaging in syringomyelia.[98]

A symptomatic syrinx should be surgically drained; this may improve neurologic defects. In Gurr's series of 15 patients treated with surgical drainage of a syrinx, 3 patients had an improvement in their curves, and in none of the remaining patients did curves progress after syrinx drainage.[70]

Surgical correction of spine deformities in patients with syringomyelia carries significant risks. Huebert reported a case of postfusion paraplegia in a patient with syringomyelia treated without spinal instrumentation.[84] Nordwall reported a case of delayed paraparesis 16 days after Harrington instrumentation.[124] With these in mind, surgery for the scoliosis in syringomyelia should be approached with caution, and only moderate curve correction should be obtained. The surgical treatment should always be preceded by syrinx drainage if the spine is to be lengthened.

SPINAL DEFORMITIES SECONDARY TO SPINAL CORD INJURY

Loss of spinal cord function is a devastating event leaving the individual with an inability to ambulate, lack of sensation in the lower extremities with a propensity toward developing pressure sores, loss of ability to control bowel and bladder function with a high probability of developing urinary tract infections, disuse osteopenia leading to hypercalcemia, kidney stones, and potential pathologic fractures in the lower extremities. Spinal cord injury can result from fractures and/or dislocations, penetrating injury, or injury to the neural structure without radiographic of bony injury.[169] Spinal cord injury in the skeletally immature patient is almost certain to lead to a paralytic spine deformity.[125] The paralytic spine deformity can lead to a pelvic obliquity, hip subluxation, loss of sitting balance, and pressure sores.

Campbell, in a study of preadolescent children who sustained spinal cord injury, documented a 91% incidence of spinal deformity after injury.[30] Kilfoyle documented a 93% incidence of spinal deformity in children who had spinal cord dysfunction.[91] Lancourt, in a review of 50 patients, newborn to 17 years of age at the time of spinal cord injury, documented an incidence of scoliosis in 100% of the children injured before the age of 10, a 19% incidence of scoliosis in children injured between 10 and 16 years of age, and a 12% incidence of scoliosis in patients aged 17 or older.[96] The age at injury was the single most important influence affecting the

development of scoliosis. Patients with neural lesions at any level of the spinal cord were at risk for development of scoliosis, and spasticity was a significant factor in the development of a spinal deformity.

Paralytic spinal deformity in these patients led to pelvic obliquity, and a study of the 10 patients who developed pressure sores revealed a scoliosis in excess of 20° in 90%. One patient, who did not have a scoliosis but who developed a pressure sore, had a large trunk shift. There were no pressure sores seen in the 8 patients who did not develop a scoliosis. Mayfield and Winter, in a review of spinal deformities caused by childhood spinal cord injury, documented a 96% incidence of spinal deformity in children injured before their adolescent growth spurt.[110] Scoliosis was seen in 23 of the 25 patients, kyphosis in 16 of the 25 patients, and lordoscoliosis in 5 of the 25 patients. In individuals injured after the adolescent growth spurt, the incidence of spine deformities was much less. Nine (60%) of 15 patients developed a kyphosis after fracture. In 47% of the injured patients, the kyphosis was progressive.

Laminectomy, when used to treat the initial spinal cord injury, was associated with an increased incidence of kyphosis and an increased severity of that kyphosis. Brown, in a review of 64 quadriplegic adolescents and children, identified a spinal deformity in 47 of the 64.[19] All children 13 years and younger at the time of spinal cord injury developed spinal deformities. The incidence of spinal deformity after spinal cord injury was 78% in 14-year-olds, 57% in 15-year-olds, and 50% in 16-year-olds. Progressive spinal deformities led to pelvic obliquity, pressure sores, and loss of sitting balance.

Treatment

Spinal orthotics have been used to treat spinal deformity after spinal cord injury. Campbell recommended external support of the spine before radiologically documented development of a fixed spinal deformity.[30] In addition to preventing or improving the degree of spinal deformity, the orthotic frequently improves function by restoring sitting balance and freeing the upper extremities.

Campbell defined the optimal characteristics of a spinal orthotic. It should be well padded to protect anesthetic skin, removable to permit frequent skin checks, easily adjusted to allow for growth, easily cleaned for adapting to incontinence, and nonrestrictive to allow chest expansion.[30]

Lancourt did not feel that bracing altered the progression of scoliosis in these patients, and Mayfield believed that orthotic management was difficult.[96, 110] In Mayfield's series, orthoses were ineffective in 5 of 6 patients, but they did serve as holding devices until the age of 10 to 12, the age at which he recommends surgery. Brown documented that early application of a spinal orthotic before the onset of a spinal deformity delayed its presentation.[19] The average time from injury to onset of a 20° scoliosis was 2.3 years in patients without braces and 3.6 years in braced patients. Brown and associates believed that bracing in a body jacket before deformity developed lessened the incidence of a significant deformity, but spinal fusion might still become necessary.

Surgical treatment of a spinal deformity after injury has been recommended. Campbell recommended a long posterior spinal fusion and Harrington rod instrumentation to the sacrum.[30] In his series, curve correction averaged 35%, but pseudarthroses rates were greater than 50% and infection was seen in 12% of patients. Surgery was performed for a spinal kyphosis of greater than 60° when rigid with an anterior spinal fusion followed by compression Harrington rod instrumentation. Lancourt reviewed 10 patients treated with Harrington rod instrumentation, and curve correction averaged 44%.[96] Fifty percent of patients had a significant improvement in their pelvic obliquity. In Mayfield's series, 68% of patients eventually required Harrington rod instrumentation.[110] Postoperative complications were frequent, with a pseudarthrosis rate of 53%. Three of 17 patients developed postoperative infection, 3 of 17 developed decubiti, and 2 patients had hook dislodgment. All patients, however, had improved sitting balance. The pseudarthrosis rate was reduced from 53% to 20% by performing a first-stage anterior spinal release and fusion, followed by a posterior Harrington rod instrumentation for large curves or those with kyphotic deformities.

In Brown's series, 11 of 33 patients required spinal instrumentation and fusion for progressive spinal deformities.[19] Scoliosis correction averaged 47%, kyphosis correction averaged 70%, lordosis correction averaged 64%, and pelvic obliquity correction averaged 37.5%. There was at least one complication in each patient. Complications included pseudarthroses, progressive kyphosis above the fusion when the instrumentation was too short, and a progressive postoperative lordosis in 11 patients.

Authors' Preferred Treatment

Preadolescent children who sustain spinal cord injury should be managed expectantly for the development of a spinal deformity. At the first sign of the development of a spinal deformity, before it becomes rigid and interferes with proper sitting, orthotic management should be implemented. A light weight, total-contact plastic orthosis that fits from the axilla to the pelvis should be used. Although the orthosis will not change the natural history of the curve, it should slow the progression of the spinal deformity. After the age of 10, a scoliosis in excess of 40° or a structural scoliosis in excess of 60° at any age should be treated with a long posterior spinal instrumentation using a segmental fixation system, instrumenting the spine from T2 to the sacrum or pelvis (Fig. 12-16).

Scoliosis that cannot be corrected on bending films to less than 30° should be treated with a first-stage anterior release and spinal fusion, followed by a posterior segmental spinal instrumentation and fusion. A kyphosis that is rigid and cannot be corrected to less than 50° on prone hyperextension should be treated with a first-stage anterior release and spinal fusion, followed by a long posterior spinal instrumentation and fusion. In patients who are ambulators and in whom adequate correction can be obtained without going to the pelvis, an effort should be made to end the instrumentation above the pelvis. This is nicely accomplished with the Cotrel–Dubousset instrumentation (Fig. 12-17). Posterior bone graft should be quite thick, and use of allograft is recommended.

SPINAL MUSCULAR ATROPHY

Spinal muscular atrophy is a genetically determined neuromuscular disorder with degeneration of the anterior horn cells of the spinal cord and, occasionally, the motor neurons of the lower bulbar nuclei. It has been shown to be inherited in an autosomal recessive manner and also occurs sporadically.[11, 131, 140, 164] Werding and Hoffman, at the turn of the century, first described the disease and emphasized its early onset and the early demise of affected children.[82, 159] In 1956, Kugelberg and Welander described the later onset and long-term survival in patients with a similar disease process.[93] In 1974, Dubowitz stated that spinal muscular atrophy was one of the more common neuromuscular disorders and asserted that the various manifestations were one disease process.[49–52] Emery, in 1975, reviewed over 500 patients, substantiating the one-disease hypothesis. He noted that over 80% of patients survived and achieved sitting balance.[55]

Spinal muscular atrophy appears to be one disease

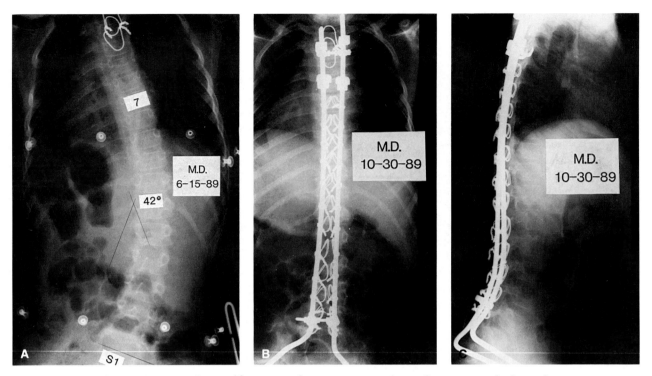

FIG. 12–16. **A.** A 7-year-old patient with a progressive scoliosis after a motor vehicle accident with resultant paraplegia. **B.** Scoliosis treated with pediatric Cotrel–Dubousset instrumentation, sublaminar wires, and Galveston technique of pelvic fixation. **C.** Sagittal contours maintained.

process, varying in onset from prenatal life to adolescence, characterized by an episode of neural destruction of relatively short duration, and followed by the development of progressive spinal and extremity deformities in surviving patients.[68, 121, 135]

In evaluating patients with spinal muscular atrophy, there seem to be three distinct autosomal recessive forms of the disease.[7] They differ in terms of the age at onset and clinical progression. Type I or infantile acute Werdnig-Hoffman disease presents with generalized weakness of the limbs, trunk and bulbar muscles. Its onset is in the first few months of life. The course of the disease is progressive, with early death caused by pulmonary insufficiency. Some children with Type I spinal muscular atrophy may have an acute period of functional deterioration followed by an arrest of the disease process and a relatively benign course.[50, 121, 131] Type II or chronic Werdnig-Hoffman disease has its onset in the first 4 years of life. Most children achieve sitting balance. Type III or Kugelberg-Welander disease begins later, usually between the ages of 2 and 15. It is more slowly progressive, and

most patients are able to ambulate independently.[51] The survival rate in Type III patients is much higher than in either Type I or Type II.

The clinical features of patients with spinal muscular atrophy include axial and proximal muscle weakness. Although most frequently described as symmetric, up to 40% have some degree of asymmetry; fasciculations of the tongue and coarse tremors of the extremities are frequently seen.[140] The patients are areflexic, and no Babinski's signs are found. The patients have normal intelligence.[20, 121] The heart remains unaffected. The cause of death is usually pulmonary insufficiency.[50, 51] Serum enzyme studies reveal normal creatinine phosphokinase levels. Electromyograms show a denervation pattern with spontaneous fibrillation potentials, isolated action potentials of increased amplitude and duration, and normal nerve conduction studies. The muscle biopsy shows a denervation pattern with atrophy of both fiber types I and II with hypertrophy of surviving fibers and evidence of fiber-type grouping.[140] Although the muscle biopsy is characteristic, it has no prognostic value.

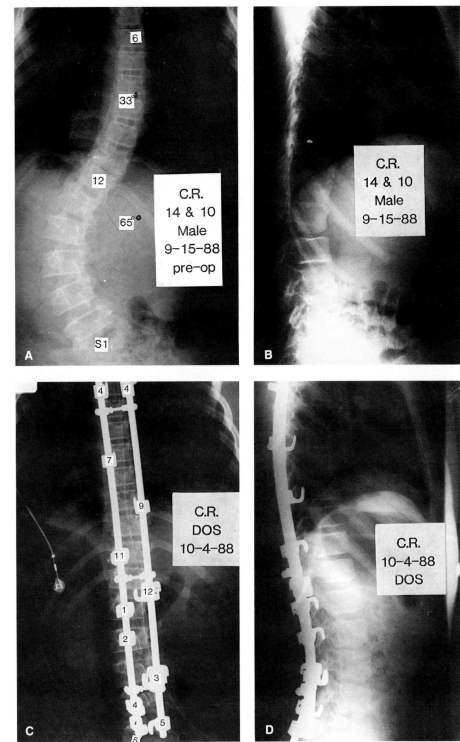

FIG. 12–17. A 14 + 10-year-old boy with a prior spinal cord injury from a gunshot wound at T11. **A, B.** Posterior-anterior and lateral sitting spine radiographs showing preoperative deformity in both planes. The curves were flexible on side bending. **C, D.** Postoperative anterior-posterior and lateral spine radiographs showing excellent correction of scoliosis and pelvic obliquity and normalization of sagittal alignment. This patient was an active user of his RGO and remained so after surgery. The curve and pelvic obliquity were corrected with Cotrel–Dubousset instrumentation without going to the pelvis.

Scolosis is frequently seen in surviving patients with spinal muscular atrophy. Hardy and Curtis, in 1971, in a review of 88 cases, found an 80% incidence of scoliosis in patients over 12 years of age.[75] In 1976, Schwentker and Gibson reviewed 57 patients, 70% of whom had a scoliosis greater than 20°. Benady, in 1978, reviewed 50 patients with spinal muscular atrophy, and scoliosis was a consistent complication of the more severe forms of the disease.[11, 140] In 1981, Evans reviewed 54 patients and found 91% had spinal deformities.[56] One year later, Riddick, in a review of 36 patients with spinal muscular atrophy, found a spinal deformity in 86% of patients.[135] Of the patients with spinal muscular atrophy who develop scoliosis, 68 to 74% develop a lumbar or thoracolumbar scoliosis that includes the sacrum and pelvis. After scoliosis occurs, it is relentlessly progressive (Fig. 12-18).[115]

A progressive scoliosis can cause major functional compromise in patients with spinal muscular atrophy.[7, 56] Ambulatory patients develop a curve that is large enough to unbalance the trunk and compromise their walking capabilities, leading to a wheelchair existence. For the patient in a wheelchair, a collapsing spinal deformity interferes significantly with the ability to sit unsupported. As the trunk collapses, the upper extremities are increasingly needed to support the

trunk in a sitting position, creating a functional quadriplegic. With curve progression the ribs may abut against the pelvis, causing pain, and the chest wall becomes progressively deformed, producing further compromise of the patient's pulmonary status.

Treatment

Spinal orthotics have been used in an attempt to control the relentless progression of scoliosis in patients with spinal muscular atrophy. Hensinger presented 2 patients treated with a Milwaukee brace.[76] In 1 patient, the brace slowed the progression of the curve, but in the second patient, the brace had to be discontinued because of interference with respiratory function and balance. Schwentker evaluated 23 patients who were treated with spinal orthoses.[140] In 18 of the 23 the curves continued to progress, and in 4 patients the follow-up was too short to evaluate the orthotic management. He concluded that orthoses, although seldom successful in preventing or controlling the scoliosis, seemed to be helping the patients to sit and to retard the rate of progression of the spinal deformity. Apirn, in a review of 15 patients with spinal muscular atrophy treated with bracing, reported that in 5 of the patients the brace had to be discontinued because of respiratory difficulties; in the remaining ten, the curves progressed despite orthotic management.[7]

Riddick reviewed 20 patients treated with orthotic management.[135] In children younger than 3 years, a chest wall deformity occurred as a result of the spinal orthosis. In the remaining patients, the orthosis slowed the progression of the curve but did not seem to prevent the need for eventual surgical intervention. Merlini reviewed 24 patients, aged 4 to 21 years, with the intermediate form of spinal muscular atrophy treated with spinal bracing.[115] Scoliosis increased an average of 8° per year while in the brace. The study concluded that total-contact, underarm plastic orthoses failed to prevent or arrest the progression. The brace did seem to give some support in the sitting position, allowing patients with more severe deformities to sit upright instead of being restricted to bed.

Orthotic management is indicated in the child with spinal muscular atrophy and a small curve. The patient who is ambulatory may not be able to tolerate the brace because it may compromise movement. Children younger than 3 years should be watched closely for the possible development of chest wall deformities. In older patients, the orthosis at best will slow the rate of

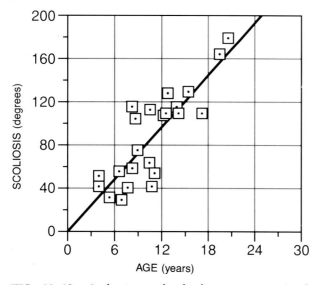

FIG. 12–18. Scoliosis is relentlessly progressive. (With permission from Merlini L, et al: Scoliosis in spinal muscular atrophy: Natural history and management. Dev Med Child Neurol 331:501, 1989)

progression but not prevent progression of the spinal deformity.

Surgery has a significant role in the management of spinal deformities in these patients.[43] Hensinger reviewed 14 patients treated with long posterior instrumentation that included the sacrum when it appeared to be part of the curve.[76] The average correction in wheelchair-bound patients was 43.2%; in ambulatory patients it was 51.5%. Riddick reviewed 16 patients treated surgically—10 with Harrington rods with a 33% correction of spinal curves, 4 with first-stage anterior instrumentation and fusion using a Dwyer apparatus followed by a posterior Harrington rod giving curve correction of 35%, 1 with a subcutaneous rod without fusion, and 1 with Luque rod instrumentation.[135] Apirn reviewed 22 surgically treated patients.[7] One patient was treated with a posterior fusion without instrumentation, 15 with Harrington rod instrumentation, and 6 with anterior Dwyer instrumentation and spinal fusion. Average curve correction in this series was 44.1%.

Brown reviewed 40 patients treated surgically.[20] Thirty-four patients were treated with posterior instrumentation and spinal fusion using Harrington rod, and 6 were treated with posterior Luque rod instrumentation and fusion. Curve correction averaged 42% in both groups of patients. The average postoperative loss of correction was greater in the Harrington rod group (9°) than in the Luque rod group (3°). The complication rate in the Harrington rod group was also greater (35%) than in the Luque rod group (17%).

In reviewing the surgically treated patients, certain common factors were noticed. These patients enter surgery with pulmonary functional compromise. They need a detailed preoperative pulmonary evaluation, including blood gases and pulmonary function studies. Two to 3 weeks of intensive out-patient pulmonary exercises may improve their preoperative pulmonary function.[56, 76] Postoperative pulmonary complications are frequent, especially in patients undergoing anterior spine surgeries. Pulmonary complications can be minimized by avoiding anterior spine surgeries and by using a posterior instrumentation system that allows early return to the upright posture.[7, 56, 115] These patients usually have very osteoporotic bone; instrumentation systems that provide only two points of fixation are associated with problems of hook cut-out, loss of correction, and erosion into the spinal canal, causing paraplegia.[20, 135] Systems that use segmental fixation lessen the incidence of these problems.[7, 20, 137] Pelvic

bone for grafting is limited, and generous use of banked bone is recommended.[36]

Postoperative functional loss occurs frequently.[7, 20, 56, 140] Limited ambulators may become nonambulators; patients who were able to manually propel their wheelchairs may require the use of an electric wheelchair postoperatively, and more upper-extremity mobile arm support may be required. It is a long-term trade-off for having a stable spine, a level pelvis, and prevention of further scoliosis with its attendant pulmonary compromise.[20] Patients and their families need to be informed of this preoperatively.

Authors' Preferred Treatment

Children with spinal muscular atrophy should be fitted with a lightweight, removable thoracolumbosacral orthosis when curves progress beyond 20° and interfere with sitting. Even with slow progression, they should be maintained in the orthosis until the curve exceeds 50°. An effort is made to delay definitive surgery until after the child is 10 years old. At any age over 6 years, a curve in excess of 50° requires definitive surgical correction with a posterior procedure using segmental instrumentation. Ambulatory patients are fused and instrumented from T1 or T2 to the lower lumbar spine if possible, and sitting patients from T2 to the pelvis (Fig. 12-19). The normal sagittal contours of the spine should be maintained. Generous use of bank bone is recommended, and postoperative immobilization is not required.

ARTHROGRYPOSIS

Arthrogryposis is characterized by multiple joint contractures that are present from birth.[46] The myopathic subtype is characterized by muscle changes similar to those found with progressive muscular dystrophy.[21, 39] The neuropathic subtype has fixed extension or flexion deformities of the limb and no obvious hereditary component, and pathologic specimens of the spinal cord show a reduction or complete lack of anterior horn cells in the cervical, thoracic, and lumbosacral segments.[21, 39, 46] Pathologic specimens of the spinal cord show no evidence of inflammatory cells. In the third subtype, joint fibrosis and contracture are the main problems.[39]

Winter has enumerated the diagnostic criteria generally accepted for arthrogryposis:[165] (1) multiple flexion or extension contracture present at birth, (2) marked limitation of active and passive motion of the

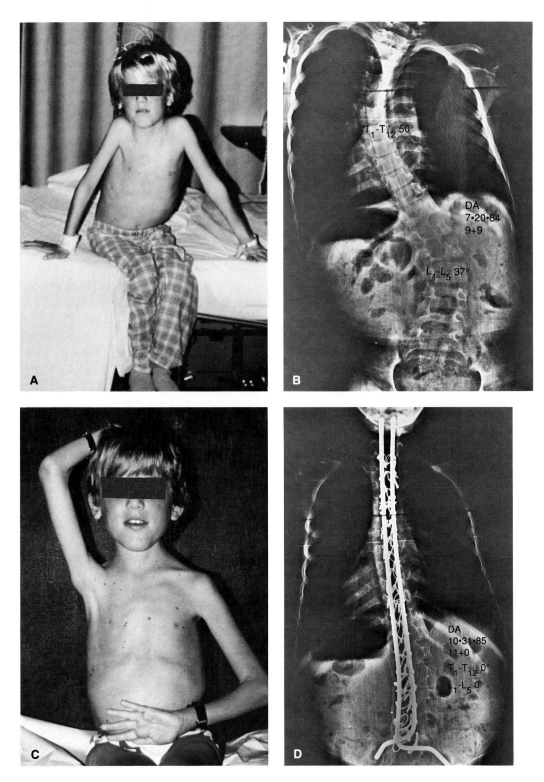

FIG. 12–19. **A.** A child with progressive scoliosis caused by spinal muscular atrophy requiring use of the hands for trunk support. **B.** Child's preoperative scoliosis of 50°. **C.** After Luque rodding, scoliosis was corrected and the hands were freed. **D.** Postoperative x-ray film showing corrected scoliosis. The rods were left too long proximally. The left-sided Galveston portion was too short, but a solid fusion was still achieved.

involved joints but relatively free motion over the small range of motion remaining, (3) cylindrical and fusiform joints, (4) intact sensation, (5) diminished or absent deep tendon reflexes, (6) nonprogressive muscular atrophy, (7) general absence of skin creases over joints, and (8) flexion contractures usually associated with skin webbing across the joint.

Scoliosis is a frequent finding in arthrogryposis. Herron, in a study of 80 patients with arthrogryposis, found 16 (20%) with structural curves greater than 15°.[78] The syndrome was noted at birth in 6 of the 16 patients, during the first 5 years of life in 5, and between the ages of 10 and 13 in 4 patients. Thoracolumbar curves were reported for all patients. The curves extended to the sacrum and were associated with increased lumbar lordosis and pelvic obliquity. No congenital curves were noted in this series. Significant deformities of the hips were noted in all patients but 1.

Drummond and MacKenzie studied 50 patients with arthrogyposis.[45] Fourteen (28%) of the patients had scoliosis. Congenital scoliosis occurred in 7, neuromuscular or long "C" curve in 4, and scoliosis secondary to femoral pelvic obliquity in 3. Daher reported 16 arthrogrypotic patients with scoliosis.[39] Scoliosis was noted at birth in 3 patients, and in the first 5 years of life in 7 others. Seventeen patients had thoracolumbar curves, and 5 patients had a decreased anterior-posterior diameter of the chest, decreasing vital capacity.

In a study of 180 patients with arthrogryposis at the Chicago Unit of Shriners Hospital for Crippled Children, 27% (49) had scoliosis. Of these, only 6 did not have all four extremities involved. Two of the 14 patients who required surgical treatment for their curves developed pseudarthrosis. These patients had posterior spinal fusions alone (Lubicky, unpublished data).

These studies demonstrate certain characteristics of scoliosis in arthrogrypotic children. They present early or during adolescent growth spurts. The syndrome may be associated with lumbar lordosis and pelvic obliquity.[39, 78] Extremity deformities are frequently seen, and when associated with progressive scoliosis, the patient's ambulatory abilities may be significantly impaired.[45, 81]

Treatment

Orthotic management has been instituted in the treatment of arthrogrypotic patients. Herron reported the use of a Milwaukee brace in 2 patients.[78] Both failed and ultimately required fusions. Three patients were treated with corrective casts and required casting essentially from birth to 8 to 10 years of age, at which time a definitive surgery was instituted. Daher reported 8 patients treated with a brace.[39] The brace controlled the curve for 1 patient. In 2 patients, the curve increased but not to a significant degree. One patient was left with a significant decrease in the anterior-posterior chest diameter because of thoracic lordosis. Four other patients were placed in braces, and brace treatment failed; ultimately the patients required surgery. Bracing may also interfere with function and inhibit motor development.

Surgical treatment of curves in arthrogryposis has met with limited success. In Herron's study 10 patients progressed to the point where surgery was recommended.[78] Only 7 patients had surgery. Three patients had posterior fusion with localized cast correction. All patients had pseudarthroses, 2 eventually requiring revision with Harrington instrumentation. Two patients were treated primarily with Harrington rods. Two patients had a posterior spinal osteotomy with intercurrent halo-pelvic or halo-femoral traction. Only 1 of 7 patients had initial fusion to the sacrum. Postoperatively the complications were frequent, occurring in 5 of 7 patients. There were 3 pseudarthroses, 4 with progression above or below the fusion, and 1 with a deep spinal infection. Daher reported on 6 patients treated with surgery.[39] One patient had a posterior fusion without instrumentation, 4 had posterior fusion with instrumentation, and 1 had posterior instrumentation without fusion. Curve correction averaged 34%.

Orthotic management can slow the progression of curves and may allow the delay of surgery until the child is older, but problems are associated with it. Progressive thoracic lordosis is associated with decreased anterior-posterior diameter of the chest, compromising pulmonary function.[39] Despite orthotic management, a progressive pelvic obliquity coupled with the scoliosis causes a decrease in ambulatory abilities.[45, 78, 81] If either of these problems is noticed, the orthotic management should be abandoned and surgery performed. The deformities are rigid and posterior surgery gives little correction.[78]

Authors' Preferred Treatment

Children with arthrogryposis should be managed expectantly. Curves that are manifested in infancy and childhood should be managed with a spinal orthosis.

Curves that progress beyond 45°, curves that are associated with an increasing thoracic lordosis, and curves associated with an increasing pelvic obliquity should be managed with posterior instrumentation and spinal fusion (Fig. 12-20). If curves are greater than 50° and rigid or if there is a spinal pelvic obliquity that does not correct on preoperative bending films, a first-stage anterior release is indicated, followed by posterior instrumentation and spinal fusion. Curves associated with a pelvic obliquity should be fused to the pelvis.

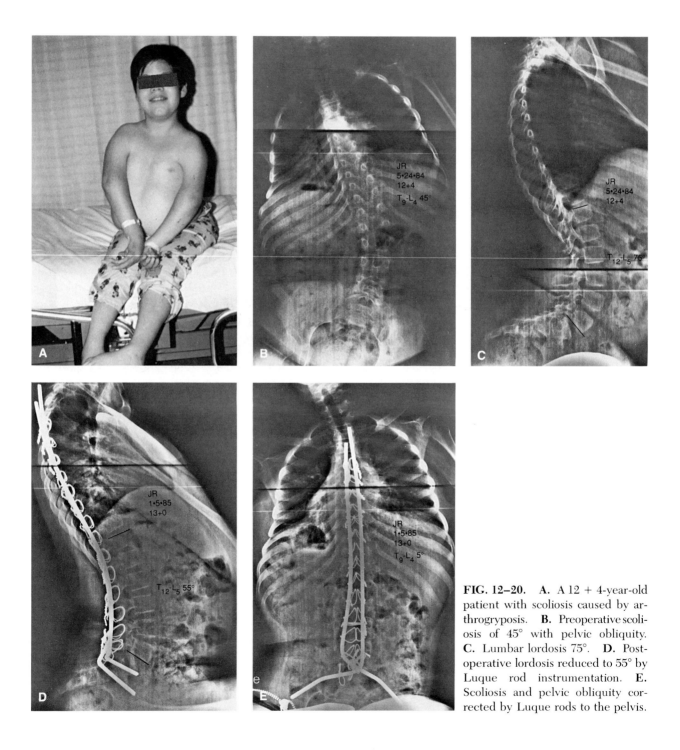

FIG. 12–20. **A.** A 12 + 4-year-old patient with scoliosis caused by arthrogryposis. **B.** Preoperative scoliosis of 45° with pelvic obliquity. **C.** Lumbar lordosis 75°. **D.** Postoperative lordosis reduced to 55° by Luque rod instrumentation. **E.** Scoliosis and pelvic obliquity corrected by Luque rods to the pelvis.

DUCHENNE'S MUSCULAR DYSTROPHY

Duchenne's muscular dystrophy is a progressive, sex-linked recessive disorder of skeletal muscle. Affected males show clinical symptoms of this disorder; females are carriers. As many as 33% of cases represent new mutations.[67]

Several clinical features suggest the diagnosis of Duchenne's muscular dystrophy. A male child presents with progressive muscular weakness manifested as progressive clumsiness. Characteristic features of pseudohypertrophy of the calf and masseter muscles are frequently seen. Chemistry studies reveal a markedly elevated level of creatinine phosphokinase—from 50 to 100 times the normal value. An electromyogram shows myopathy, and muscle biopsy shows characteristic findings of variations in fiber size with internal nuclei, split fibers, degenerating or regenerating fibers, and a fibrous tissue deposition.[143]

There are few disease processes that are as predictable as Duchenne's muscular dystrophy.[157] The typical child presents with mildly delayed motor milestones, but he begins to walk at approximately 18 months to 2 years of age. Weakness is usually evident by the age of 3 to 5, and definite difficulties with "keeping up" with his peers are seen by the age of 5 to 7. By the age of 8 to 10 years, walking becomes progressively more difficult, with increased tripping and falling. Eventually, the gait becomes unstable enough that a wheelchair is required. Approximately 2 years later, a significant scoliosis is detectable. Spinal deformity continues to progress throughout the adolescent growth spurt. By the time the curve gets to be 40°, it has progressed enough that trunk balance is lost, and the child has to use his hands or elbows to support his trunk in the upright posture.[83] The curve progresses until it becomes approximately 80°, and the ribs are usually abutting against the iliac crest. The young man can usually only be up for short periods of time without having severe discomfort from the rib-pelvic impingement and increased buttock pressure caused by pelvic obliquity. From the time the child becomes wheelchair dependent until his curve is severe, at approximately 80°, the progressive myopathic process leads to progressive respiratory insufficiency.[116] Most males affected with this disorder die between 17 and 20 years of age from progressive pulmonary insufficiency and cardiomyopathy.[67, 143]

Several studies following the progressive pulmo-

nary dysfunction in these patients have shown that forced vital capacity (FVC) is perhaps the best single measure of the patient's pulmonary capabilities.[86, 94, 116] Patients eventually develop a restrictive pulmonary disease caused by muscle weakness, muscle fibrosis, and contracture and severe spinal deformity. The patient's pulmonary function peaks at about the age when standing ceases, thereafter declining rapidly by approximately 4° each year.[94] Pulmonary function deteriorates because of progressive muscle weakness, and progressive spinal deformity seems to have little effect on decreasing pulmonary function further (Fig. 12–21).[116]

Treatment

In 1964, Dubowitz suggested that patients be fitted with a lightweight body jacket as soon as they become wheelchair bound.[48] It was his hope that by preventing the development of a spinal deformity, the patient's quality of life would be improved.

Wilkins and Gibson, in a study of patients with Duchenne's muscular dystrophy felt that there was a stable and an unstable pathway for the progressive spinal deformity.[66, 161] They observed that spines that adopted an extended lordotic posture developed much less scoliosis and much less pelvic obliquity than curves that fell into a kyphotic pattern. Kyphosis was thought to be associated with unlocking of the posterior facet joints, creating an unstable condition in which the

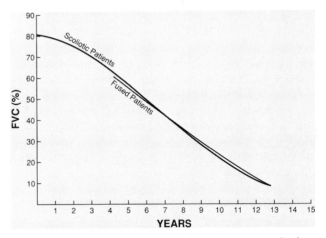

FIG. 12–21. Spine stabilization does not prevent further pulmonary deterioration in patients with Duchenne's muscular dystrophy. (With permission from Miller F et al: Pulmonary function and scoliosis in Duchenne dystrophy. J Pediatr Orthop 8:133, 1988)

spine could fall into a significant scoliosis and accompanying pelvic obliquity. Wilkins and Gibson suggested a seating spinal support system that would endeavor to position the spine in a lordotic posture, thereby placing the spine in a stable configuration.[161] Smith, in 1989, reviewed 33 patients treated with the custom seating system; 13 had to abandon the seating system because of skin breakdown or pain.[145]

Thoracolumbosacral orthoses have been used in the treatment of progressive spinal deformity in patients with Duchenne's muscular dystrophy. Seeger reviewed 24 patients with Duchenne's muscular dystrophy.[141] He found that during the 3.7 years when the curves were followed, they progressed more than 1° each month between 14 and 18 years of age, whether or not the patients used a brace, custom-molded seating, or a modified wheelchair. Cambridge reviewed 32 patients treated with spinal orthosis.[29] Initially, the spinal orthosis seemed to control the curve, but over a long period, there was continued slow progression; ultimately the curve averaged 75° whether or not a patient was braced. Bracing was discontinued in 8 of 32 patients because of severe discomfort or skin compromise. Smith, in a review of 33 patients whose curves were greater than 30°, demonstrated that the use of spinal orthosis or spinal support systems did not seem to influence the final magnitude of the spinal deformity.[145]

As late as 1970, surgical treatment of spinal deformities in Duchenne's muscular dystrophy patients was not recommended.[36] As a result of excellent results achieved by spinal stabilization of other paralytic neuromuscular disorders, physicians at Rancho Los Amigos Hospital began to stabilize the collapsing spinal deformities in patients with Duchenne's muscular dystrophy. Swank, in 1982, reported 13 patients treated with dual Harrington rods from the upper thoracic spine to the sacrum.[152] Spinal deformity averaged 39° before surgery and 15° postoperatively, for a 38% correction. Pelvic obliquity improved from 10 to 4°, for an average 60% correction. There were major or minor complications in 8 of 13 patients. Weimann, in 1983, reviewed 24 patients treated with posterior Harrington rod instrumentation and spinal fusion. Preoperative curves averaged 49° and postoperative curves 22°, for an average correction of 55%.[157] There was a 29% failure rate for instrumentation: 1 rod fracture, 5 rod-hook dislodgments, and 1 superior hook cut-out.

Cambridge, in 1987, reported 13 patients treated with segmental spinal instrumentation.[29] The study recommended spinal fusion when there was evidence of a progression of a spinal deformity greater than 30°. Sussman, in 1987, presented two groups of patients treated with segmental spinal instrumentation and fusion using Luque rod instrumentation.[149] Three patients had curves in excess of 82° and a pelvic obliquity of 27°. Their preoperative vital capacities were 39%. Postoperative correction of spinal deformity was 35%, and correction of pelvic obliquity was 40%. The patients required prolonged postoperative intubation, and the average hospitalization of these 3 patients was 39 days. In a second series treated with segmental spinal instrumentation using Luque rod instrumentation were 5 patients with curves averaging 46°, pelvic obliquities averaging 10°, and vital capacities averaging 66%. Postoperative correction of spinal deformity was 60%. Postoperative improvement in pelvic obliquity was 75%. All patients were extubated on the day of surgery, and hospitalization averaged 8 days.

From these studies, several points can be made. All curves that progress to 30° continue to progress. Instrumentation systems that rely on two to four points of stabilization between the spine and the rod (e.g., Harrington rod instrumentation) are associated with a significant postoperative failure, with hook-rod uncoupling and hook cut-out.[152, 157] Instrumentation failures are significantly less when a segmental spinal instrumentation is used. The worse the preoperative vital capacity, the greater the chance of postoperative pulmonary problems and prolonged hospitalization. If surgery is to be performed, it should be done when the curves are small (30–40°) and before pulmonary deterioration.[150]

In reviewing patients who have had surgical stabilization of their progressive spinal deformities, it is apparent that controlling curve progression does not increase lifespan.[29] It does, however, improve the quality of life.[150, 152] Preoperative back pain is alleviated, and pain in the buttock from a pelvic obliquity is eliminated. The patient's body image is much improved, and stabilization of a spinal deformity to create a level pelvis frees the upper extremities to be used in more meaningful activities than trunk support.

Before considering surgical intervention for a progressive deformity in the patient with Duchenne's muscular dystrophy, a detailed medical evaluation of the patient should be performed. He should be asked about repeated episodes of pneumonitis in the previous year. The patient should be observed for mechanics of respiration, including the use of accessory

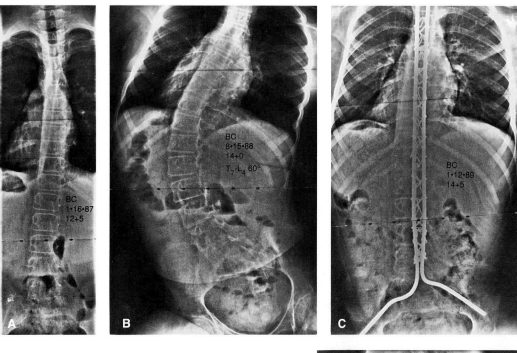

FIG. 12–22. A. A 12 + 5-year-old patient with Duchenne's muscular dystrophy in a wheelchair on sitting x-ray film. **B.** Curve has progressed to 60° with a pelvic obliquity 17 months later. **C.** Curve straightened with Luque rod instrumentation to the pelvis. **D.** Sagittal curves maintained by rod contouring. Spina bifida occulta at L5 prevented by sublaminar wiring at this level.

muscles and diaphragmatic breathing. In addition, the patient should demonstrate a functional cough. A chest x-ray film and an electrocardiogram should be obtained to search for cardiac conduction defects, dysrhythmias, and ventricular hypertrophy. Arterial blood gases should be obtained; if hypercarbia is demonstrated, the patient is an extremely poor candidate for surgery.[85] Pulmonary function tests should be obtained, and a forced vital capacity of greater than 35% of the predicted normal value should allow the patient to safely undergo a general anesthetic, although in certain cases patients in the 20% to 35% predicted range may be candidates.[29, 117]

Authors' Preferred Treatment

After a patient is forced to resort to a wheelchair, his spine should be followed expectantly. Clinical examinations every 3 to 6 months should be performed, and if a spinal deformity is detected, x-ray films should be taken. Specially designed seating systems are more for the patient's ease and comfort in transportation rather than control of a spinal deformity. If a spinal deformity develops and reaches 30°, the patient should be considered for surgical intervention. The surgical procedure of choice is a posterior instrumentation and spinal fusion using a segmental instrumentation system. If there is a preexistent pelvic obliquity, the instrumentation and fusion should go from the upper thoracic spine to the pelvis (see Fig. 12-19). If there is no preoperative pelvic obliquity, inferior instrumentation can stop at L5. However, our preference is to instrument all patients from the upper thoracic spine to the pelvis, taking care to preserve normal sagittal contours. Within 5 to 7 days of surgery, the patient should be mobilized; external support is not necessary. Extubation after surgery should be done promptly to prevent the patient from becoming dependent on the ventilator.

References

1. Adams FH, Emmanouilides GC, Rienenschnuda TA: Moss Heart Disease in Infants and Children, pp 785–790. Baltimore, Williams and Wilkins, 1989
2. Allen BL, Ferguson RL: L-rod instrumentation for scoliosis in cerebral palsy. J Pediatr Orthop 2:87, 1982
3. Allen BL, Ferguson RL: The Galveston technique of pelvic fixation with L-rod instrumentation of the spine. Spine 9:388, 1984
4. Allen BL, Ferguson RL: Neurologic injuries with the Galveston technique of L-rod instrumentation for scoliosis. Spine 11:14, 1986
5. Allen BL, Ferguson RL: A 1988 perspective on the Galveston technique of pelvic fixation. Orthop Clin North Am 19:409, 1988
6. Anderson RH, MaCartney FJ, Sphinebourne EA, Tynan M: Pediatric Cardiology, pp 1256–1260. London, Churchill Livingstone, 1987
7. Aprin H, Bowen H, MacEwen GD, Hall JE: Spine fusion in patients with spinal muscular atrophy. J Bone Joint Surg [Am] 64:1179, 1982
8. Baker AS, Dove J: Progressive scoliosis as the first presenting sign of syringomyelia. J Bone Joint Surg [Br] 65:472, 1983
9. Balmer GA, MacEwen GD: The incidence and treatment of scoliosis in cerebral palsy. J Bone Joint Surg [Br] 52:134, 1970
10. Bell GR, Gurd AR, Orlowski JP, Andrish JT: The syndrome of inappropriate antidiuretic-hormone secretion following spinal fusion. J Bone Joint Surg [Am] 68:720, 1982
11. Benady SG: Spinal muscular atrophy in childhood: Review of 50 cases. Dev Med Child Neurol 20:746, 1978
12. Ben-David B: Spinal cord monitoring. Orthop Clin North Am 19:427, 1988
13. Berquist WE, Rachelefsky GS, Kadden M, et al: Gastroesophageal reflux-associated recurrent pneumonia in chronic asthma in children. Pediatrics 68:29, 1981
14. Bonnett C, Brown JC, Perry J, et al: Evolution of treatment of paralytic scoliosis at Rancho Los Amigos Hospital. J Bone Joint Surg [Am] 57:206, 1975
15. Bonnett C, Brown JC, Grow T: Thoracolumbar scoliosis in cerebral palsy. J Bone Joint Surg [Am] 58:328, 1976
16. Bradford DS: Neuromuscular spinal deformity. In Bradford DS, Lonstein JE, Moe JH, et al (eds): Moe's Textbook of Scoliosis and Other Spinal Deformities, 2nd ed, pp 271–305. Philadelphia, WB Saunders, 1987
17. Brown JC, Swank S., Specht L: Combined anterior and posterior spine fusion in cerebral palsy. Spine 7:570, 1982
18. Brown JC, Swank SM: Paralytic spine deformity. In Bradford D, Hensinger R (eds): The Pediatric Spine, pp 251–272. New York, Thieme, 1985
19. Brown JC, Swank SM, Matta J, Barras D: Late spinal deformity in quadriplegic children and adolescents. J Pediatr Orthop 4:456, 1984
20. Brown JC, Zeller JL, Swank SM, et al: Surgical and functional results of spine fusion in spinal muscular atrophy. Spine 14:763, 1989
21. Brown LM, Robson MJ, Sharrard WJW: The pathophysiology of arthrogryposis. J Bone Joint Surg [Br] 62:291, 1980
22. Bunch WH: Treatment of the paralytic spine. In AAOS Atlas of Orthotics, pp 402–406. St. Louis, CV Mosby, 1975
23. Bunch WH: The Milwaukee brace in paralytic scoliosis. Clin Orthop Rel Res 110:63, 1975

24. Bunch WH, Keagy RD: Principles of Orthotic Treatment, pp 77–99. St. Louis, CV Mosby, 1976

25. Bunch WH, Smith D, Hakala M.: Kyphosis in the paralytic spine. Clin Orthop Rel Res 128:107, 1977

26. Bunnell WP, MacEwen GD: Non-operative treatment of scoliosis in cerebral palsy: Preliminary report on the use of a plastic jacket. Dev Med Child Neurol 19:45, 1977

27. Cadman D, Richards J, Feldman W: Gastroesophageal reflux in severely retarded children. Dev Med Child Neurol 20:95, 1978

28. Cady RB, Bobechko WP: Incidence, natural history and treatment of scoliosis in Friedreich's Ataxia. J Pediatr Orthop 4:673, 1984

29. Cambridge W, Drennan JC: Scoliosis associated with Duchenne muscular dystrophy. J Pediatr Orthop 7:436, 1987

29a. Camp JF, Caudles R, Ashmun RD, Roach J: Immediate complications of Cotrel–Dubousset instrumentation of the sacra-pelvis: A clinical and biomechanical study. Spine 15:932, 1990

30. Campbell J, Bonnett C: Spinal cord injury in children. Clin Orthop Rel Res 112:114, 1975

31. Carlson JM, Winter R: The "Gillette" sitting support orthosis for non-ambulatory children with severe cerebral palsy or advanced muscular dystrophy. Minn Med 61:469, 1978

32. Casey MP, Asher MA, Jacobs RR, Orrick JM: The effect of Harrington rod contouring on lumbar lordosis. Spine 12:750, 1987

33. Colonna PC, VomSaal F: A study of paralytic scoliosis based on five hundred cases of poliomyelitis. J Bone Joint Surg 23:335, 1941

34. Coonrad RW, Richardson WJ, Oakes WJ: Left thoracic curves can be different. Presented at 19th Annual Meeting of the Scoliosis Research Society, Orlando, FL, 1984

35. Cote CJ: Blood replacement and blood product management. In Ryan JF, Cote CJ, Todres ID, Goudsouzian N (eds): A Practice of Anaesthesia for Infants and Children, pp 123–132. Orlando, FL, Grune and Stratton, 1986

36. Curtis BH: Orthopedic management of muscular dystrophy and related disorders. In AAOS Instructional Course Lectures, vol 19, pp 78–89. St. Louis, CV Mosby, 1970

37. Daher YH, Lonstein JE, Winter RB, Bradford DS: Spinal surgery in spinal muscular atrophy. J Pediatr Orthop 5:391, 1985

38. Daher YH, Lonstein JE, Winter RB, Bradford DS: Spinal deformities in patients with Friedreich ataxia: A review of 19 patients. J Pediatr Orthop 5:553, 1985

39. Daher YH, Lonstein JE, Winter RB, Moe JH: Spinal deformities in patients with arthrogryposis. A review of 16 patients. Spine 10:609, 1985

40. Daher YD, Lonstein JE, Winter RB, Bradford DS: Spinal deformities in patients with Charcot-Marie-Tooth disease. Clin Orthop Rel Res 202:219, 1986

41. Darling DE, McCauley RGK, Leonidas JC, Swartz AM: Gastroesophageal reflux in infants and children: Correlation of radiological severity and pulmonary pathology. Radiology 127:735, 1978

42. DeWald RL, Faut MM: Anterior and posterior spinal fusion for paralytic scoliosis. Spine 4:401, 1979

43. Dorr JR, Brown JC, Perry J: Results of posterior spine fusion in patients with spinal muscular atrophy. A review of 25 cases. J Bone Joint Surg [Am] 55:436, 1973

44. Drummond D, Guadagni J, Keene JS, et al: Interspinous process segmental spinal instrumentation. J Pediatr Orthop 4:397, 1984

45. Drummond DS, MacKenzie DA: Scoliosis in arthrogryposis multiplex congenita. Spine 3:146, 1978

46. Drummond DS, Siller TN, Cruess RL: Management of arthrogryposis multiplex congenita. In AAOS Instructional Course Lectures, vol 23, pp 79–95. St. Louis, CV Mosby, 1974

47. Drvaric DM, Roberts JM, Burke SW, et al: Gastroesophageal evaluation in totally involved cerebral palsy patients. J Pediatr Orthop 7:187, 1987

48. Dubowitz V: Progressive muscular dystrophy prevention of deformities. Clin Pediatr 3:323, 1964

49. Dubowitz V: Recent advances in neuromuscular disorders: spinal muscular atrophy. Rheum Phys Med 11:126, 1971

50. Dubowitz V: Infantile spinal muscular atrophy: A progressive study with particular reference to a slowly progressive variety. Brain 57:767, 1974

51. Dubowitz V: Benign infantile spinal muscular atrophy. Dev Med Child Neurol 16:672, 1974

52. Dubowitz V: Muscle Disorders in Childhood. Philadelphia, WB Saunders, 1978

53. Dwyer AF, Schafer MF: Anterior approach to scoliosis. J Bone Joint Surg [Br] 56:218, 1974

54. Eberle CF: Failure of fixation after segmental spinal instrumentation without arthrodesis in the management of paralytic scoliosis. J Bone Joint Surg [Am] 70:696, 1988

55. Emery AEH, Hausmanowa-Petrusewics I, Davie AM: International collaborative study of the spinal muscular atrophies: I. Analysis of clinical data. J Neurosurg 29(1):83, 1976

56. Evans GA, Drennan JC: Functional classification and orthopedic management of spinal muscular atrophy. J Bone Joint Surg [Br] 63:516, 1981

57. Ferguson RL, Allen BL: Staged correction of neuromuscular scoliosis. J Pediatr Orthop 3:555, 1983

58. Ferguson RL, Allen BL: Considerations in the treatment of cerebral palsy patients with spinal deformities. Orthop Clin North Am 19:419, 1988

59. Fisk JR, Bunch WH: Scoliosis in neuromuscular disease. Orthop Clin North Am 10:863, 1979

60. Floman Y, Micheli LJ, Penny JN, et al: Combined anterior and posterior fusion in seventy-three spinally deformed patients. Clin Orthop Rel Res 164:110, 1982

61. Friedlander GE: Current concepts review: Bone grafts. J Bone Joint Surg [Am] 69:786, 1987

62. Garrett AL, Perry J, Nickel V: Stabilization of the collapsing spine. J Bone Joint Surg [Am] 43:474, 1961

63. Garrett Al, Perry J, Nickel VL: Paralytic scoliosis. Clin Orthop Rel Res 21:117, 1961

64. Geoffroy G, Barbeau A, Breton G, et al: Clinical description and roentgenologic evaluation of patients with Friedreich's ataxia. Can J Neurol Sci 3:279, 1976

65. Gersoff WK, Renshaw TS: The treatment of scoliosis in cerebral palsy by posterior spinal fusion with Luquerod segmental instrumentation. J Bone Joint Surg [Am] 70:41, 1988

66. Gibson DA, Wilkins KE. The management of spinal deformities in Duchenne muscular dystrophy. Clin Orthop Rel Res 108:41, 1975

67. Glasberg MR: Myopathies. Neurosurgery 5:747, 1979

68. Granata C, Merlini L, Magni E, et al: Spinal muscular atrophy: Natural history and orthopedic treatment of scoliosis. Spine 14:760, 1989

69. Gucker T: Experiences with poliomyelitic scoliosis after fusion and correction. J Bone Joint Surg [Am] 38:1281, 1956

70. Gurr KR, Taylor TKF, Stobo P: Syringomyelia and scoliosis in childhood and adolescence. J Bone Joint Surg [Br] 70:159, 1988

71. Haas SL: Spastic scoliosis and obliquity of the pelvis. J Bone Joint Surg 24:774, 1942

72. Hahn Th, Avioli LV: Anticonvulsant osteomalacia. Arch Intern Med 135:997, 1975

73. Hale KA, Rasp FL: Pulmonary function testing. In Bradford DS, Lonstein JE, Moe JH, et al (eds): Moe's Textbook of Scoliosis and Other Spinal Deformities, 2nd ed, pp 585–592. Philadelphia, WB Saunders, 1987

74. Hall JE: Current concepts review: Dwyer instrumentation in anterior fusion of the spine. J Bone Joint Surg [Am] 63:1188, 1981

75. Hardy JH, Curtis BH: Neuromuscular scoliosis. J Bone Joint Surg [Am] 53:1021, 1971

76. Hensinger RN, MacEwen GD: Spinal deformity associated with heritable neurological conditions: Spinal muscular atrophy, Friedreich's ataxia, familial dysautonomia and Charcot-Marie-Tooth disease. J Bone Joint Surg [Am] 58:13, 1976

77. Herring JA, Wenger DR: Segmental spinal instrumentation. Spine 7:285, 1982

78. Herron LD, Westin GW, Dawson EG: Scoliosis in arthrogryposis multiplex congenita. J Bone Joint Surg [Am] 60:293, 1978

79. Hewer RL: A study of fatal cases of Friedreich's ataxia. Br Med J 3:649, 1968

80. Hodgson AR, Stock FE: Anterior spinal fusion. A preliminary communication on the radical treatment of Pott's disease and Pott's paraplegia. Br J Surg 44:266, 1956

81. Hoffer MM, Swank S, Eastman F, et al: Ambulation in severe arthrogryposis. J Pediatr Orthop 3:293, 1983

82. Hoffman J: Uber chronische spinale Muskelatrophie in Kindesalter, auf familiarer Basis. Deutsch Z Nervenheilk 3:427, 1983

83. Hsu J: The natural history of spine curvature progression in the nonambulatory Duchenne muscular dystrophy patient. Spine 8:771, 1983

84. Huebert HT, MacKinnon WB: Syringomyelia and scoliosis. J Bone Joint Surg [Br] 51:338, 1969

85. Hunsaker RH, Fulkerson PK, Barry FJ, et al: Cardiac function in Duchenne's muscular dystrophy: Results of a 10-year follow-up study and noninvasive tests. Am J Med 73:235, 1982

86. Inkley SR, Oldenburg FC, Vignos PJ: Pulmonary function in Duchenne muscular dystrophy related to stage of disease. Am J Med 56:297, 1974

87. Irwin CE: The iliotibial band: Its role in producing deformity in poliomyelitis. J Bone Joint Surg [Am] 31:141, 1949

88. James JP: Paralytic scoliosis. J Bone Joint Surg [Br] 38:660, 1956

89. Jensen JE, Jensen TG, Smith TK, et al: Nutrition in orthopedic surgery. J Bone Joint Surg [Am] 64:1268, 1982

90. Jolley SG, Herbst JJ, Johnson DG, et al: Surgery in children with gastroesophageal reflux and respiratory symptoms. J Pediatr 96:194, 1980

91. Kilfoyle RM, Foley JJ, Norton PL: Spine and pelvic deformity in childhood and adolescent paraplegia. J Bone Joint Surg [Am] 47:659, 1965

92. Krlegn I: Pediatric Disorders of Feeding, Nutrition, and Metabolism, pp 94–96. New York, John Wiley, 1982

93. Kugelberg E, Welander L: Heredofamilial juvenile muscular atrophies simulating muscular dystrophy. AMA Arch Neurol Psychiatry 75:500, 1956

94. Kurz LT, Mubarak SJ, Schultz P, et al: Correlation of scoliosis and pulmonary function in Duchenne muscular dystrophy. J Pediatr Orthop 3:347, 1983

95. Labelle H, Tohme S, Duhaime M, Allard P: Natural history of scoliosis in Friedreich's ataxia. J Bone Joint Surg [Am] 68:564, 1986

96. Lancourt JE, Dickson JH, Carter RE: Paralytic spinal deformity following traumatic spinal cord injury in children and adolescents. J Bone Joint Surg [Am] 63:47, 1981

97. Law DK, Dudrick SJ, Abdoll NI: The effects of protein calorie malnutrition on immune competence of the surgical patient. Surg Gynecol Obstet 139:459, 1968

98. Lee BCP, Zimmerman RD, Manning JJ: MR imaging of syringomyelia and hydromyelia. AJNR 6:221 1985

99. Leong JCY, Wilding K, Mok CK, et al: Surgical treatment of scoliosis following poliomyelitis. J Bone Joint Surg [Am] 63:726, 1981

100. Letts M, Shapiro L, Mulder K, Klassen O: The windblown hip syndrome in total-body cerebral palsy. J Pediatr Orthop 4:55, 1984

101. Lonstein JE, Akbarnia BA: Operative treatment of spinal deformities in patients with cerebral palsy or mental retardation. J Bone Joint Surg [Am] 65:43, 1983

102. Lonstein JE, Renshaw TS: Neuromuscular spine deformities. In Griffin PP (ed): AAOS Instructional Course Lectures, vol 36, pp 285–304. St. Louis, CV Mosby, 1986

103. Luque ER: Segmental spinal instrumentation for correction of scoliosis. Clin Orthop Rel Res 163:192, 1982

104. MacEwen GD: Operative treatment of scoliosis in cerebral palsy. Reconstr Surg Traumatol 13:58, 1972

105. Madigan RR, Wallace SL: Scoliosis in institutionalized cerebral palsy population. Spine 6:583, 1981

106. Makley JT, Herndon C, Inkley S, et al: Pulmonary

function in paralytic and non-paralytic scoliosis before and after treatment. J Bone and Joint Surg [Am] 50:1379, 1968

107. Matthews SJ, Versfeld GA: Rickets in cerebral palsied children. J Pediatr Orthop 6:717, 1986
108. Mayer L: Further studies of fixed paralytic pelvic obliquity. J Bone Joint Surg 18:87, 1936
109. Mayer PJ, Dove J, Ditmansor M, Shen YS: Post-poliomyelitis paralytic scoliosis: A review of curve patterns and results of surgical treatments in 118 consecutive patients. Spine 6:573, 1981
110. Mayfield JK, Erkkila JC, Winter RB: Spine deformity subsequent to acquired childhood spinal cord injury. J Bone Joint Surg [Am] 63:1401, 1981
111. McAffee PC, Lubicky JP, Werner FW: The use of segmental spinal instrumentation to preserve longitudinal spinal growth. J Bone Joint Surg [Am] 65:935, 1983
112. McCarthy RE, Peek RD, Morrissy RT, Hough AJ: Allograft bone in spinal fusion for paralytic scoliosis. J Bone Joint Surg [Am] 68:370, 1986
113. McIlroy WJ, Richardson JC: Syringomyelia: A clinical review of 75 cases. Can Med Assoc J 93, 1965
114. McRae DL, Standen I: Roentgenologic findings in syringomyelia and hydromyelia. AJR 98:695, 1966
115. Merlini L, Granata C, Bonfiglioli S, et al: Scoliosis in spinal muscular atrophy: Natural history and management. Dev Med Child Neurol 31:501, 1989
116. Miller F, Moseley CF, Koreska J, Levison H: Pulmonary function and scoliosis in Duchenne dystrophy. J Pediatr Orthop 8:133, 1988
117. Milne B, Rosales JK: Anaesthetic considerations in patients with muscular dystrophy undergoing spinal fusion and Harrington rod insertion. Can Anaesth Soc J 29:250, 1982
118. Moe JH, Kharrat K, Winter RB, Cummine JL: Harrington instrumentation without fusion plus external orthotic support for the treatment of difficult curvature problems in young children. Clin Orthop Rel Res 185:35, 1984
119. Morrissy RT, Busch MT: Neuromuscular scoliosis. State Art Rev 1:283, 1987
120. Mullen JL, Gertner MH, Buzby GP, et al: Implications of malnutrition in the surgical patient. Arch Surg 114:121, 1979
121. Munsat TL, Woods R, Fowler W, Pearson CM: Neurologic muscular atrophy of infancy with prolonged survival. The variable course of Werdnig-Hoffman disease. Brain 92:9, 1969
122. Nash CL: Scoliosis bracing. J Bone Joint Surg [Am] 62:848, 1980
123. Nickel VL, Perry J, Affeldt JE, Dail C: Elective surgery on patients with respiratory paralysis. J Bone Joint Surg [Am] 39:989, 1957
124. Nordwall A, Wikkelso C: A late neurologic complication of scoliosis surgery in connection with syringomyelia. Acta Orthop Scand 50:407, 1979
125. Norton PL, Foley JJ: Paraplegia in children. J Bone Joint Surg [Am] 41:1291, 1959
126. O'Brien JP, Dwyer AP, Hodgson AR: Pelvic obliquity: Its prognosis and management and the development of a technique for full correction of the deformity. J Bone Joint Surg [Am] 57:626, 1975
127. O'Brien JP, Yau ACMC: Anterior and posterior correction and fusion for paralytic scoliosis. Clin Orthop Rel Res 86:151, 1972
128. OBrien JP, Yau ACMC, Gertzbein S, Hodgson A: Combined staged anterior and posterior correction and fusion of the spine in scoliosis following poliomyelitis. Clin Orthop Rel Res 110:81, 1975
129. Palmer S, Ekvall S: Pediatric Nutrition in Developmental Disorders, pp 42–49. Springfield, IL, Charles C Thomas, 1978
130. Pavon SJ, Manning C: Posterior spinal fusion for scoliosis due to anterior poliomyelitis. J Bone Joint Surg [Br] 52:420, 1970
131. Pearn JH, Wilson J: Chronic generalized spinal muscular atrophy of infancy and childhood. Arch Dis Child 48:768, 1973
132. Pennet A: Congenital and developmental anomalies. Skeletal and clinical manifestation anomalies and defects of the neuraxis. Clin Orthop Rel Res. 27:9, 1963
133. Radin EL, Simon SR, Rose RM, Paul IL: Practical Biomechanics for the Orthopedic Surgeon, pp 24–25. New York, John Wiley, 1979
134. Rang M, Silver R, Garza J: Cerebral palsy. In Lovell WW, Winter RB (eds): Pediatric Orthopedics, 2nd ed, pp 345–396. Philadelphia, JB Lippincott, 1986
135. Riddick MF, Winter RB, Lutter LD: Spinal deformities in patients with spinal muscular atrophy: A review of 36 patients. Spine 7:476, 1982
136. Rinsky LA, Gamble JG, Bleck EE: Segmental instrumentation without fusion in children with progressive scoliosis. J Pediatr Orthop 5:687, 1985
137. Roaf R: Paralytic scoliosis. J Bone Joint Surg [Br] 38:640, 1956
138. Rosenthal RK, Levine OB, McCarver CL: The occurrence of scoliosis in cerebral palsy. Dev Med Child Neurol 16:664, 1974
139. Samilson RL, Tsou P, Aamoth G. Green WM: Dislocation and subluxation of the hip in cerebral palsy. Pathogenesis, natural history and management. J Bone Joint Surg [Am] 54:863, 1972
140. Schwentker EP, Gibson DA: The orthopedic aspects of spinal muscular atrophy. J Bone and Joint Surg [Am] 58:32, 1976
141. Seeger BR, Sutherland Ad'A, Clark MS: Orthotic management of scoliosis in Duchenne muscular dystrophy. Arch Phys Med Rehab 65:83, 1984
142. Shands AR, Eisberg HB: The incidence of scoliosis in the state of Delaware. A study of 50,000 minifilms of the chest made during a survey for tuberculosis. J Bone Joint Surg [Am] 37:1243, 1955
143. Shapiro F, Bresnan MJ: Orthopedic management of childhood neuromuscular disease. J Bone Joint Surg [Am] 64:785, 1982
144. Sladen RN: Inadvertent hypothermia: Risks and prevention. Presented at American Society of Anaesthesiologists, New Orleans, October 1989
145. Smith AD, Koreska J, Moseley CF: Progression of scoliosis in Duchenne muscular dystrophy. J Bone Joint Surg [Am] 71:1066, 1989

146. Sondheimer JM, Morris BA: Gastroesophageal reflux among severely retarded children. J Pediatr 94:710, 1979

147. Sponseller PD, Wiffen JR, Drummond DS: Interspinous process segmental spinal instrumentation for scoliosis in cerebral palsy. J Pediatr Orthop 6:559, 1986

148. Stagnara P, DeMauray JC, Gonon G, Campo-Paysaa A: Scolioses cyphosantes de l'adulte et greffes anterieures. Int Orthop 2:149, 1978

149. Stanitski CL, Micheli LJ, Hall JE, Rosenthal RK: Surgical correction of spinal deformity in cerebral palsy. Spine 7:563, 1982

150. Sussman MD: Advantage of early spinal stabilization and fusion in patients with Duchenne muscular dystrophy. J Pediatr Orthop 4:532, 1984

151. Swank S, Lonstein JE, Moe JH, et al: Surgical treatment of adult scolioses. A review of two hundred and twenty-two cases. J Bone Joint Surg [Am] 63:268, 1981

152. Swank SM, Brown JC, Perry RE: Spinal fusion in Duchenne's muscular dystrophy. Spine 7:484, 1982

153. Swank SM, Cohen DS, Brown JC: Spinal fusion in cerebral palsy with L-rod segmental spinal instrumentation. A comparison of single and two-stage combined approach with Zielke instrumentation. Spine 14:750, 1989

154. Taddonio RF: Segmental spinal instrumentation in the management of neuromuscular spinal deformity. Spine 7:305, 1982

155. Thometz JG, Simon SR: Progression of scoliosis after skeletal maturity in institutionalized adults who have cerebral palsy. J Bone Joint Surg [Am] 70:1290, 1988

156. Tolman KG, Jubiz W, Sannella JJ, et al: Osteomalacia associated with anticonvulsant drug therapy in mentally retarded children. Pediatrics 56:45, 1975

157. Weiman RL, Gibson DA, Moseley CF, Jones DC: Surgical stabilization of the spine in Duchenne muscular dystrophy. Spine 8:776, 1983

158. Wenger DR, Carollo JJ, Wilkerson JA: Biomechanics of scoliosis correction by segmental spinal instrumentation. Spine 3:260, 1982

159. Werding G: Zwei fruhinfatile hereditare Falle von progressiver Muskelatrophie unter dem Balde der Dystrophie, aber auf neurotischer Grundlage. Arch Psychiatry Nervenkrank 22:237, 1981

160. White AA, Panjabi MM: Clinical Biomechanics of the Spine, pp 91–114. Philadelphia, JB Lippincott, 1978

161. Wilkins KE, Gibson DA: The patterns of spinal deformity in Duchenne muscular dystrophy. J Bone Joint Surg [Am] 58:24, 1976

162. Williams B: Orthopedic features in the presentation of syringomyelia. J Bone Joint Surg [Br] 61:314, 1979

163. Wilber RG, Thompson GH, Shaffer W, et al: Postoperative neurological defects in segmental spinal instrumentation. J Bone Joint Surg [Am] 66:1178, 1984

164. Winson EJ, Murphy EG, Thompson MW, Reed TE: Genetics of childhood spinal muscular atrophy. J Med Genet 8:143, 1971

165. Winter RB: Arthrogryposis. In Bradford DS, Lonstein JE, Moe JH, et al (eds): Moe's Textbook of Scoliosis and Other Spinal Deformities, pp 561–567. Philadelphia, WB Saunders, 1987

166. Winter RB, Carlson JM: Modern orthotics for spinal deformities. Clin Orthop Rel Res 126:74, 1977

167. Winter RB, Carvalho W: Pelvic obliquity: Its causes and its treatment. Spine 11:225, 1986

168. Winter RB, Koop SE, Lonstein JE, Vanden Brink KD: Spinal instrumentation without fusion in progressive spinal deformity of childhood. Presented at Pediatric Orthopedic Society of North America Annual Meeting, Colorado Springs, Colorado, 1988

169. Yngve DA, Harris WP, Herndon WA, et al: Spinal cord injury without osseous spine fracture. J Pediatr Orthop 8:153, 1988

Color Section Two

CONGENITAL SCOLIOSIS AND MYELOMENINGOCELE DEFORMITY

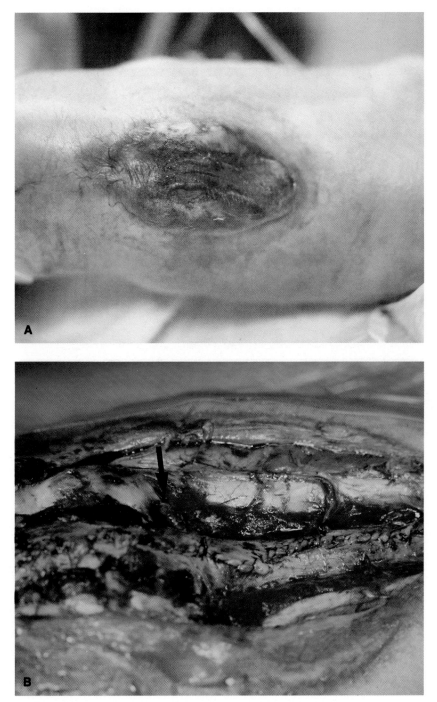

COLOR PLATE 6. Neonatal verte-brectomy for severe kyphosis noted at birth. **A.** Neonate with myelomenin-gocele prior to sac closure showing large defect associated with kyphosis. **B.** The same patient after the neurosurgeons closed the dural tube (*arrow*). (See also Fig. 13-18.)

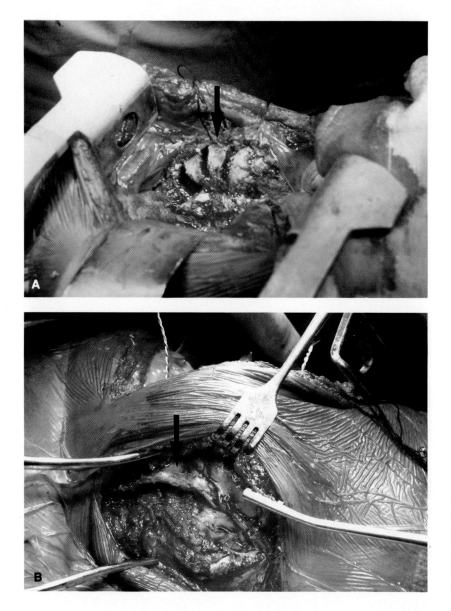

COLOR PLATE 7. A. Simultaneous anterior and posterior exposures. The anterior procedure is done through the usual thoracolumbar approach. **B.** The entire patient was widely prepared and draped so that the posterior exposure could be made as well.

CHAPTER
13

The Myelomeningocele Spine

John P. Lubicky

The myelomeningocele patient with a spinal deformity has unusual and significant problems. These children have multiple-system dysfunctions that influence the treatment plans for their deformity and present challenging problems for the spinal surgeon.

Several series have delineated the natural history and incidence of spinal deformity in patients with myelomeningocele.[4, 19, 20, 29, 33] The higher the neurologic level of the lesion, the higher the incidence of spinal deformity. In a study of 268 patients, Banta and colleagues found that the incidence of scoliosis increased with increasing age and neurologic level, such that patients with thoracolumbar spina bifida have essentially a 100% incidence of spinal deformity by age 14.[4] Similar findings were found by Bradford and colleagues, Mackel and Lindseth, and Raycroft and Curtis.[6, 20, 30] Raycroft and Curtis stressed that the cause of the spinal deformity may be paralytic and/or congenital. Eighty of 130 patients in their series had spinal deformity; one-third had congenital deformity in addition to their spina bifida anomaly. The researchers found that the severity of the curve correlated with the severity of the neurologic deficit. Therefore, spinal deformity is a common and potentially difficult aspect of the overall problem of the myelomeningocele.

Evaluating and treating the spinal deformity cannot be done without considering associated factors, such as shunt and spinal cord function. At least two studies have demonstrated that abnormalities of the spinal cord and increased intracranial pressure may cause a rapid increase in spinal curvature beyond that which would be expected with growth.[12, 29] Correction of these problems should stop the rapid progression; in some cases, correction may effect regression of the deformity. Similarly, spinal cord tethering may be associated with the abnormally rapid increase in the size of the curve.[14] However, most patients with myelomeningocele have radiographic tethering of the spinal cord at the site of the sac closure, and the mere presence of the radiographic tethering does not imply traction on the cord. On the other hand, clinical signs and symptoms of cord tethering, such as back pain, new or increased spasticity, changes in muscle strength, difficulty with gait, changes in bowel or bladder function, and the appearance of lower-extremity deformities, may indicate traction on the spinal cord, which may be aggravating the spinal deformity. These clinical changes are more commonly seen in patients with lower neurologic levels, but some patients with high-level abnormalities have developed increasing lower-extremity spasticity, which interfered with bracing and responded to untethering of the cord.

In patients with a lower lumbar level who have curves that require surgical treatment, evaluation of the spinal canal before surgical correction should be done whether or not the patients have clinical symptoms of cord tethering. Similarly, those who have clinical evidence of cord tethering—no matter what their neurologic level of involvement—and who have rapidly increasing spinal deformity should have their spinal canals evaluated. Magnetic resonance imaging (MRI) or computed tomography (CT) myelography are methods available for imaging the spinal canal. However, severe deformity makes interpretation of the MRI difficult; in these situations CT myelography is more reliable (Fig. 13-1).

If cord tethering is found in patients who are ambulatory and spinal corrective surgery is planned, release of the tether should be done before or concomitant with that surgery to prevent neurologic deficit when straightening the spine. Patients who have a high neu-

rologic level of involvement (nonambulatory) and who have no particular problems with spasticity or other clinical signs of cord tethering probably do not need preoperative evaluation of the spinal canal, because their neurologic function will not be affected by surgical manipulation of the spine. Although there is some evidence for curve regression after correction of abnormalities of the brain or spinal cord, it is unrealistic to think that a stiff 90° curve will regress without other treatment.[11, 14, 28]

Treatment is required for large and progressive spinal deformities. Therefore, not every child with myelomeningocele and spinal deformity needs surgery or brace treatment. However, large curves are associated with abnormal sitting posture, the need to use the upper extremities for balance while sitting, pelvic obliquity and concomitant pressure sores, and decreased pulmonary function.[5] For patients with lower extremity orthoses, severe deformity also interferes with trunk posture in the standing position. Treatment options are bracing and surgery.

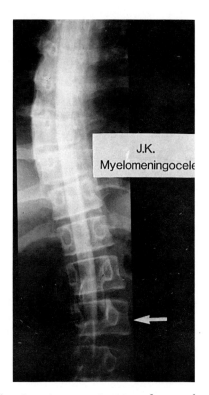

FIG. 13-1. Anterior-posterior view of a complete myelogram showing low-lying cord (*arrow*) in a teenager with progressive scoliosis and functioning quads.

TREATMENT

It is known that the natural history of paralytic curves is not changed by bracing.[6, 20, 21] However, bracing can make a significant difference in the sitting and standing posture, even with large curves if they are flexible. Straightening the trunk increases torso height and improves sitting and standing posture. Bracing can help delay spinal fusion until the patients are older and larger while providing improved spinal alignment in the interim. A bivalved plastic TLSO is the brace most widely used for this purpose. It probably should be separate from the patient's lower extremity orthoses so that he or she can wear it alone. Contraindications to bracing are obesity because of poor fit and hindrance of function, parents who cannot manage the orthosis, or repeated problems with skin breakdown with an apparently properly fitted and padded brace. The TLSO works best and the patient benefits most if the curve is flexible. The patient and his or her parents need to understand that the brace is not definitive treatment for the curve. Bracing does not need to be instituted until the curve is beginning to cause clinical problems, and it should be worn only when the patient is upright.

Bracing should be discontinued if the curve is progressing, if the patient cannot tolerate it, or when the child reaches 10 or 12 years old. At this point surgery should be performed, because children of this age have reached a significant amount of their adult trunk height, and arrest of further growth from the arthrodesis will not make their trunk-to-total-height measurement disproportionate. I do not routinely recommend or prescribe the suspension orthosis.[8]

Surgery on the myelomeningocele spine is and has been accompanied by numerous and serious complications.[9, 16, 20, 23, 27, 34] Although there are newer techniques of surgery and instrumentation, bank bone, and

antibiotics, the problems have not been eliminated. The patient's parents must be made aware of this before surgery and must accept these potential problems as part of the treatment. However, certain measures can be taken to minimize the chances of these complications. In addition to evaluating shunts and spinal canals preoperatively, sac penetration during surgery can be avoided by staying away from the midline in the area of the defect. The inverted Y incision is very useful for this (Fig. 13-2).[6, 20, 21] There is no advantage to exposing the midline in the area of the sac in these patients. The

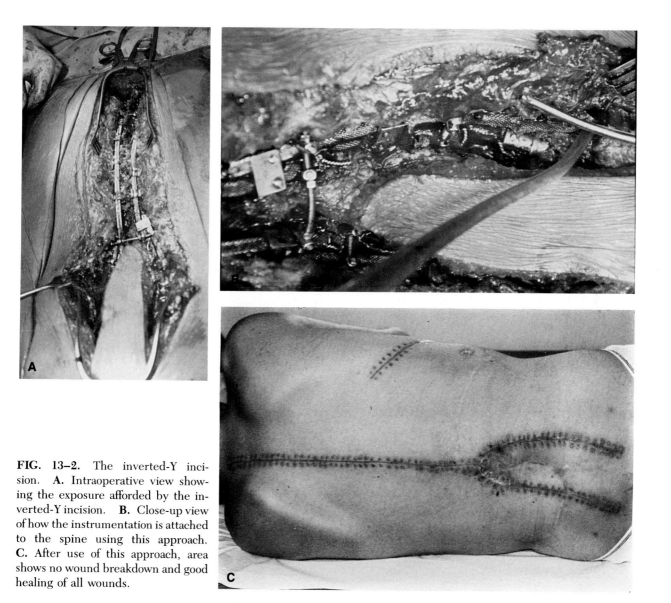

FIG. 13–2. The inverted-Y incision. **A.** Intraoperative view showing the exposure afforded by the inverted-Y incision. **B.** Close-up view of how the instrumentation is attached to the spine using this approach. **C.** After use of this approach, area shows no wound breakdown and good healing of all wounds.

vertebrae are splayed out, and the bone available for instrumentation and fusion is lateral. Dural tears are more likely to occur with a midline approach. Adequate soft tissue coverage of the bone and instrumentation is needed, and this should consist of more than just skin. Because mobilization of muscle or myocutaneous flaps may be necessary, the spinal surgeon should be proficient in the use of these techniques or have a plastic surgeon available.

The major problem with the myelomeningoceles and their spinal deformities is the lack of normal posterior vertebral elements, which makes achieving a solid fusion difficult (Fig. 13-3). This situation is coupled with abnormal placement of the paraspinal muscles, with the resultant lack of the usual soft tissue coverage of the spine and correct function of these muscles to aid in extension of the spine. Few of these patients can be adequately handled by posterior fusion and instrumentation alone.[6, 20, 21, 27] Taking this shortcut in an effort to minimize the number of operations often results in a pseudarthrosis or instrument failure, requiring more operations than would have been needed if proper anterior and posterior surgery had been done in the first place. High pseudarthrosis rates have plagued series of patients requiring myelomeningocele spinal surgery through the years; several studies have reported rates of 20 to 44%.[21, 28, 34] Therefore, every effort should be made to maximize the ability to achieve a solid fusion, and that requires anterior and posterior fusion.

An adequate supply of bank bone is essential to achieve a fusion. The iliac bone in these patients is not sufficient to provide the amount of bone graft needed, particularly because most of them need long fusions. Harvesting iliac bone should be avoided to maximize the bone stock of the ilium into which the rods are inserted, especially if the Galveston technique is used. Despite one report of poor results with the use of bank bone in cervical spine fusions in children, the use of bank bone has been generally successful.[10, 16, 23, 35]

Significant contractures around the hips can magnify the pelvic obliquity or influence the lumbar lordosis to such a degree that preliminary releases may be needed. In walkers, an effort should be made to limit the distal extent of the fusion, ending it above the pelvis. This eliminates the stresses on the instrumentation and fusion areas at the lumbosacral junction and allows some motion there for the adjustment of the lordosis in those who have mild, residual hip flexion contractures (see Fig. 13-14).

Infection remains a significant problem in these patients. Poor soft tissue coverage of the spine may lead to wound breakdown and superficial or deep infection. The incidence of wound infection in these patients is higher than it is for idiopathic scoliosis. Although Mayfield reported no wound infections in 20 patients undergoing anterior and posterior fusions after preliminary treatment of urinary tract infections, others have had different results.[21] Osebold and colleagues had an 8% incidence.[28] Sriram and associates had a 22% incidence.[34] Hull and colleagues had an unacceptable rate of infection of 67%.[16] The urine of these patients is often contaminated, and positive cultures in patients to be operated upon should be treated. In my opinion, cystitis or a positive urine culture without symptoms of fever or upper tract findings may be treated with anti-

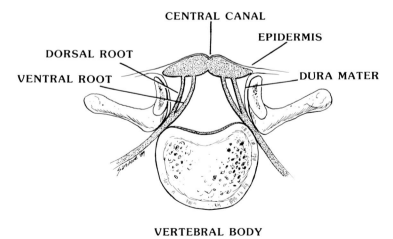

FIG. 13–3. Defects encountered in the area of the spina bifida showing the deficient posterior elements and the exposed, untubulated spinal cord.

biotics concomitant with surgery but started preoperatively. Using this regimen, I have not encountered any problems directly associated with urinary tract infections. Upper tract infection, however, needs to be eradicated preoperatively. An effort is also made to discontinue indwelling urinary catheters as soon as possible postoperatively and to resume intermittent catheterizations to decrease the possibility of causing a urinary tract infection.

SCOLIOSIS

Although all patients with myelomeningocele have congenital vertebral anomalies as a result of their dysraphism, some also have abnormalities that add the effects of congenital spinal deformity to the paralytic component. Therefore, scoliosis in the patient with myelomeningocele can be classified as congenital, paralytic, or combined. Congenital abnormalities other than those from the dysraphism can be problematic and cause a relentless progression of deformity in a very small, stunted spine. These congenital anomalies are like those in the usual cases of congenital scoliosis. However, many of these children have large, stiff curves at birth but do not undergo severe, rapid progression of the curve during early childhood because of poor growth potential in the abnormal segment. These particular patients represent a therapeutic dilemma, because even if a fusion in situ were to keep the curve from progressing, the child would still have a very significant deformity that requires correction to improve posture and trunk alignment. Surprisingly, many of these children have good neurologic function below the deformed level and have complex, stiff curves that would require osteotomies to correct, introducing the possibility of an unacceptable risk for neurologic complications.

The parents of many of these children are unwilling to accept the risk for complicated spinal corrective surgery when the children are young. Even if corrective surgery were attempted, the vertebrae are too small and weak to accommodate the internal fixation necessary to achieve the desired correction. Although turnbuckle casts may be an alternative, they may also cause serious complications, such as decubiti and interference with the child's development. However, in a situation in which there is a more isolated congenital anomaly (such as a hemivertebra or a congenital bar)

that has a significant risk of progression or that has demonstrated progression, the usual means of managing congenital scoliosis should be used to control that portion of the spine (Fig. 13-4).

Paralytic scoliosis is the most common spinal deformity, and lordoscoliosis is the most common subgroup. Although these curves can become quite large, many of them remain flexible for prolonged periods. This is helpful when the surgery becomes necessary and also preoperatively, when bracing may be appropriate. Children with large curves as youngsters may be managed with bracing until 10 or 12 years of age, at which time definitive surgery should be done to correct and stabilize their spines. Because the children are older when surgery becomes necessary, their vertebrae are of adequate size for accepting the more standard types of instrumentation. Preoperatively, these children need to have their ventricular-peritoneal shunts evaluated for function and their genitourinary tracts examined to rule out active infection. Some of these patients also need evaluation of their spinal canals, as was previously mentioned.

When both anterior and posterior fusions are planned—and almost every patient requiring surgery for myelomeningocele needs both—the anterior fusion should be done first. Adequate exposure and meticulous discectomies must be performed. I perform my own chest and abdominal approaches, but routine assistance of a pediatric or general surgeon may be preferred. Involvement of another surgeon, however, often complicates scheduling, and for orthopedic surgeons experienced in these approaches, another surgeon's presence is not usually necessary. In certain situations, however, such as reoperations or surgery for patients who have had multiple abdominal procedures, their help may be required.

The eventual distal level of instrumentation posteriorly should be decided before the anterior fusion, because the anterior and posterior fusions should extend, ideally, to the same level. Therefore, if a fusion to the sacrum is planned with instrumentation posteriorly, the discectomies must be carried down to the L5–S1 level. This level is almost always accessible, at least for discectomy, after the ascending lumbar vein is ligated and divided.

The discectomy should be thorough. Careful assessment of the rotation of the spine is needed intraoperatively to determine the position of the spinal canal so that it is not entered. Subperiosteal exposure

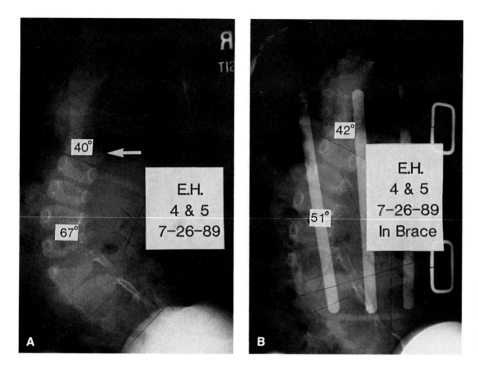

FIG. 13–4. A 4-year-old girl with myelomeningocele associated with congenital spinal deformities. **A.** Posterior-anterior (PA) sitting roentgenogram out of the brace showing the multiple abnormal vertebrae in this child's spine. There is a fully segmented hemivertebra (*arrow*) at the end of a segment of the spine with numerous congenital anomalies. **B.** An upright sitting PA roentgenogram in her brace showing some correction of the paralytic portion of her curve. Pelvic obliquity has been corrected to some degree because of the brace.

of the vertebrae facilitates discectomy and aids in achieving an arthrodesis. The periosteum and anterior longitudinal ligament are reflected with electrocautery and periosteal elevators; they are later reapproximated after the discs are filled with bone graft. The discs are removed with osteotomes, rongeurs, and curettes. Spreading the disc space open with a lamina spreader helps in removing the part of the disc over the posterior longitudinal ligament and facilitates a complete discectomy. Retraction of the psoas muscle is aided by stay sutures placed in the medial edge of the muscle; they are then attached to hemostats. An additional maneuver to aid retraction of the wound during a thoracoabdominal approach without the use of a large chest retractor is to suture the everted abdominal muscle and skin edge to the flank. This frees the assistant's hands and keeps unnecessary instruments out of the wound.

During the anterior procedure, the anesthesiologist should be allowed to expand the lungs periodically to avoid atelectasis. Although a rib is usually removed at the time of exposure, it may not provide enough bone for bone graft; bank bone is necessary to augment the available rib.

A small number of patients (mid to low lumbar level, ambulatory) may be candidates for anterior spinal fusion with instrumentation alone. The Dwyer or Zielke instrumentation may afford excellent correction and allow mobile segments below the fusion (Fig. 13-5). In patients who also need posterior fusion and instrumentation, however, anterior instrumentation may not always be absolutely necessary, especially if the posterior fusion will be taken down to the pelvis. It is very difficult to instrument to the sacrum anteriorly; therefore, using anterior instrumentation that ends two or three levels above the eventual posterior instrumentation may cause a stress riser effect and be detrimental to a solid posterior fusion at those lower levels (Fig. 13-6). Proper discectomies will loosen up the spine, and some immediate correction will occur even without the instrumentation.

If anterior instrumentation is used, care must be taken not to kyphose the lumbar spine. This is easy to do, especially with the Dwyer instrumentation. The sagittal contour of the spine should be normalized for proper weight bearing on the ischium and posterior thighs, which a kyphotic lumbosacral spine prevents.

Various types of instrumentation can be used poste-

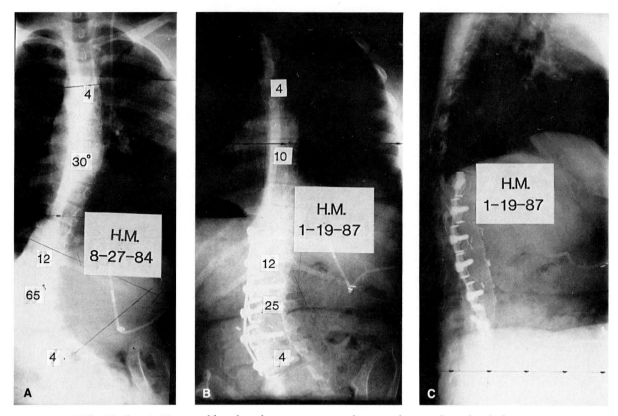

FIG. 13–5. A 10-year-old girl with progressive scoliosis with neurologic level about L3–L4. **A.** Posterior-anterior sitting roentgenogram of the spine showing her curves preoperatively with significant pelvic obliquity. **B.** Postoperative film taken over 2.5 years after her surgery, showing the presence of Dwyer instrumentation, correction of her scoliosis with fairly good balance of the trunk, and significant correction of her pelvic obliquity. **C.** Lateral sitting roentgenogram showing that the lumbar lordosis has been somewhat flattened with the instrumentation.

riorly. Actually, this may require creative hybrids to obtain the desired correction and fixation (Fig. 13-7). It must be remembered that a variable number of vertebrae have deficient posterior elements that can limit the usual fixation sites. I prefer the inverted Y incision posteriorly; this allows good exposure of the available bone while minimizing the risk of entering the dural sac. With this approach, the dissection can be performed out to the tips of the transverse processes alongside the rudimentary lamina. The lamina, pars, and pedicles can be located and used for fixation sites. The lamina can be used to anchor Drummond wires from inside out, and the pars can be encircled by wires as well.

Cotrel–Dubousset instrumentation with pedicle fixation into the lumbar vertebra has been used and is especially useful when fusion to the pelvis can be avoided (Fig. 13-8).

Pelvic fixation is still best achieved by the Galveston technique or one of its modifications. If the curve is fairly flexible and pelvic obliquity is easily correctable by straightening the curve, the standard Luque construct can be used (Fig. 13-9).[8, 9] However, if pelvic obliquity is a major problem in addition to the curve and if some distraction force on the concave side of the curve is desirable to achieve and maintain correction, Cotrel–Dubousset instrumentation to the pelvis in the Galveston configuration can be achieved by using one long rod into the pelvis or two rods joined

(*text continues on page 332*)

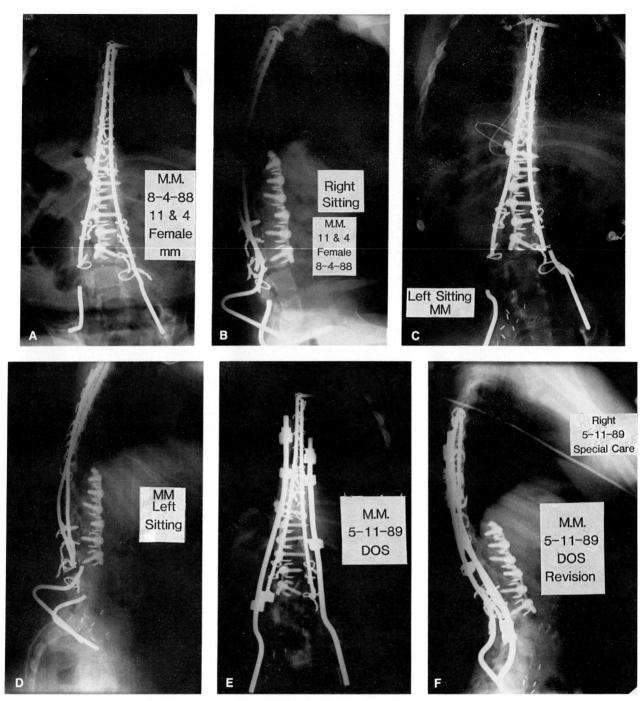

FIG. 13–6. An 11 + 4-year-old girl with lower thoracic level myelomeningocele after anterior and posterior spinal fusions. **A,B.** Posterior-anterior and lateral sitting roentgenograms showing broken Luque rods and the relative kyphosis of the lumbar spine under the Dwyer instrumentation done at another institution. Although excellent correction was obtained in the segment that incorporated the Dwyer instrumentation, no anterior fusion was done below the Dwyer instrumentation. **C,D.** Anterior-posterior and lateral postoperative roentgenograms after doing an anterior interbody spinal fusion from the last level of the Dwyer instrumentation down to the sacrum. **E,F.** Anterior-posterior and lateral postoperative roentgenograms after revision of the posterior instrumentation using Cotrel–Dubousset instruments into the pelvis in the Galveston configuration.

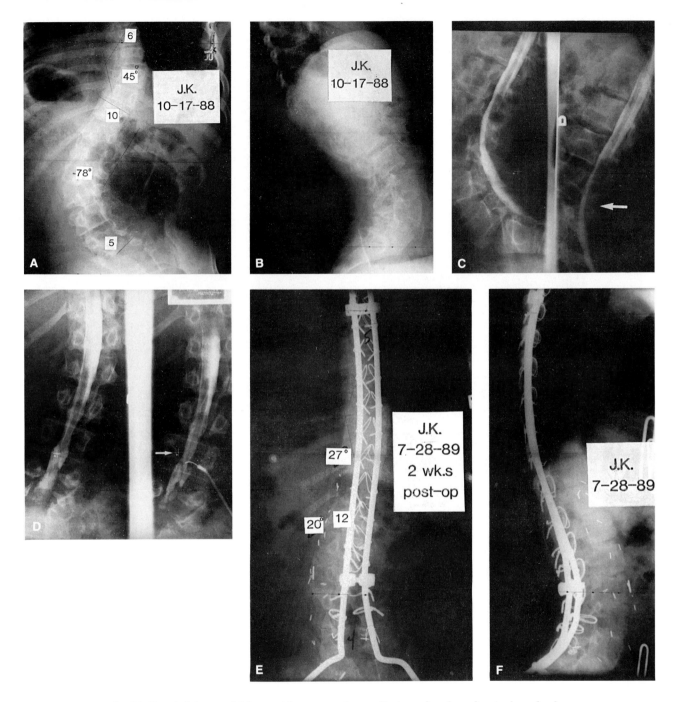

FIG. 13–7. A 14-year-old boy with progressive scoliosis and tethered spinal cord whose neurologic level was L3–L4. **A,B.** Posterior-anterior and lateral sitting roentgenograms of the thoracolumbar spine showing severe left thoracolumbar curve. **C,D.** Myelogram showing low-lying conus (*arrows*). This patient had his tethered cord released before the corrective surgery. **E,F.** Sitting posterior-anterior and lateral thoracolumbar spine roentgenograms after anterior or posterior surgery showing presence of Luque instrumentation attached to the spine with sublaminar wires and Drummond wires in the area of the spina bifida defect, with the rods coupled with the Texas Scottish Rite Crosslink™ System.

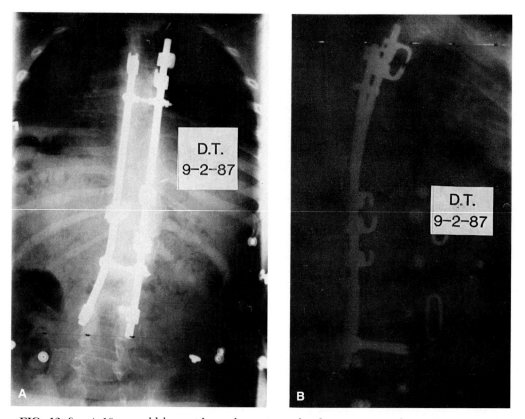

FIG. 13–8. A 10-year-old boy with myelomeningocele after anterior and posterior surgery with posterior Cotrel–Dubousset instrumentation incorporating both hooks and pedicle screws. Postoperative anterior-posterior (**A**) and lateral (**B**) sitting thoracolumbar spine roentgenograms depict anterior and posterior spinal fusion and instrumentation.

by connectors such as Cotrel–Dubousset dominoes and axial connectors (Stuart, Greensburg, PA) or the Texas Scottish Rite Crosslink™ System (Danek, Memphis, TN) (Fig. 13-10).[30] Experience with dominoes and cross-links in paralytic scoliosis is limited. Although using them bilaterally at the same level may pose no problem, it may be better to stagger the connections by a couple of segments to reduce the potential stress riser.

The Cotrel–Dubousset system offers the advantage of being able to apply distraction force along the rod while still being able to connect with the pelvis. When using this system with two rods on each side, the long rod should be attached to the spine as far down as possible. Whether the derotation maneuver can be used to achieve the correction is determined by the stiffness of the curve. The second rod should overlap the first enough to get firm fixation and to prevent a junctional kyphosis if the dominoes or crosslinks are used. The second rod is contoured to fit into the ilium according to the Galveston concept and connected to it as mentioned. Vertebrae that do not accept a Cotrel–Dubousset hook can be connected to the rods with wires passed around the pars or pedicles or with Drummond wires that are passed through the rudimentary lamina (Fig. 13-11). Alternatively, pedicle screws can be used in the lower lumbar vertebrae. The cannulated Cotrel–Dubousset Iliosacral screws are also helpful for spinopelvic fixation. The Cotrel–Dubousset alar staples alone are probably not reliable. Pelvic fixation by means of sacral pedicle screws is also probably not reliable in these small osteopenic patients either.[6a]

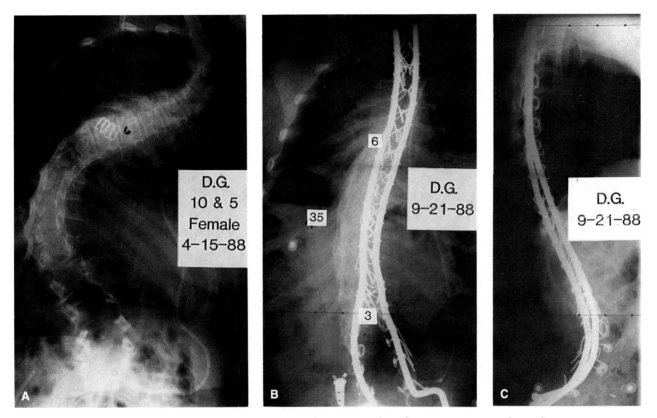

FIG. 13–9. A 10 + 5-year-old girl with myelomeningocele and progressive severe thoracolumbar scoliosis. **A.** Preoperative sitting posterior-anterior thoracolumbar spine film showing the severe scoliosis. This patient also had a relatively severe preoperative lumbar lordosis. **B, C.** Postoperative sitting posterior-anterior and lateral thoracolumbar spine roentgenograms showing the Luque instrumentation in place with a nearly level pelvis and excellent correction of her scoliosis.

Although various types of hooks for Moe rods have been used successfully to instrument and fuse to the pelvis in some patients, this configuration does not adequately immobilize the lumbosacral junction. The construct is analogous to trying to achieve a knee fusion by placing one pin of the compression clamp through the distal femur and resting the other on the top of the tibial plateau. More secure types of fixation are desirable.

Attention to sagittal contour of the spine while correcting the scoliosis is very important (Fig. 13-12). Even though many of these patients do not walk, maintenance of the lumbar lordosis is important. By producing lumbar lordosis, the distribution of weight while sitting is extended over the ischia and the posterior thighs. If the lumbar lordosis is flattened, it tends to rotate the pelvis and direct much of the sitting weight on the ischia, encouraging the development of pressure sores. It is important to lock together solidly the two rods, whether using the Cotrel–Dubousset system or the Luque system. This can be done very nicely using the Texas Scottish Rite Crosslink™ System or the Cotrel–Dubousset devices for transverse traction (DTT).

The surgeon who manages myelomeningocele spinal deformity must have the ability to use many kinds of instrumentation and the availability in the operating room of various instrumentation systems. Even though

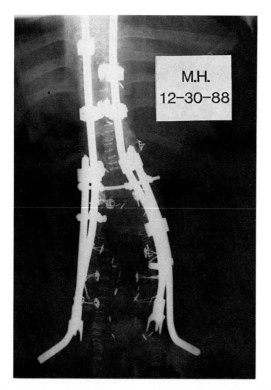

FIG. 13–10. An anterior-posterior roentgenogram of the lumbosacral spine showing Cotrel–Dubousset (CD) instrumentation used down to the pelvis. The long rods that extended throughout the thoracolumbar spine were secured to the spine by the CD hooks and Drummond wires and anchored to the ala of the sacrum with the CD sacral staples. Shorter rods were contoured to fit into the ilium by the Galveston technique and were secured to the two long rods with dominoes and DTTs.

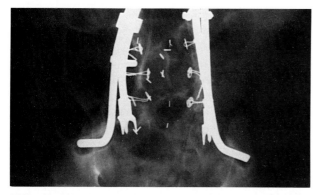

FIG. 13–11. An anterior-posterior roentgenogram of the lumbosacral spine. The rods are attached to the spine in the area of deficient posterior elements by Drummond wires passed from the undersurface of the lamina outward to the rods.

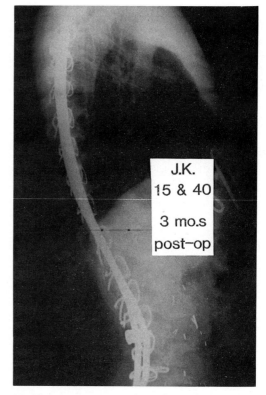

FIG. 13–12. Postoperative lateral sitting thoracolumbar spine roentgenogram showing excellent sagittal contour.

there may be adequate preoperative planning, intraoperative events may dictate a change in instrumentation. If alternatives are not available in the operating room, compromises will have to be made.

Because most of these patients require instrumentation to the ilium and because the ilia are small, bank bone is used to achieve a fusion. Commercially available bank bone can be stored on the shelf in the operating room. This bone is harvested under sterile conditions, and testing of donors for hepatitis and HIV and other diseases is now routinely done. Usually morselized cancellous or cortical cancellous preparations are used. Other specific forms are also available, such as rib or fibular struts.

I have used postoperative orthoses for these patients, although others do not (Fig. 13-13). Even though the fixation is designed to be as secure and as rigid as possible, the additional external support protects the instrumentation from extremes of trunk motion and often gives the parents, patients, and surgeons an additional sense of security.

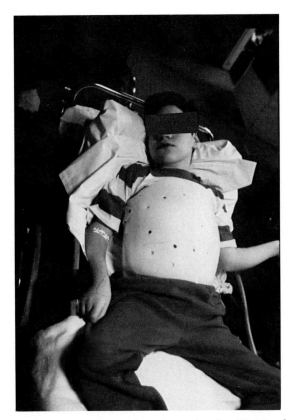

FIG. 13–13. Patient in his plastic bivalve TLSO after surgery.

If during the postoperative period a problem develops with the instrumentation or it becomes obvious that a pseudarthrosis is forming, corrective action should be considered, even in the absence of clinical symptoms (Fig. 13-14).

Halo traction for patients with myelomeningocele may be dangerous. Even though care may prevent placing a pin in the shunt reservoir, the stretching of the neck may have an adverse effect on the shunt or the Arnold-Chiari malformation. Therefore, I have abandoned its use in treating the myelomeningocele patient. There is enough potential for postoperative complications without encouraging more.

KYPHOSIS

Kyphosis in the myelomeningocele can be classified as paralytic or congenital. Regardless of the type, severe kyphosis can have a detrimental effect on function. The child with severe collapsing kyphosis must use his arms to support himself while sitting. If these curves are flexible, orthoses can help realign the spine and improve sitting posture, but the orthosis cannot change the natural history of the curve.[6]

Congenital kyphosis in the myelomeningocele represents the full expression of severe spinal dysraphism.[15, 32] These children usually have high neurologic levels of involvement, significant hydrocephalus, problems with skin breakdown over the kyphosis, and abnormal sitting posture.[3, 7, 13, 17, 18, 26] The displacement of the paraspinal muscles anteriorly and laterally makes them perverted flexors of the spine. The psoas is displaced anteriorly and is bow-strung across the concavity of the curve. All these factors contribute to a rigid curve.

In a patient with a very severe acute kyphus, the underlying sac may actually undergo attrition from pressure on it. The child with a severe congenital kyphosis is difficult to brace with a parapodium or HKAFOs and so may be unable to be placed in the upright position. In Raycroft and Curtis' series, 12 of 80 patients with spinal deformity had primarily kyphotic deformities.[30] Other series have reported incidences of between 8 and 15%.[9, 15, 29, 33]

Paralytic Kyphosis

Paralytic kyphosis with or without scoliosis can be treated by standard means of anterior spinal fusion followed by posterior spinal fusion and instrumentation. The kyphosis may be stiff or relatively flexible although its magnitude is large. The younger children may be managed initially with a TLSO to facilitate better upright posture. When surgery becomes necessary, an anterior spinal fusion over the area of the apex and all levels with deficient posterior elements to be instrumented posteriorly should be done. This is followed by a posterior spinal fusion with appropriate instrumentation. The Cotrel–Dubousset instrumentation is particularly good for this because of its ability to compress across the apex. The compression is provided by hooks in a compression construct or by the use of pedicle screws in areas where the posterior elements are deficient. The distal extent of the fusion is dictated by the position of the curve and the patient's ambulatory status. If the fusion needs to extend to the pelvis,

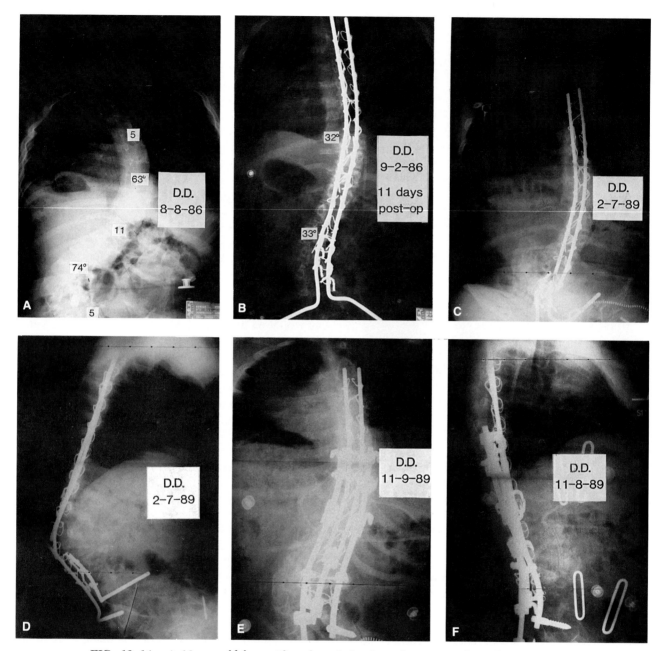

FIG. 13–14.   A 16-year-old boy with a thoracic-level myelomeningocele with progressive severe scoliosis.   **A.**   Posterior-anterior (PA) sitting thoracolumbar spine roentgenogram showing severe scoliosis.   **B.**   Postoperative PA sitting thoracolumbar spine film after anterior and posterior fusion with instrumentation using the ³/₁₆-in Luque rods posteriorly.   **C,D.**   Sitting PA and lateral thoracolumbar spine roentgenograms 3 years postoperatively showing breakage of the Luque rods, loss of correction, particularly in the sagittal plane, and formation of hypertrophic bone. This patient also had severely limited hip flexion. He used the pseudarthrosis in his spine to allow himself to sit.   **E,F.**   Sitting PA and lateral thoracolumbar spine roentgenograms after revision of the pseudarthrosis front and back using Cotrel–Dubousset instrumentation posteriorly. After these procedures were completed, the patient returned for flexion-shortening osteotomies of the femurs, which allowed his hips to flex at least 100° bilaterally. This took the stress off the spinal pseudarthrosis.

then the four-rod construct can be used (Fig. 13-15A–H). A postoperative TLSO is recommended to decrease gross motion of the spine. As in all cases of myelomeningocele spinal surgery, adequate amounts of bank bone will be needed.

Congenital Kyphosis

The congenital kyphotic spine in the myelomeningocele is a more difficult problem than the paralytic kyphotic spine and requires a different approach. The usual methods to correct a kyphosis do not work well in this situation. Any significant residual kyphosis predisposes the patient to recurrent deformity. Early attempts to decrease the kyphosis by resecting the apex of the curve and implantation of inadequate or inappropriate fixation failed.[25, 31] Although strut grafting across the concavity of the curve may arrest the initial kyphosis, as the child grows, fall-off over the top of the fused segment often occurs. Moreover, it does not correct the curve or elongate the trunk. Lindseth and Stelzer made a significant contribution to the treatment of this problem.[18] Although they used minimal fixation and a pantaloon cast postoperatively, they found that excising the upper lordotic portion of the kyphus yielded better correction and fewer recurrent deformities (Fig. 13-16). Christopherson and Brooks, using prolonged postoperative casting, reported a 50% loss of correction in 3 of their 9 patients.[7] Although good correction can be achieved initially by the proper resection level, minimal internal fixation, and prolonged use of a pantaloon cast, in these patients this technique has its disadvantages, with loss of correction and the complications associated with prolonged casting.

I feel that rigid fixation, coupled with the use of a postoperative brace, allows the children to resume their upright activities as soon as possible while still maintaining good alignment and minimizing the risk of recurrent deformity. In support of this, McMaster showed that long fusions with rigid internal fixation had the best results.[27] Similarly, Heydemann and Gillespie, using Luque rods with special lower end contouring, corrected the deformities from an average preoperative measurement of 124° to 32.8°.[13] Half of their patients had had prior strut grafts that failed. The average age at surgery for these series was 10 to 11 years old.

Various types of instrumentation systems have been described to achieve and maintain correction in these patients. The Harrington compression system, a special hook cable system described by Mayfield, and the McKay plate have all been used in various series.[22, 25] However, I believe that Luque rods with the special lower-end contouring, as described by Heydemann and Gillespie, achieve the best correction and fixation (Fig. 13-17).[13] Although it is technically possible to do a vertebral resection without excising the overlying spinal cord and dural sac, it seems much better to do so and remove the sac from danger of perforation. This also facilitates the bony work and provides more area for bone grafting. A prerequisite for this technique of vertebral resection is good hip flexion. The technique uses extension of the lumbosacral spine, pelvis, and hips during the correction, and if hip flexion is poor the patient will not be able to sit after surgery.

Other than neonatal vertebrectomy, the timing of such a procedure is difficult to determine. Bracing is not effective in these situations, and therefore the procedure is indicated when the kyphos is progressing or causing problems such as skin breakdown. In children with a large, congenital kyphosis at birth, neonatal vertebrectomy at the time of sac closure may be helpful in eliminating or minimizing the risk of kyphosis in the future. Unfortunately, orthopedic surgeons are usually not involved in the sac closure, and although neurosurgeons may find it difficult to close the soft tissues on such patients, vertebrectomy usually is not considered.

The surgery involved in accomplishing neonatal vertebrectomy is not particularly difficult and can be done with or without cord sacrifice. The osteotomized spine is stabilized with wires or heavy sutures around the adjoining pedicles or through the vertebral bodies (Fig. 13-18; see also Color Plate 6). Soft tissue coverage should consist of swinging muscle over the posterior aspect of the spine, to aid in better soft tissue coverage and to provide some extensor muscle function for the spine. Simple positioning of the infant in the prone position postoperatively is used. Perhaps more frequent use of this approach may decrease the incidence of severe kyphosis later on; in the past, however, this approach has not been consistently beneficial.[31] In older children, the procedure becomes a bit more complicated, but rigid fixation with resumption of upright activities as soon as possible is desirable.

The operation should be done in a step-wise fashion so that the procedure can be aborted easily if problems

(text continues on page 341)

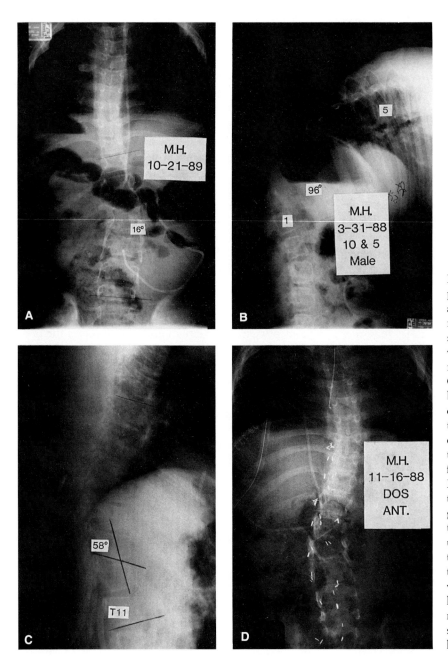

FIG. 13–15. A 10-year-old boy with paralytic kyphosis. **A,B.** Posterior-anterior (PA) and lateral sitting thoracolumbar spine roentgenograms showing the lack of severe scoliosis but wide open posterior elements and the rather severe collapsing kyphosis. **C.** Hyperextension lateral thoracolumbar spine roentgenogram showing good correction of the kyphosis. **D.** An AP thoracolumbar roentgenogram immediately after the anterior fusion showing the extent of anterior discectomy and fusion as indicated by the hemoclips. **E,F.** Postoperative PA and lateral sitting thoracolumbar spine roentgenograms showing excellent correction of the lateral contour of the spine after the use of Cotrel–Dubousset instrumentation with the four-rod construct and attachment to the pelvis with the Galveston technique. **G,H.** PA and lateral sitting thoracolumbar spine roentgenograms 8 months after surgery showing no loss of correction and excellent maintenance of the sagittal contour.

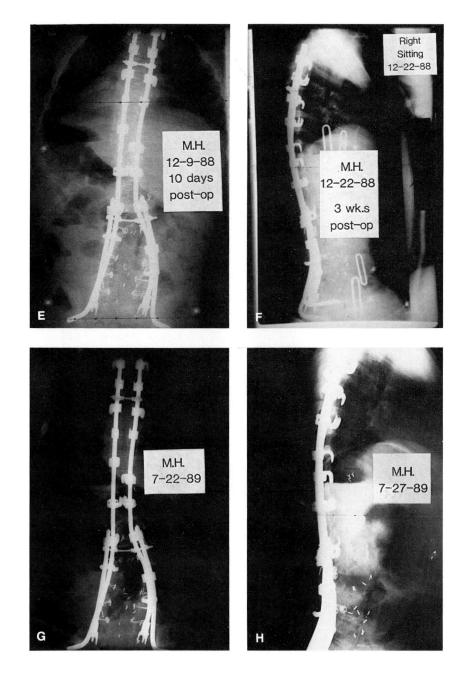

FIG. 13–15. *(continued)*

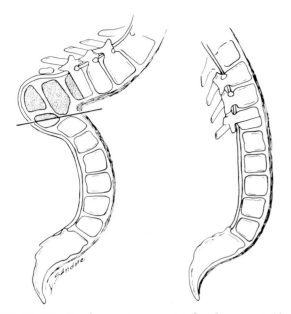

FIG. 13–16.   Kyphotic spine associated with congenital ky-phosis in the myelomeningocele showing the extent of resec-tion necessary for adequate correction of the deformity. This involves the upper lordotic limb of the kyphosis.

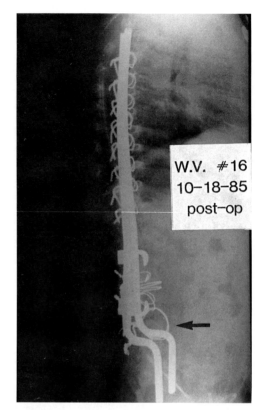

FIG. 13–17.   Rod contouring of the Luque rods used for correction of congenital kyphosis.

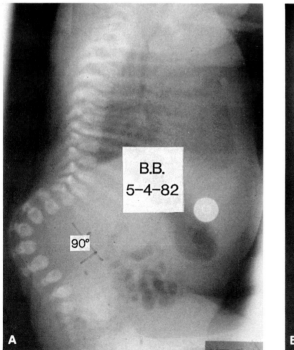

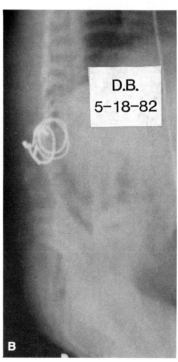

FIG. 13–18.   Neonatal ver-tebrectomy for severe kyphosis noted at birth. **A.** Lateral thoracolumbar spine roent-genogram showing the rather severe lumbar kyphosis. **B.** Postoperative lateral tho-racolumbar roentgenogram showing correction of the ky-phosis and fixation with wire. The skin was approximated pri-marily after resection of the ver-tebrae and the paraspinal mus-cles and was swung over the spine before the skin closure. (See also Color Plate 6.)

arise, although this has been necessary in only a few cases in my experience. These operations are potentially bloody and the patients are often frail to begin with. Their lack of sympathetic function in the lower extremities makes their blood pressures labile. I recommend using a cell saver (Haemonetics, Braintree, MA) to salvage blood during the procedure.

The procedure should start with exposure (Fig. 13-19A–C) of the normal thoracic spine, with exposure of the posterior elements according to whether fusion will be done in that area. This also involves removal of the ligamentum flavum in preparation for the passage of the sublaminar wires.

The next step is cord and dural division. This is a critical part of the procedure and is often unavoidably bloody. The area just above the dilated sac is selected for durotomy. Stay sutures should be placed before the opening of the dura, and circumferential mobilization of the dural tube should be done before opening it. Bleeding is controlled by bipolar cautery, gelfoam (Upjohn, Kalamazoo, MI), and cottonoids. Avitine (Alcon Labs, Ft. Worth, TX) is useful in this situation but cannot be used with the cell saver. The dura is opened transversely. The spinal cord is divided after coagulation of the vessels and allowed to retract upward (see Fig. 13-19). After all bleeding from the cord is controlled, the durotomy is completed and the dura closed below the divided cord with running or interrupted sutures. Circumferential ligatures of the cord and dura together should not be done, to avoid hypertensive crisis caused by acute hydrocephalus.[36] The area can then be sealed off further with gelfoam after testing the closure with a Valsalva maneuver performed by the anesthesiologist. The distal sac is removed, using cautery and bone wax to control bleeding (see Fig. 13-18).

Once the sac has been removed, circumferential dissection of the spine is necessary, particularly at the apex and around the upper lordotic aspect of the kyphos (see Fig. 13-19F). After this is done, the spine can be divided at the apex, and the two sections are overlapped to determine the appropriate level of the second osteotomy. The excised segment can be used to supply some bone graft (Fig. 13-19G). An effort should be made to leave the anterior longitudinal ligament in place in front of the spine; bone graft can then be placed between it and the spine.

Instrumentation is the next step. Many different types of constructs have been used, but I have found that Luque rods contoured distally, similar to those described by Heydemann and Gillespie, work best.[13] This construct aids in the intraoperative correction of the deformity and the maintenance of that correction after surgery. The distal ends of the rods should be placed through sacral foramina and lie anterior to the sacrum. By pushing forward on the rods above, the lower lumbar spine, sacrum, and pelvis are rotated (extending the spine) until the osteotomy site closes. Sublaminar wires in the more normal thoracic spine are passed in the usual fashion. In the lower segment, wires are passed around the pedicles, through foramina, and even circumferentially around the entire vertebral bodies to achieve as rigid a construct as possible (Fig. 13-19H,I). In some cases, a two-hook Harrington compression system (Fig. 13-20) or a Cotrel–Dubousset compression construct (Fig. 13-21) has been used to compress across the osteotomy. The pediatric Cotrel–Dubousset system is useful when there are few fixation sites even for wires. In this situation the lower parts of the rods are bent in the usual fashion, and upper fixation is achieved with hooks. Pedicle screw systems may be useful in this situation, but they are probably too large and prominent for most of these patients.

After the instrumentation has been secured, decortication is performed and autogenous and bank bone graft is inserted posteriorly and anteriorly around the osteotomy site of vertebral bodies. Whether or not to fuse the upper part of the spine is up to the surgeon. I have found a modest degree of growth in this area when it is not fused.

Closure is very important. Muscle should be swung over the spine and the instrumentation to add soft tissue coverage. This is accomplished by undermining the skin and freeing the latissimus dorsi and the displaced paraspinal muscles. These are displaced medially and sutured over the spine. It is important that they be dissected enough so that there is essentially no tension on the suture lines. The skin can then be closed with interrupted sutures. It has been necessary to mobilize formal myocutaneous flaps in a few cases, but this step is usually not needed. Preliminary use of tissue expanders can also be helpful but probably is not necessary in the majority of cases. I prefer to close the skin over Jackson Pratt drains (American V. Mueller, Chicago, IL).

The child should be nursed in a prone or decubitus position so as not to interfere with the blood supply of

(text continues on page 344)

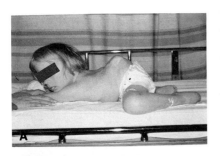

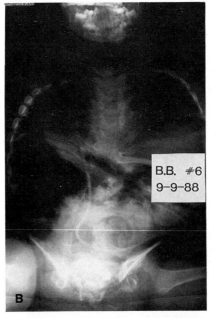

B.B. #6
9-9-88

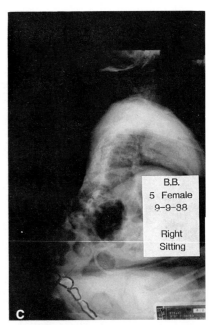

B.B.
5 Female
9-9-88

Right
Sitting

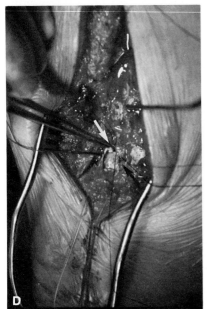

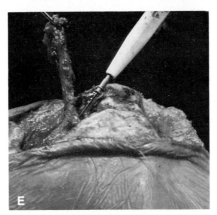

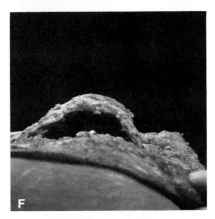

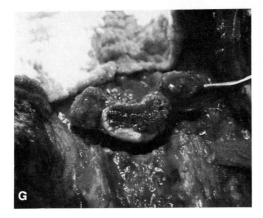

FIG. 13–19.

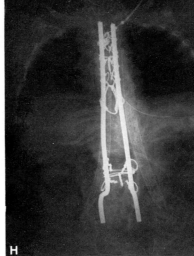

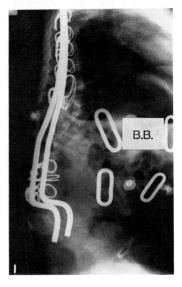

B.B.

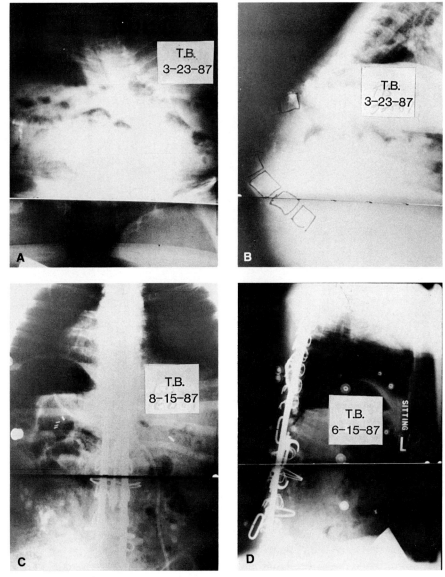

FIG. 13–20. A 10-year-old girl with congenital kyphosis and spina bifida. **A,B.** Posterior-anterior and lateral sitting thoracolumbar films preoperatively showing a very severe kyphosis. **C,D.** Postoperative sitting posterior-anterior and lateral thoracolumbar spine roentgenograms showing excellent correction of the kyphosis. Two Luque rods and a midline Harrington compression device were used for the construct.

◀ **FIG. 13–19.** A young child with congenital kyphosis. **A.** Clinical photograph of the patient preoperatively showing the very severe angular kyphosis. **B,C.** Posterior-anterior and lateral sitting thoracolumbar spine roentgenograms showing the severe spinal dysraphism and severe kyphosis. **D.** Intraoperative photograph at the time of durotomy and spinal cord transection. The *white arrow* points to the forceps holding the end of the spinal cord after it has been transected. The *black arrow* points to the open dura and the subarachnoid space. Stay sutures are present in preparation for closure of the dura. **E.** Resection of the sac after spinal cord transection. **F.** Photograph of the exposed kyphotic area of the spine after complete circumferential dissection. **G.** Intraoperative photograph after transection of the spine and resection of the upper lordotic portion of the kyphosis. Although the posterior elements are quite deficient, the vertebral bodies are relatively normal. **H,I.** Anterior-posterior and lateral thoracolumbar spine roentgenograms postoperatively showing excellent correction of the kyphosis.

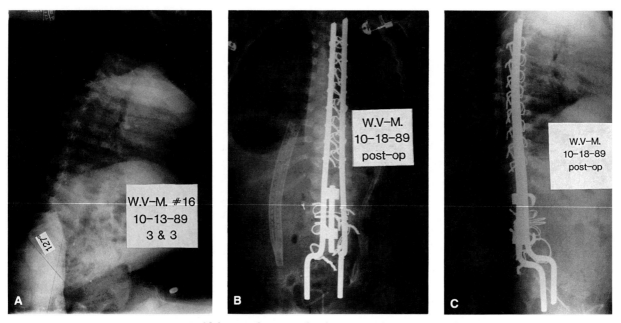

FIG. 13–21. A 3-year-old boy with severe kyphosis. **A.** Preoperative lateral sitting thoracolumbar spine roentgenogram showing very severe kyphosis. **B,C.** Anterior-posterior and lateral thoracolumbar spine roentgenograms showing two Luque rods and a midline pediatric Cotrel–Dubousset compression system offering excellent correction of the kyphosis.

the skin and muscle. Drains are left in place until there is no more drainage. After they are out, the child may sit up in bed and be molded for his or her TLSO. Once the TLSO is delivered, all usual wheelchair activities may be resumed.

The surgical treatment of congenital kyphosis in the myelomeningocele is one of the most difficult in spinal surgery. Because the potential risks are great, this is a procedure only for experienced spinal surgeons. To make it as safe as possible, appropriate anesthesia and postoperative support personnel are essential.

References

1. Allen BL Jr: The operative treatment of myelomeningocele spinal deformity. Orthop Clin North Am 10:845, 1979
2. Allen BL Jr, Ferguson RL: The place for segmental instrumentation in the treatment of spinal deformities. Orthop Trans 6:21, 1982
3. Banta JV, Hamada JS: Natural history of the kyphotic deformity in myelomeningocele. J Bone Joint Surg [Am] 55:279, 1976
4. Banta JV, Whiteman S, Dych PM, et al: Fifteen-year review of myelodysplasia. J Bone Joint Surg [Am] 58:726, 1976
5. Banta JV, Park SM: Improvement in pulmonary function in patients having combined anterior and posterior spine fusions for myelomeningocele scoliosis. Spine 8:765, 1983
6. Bradford DS, Lonstein JE, Ogilvie JW, Winter RB (eds): Moe's Textbook of Scoliosis and Other Spinal Deformities, 2nd ed. Philadelphia, WB Saunders, 1987
6a. Camp JF, Caudle R, Ashmun RD, Roach J: Immediate complications of Cotrel–Dubousset instrumentation to the sacropelvis: A clinical and biomechanical study. Spine 15:932, 1990
7. Christopherson MR, Brooks AL: Excision and wire fixation of rigid myelomeningocele kyphosis. J Pediatr Orthop 5:717, 1985
8. Drennan JC, Renshaw TS, Curtis BH: The thoracic suspension orthosis. Clin Orthop 139:33, 1979
9. Eyring EJ, Wonhen JJ, Sayers MP: Spinal osteotomy for kyphosis in myelomeningocele. Clin Orthop 88:24, 1972
10. Goldberg VM, Stevenson S: Natural history of autografts and allografts. Clin Orthop 225:7, 1987
11. Hall JE, Poitras B: The management of kyphosis in patients with myelomeningocele. Clin Orthop 128:33, 1977
12. Hall PV, Lindseth RE, Campbell RL, Kalsbeck JE: Myelodysplasia and development of scoliosis: a manifestation of syringomyelia. Spine 1:48, 1976
13. Heydemann JS, Gillespie R: Management of myelomeningocele kyphosis in the older child by kyphectomy and segmental spinal instrumentation. Spine 12:37, 1987

14. Holtzman RN, Stein BM (eds): The Tethered Spinal Cord. New York, Thieme-Stratton, 1985
15. Hoppenfeld S: Congenital kyphosis in myelomeningocele. J Bone Joint Surg [Br] 49:276, 1967
16. Hull WJ, Moe JH, Loi C, Winter RB: The surgical treatment of spinal deformities in myelomeningocele. J Bone Joint Surg [Am] 57:1767, 1974
17. Knapp DR Jr, Jones ET: Use of cortical-cancellous allograft for posterior spinal fusion. Clin Orthop 229:99, 1988
18. Lindseth AE, Stelzer L: Vertebral excision for kyphosis in children with myelomeningocele. J Bone Joint Surg [Am] 61:699, 1979
19. Lubicky JP, Fredrickson BE: Combined use of vertebral resection, spinal cord excision, Luque instrumentation and myocutaneous flaps for the treatment of severe kyphoses in the myelomeningocele. Paper presented at 18th annual meeting of Scoliosis Research Society, New Orleans, 1983
20. Mackel JL, Lindseth RE: Scoliosis in myelodysplasia. J Bone Joint Surg [Am] 57:1031, 1975
21. Mayfield JK: Severe spinal deformity in myelodysplasia and sacral agenesis—an aggressive surgical approach. Spine 6:498, 1981
22. Mayfield JK: Spinal deformity in myelomeningocele. In Bradford DS, Hensinger RN (eds): The Pediatric Spine. New York, Thieme, 1985
23. Mayfield JK, King H: Congenital lumbar kyphosis—an alternative instrumentation system. Paper presented at 18th annual meeting of Scoliosis Research Society, New Orleans, 1983
24. McCarthy RE: Allograft bone in spinal fusion for paralytic scoliosis. J Bone Joint Surg [Am] 68:370, 1986
25. McKay DW: Use of the McKay plate in kyphosis. Orthop Trans 6:70, 1982
26. McLauren RL: Myelomeningocele. New York, Grune & Stratton, 1976
27. McMaster JJ: The long-term results of kyphectomy and spinal stabilization in children with myelomeningocele. Spine 13:417, 1988
28. Osebold WR, Mayfield JK, Winter RB: Surgical treatment of paralytic scoliosis associated with myelomeningocele. J Bone Joint Surg [Am] 64:841, 1982
29. Park TS, Coil WS, Maggio WM, Mitchell DC: Progressive spasticity and scoliosis in children with myelomeningocele. J Neurosurg 62:367, 1985
30. Raycroft JE, Curtis BH: Spinal curvature in myelomeningocele: Natural history and etiology. In AAOS Symposium on Myelomeningocele. St. Louis, CV Mosby, 1972
31. Sharrard WJ: Spinal osteotomy for congenital kyphosis in myelomeningocele. J Bone Joint Surg [Br] 50:466, 1968
32. Sharrard WJ: The kyphotic and lordotic spine in myelomeningocele. In AAOS Symposium on Myelomeningocele. St. Louis, CV Mosby, 1972
33. Shurtleff DB, Bourney R, Gordon LH, Livermore N: Myelodysplasia: The natural history of kyphosis and scoliosis, a preliminary report. Dev Med Child Neurol 18:126, 1976
34. Sriram K, Bobechko WP, Hall JE: Surgical management of spinal deformities in spina bifida. J Bone Joint Surg [Br] 54:666, 1972
35. Stabler CL, Eismont FJ, Brown MD, et al: Failure of posterior cervical fusion using cadaveric bone graft in children. J Bone Joint Surg [Am] 67:371, 1985
36. Winston K, Hall JE, Johnson D, Micheli L: Acute elevation of intracranial pressure following transection of nonfunctioning spinal cord. Clin Orthop 128:41, 1977

CHAPTER 14

Cotrel–Dubousset Instrumentation for Paralytic Neuromuscular Spinal Deformities with Emphasis on Pelvic Obliquity

Jean Dubousset

The treatment of paralytic spinal deformities must reflect the patient's overall medical and functional conditions. In particular, certain factors, such as cardiorespiratory function and nutrition, must be evaluated. There are three main goals of treatment:

1. To improve cardiorespiratory function or prevent worsening of it by correction of the spinal deformity
2. To provide trunk realignment and balance to enhance ambulation or sitting ability through adequate correction of the curve
3. To assure permanent improvement by achieving a solid fusion.

Ideally, these goals should be achieved without immobilizing the patients for prolonged periods of bedrest and allowing them to resume their usual activities as soon as possible. Stable internal fixation allows this with minimal or no postoperative bracing. The Cotrel–Dubousset instrumentation is particularly well suited for these problems.

ETIOLOGIC CONSIDERATIONS

Paralytic spinal deformities are associated with many different neuromuscular diseases, including abnormalities of the peripheral and central nervous systems. Detailed discussions of the particular disease entities are found elsewhere in this volume.

OVERALL STRATEGIES FOR TREATMENT

The general strategy for treatment depends on three factors. First, define the goals and abilities of the patient. Is he a community or household ambulator, or is he wheelchair bound? The second factor is the age of the patient. Although I feel that a patient should have a trunk height of greater than 70 cm before arthrodesis, surgical intervention may be necessary before that. In those cases, subcutaneous rodding and bracing may control the curve temporarily. Posterior fusions alone in very young children may undergo the crankshaft phenomenon, with continued increase in the curve from persistent anterior element growth.

The third factor is the general medical status of the patient. Proper evaluation of heart and lung function are necessary before surgical intervention. Poor pulmonary function may signal postoperative ventilatory problems. This is especially true in cases of polio or spinal muscular atrophy. Patients with muscular dystrophy, for example, may have cardiomyopathy, and they should be evaluated for this. Patients with cerebral palsy, especially those with total-body involvement, often are nutritionally depleted. They also may have gastroesophageal reflux, which interferes with normal enteral feedings and may contribute to aspiration pneumonia.

Local Strategy for Treatment

The local strategy should be planned in conjunction with the general goals of treatment and the functional goals and age of the patient. For very young children, when nonsurgical treatment does not control progression of the curve, Cotrel–Dubousset instrumentation can be performed in young children without fusion. The diamond points of the rods are imbedded in Silastic to prevent fibrosis around the rods. A few points of fixation were initially achieved at either end of the rods and at one intermediate vertebra on each side. The correction obtained was generally good; in some cases, when the deformity was not very severe, further lengthening at the upper ends every 6 months was performed as the child grew. This technique was used without external bracing in some cases. One patient, however, developed a spontaneous posterior fusion; other patients demonstrated the crankshaft phenomenon.

For children younger than 7 years, my treatment of choice is Cotrel–Dubousset instrumentation with rods imbedded in Silastic in a subcutaneous fashion, with one grip at each end, leaving the intermediate part free. Because the rod is used only to help prevent collapse, an external brace is always needed.

When the patient is old enough to proceed directly to fusion, the strategy chosen falls within the global strategies of spinal correction, taking into account the expected functional goals of the patient. This local strategy depends on three elements: three-dimensional analysis of the deformity, analysis of the pelvic obliquity, and analysis of any deformities of the lower extremities that may affect control of the pelvis or the spine.

Cotrel–Dubousset Instrumentation in Paralytics

The application of Cotrel–Dubousset instrumentation to paralytic deformities is not much different from its other applications, but usually the upper thoracic spine must be included, and it is often necessary to end the instrumentation with a claw grip. This can be accomplished with a pedicle hook at T2 and a special laterally tilted laminar hook over the top of the lamina of T1.

Another important point is the mixture of hooks and pedicle screws in the lumbar spine, especially when posterior elements are missing (e.g., myelomeningocele) or when maximal ability to correct by having a lateral apical force on a severely rotated vertebra is desired. This combination is also useful when the construct is short and located close to the lumbosacral junction.

PELVIC OBLIQUITY AND COTREL–DUBOUSSET INSTRUMENTATION

Since 1973, my colleagues and I at the Hopital St. Vincent de Paul have developed the concept of the "pelvic vertebra."[2] Since that time, the treatment of pelvic obliquity has become more effective because of a better understanding of the deformity in three-dimensional space.[1]

The pelvic obliquity of interest is a *fixed structural deformity* existing between the spinal axis and the pelvic axis. Postural deformities that are not fixed and that are easily changed are not germane to this discussion. The classical definition of pelvic obliquity usually speaks only to what is happening in the frontal plane. However, both the spine and the pelvis are three-dimensional, and abnormalities of alignment can occur in any of these planes. Therefore, the complete definition of pelvic obliquity is a fixed malalignment existing between the spinal and pelvic structures in the frontal, sagittal, or horizontal plane.

THE PELVIC VERTEBRA

The pelvic unit should be considered as one unique vertebra (Fig. 14-1). In fact, the sacrum and the iliac wings are united by the two sacroiliac joints and the pubic symphysis. Very little motion occurs physiologically through these joints, so that the construct of the sacrum and the pelvis can be considered as a unique vertebra—the pelvic vertebra.

The only exception to this concept is sacroiliac joint abnormality in which the iliac bones rotate independently of the sacrum (e.g., chondrodysplasias, congenital abnormalities, or infectious diseases). In some

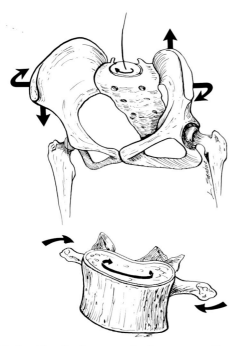

FIG. 14–1. The "pelvic vertebra" concept. The entire pelvis can be considered as one unique vertebra and can be displaced in the three dimensions of space like any vertebra of the spine.

chondrodystrophies, the sacrum appears to be horizontal both in the anterior-posterior and lateral views, although the ilia look vertical. Another way to evaluate pelvic obliquity is to observe the appearance of the obturator foramina on roentgenograms. In the normal orientation, the long axis of the obturator foramina is horizontal. Rotation of the pelvis in the sagittal plane changes this appearance.

The pelvic vertebra can be displaced in three dimensions. This displacement is not similar in all cases. In some cases, the major pelvic obliquity is in the frontal plane, while in others it is in the sagittal plane. This stresses the need to fully evaluate the deformity in three dimensions to properly correct it.

Another conception of the pelvic vertebra is that this pelvic vertebra is an intercalary bone between the trunk and the lower extremities (Fig. 14-2). There are three areas of motion between the pelvic vertebra and the structures around it. These points of motion exist at the lumbosacral junction and at each hip joint, and each has six degrees of freedom. In terms of the intercalary bone concept of the pelvic vertebra, one can see how the entire pelvis adjusts to balance the body on

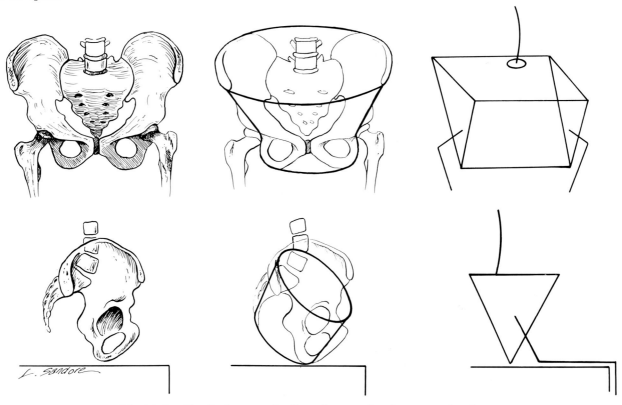

FIG. 14–2. The "pelvic vertebra" can be considered an intercalary bone.

one foot through the pelvis to the trunk. For double limb stance, balance is achieved through adjustment of the position of the pelvic vertebra for such things as hip flexion contractures, hip abduction contracture, and lordosis of the lumbar spine (Fig. 14-3).

In sitting, the pelvic vertebra tilts forward or backward, depending on the alignment of the trunk above and the mobility and position of the hips below.

The third conception of the pelvic vertebra is that it is a plastic bone that can be distorted in its shape if muscle imbalance or a congenital anomaly exists during growth. In these situations, if abnormal forces exist in a growing child, distortion of the pelvis can occur just as it can in any other bone subjected to abnormal forces. The pelvis can be distorted in different axes.

Analysis of the Pelvic Obliquity

From the concept of the pelvic vertebra, it is easy to understand that the causes of pelvic obliquity are nu-

merous and can be divided into three areas: infrapelvic, pelvic, and suprapelvic (Fig. 14-4).

In the infrapelvic category, disorders of the lower extremities, especially the hip joints, that cause contracture, paralysis, or deformity can limit the six degrees of freedom normally available and can displace the pelvis. For example, hip flexion contractures cause the pelvis to rotate anteriorly while the patient is standing, increasing lumbar lordosis. Conversely, tight hamstrings and glutei tilt the pelvis posteriorly during the transition from standing to sitting. Tight hip abductors and adductors have similar effects in the coronal plane. Most of these kinds of deformities of the pelvis can be corrected with proper soft tissue releases or osteotomies to realign the legs with respect to the pelvis.

In the pelvic category of pelvic obliquity, the pelvis itself is distorted as a result of malunion after a fracture, injury to growth centers of the pelvis from trauma or infection, or congenital or metabolic bone disease that causes malformation of the pelvis.

In the suprapelvic category, the spinal deformity is the primary cause of the pelvic obliquity. Most forms of spinal deformity can cause pelvic obliquity. Although many curves end above the lumbosacral junction, they can still cause pelvic obliquity by the nature of their size, stiffness, inability to create a compensatory lumbosacral curve below, tightness of the iliolumbar ligaments, or asymmetric function of the erector spinae muscles. This category of pelvic obliquity most often

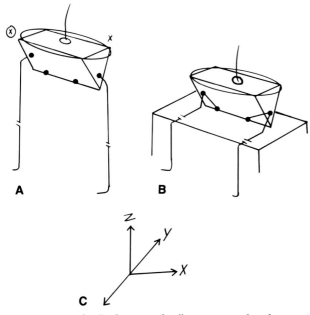

FIG. 14–3. The "pelvic vertebra" is an intercalary bone in the standing posture **(A)** and in the sitting position **(B)**. Notice the important role of the posterior aspect of both thighs linked by the pelvis. The balanced sitting base is constructed by both ischial tuberosities and the posterior aspect of both thighs. **C.** Notice the different degrees of freedom of the pelvic vertebra made possible by the motion of the lumbosacral joint, both ischial tuberosities, and both hip joints.

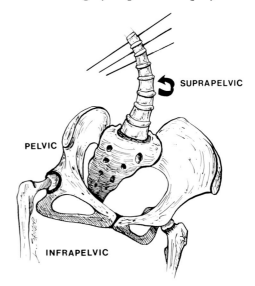

FIG. 14–4. There are three possible causes of pelvic obliquity: suprapelvic, pelvic, and infrapelvic levels.

concerns the spinal surgeon, and its resolution depends on how well he or she can correct the spinal deformity.

Practical Consequences of the Pelvic Vertebra Concept

What follows is an analysis, based on treatment of pelvic obliquity over the past 20 years, of 215 cases of pelvic obliquity caused by various abnormalities but most commonly due to paralytic problems.

If the pelvis is considered a pelvic vertebra and can be displaced in three planes, then a classification of pelvic obliquity can be developed (Fig. 14-5). When the infrapelvic and pelvic causes of the pelvic obliquity have been corrected, only the suprapelvic cause remains to be solved. The residual deformity then should be analyzed by looking at the thoracolumbar component and the lumbosacral junction. If the spine and the

pelvis are continuous (i.e., the pelvis directly follows the spine) in all three planes, this is called *regular pelvic obliquity*. However, there are instances in which the displacement of the pelvis does not follow the spine in at least one dimension; this is called *opposite pelvic obliquity*.

Regular pelvic obliquity occurs in the frontal plane if the pelvic tilt is in the same direction as the lumbar spine and in the sagittal plane if the pelvis follows the same lordotic inclination as the lumbar spine (Fig. 14-6). Regular pelvic obliquity exists also if the tilt in the frontal plane is continuous and if a kyphotic pelvic tilt follows a kyphotic tilt of the lumbar spine (Fig. 14-7).

Opposite pelvic obliquity occurs if, in the frontal plane, the pelvic vertebra is displaced in the opposite direction from that of the lumbar spine. Numerous variations can occur in three planes at each level of the lumbar spine and pelvis. Understanding the type of

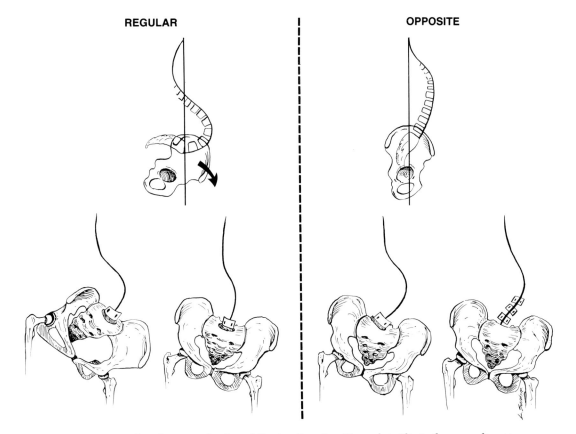

FIG. 14–5. Classifications of pelvic obliquity. Regular: The pelvis tilts in the same direction as the spine in the frontal and sagittal planes. Opposite: The pelvis tilts in the opposite direction from the spine in any plane.

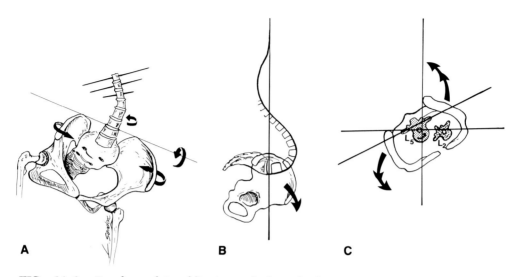

FIG. 14–6. Regular pelvic obliquity with hyperlordosis. **A.** Frontal projection. **B.** Sagittal projection. **C.** Horizontal projection (top view). Compare the position of L2 with L5 and the posterior positioning of the left iliac wing.

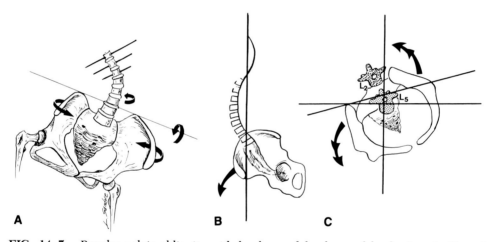

FIG. 14–7. Regular pelvic obliquity with lumbar and lumbosacral kyphosis. **A.** Frontal projection. **B.** Sagittal projection. **C.** Horizontal projection (top view).

pelvic obliquity is of considerable importance in correcting the deformity with Cotrel–Dubousset instrumentation.

The pelvic vertebra must be considered as an intercalary bone. The practical consequence is functional and determines whether instrumentation and fusion is carried to the pelvis (Fig. 14-8). Whether the patient stands or is only a sitter, the pelvis should be balanced in three planes in the appropriate functional positions. If the motor function is good and postural balance is operative, it may be possible to correct the spine without extending the instrumentation to the pelvis. How-

ever, if the intercalary pelvic vertebra cannot be balanced because of paralysis or postural deformity, there exists a sort of instability between the pelvis and the spine, and the instrumentation must be extended to the pelvis to insure a good result.

Although it has been said that fusion to the pelvis may impair ambulatory function (e.g., in the polio patient), this is not necessarily true. Some patients are able to ambulate only when there is some stabilization of the spine, especially in the sagittal plane. Stabilization is also important for sitting. The sitting base in the human is the surface provided by both ischial tuber-

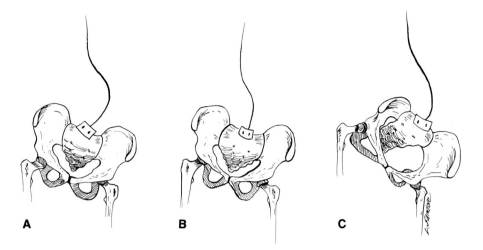

FIG. 14–8. To fuse or not to fuse to the sacrum? Fusion to the sacrum is recommended if (**A**) the pelvic obliquity is opposite or (**C**) if the pelvic obliquity is regular but tilts more than the lumbar curve itself can account for (rare condition). **B.** If correction of the lumbar spine produces a pelvis that is balanced with the spine in three dimensions, fusion does not have to be carried to the sacrum.

osities and the posterior aspects of the thighs. The proper orientation of the hip joints, and thus the legs, is important in achieving this.

Based on 20 years' experience, I maintain that it is mandatory to fuse to the pelvis in any patient in whom there exists an immediate or potential instability at the lumbosacral junction in any plane. If this is to be done, the alignment achieved at surgery must achieve proper alignment in all three planes for ambulation and sitting. On the other hand, it is not necessary to fuse to the pelvis if the pelvis is well balanced below the fusion and has sufficient muscle and postural control to allow the patient stable sitting and standing balance.

The third practical consequence of the concept of the pelvic vertebra is that it can be distorted. Therefore, there are limits to correction of the pelvic obliquity. Even though the suprapelvic and infrapelvic deformities can be corrected, the pelvic causes may still exist and may not be able to be corrected. Sometimes these deformities are compensatory, but if not, the only way to correct them is by an osteotomy to achieve the best possible position. These osteotomies are often difficult but may be of great help to the patient.

STRATEGY FOR CORRECTION

Preoperative Surgical Planning

In order to achieve the best surgical correction of pelvic obliquity, it is necessary to determine the flexibility of the curve. This can be done by bending films or films using traction on one or both legs. This ability to correct with bending or traction should be assessed for

sagittal and frontal deformities. These studies should be able to determine the flexibility of the curve and the location of the stiffest part of the curve. The growth potential of the patient should also be taken into account for surgical planning.

It must first be decided whether an anterior approach will be useful. There are two reasons to do an anterior approach. The first is to address the problem of significant growth potential. The anterior approach and fusion, which acts as an epiphysiodesis, is necessary to prevent the crankshaft phenomenon. The phenomenon is produced by continued growth in the anterior part of the still distorted spine in the presence of a posterior fusion. This is a common occurrence after an early fusion is done, with or without instrumentation. This crankshaft phenomenon is prevented by removal of the anterior growth potential at the level of the growth plate of the vertebral body and adequate anterior fusion done at the same time or very close to the posterior spinal fusion.

The second reason for an anterior approach is to "loosen" the spine if it is very stiff. In such cases, discectomy enhances correction of the spinal deformity and the pelvic obliquity. Occasionally, anterior instrumentation is indicated, but this instrumentation should be short, located at the apex of the curve, and designed to maintain lordosis in the lumbar spine, which is difficult to achieve even with Zielke VDS instrumentation. Long anterior instrumentation should not be used because it impedes subsequent correction with posterior instrumentation, especially in the sagittal plane.

Surgical planning should be done for the posterior instrumentation. Cotrel–Dubousset instrumentation is well suited for these problems. The principles are the same as for any scoliosis curve located at any level. Compression and distraction force at appropriate levels, as well as rotation, are used to correct the deformities in three planes.

Preoperative planning should divide the spine and the pelvis into different segments to correct selectively each segment, using the basic principles of Cotrel–Dubousset instrumentation. These should include a compression configuration to achieve lordosis and to correct kyphosis and a distraction force configuration to produce kyphosis or decrease lordosis. These effects can be obtained at successive levels or selectively at only one functional unit. The effect can be selectively obtained at the lumbosacral junction, if one considers the pelvis as a pelvic vertebra.

Another point to consider is the pelvic fixation. Pelvic fixation can be achieved by Cotrel–Dubousset instrumentation in a number of ways. Alar staples (Fig. 14-9) are used only when distraction is needed between the spine and the pelvis. One or two rods can be placed into the staples. They must be implanted only in the ala of the sacrum, which requires exposing the lumbosacral facet joint before going laterally to expose the superior aspect of the ala. It is here that the staples are to be inserted. It is mandatory that a permanent distraction exists in any position of the spine relative to the pelvis. Dislodgment can occur because transverse, rotary, and flexion stability is poor with a staple. Addi-

tionally, the alar staple does not allow any compression through it between the spine and the pelvis. In my opinion, alar staples should be used only in addition to another kind of pelvic fixation on the other side.

An alternative for instrumenting the pelvis is the use of sacral screws (Fig. 14-10). These are available in closed or open varieties, with long or short necks; these variations help in passing the rod through them. The best area for fixation in the sacrum is the body of the sacrum. Often the ala are weak, especially in older or osteoporotic patients. A number of biomechanical studies have shown that the strongest fixation is achieved when the screw enters the superior endplate of the S1 body. The entrance point must be at the base of the superior facet of S1, with the screw directed medially (Fig. 14-11). Screws can also be used in a divergent manner on each side of the sacrum. The first one should be 30 mm long and have an anterior-posterior direction but be slightly medial. The second screw is inserted more distally and tilted 30° laterally (see Fig. 14-10). In the horizontal plane, the screw is entirely within the ala and not through the SI joint. The screws can be inserted with a special jig that helps to align the screws to make rod insertion easier. In some cases, a short (20-mm) sacral screw can also be placed in the pedicle of S2.

When using sacral screws, compression and distraction can be applied across the lumbosacral junc-

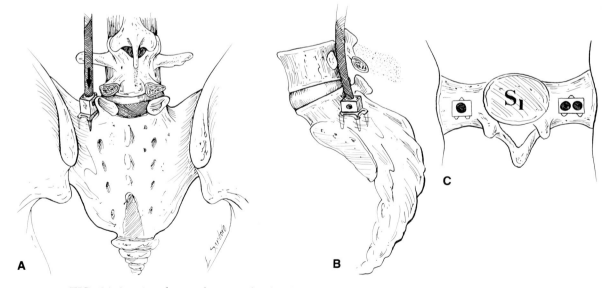

FIG. 14–9. A. Alar staples must be fitted onto the ala of the sacrum.   **B.** Seen from the lateral view, the staple is anterior to the S1 facet.   **C.** Seen from the top, it is possible to use a single-hole or double-hole staple.

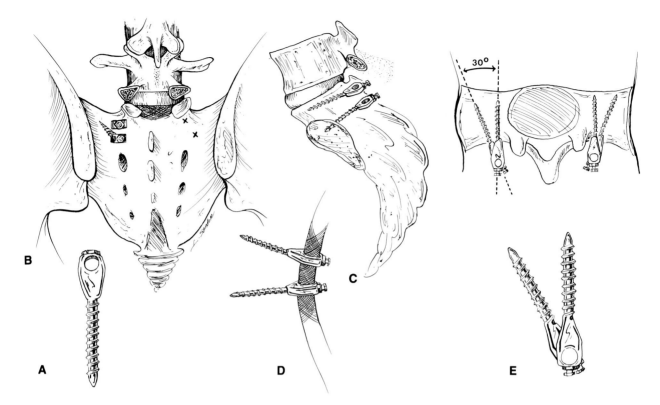

FIG. 14–10. Sacral screws. **A.** The sacral screw can be placed in a strictly anterior-posterior direction, using a 30-mm length entering at the junction of the S1 facet cartilage in the posterior bone of S1 above the first posterior sacral foramen. **B–D.** The second screw can be tilted laterally, 30° from the first, entering distally (7 mm) and laterally (7 mm) from the first one, avoiding entrance into the sacroiliac joint. **E.** The openings to the screws should be concentric to facilitate entrance of the rod.

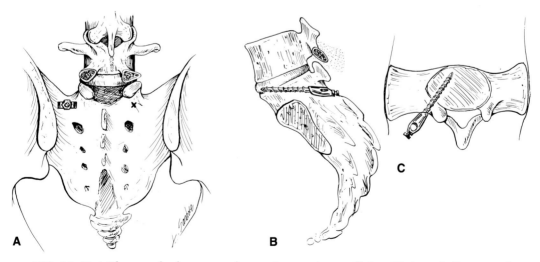

FIG. 14–11. The use of only one sacral screw is sometimes sufficient if it is medially oriented and goes through the superior endplate of S1. This provides firm fixation, especially in osteoporotic bone.

tion. However, two problems can occur with the use of these implants. The first is poor quality of bone, making the fixation tenuous; the second is insufficient soft tissue coverage of the implant, such as in myelomeningocele. Because of these problems, another form of fixation to the pelvis may be needed.

In patients in whom the bone stock is poor or soft tissue coverage is lacking, the procedure can be achieved by the use of a cannulated iliosacral screw (Fig. 14-12). My colleagues and I have used this type of screw fixation for over 20 years with Harrington instrumentation, even before Cotrel–Dubousset instrumentation. The screw, which is 7 mm in diameter, slides over a K-wire, which is inserted under x-ray control. The K-wire is inserted from the level of the posterior superior iliac spine, appearing just at the base of the S1 facet joint, and then entering the sacrum just lateral and distal to this facet, to end up in the body of S1.

Sometimes it is necessary to make a hole in the superior aspect of the ala to accommodate the hook used to connect the screw with the rod. This screw does not cross through the SI joint. It is posterior to the joint, and the strong fixation is achieved by the length of the screw that is inserted through the sacrum to the middle of the body of S1. In general, the length of the iliosacral screw is between 6 and 8 cm. The fixation of the rod to the iliosacral screw can be accomplished by any laminar hook. Because rotation of the hook around the screw can cause dislodgment, it is probably better

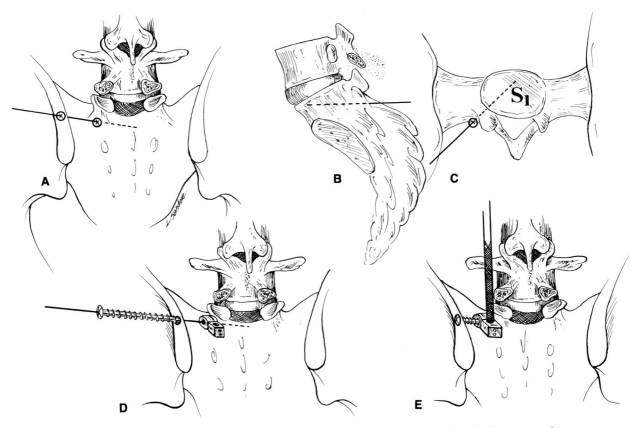

FIG. 14–12. Iliosacral cannulated screw with the cylindrical or cardan hook. **A,B.** The entering point of the guidewire is at the posterior and superior part of the iliac crest, coursing posterior to the sacroiliac joint, entering the sacrum distal and lateral to the superior facet of S1, and then passing through the S1 pedicle to the center of the S1 body. **C.** Lateral view of the guidewire. **D.** Top view of the guidewire. If using a cylindrical hook, it must be placed on the guidewire before being inserted into the sacrum. The cannulated iliosacral screw is placed on the guidewire after its position is checked radiographically. The screw is then threaded over the wire, through the hook, and into the sacrum. **E.** The final construct with the rod inside the superior hole of the hook.

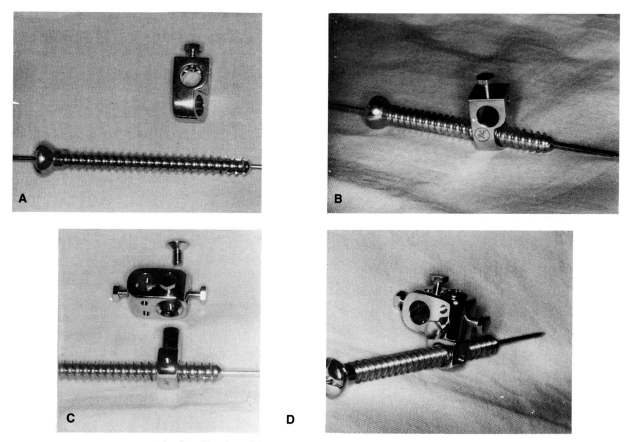

FIG. 14–13. Cylindrical hook and iliosacral screw. **A,B.** Notice the two holes with directions almost orthogonal from each other. One is for the iliosacral screw, and the other is for the rod. **C,D.** Cardan hook and iliosacral screw.

to use the cylindrical hook (Fig. 14-13A,B) that is placed at the same time the K-wire is inserted. The cannulated screw is then passed over the K-wire, through the cylindrical hook, and on into the sacrum. Proper bending of the rod is needed to allow easy entrance of the rod into the canal of the hook. Compression and distraction forces can be applied through this construct.

It is not always possible to use a single long rod from the upper thoracic spine to the sacrum, and often it is not possible to rotate the rod after insertion into the hook. For that reason, a special hook (the cardan hook; Fig. 14-13C,D) has been designed. It is made in two parts and used in the same way as the usual cylindrical hook, except that the canal for the iliosacral screw is a separate piece that is attached to the rest of the hook by a bolt. This junction can be adjusted through the axis of the connecting bolt. Motion is possible around the iliosacral screw and through this connection of the two

parts of the cylindrical hook, making it easier to insert and fix the final construct.

It must be remembered that after any pelvic fixation it is necessary to form a rectangular construct by adding devices for transverse traction (DTT). The DTT should exert a distraction between the rods at the lumbosacral junction area.

Cotrel–Dubousset instrumentation can also be fixed to the pelvis via the Galveston technique. This is done in the same way as for Luque instrumentation. A single rod can be used on either side, or two separate rods can be used on either side, and connected with dominoes or an axial connector. In long instrumentation constructs, the use of two rods on each side is often easier.

Other important considerations are the proper bending of rods and the use of linking systems (i.e., the dominoes or axial connectors). The proper amount of lordosis in the lumbosacral spine and the lumbosacral junction must always be obtained. This is especially important in paralytic curves extending from the upper thoracic spine to the pelvis. It is often helpful to use a single short rod temporarily close to the pelvis; it is placed on the convex side and then rotated to restore the lumbar lordosis. The permanent rods can then be inserted into the pelvis in whatever configuration has been selected. It is easier in many cases to perform the instrumentation in the same way as it is used in idiopathic scoliosis down to L4 and then extend the instrumentation to the pelvis with a short, contoured rod that is attached to the main rod with some linking system. I prefer to use only one rod on either side. If this is not possible, two rods are used on one side and a single one is used on the other (D. Chopin, personal communication).

Surgical Technique

I prefer to operate on patients with paralytic scoliosis on a special traction table, which allows traction to be applied selectively on the leg on the high side of the pelvic obliquity. This maneuver helps to obtain both frontal- and sagittal-plane correction and decreases the stresses on the rods.

Subperiosteal exposure of the posterior elements of the spine is performed in the usual way, out to the tips of the transverse processes. After proper insertion of

the hooks, facet excision is performed, and facet fusion is done by impacting iliac or bank bone into each joint. The rods are inserted and may or may not be rotated to achieve correction.

If the patient has very little iliac crest bone, I prefer to harvest an autologous tibial cortical bone strut (1 cm wide and as long as the tibia) at the start of the operation. This is taken from the wider cortex of the tibia, leaving intact the anterior tibial crest to prevent fracture. After insertion of the rods and before placing the DTTs, the tibial bone graft is inserted and the DTTs are applied over it, securing it into place. This tibial bone graft is flexible, conforms to the lumbar lordosis, and is usually sufficiently long to bridge from the lower thoracic spine to across the lumbosacral junction.

Suction drainage is always used and is placed in the subcutaneous layer.

EXAMPLES

Regular Pelvic Obliquity with Hyperlordosis

In a regular pelvic obliquity with increased lordosis, it is logical to start by applying distraction forces on the concave side that will correct the frontal- and sagittal-plane deformity (Fig. 14-14). After that, compression is used on the convex side to supplement frontal-plane

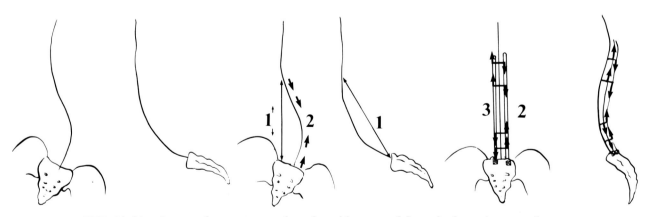

FIG. 14–14. Strategy for treating regular pelvic obliquity with hyperlordosis. *Arrows* indicate positioning and direction of the hooks and the pedicle screws. (1) Temporary distraction force is applied on the concave side between the sacrum and the thoracolumbar spine in an effort to correct the frontal and sagittal alignments. (2) Compression is applied on the convex side of the lumbar spine and the lumbosacral junction in an effort to improve the correction in the frontal plane without causing increase in the hyperlordosis. (3) The temporary corrective rod is removed, and the final long rod replaces it, completing the instrumentation.

correction, but not to change the sagittal alignment that has already been achieved by the first rod, which has stabilized the lumbar lordosis.

The concave rod should be placed first, with hooks placed between the pelvis and the upper lumbar spine in a distraction configuration to correct the scoliosis and decrease the lordosis. If the curve is very stiff, a short rod can be used in the apex, and a long one can then span the entire thoracolumbar spine. On the convex side, hooks or screws are used around the apex in a compression configuration. The instrumentation is then continued down to the pelvis and upward to the thoracic spine. If it is too difficult to use a single rod for this purpose, two rods can be used and connected with the appropriate linking system.

Regular Pelvic Obliquity with Kyphosis

In a spine in which the sagittal deformity is kyphotic, it is not logical to start with a concave distraction construct because this tends to increase the kyphosis (Figs. 14-15 and 14-16). Therefore, it is necessary to insert the convex instrumentation first, using compression to correct the kyphosis across the lumbar spine and the lumbosacral junction. The concave rod can then be inserted without increasing the kyphosis,

because this has already been corrected and fixed by the convex instrumentation (Figs. 14-17 and 14-18).

Opposite Pelvic Obliquity

In opposite pelvic obliquity, the strategy is to correct the problem of the pelvic obliquity itself first with the appropriate instrumentation and then correct the rest of the thoracolumbar deformity, linking the two systems together (Fig. 14-19).

Opposite Pelvic Obliquity with Lumbosacral Kyphosis

The preoperative planning must devise a construct that starts with correction of the lumbosacral kyphosis with compression on the convex side of the scoliotic component of the deformity (Fig. 14-20). The second rod is used in a distraction configuration on the other side. After the lumbosacral part is corrected, the thoracolumbar component of the deformity can be corrected by separate rods, which are then connected to the lumbosacral construct with a linking system. Alternatively, a temporary short rod can be placed on one side, the opposite rod is then inserted, and the short rod is replaced with a single long rod. The ability to correct two areas of the spine separately and then join

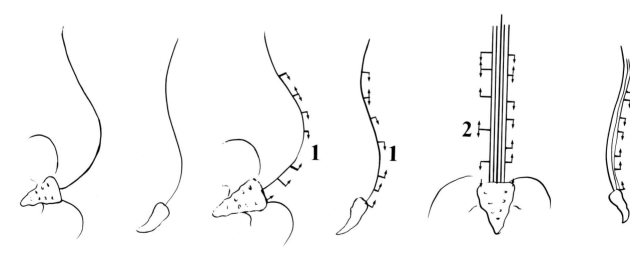

FIG. 14–15. Strategy for treating regular pelvic obliquity with kyphosis. (1) It is mandatory to start on the convex side from the pelvis. Notice the upper claw on the upper-end vertebra, the compression forces centered on the apex of the lumbar curve, and compression from the pelvis. (2) The second rod is placed on the concave side, applying distraction to the frontal plane without disturbing the lumbosacral lordosis already achieved from the other side.

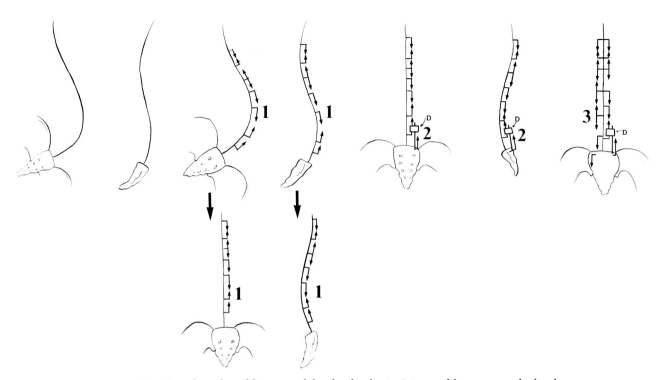

FIG. 14–16. Regular pelvic obliquity with lumbar kyphosis. It is possible to correct the lumbar curve on the convex side first (1) and then extend the instrumentation to the pelvis (2) using a domino (D). This gives almost complete correction. The construct is completed by inserting a long rod on the the other side (3) that spans top to bottom. Notice the double claw at the upper part of the construct.

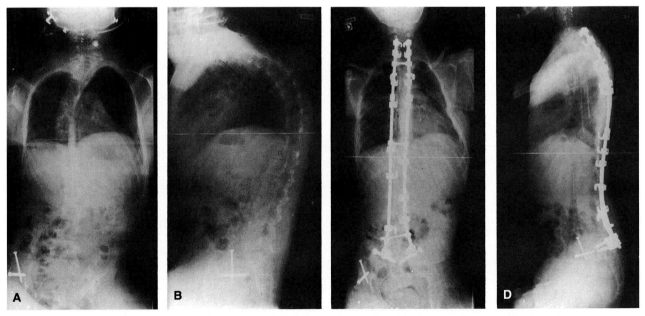

FIG. 14–17. Patient with trauma to the cervical spine and cord with incomplete paraplegia and with a large kyphoscoliosis and sagittal pelvic obliquity after laminectomy. **A.** Preoperative frontal view in traction. **B.** Sagittal view demonstrating the thoracic kyphosis and vertical sacrum. **C.** Postoperative frontal view after anterior release and fusion in the thoracic spine with Cotrel–Dubousset instrumentation using iliosacral screws and carden hooks. **D.** Postoperative sagittal view illustrating the anterior thoracic fusion with a strut graft.

360

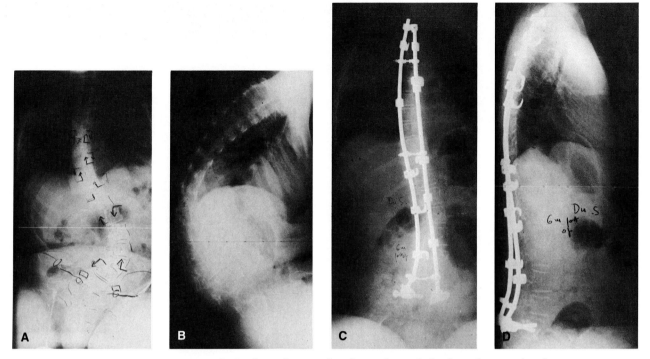

FIG. 14–18. Patient with Duchenne's muscular dystrophy with kyphoscoliosis and pelvic obliquity. **A, B.** Preoperative frontal and sagittal views. **C, D.** Postoperative views after Cotrel–Dubousset instrumentation.

the two constructs is an example of the flexibility and versatility of Cotrel–Dubousset instrumentation.

PARTICULAR SITUATIONS

Pelvic Obliquity Progression Below an Insufficiently Long Fusion

There are cases in which paralytic curves were fused short of the pelvis and the deformity progressed below the fused level, either in the frontal or sagittal planes.

Using the modular features of the Cotrel–Dubousset instrumentation, the instrumentation and fusion can easily be extended to the pelvis to correct the deformity. The added instrumentation should overlap the original instrumentation, if possible, and be attached by two connectors on either side to avoid junctional motion and the possibility of the development of a pseudarthrosis.

Pelvic Obliquity Recurrence After Posterior Spinal Fusion in a Growing Child

The recurrence of pelvic obliquity after posterior spinal fusion demonstrates the effect of the crankshaft phenomenon. The posterior fusion mass is solid and acts as a tether while growth continues anteriorly, leading to torsion of the spine with increased curvature and pelvic obliquity in many cases, even though the previous fusion extended to the pelvis. To correct this problem, anterior release and fusion without instrumentation are the first steps. Then multiple osteotomies of the fusion mass are done, and the spine is reinstrumented. Instrumentation may be pedicle screws (using x-ray films to insure proper placement) or hooks anchored in the fusion mass. The blade of the hook should enter the spinal canal and not just rest on the fusion mass alone, to afford a better purchase for the hook.

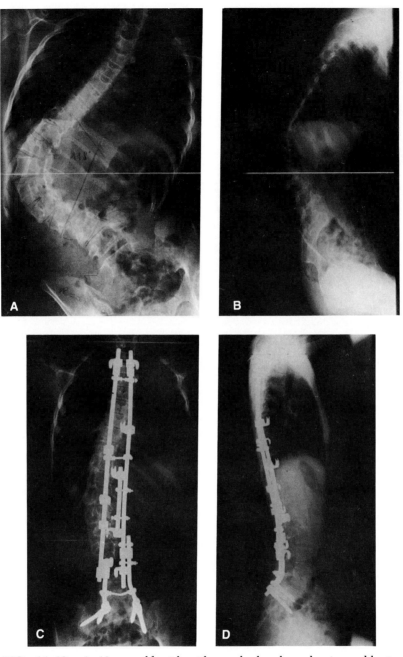

FIG. 14–19. A 13-year-old girl with cerebral palsy who is unable to walk. **A.** Frontal view taken preoperatively. **B.** Sagittal view taken preoperatively. **C.** After anterior release from T10 to L4 and Cotrel–Dubousset instrumentation with the use of sacral screws and dominoes. **D.** Sagittal view taken postoperatively.

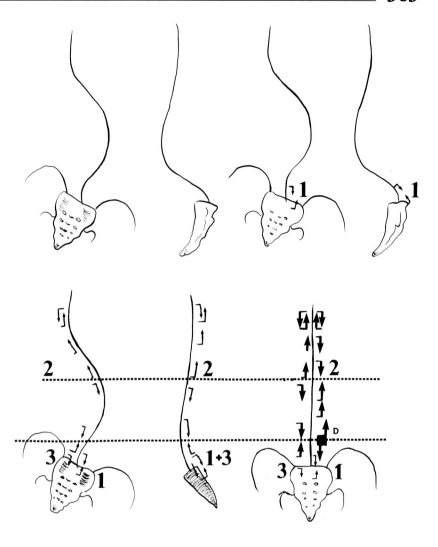

FIG. 14–20. Strategy for opposite pelvic obliquity. (1) The kyphotic lumbosacral junction is compressed on the concave side in an effort to decrease the iliolumbar angle. When observed in the frontal plane, this iliolumbar angle is greater than 90°. Compression of the instrumentation allows restoration of lumbosacral lordosis. (2) The next step includes applying distraction to the concave lumbar curve from the apex of the lordotic lumbar curve (*upper dotted line*). (3) Selective correction of the lumbosacral junction is performed on the side when the iliolumbar angle is less than 90° in the frontal plane. Just caudal to the main concavity of the lumbar curve and just cephalad to the lower iliolumbar angle is the short convex region. This apical region is placed under localized compression during instrumentation (*lower dotted line*). (4) Compression and rotation of the convex side of the lumbar curve is performed. This convex lumbar rod is lengthened to the lumbosacral rod previously placed by using a connecting device like a domino (D).

Short Spans of Instrumentation for Spondylolisthesis

Using the same type of preoperative planning, the instrumentation for degenerative or congenital spondylolisthesis is carried out with pedicle screws on the spinal side and appropriate fixation on the pelvic side, as previously described. The upper pedicular screw should be protected by a special three-directional hook, which is inserted over the lamina of the vertebra immediately above the last one with the pedicle screw. This helps to produce or maintain lordosis and protects the screw from acute and chronic stress. It acts as a shock absorber and provides some flexibility to the transitional disc space.

POSTOPERATIVE CARE AND RESULTS

All of the techniques discussed here have been used effectively in cases of paralytic, congenital, postural, and degenerative pelvic obliquity. In most cases no external support has been used in the ambulatory or nonambulatory patients.

In a study of 80 patients with Cotrel–Dubousset instrumentation for pelvic obliquity, most were paralytic. Diagnoses included Duchenne's muscular dystrophy, congenital scolioisis, cerebral palsy, myelomeningocele, polio, spinal muscular atrophy, post-traumatic paraplegia, and postradiation deformity.[3] Several types of pelvic fixation were used: staple in 9 cases, sacral screws in 25 cases, iliosacral screws in 45 cases, and

Galveston in 1 case. The correction of the frontal-plane deformity was 80%, with most patients having no residual pelvic obliquity. The most striking improvement in alignment compared with previous instrumentation techniques (e.g., Harrington and Luque instrumentation) was in the sagittal plane. The mean preoperative lumbar hyperlordosis was 80° and 40° after surgery. The mean lateral preoperative hyperkyphosis of the lumbar spine was 30°; postoperative lordosis was 36° (i.e., 66° correction). The horizontal-plane deformity (i.e., viewing the pelvis from above) did not correct as well as the coronal- and sagittal-plane deformities in these severe cases. It is because of this that the special cardan hook was developed.

When correcting pelvic obliquity, technically the most difficult part is to achieve what was planned, especially in the sagittal plane. The planned correction must take into account the needs of the patient and his or her balance and muscle function, especially for ambulators. Unfortunately, in this series of patients with poor muscle strength, the standing balance obtained was not always good enough to foster ambulation.[3] For example, if the lordosis was corrected too much in those with poor or no gluteal muscles, the gravity line fell in front of the femoral heads, and good standing balance could not be achieved. In two cases, this situation was salvaged with bilateral innominate osteotomies, which allowed readjustment of the sagittal-plane alignment.

COMPLICATIONS

Infection

There were 7 cases of infection, 3 of them deep, requiring debridement and drainage. The instrumentation had to be removed completely 1 year after surgery from 1 patient with myelomeningocele and 1 with posttraumatic paraplegia.

Skin Necrosis Without Infection

Skin necrosis without infection occurred in 9 patients, 2 of whom required plastic surgery. However, these problems had no effect on the spinal correction or the fusion.

Mechanical Problems

There were 3 patients with staple dislodgments, 3 sacral screw pull-outs, and 1 sacral screw fracture.

Three iliosacral screws backed out, necessitating retightening or longer screw insertion, which is easily done over guidewires. In 1 case, the iliosacral screw failed completely, and the situation was salvaged using the Galveston method.

Suprapelvic complications included 1 patient with a fractured rod and 2 with linking-system (dominoes) failures secondary to pseudarthrosis. These were managed by pseudarthrosis repair and reinstrumentation with dominoes.

CONCLUSIONS

I have found the Cotrel–Dubousset instrumentation to be the most effective method of correcting pelvic obliquity. It is necessary to analyze the deformity in three planes and plan the instrumentation to correct it effectively. The surgery is time-consuming and can be technically difficult; two well-trained surgeons working together can facilitate the procedure. However, the resulting quality of the correction and elimination of postoperative external support confirms the efficacy of this method.

Acknowledgment

Thanks to Laura Sandore (Shriners Hospital, Chicago) for redoing the original illustrations for this chapter.

References

1. Dubousset J: Pelvic obliquity, a three-dimensional entity. Proceedings of the Groupchide Scoliose Berck, Paris, 1973
2. Dubousset J: The pelvic vertebra: Three-dimensional concept for the pathophysiology, classification and management of pelvic obliquity. Presented at the Zielke Farewell Meeting, Badwildungen, Germany, October 1989
3. Dubousset J, Guillaumat M, Cotrel Y: Correction of pelvic obliquity and fusion to the sacrum with Cotrel–Dubousset instrumentation in children and adults. Presented to the Scoliosis Research Society meeting, Bermuda, 1986
4. Dubousset J, Herring JA, Shufflebarger H: The crankshaft phenomenon. J Pediatr Orthop 9:541, 1989
5. Guillaumat M, Tassim JL: Cotrel–Dubousset instrumentation for pelvic obliquity. Proceedings of the Groupchide Scoliose Berck, Paris, 1989

CHAPTER
15

■ ■ ■

Congenital
Spinal Deformity

John P. Lubicky
James E. Shook

■

CONGENITAL SCOLIOSIS
AND CONGENITAL KYPHOSIS

JOHN P. LUBICKY

Despite the amount of literature about congenital spinal deformity, including Winter's superb book, this area of spinal deformity remains challenging.[12, 34] Both surgical treatment and decision making can be problematic for the surgeon. To say that each case must be evaluated individually may seem like a cliché, but it is nonetheless true. Although the literature has provided general information about how certain abnormalities behave, these data must be put into perspective along with factors such as age, associated conditions, general health of the child, and the behavior of the curve. One thing that should be avoided is "reinventing the wheel." For example, there is no justification for allowing a congenital curve to relentlessly progress in the mistaken belief that trunk height should increase before correcting or arresting the condition.

The experienced spinal surgeon should have at his or her disposal a variety of techniques to achieve curve control. The in situ fusion is the gold standard for the care of these problems, and in many cases, it is the most appropriate procedure. For some patients, however, procedures like vertebrectomy and osteotomy may produce better overall results. With some of the newer procedures, the result may actually be better correction and less loss of trunk height than with some of the more traditional ones. Of course, proper training and experience and the availability of ancillary support, such as spinal cord monitoring, are necessary to ensure that these more complicated procedures are as safe as possible.

In this chapter, the classification, behavior, evaluation, and treatment of congenital spinal deformities are discussed.

CONGENITAL SCOLIOSIS

Classification and Natural History

Because not all congenital spine abnormalities are the same, a classification system is appropriate. Congenital spine abnormalities can be grouped into failures of formation, failures of segmentation, a mixture of formation and segmentation failures, and rib abnormalities. This classification is based on the appearance of the

365

spine on a roentgenogram, but the differences in appearance are also associated with differences in the natural history. Special studies (e.g., tomography) are often necessary to fully elucidate the anatomy of the abnormality. The location of the abnormality is also important. A hemivertebra in the thoracic spine causes a curve that, with a compensatory curve above and below, may remain fairly well balanced. However, a similar hemivertebra at the lumbosacral junction may cause severe trunk shift and promotes the development of a rather large structural compensatory thoracolumbar curve.

Failures of Formation

Failures of formation range from a typical hemivertebra with one pedicle that is fully segmented to a wedged vertebra that is fused to its neighbor. The behavior of these different failures of formation is also different. A hemivertebra may be incarcerated in the confines of the curve and vertebral column or unincarcerated, not fitting within the contour of the curve. The incarcerated hemivertebra has, in a sense, a space shaped for it and is contained by it. Because of this, its potential for curve progression is less than that of the unincarcerated hemivertebra (Fig. 15-1A–C).

Increased curvature in the spine with congenital anomalies is caused by asymmetric growth. Therefore, the potential for growth of a particular hemivertebra is important for the prediction of progression. Each vertebral body has a growth plate located at its superior and inferior ends. If there is a good disc space between the hemivertebra (i.e., fully segmented from its neighbor), the implication is that there is also a good growth plate. If this is the case, one would expect active growth

of the hemivertebra to increase the deformity. A hemivertebra that is fused to its neighbor vertebra above and below does not have open growth plates, and the risk for hemivertebra growth and an increase in the curve is significantly less. Therefore, the concepts of incarcerated, unincarcerated, segmented, and unsegmented vertebra are important in evaluating the effects of hemivertebra.

A situation known as hemimetameric shift can occur in which two hemivertebrae are present on opposite sides of the spine, separated by at least one normal vertebra (Fig. 15-1D). The hemimetameric shift is often benign as far as progression is concerned, but it becomes more of a problem depending on the separation between hemivertebrae and the nature of the hemivertebrae involved.

In looking at the natural history of failures of formation, some general statements can be made. Fully segmented, unincarcerated hemivertebrae have the most potential for progression. Hemivertebrae, even if unincarcerated, that are only partially segmented have a more benign course. Totally incarcerated, unsegmented hemivertebrae are probably benign. Lumbosacral hemivertebrae cause significant problems with spinal balance and curve progression unless there is an abnormality of the sacrum that compensates. Although there is a high likelihood of progression for unbalanced hemivertebrae overall, progression is probably slow until the adolescent growth spurt.

Failures of Segmentation

Failures of segmentation, like failures of formation, vary in degree. A block vertebra would be one extreme of this situation, in which the vertebrae are fused com-

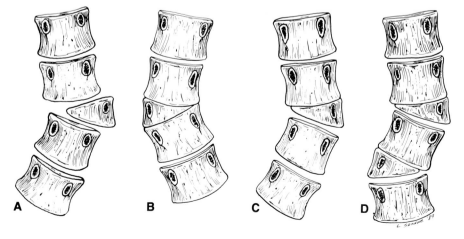

FIG. 15–1. Failure of formation Type I congenital vertebral anomalies. **A.** Unincarcerated fully segmented hemivertebra. **B.** Incarcerated unsegmented hemivertebra. **C.** Incarcerated partially segmented hemivertebra. **D.** Hemimetameric shift.

pletely across the adjacent disc. The typical unsegmented bar, however, occurs only on one side, and a well-formed disc beyond the bar occurs between the two adjacent vertebrae (Fig. 15-2A). The bar may span two or more vertebrae. The progression of the curve caused by an unsegmented bar depends on the quality of convex growth. Therefore, an unsegmented bar associated with a wide open disc space between the adjacent vertebrae has a high likelihood of progresion, but one in which the disc space is narrow has a more benign course. Unsegmented bars are most commonly seen in the thoracic spine. The posterior location of a bar increases the likelihood that associated lordosis will occur with the scoliosis. If there are bilateral bars spanning the same number of vertebral levels, pure lordosis occurs (Fig. 15-2C). Pelvic obliquity that is associated with an unsegmented bar is not associated with hip subluxation or dislocation on the high side unless some neurologic abnormality exists that causes muscle imbalance around that hip.[34]

Although failures of formation and failures of segmentation have been separated for discussion, they can occur together. In fact, the situation in which a bar is present with an intervening hemivertebra on the opposite side represents the worst scenario for progression (Fig. 15-2B). Radiographic studies may be necessary to delineate the true anatomic abnormality.

Although the threat of progression of a curve is of the utmost importance and therapeutic decisions should be made before the development of a severe

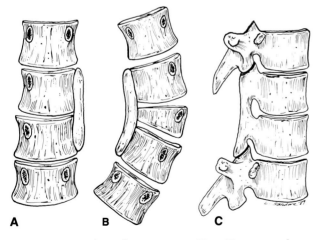

FIG. 15–2. Failure of segmentation Type II congenital vertebral anomalies. **A.** Unilateral unsegmented bar. **B.** Unilateral unsegmented bar with contralateral hemivertebra. **C.** Bilateral posterior unsegmented bars.

curve, a "knee jerk" reaction to congenital spinal deformity should be avoided. Sometimes the risk of progression for a curve is not clear when the patient is first seen. For example, a patient may present with multiple anomalies in one segment of the spine, including hemivertebrae, bars, and fused ribs. The segment may contain a curvature as well, but this particular spine may actually have little potential for curve progression because the abnormalities are balanced and cancel out each other's effects. The major problem with a spine like this is stunted growth through that segment. Female patients are more likely than males to have larger curves, and thoracic curves have a greater tendency to progress than those located in other parts of the spine.

"Controlled observation," as Winter calls it, is often required before a definitive therapeutic decision is made.[34] Winter, in his review of the patients from the Twin Cities Scoliosis Center, put the natural history in perspective. Twenty-five percent of his patients showed no progression, 25% had mild progression (less than 30°), and 50% had significant progression (more than 30°).[34]

Genetics

The classic study of the heredity of congenital spinal deformity was done by Wynne-Davies.[43] Her analysis of the families of 337 patients showed that isolated hemivertebrae or anterior failures of formation of one or two vertebrae was a sporadic anomaly and did not indicate increased risk for siblings. She felt, however, that multiple anomalies were somehow related to spina bifida cystica and anencephaly, and that there was a 5 to 10% risk for future siblings.

Many other anecdotal reports for congenital scoliosis in siblings and twins and other relatives have been reported, but they do not elucidate the heredity puzzle. In reviewing 1250 patients with congenital spinal deformity, Winter found only 13 patients with one relative with a congenital spinal deformity.[34] He concluded that isolated lesions like hemivertebrae have 1 chance in 100 of occurring in first-degree relatives. He did not find a relationship between multiple areas of involvement and spina bifida cystica.

Patient Evaluation

Clinical Presentation

Children with congenital spinal deformities have often been diagnosed before referral to the spinal surgeon or pediatric orthopedic surgeon by pediatricians, general practitioners, or other orthopedic surgeons. However, a careful history and physical examination are essential. A good axiom to follow is: If there is one congenital abnormality, search for others.

The history should begin with a review of the child's birth, growth, and development, as well as the family history, probing especially for various musculoskeletal problems. Delay in motor milestones in a child not otherwise at risk for cerebral palsy or who has normal intelligence may be a clue that there is some spinal cord malfunction. As the child gets older, other questions should be asked, particularly those exploring neurologic dysfunction. Does the child have back pain, a painful limited range of motion of the spine, weakness, numbness, or bowel or bladder incontinence? Has the patient had recurrent foot deformities despite prior adequate treatment? Does the child have a leg-length discrepancy or unequal foot sizes?

It should be kept in mind that one third of patients with congenital scoliosis have genitourinary tract abnormalities.[23] Twenty-five percent have Klippel-Feil syndrome.[39] Intraspinal abnormalities occur in about 15% of these patients, which is much higher than in the general population or in those who have other forms of spinal deformity.[11] Congenital heart disease can also be found in about 10% of patients.[29, 30] Abnormalities of the ear, nose, and throat system may also be seen.[34]

A general medical history among family members is also important because some of these conditions may be associated with the birth of a child with musculoskeletal problems. For example, sacral agenesis is associated with maternal diabetes.

The physical examination should be "from stem to stern." The child should be undressed completely except for underpants and examining gown. It is a mistake to examine a partially clothed child who is coming in for the initial comprehensive examination by the spinal surgeon. Missing a telltale finding hidden under clothes represents poor medicical practice. The physical examination should start with the head, looking at the range of motion of the neck, at the hairline, and for any eye or ear abnormalities. The spinal examination should be well known to all spinal surgeons, but trunk shift and decompensation is often more of a problem for these patients than the size of the curve alone, and it may indicate the major clinical problem caused by the abnormality seen on the roentgenogram. The skin of the back and buttocks should be examined for masses, dimples, and hairy patches, all of which may be stigmata of intraspinal abnormalities.

A good neurologic examination should be done and documented to serve as a baseline for future deterioration or improvement. As a part of the neurologic examination, a rectal examination should be done on all preoperative patients, looking for rectal tone and sensation and voluntary control (if that can be tested). The lower-extremity examination should look for abnormalities like leg-length discrepancy, which is usually associated with a recognizable pelvic obliquity. Subtle signs of neurologic dysfunction may present as a small or deformed foot or leg or a gait abnormality.

Signs of skeletal maturation should be evaluated, such as pubic hair development in boys and girls and breast development in girls. This information should be coupled with details of growth spurts and the onset of menarche.

Radiographic Evaluation

The classification of congenital scoliosis and the assessment of risk of progression for clinical purposes are based on the radiographic appearance of the vertebrae and the spine as a whole. Therefore, it is important that appropriate roentgenograms be obtained. The plain posterior-anterior and lateral roentgenograms provide a great amount of information about a particular child's spine. They demonstrate the location, size, and number of curves and indicate the patient's balance, trunk shift, and pelvic obliquity. Much of the anatomy can be seen on plain films, especially in the very young child, because they are taken supine and in the AP direction. Although the standard method of evaluating curve size is on a standing or sitting film, obviously an infant cannot sit upright and the roentgenograms are necessarily taken while he or she is recumbent. As soon as the child is able to stand or sit, the films should be taken in the upright position so that proper comparisons can be made from one film to another after that.

In changing from upright to recumbent, the congenital curve may not change much in its magnitude, but the compensatory curve does. It is surprising how often patients are referred because of apparent progression of their curves, because the film that prompted the referral was an upright film that was compared to a previous, recumbent one. The reason for doing routine scoliosis films PA is to decrease the radiation dose to the breasts. Usually, the detail is reasonably good, but because the spine is further from the film cassette and there is magnification, decreased detail often results.

Bending films to demonstrate curve flexibility may be done supine or standing with voluntary bending.

My colleagues and I prefer the supine variety with forced bending of the patient. In general, these films are not done routinely but are done preoperatively to aid in surgical planning.

Tomography is helpful in detailing the anatomy of a spinal abnormality (Fig. 15-3). By doing the anterior-posterior and lateral tomograms, much can be learned about the particular abnormality. Athough there are other techniques that may also provide similar information, tomography remains the standard. The disadvantage of conventional tomography is radiation exposure.

Computed tomography (CT) may be useful in conjunction with myelography, but alone it is usually not very helpful in determining the anatomy of the abnormal vertebrae. It is especially weak in the sagittal and

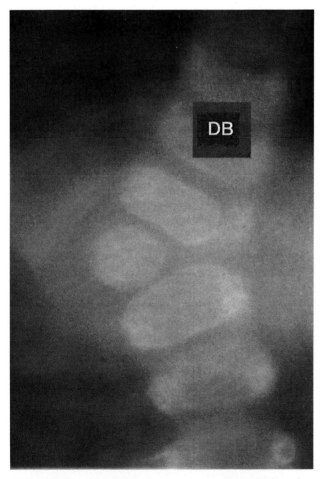

FIG. 15–3. Anterior-posterior tomogram of the thoracolumbar junction shows that the isolated hemivertebra at the thoracolumbar junction is fully segmented.

coronal reconstructions of the images, which are most valuable in evaluating the anatomy. It can, however, nicely demonstrate the anatomy of the spinal canal, and it may demonstrate clefts in the vertebral bodies that are seen with butterfly vertebrae and any bony spurs or septae associated with diastematomyelia.

Myelography is the standard for investigating intraspinal pathology. Water-soluble contrast agents used in complete spinal myelograms can demonstrate intraspinal abnormalities (Fig. 15-4). A CT scan can add more information about abnormal areas and the areas around the conus. The myelogram can be performed with the child under sedation, but some may require general anesthesia. An evaluation of the spinal canal should be done if the child has demonstrated neurologic abnormalities or problems that could be related to spinal cord dysfunction or if there are plans to correct the curve surgically. Routine evaluation of the spinal canal in the absence of these factors is probably unnecessary, because treatment of intraspinal abnormalities is usually indicated for clinical problems, not merely a radiographic abnormality.

Magnetic resonance imaging (MRI) can provide information about the neural tissues and the spinal anatomy without the use of ionizing radiation or contrast agents. Depending on the equipment used, particularly the availability of high-quality surface coils, very detailed images can be produced (Fig. 15-5). However, the child must be absolutely still while undergoing the examination because motion artifacts ruin the images. Except for pure kyphosis, the images of a severely deformed spine may be difficult to evaluate; for the sagittal and coronal images, segments of the spine may not appear on every cut of the scan because the deformity moves in and out of the plane of the cut. However, for the less-deformed spine and for purely kyphotic deformities, MRI evaluation of the intraspinal contents has the advantages of using no radiation, providing multiplanar imaging with good resolution, and being noninvasive. In my experience, reading MRIs of severely deformed spines is often equivocal, and even after MRI a myelogram may be necessary to resolve the issue.

Other methods of evaluating spinal deformity are available. Integrated Surface Imaging Systems (Oxford Metrics, Oxford, England) is another method of evaluating the magnitude of a curve without the use of radiation. The system can measure back shape, and from this data it can semiquantitatively measure the curve and rib hump. However, there are many shortcomings to this system, and for the patient with con-

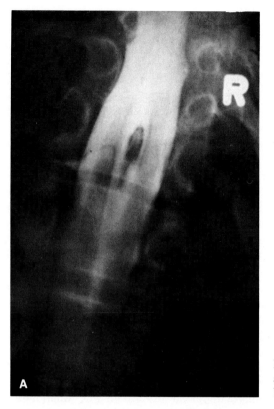

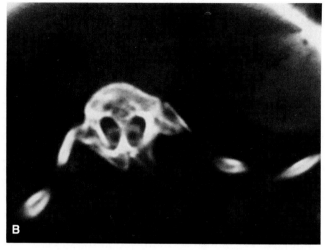

FIG. 15–4. **A.** A metrizamide myelogram showing a split cord and a diastematomyelia.   **B.** Axial CT scan showing a complete bony septum separating two hemicords.

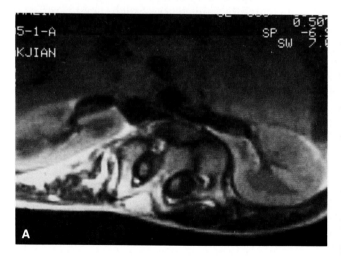

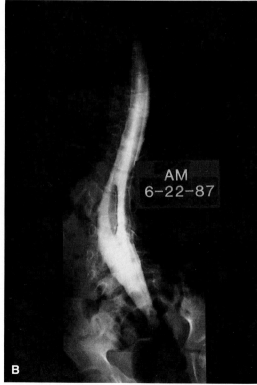

FIG. 15–5. **A.** Magnetic resonance image, axial cut, of a diastematomyelia showing the completely separated spinal canal, the bony septum, and the two hemicords.   **B.** Metrizamide myelogram of the same patient showing the split in the cord and the large bony septum.

genital scoliosis, it probably adds little in the evaluation other than analysis of back shape.

Because there is an increased incidence of genitourinary tract abnormalities, imaging of the kidneys, the collecting systems, and the bladder should be done for every patient with congenital spinal deformities. The screening examination can be done noninvasively and without radiation by using ultrasound.[1] This method is highly accurate in defining major abnormalities. If any question still exists about an abnormality, it can be further evaluated with an intravenous pyelogram.

Treatment

After a thorough evaluation of the patient, the appropriate form of treatment can be chosen. Additional factors, such as the patient's age and general health, available medical facilities, and potential risks, should be considered and discussed with the patient or the parents. The information available should be assessed to determine the risk of progression and the relative urgency of initiating treatment.

Nonsurgical Treatment

For a particular treatment to be effective, it must alter the natural history of the condition. Some excellent reviews of brace treatment and of electrical stimulation to correct idiopathic scoliosis have documented their efficacy in altering its natural history.[2, 20, 21, 28, 31] Exercises alone, spinal manipulation, electrical stimulation, various special diets, and shoe lifts are not effective treatment methods for congenital scoliosis. Braces, although they have been shown to be effective in idiopathic scoliosis, have a limited role to play in congenital scoliosis.[2, 20, 21] Bracing cannot control a short, angular, congenital curve. If a vertebral anomaly produces a long, generally flexible curve around it, it may be possible to control the curve temporarily to allow spinal growth.

Bracing may also be effective in some structural compensatory curves above or below the congenital curve. It is important, however, to cease bracing in the face of continued progression. Compensatory curves above or below congenital ones arise because of the need to balance the spine over the pelvis. To avoid increasing the compensatory curve, progression of the congenital curve must be arrested. Bracing may be indicated to treat compensatory structural curves after surgery on the congenital part.

Surgical Treatment

A number of procedures are available in the surgical treatment of congenital scoliosis. Appropriately aggressive, early intervention may allow a simpler procedure to produce a satisfactory result without the risks involved with a more complicated one. Although parents may feel that operating on a 1-year-old's spine is too aggressive, there is little justification today in permitting relentless progression of a congenital curve to occur because of the fear of surgery itself or because of the concern of causing stunted growth of the spine. Complex procedures needed to correct severe congenital scoliosis cannot restore normal height to the spine that was lost through progression of the curve.

Congenital spinal anomalies that are known to cause progression, have a high likelihood of causing progression, or have had documented progression should have early surgery to avoid the development of a severe deformity. Roentgenograms and tomograms can help in making these decisions. Good information regarding spinal growth and the effect of early fusion on the height and body proportions is available to reassure the parents that early fusion will probably not cause their child to look disproportionate.[36, 37, 42] Cooperation and help from the young child's pediatrician may be essential because many of these children have multiple congenital anomalies, some of which may influence the decision on what or when surgery may be performed.

Parents should know that nothing works 100% of the time. Until the child is fully grown, the forces of continued growth may affect the previously operated spine, making additional surgery necessary. Procedures that effect correction of the spine may be associated with neurologic deficit from stretching or direct injury to the spinal cord. Spinal cord monitoring with or without the wake-up test should be done to minimize these problems.[22, 33]

Fusion in Situ

Posterior fusion in situ remains the cornerstone of surgical treatment for congenital scoliosis. It has been shown in a number of articles that the results are very acceptable and reliable.[18, 38, 42, 34] This procedure is relatively simple and safe and most children tolerate the surgery well, even very young ones (Fig. 15-6). The key to successful in situ fusion seems to be a thick, wide fusion mass. This may require bank bone in addition to autogenous iliac bone. It is also important that the fusion be bilateral and span the entire curve. Following these guidelines minimizes the chance of the fusion

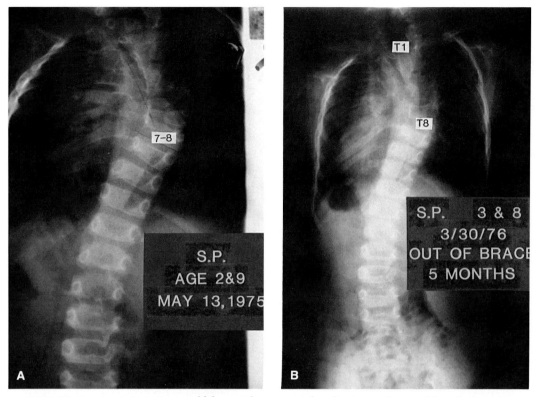

FIG. 15–6. A. A 2 + 9-year-old boy with congenital scoliosis consisting of fused ribs and unsegmented bar and hemivertebra underwent in situ fusion. **B.** Same patient 11 months after surgery showing no deterioration of the curve.

mass bending and causing progression of the curve. However, bending may result from the "crankshaft phenomenon," which is discussed later. In Winter's series, progressive lordosis and disproportionate stature did not occur when fusion was done in young patients.[42]

The disadvantage of a fusion in situ is the need to fuse a relatively long segment of the spine, which may not be much of a problem in the thoracic area, but which influences spinal motion and decreases trunk height if it involves a large segment of the lumbar spine. A posterior fusion in situ, in itself, does not produce immediate correction of the curve, nor does it effect gradual spontaneous correction with time. Moreover, it may not be a good procedure for patients with very severe kyphoscoliotic deformity, because it may not control the deformity. My colleagues and I do not recommend fusion in situ for lumbosacral hemivertebrae with significant trunk shift and a large compensatory thoracolumbar curve; this problem is better

handled by hemivertebra excision.[26] If the curve size increases in a spine that previously had an in situ fusion, the cause may not be bending of the fusion mass but pseudarthrosis or the crankshaft phenomenon.[10] This phenomenon results from tethering of the posterior aspect of the spine by the fusion mass, while the vertebral bodies continue to grow. Since the spine cannot lengthen in this situation, the vertebrae begin to rotate with the posterior elements and the fusion mass as the axis of rotation, resulting in an apparent increase in the curve (Fig. 15-7). This may also explain why progressive lordosis does not occur in the child whose spine has been fused at a young age.

A recent review of patients who had surgery for congenital scoliosis at age less than 10 years showed that this phenomenon did occur.[32] Six of 22 patients demonstrated the crankshaft phenomenon after an apparently successful posterior surgery; all 6 had only posterior surgery. This raises the issue of the necessity of an anterior spinal fusion in addition to the posterior

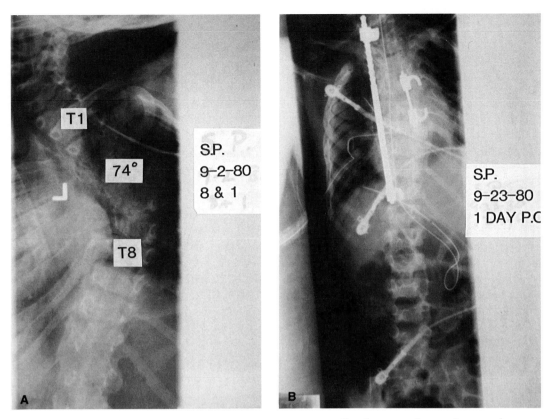

FIG. 15–7. Same patient as in Fig. 15-6. **A.** Five years after the in situ fusion, the curve has increased and cosmetic appearance is poor. **B.** Roentgenogram of the spine after a two-stage correction, an anterior wedge osteotomy followed by a posterior wedge osteotomy, instrumentation, and fusion.

in situ fusion in young patients with significant growth remaining.

My colleagues and I believe that a patient who has an in situ fusion should be placed in a cast or brace, at least until the fusion heals. Whether prolonged full- or part-time bracing afterwards is helpful is not clear.

Although correction of most curves appears to be desirable, in some areas, such as the cervical-thoracic area, attempts at correction probably represent an unacceptable risk; in these situations, the in situ fusion is probably the procedure of choice.

Two final points are important. Unilateral convex posterior in situ fusions alone are ineffective for curve control and for effecting spontaneous correction of a congenital curve, and therefore they should not be done. Imaging of the spinal canal before in situ fusion is unnecessary unless there are neurologic deficits or other stigmata of intraspinal pathology.

Posterior Fusion and Instrumentation

The usual methods of instrumenting scoliotic spines can be used in congenital scoliosis, but because of the decreased flexibility typical of these curves, the amount of correction that can be achieved is less than in idiopathic scoliosis. Often, only a modest amount of correction will occur, but the internal fixation may insure a solid fusion and yield better balance of the spine.[12] Evaluation of the spinal canal by myelography or MRI is necessary before such instrumentation. If a diastematomyelia is recognized, excision is probably needed if correction is planned. This may be done at the same time as the spinal fusion.

Various kinds of instrumentation can be used. The safest one is probably the most appropriate. The use of sublaminar wires should be avoided if possible. Because these curves are stiff, Cotrel–Dubousset instrumentation using the derotation maneuver may not work. However, Cotrel–Dubousset instrumentation can be used like a Harrington rod, and it has the advantage of being able to apply distraction and compression forces along the same rod and provide segmental fixation (Fig. 15-8).

An associated kyphosis must be recognized, and proper rod contouring should be done to prevent instrument cut-out. Pure distraction forces used in this situation to effect correction may be dangerous. If the kyphosis is large, anterior spinal fusion should be considered to achieve better correction and ensure a solid arthrodesis.

Posterior fusion and instrumentation for the purpose of correction is indicated most often for patients who have failed prior in situ fusion or for those with neglected congenital deformities with no prior treatment. Instrumentation may be used as a method of fixation, rather than correction, for patients with lesser degrees of curvature who are having an in situ fusion. In them, the instrumentation is used for stabilization and to help maximize the chances of an arthrodesis. With the Cotrel–Dubousset instrumentation, stabilization of the curve without external immobilization can be achieved because the instrumentation can be securely attached to the spine without changing the spinal alignment (Fig. 15-9).

Hemiepiphysiodesis
Hemiepiphysiodesis has been used in the extremities to correct angular deformities. Although McCarroll and Costen's report of hemiepiphysiodesis (actually, anterior hemiarthrodesis) noted failures in all four patients treated, more recent reports show that its use in the spine is effective.[4, 25, 35] Winter and Moe reviewed patients with congenital kyphosis who had posterior spinal fusion.[42] In the patients who had congenital kyphosis, at least modest amounts of correction occurred spontaneously if there was growth potential for the vertebrae anteriorly and if they achieved a thick, solid posterior fusion.

Congenital scoliosis can be managed in a similar way, provided that the hemiepiphysiodesis is done anteriorly and posteriorly and that there is some growth potential in those segments. Gradual correction does not work if the offending abnormality is an unsegmented bar. Instead, it is indicated for curves caused by failures of formation, and the procedure should probably extend two levels above and two below the hemivertebra on the convex side to maximize the chances of spontaneous correction from continued growth on the concave side. The technique affords maximal correction and improvement in a deformity if the initial curvature is not severe (Fig. 15-10). Therefore, it is not an appropriate procedure for a very severe curve that extends over many segments, which requires a long arthrodesis and instrumentation. If there is an associated compensatory curve above or below, it decreases in size as the congenital curve decreases in size. Bradford combined the technique with the use of supplementary subcutaneous rodding.[4]

The advantage of the hemiepiphysiodesis technique is the possibility of spontaneous correction along with curve control, without the use of forceful, acute correction with instrumentation. The disadvantage is the need for anterior and posterior approaches to the spine for a formal type of epiphysiodesis. However, the anterior and posterior parts can be done at the same sitting because there is only minimal blood loss from these procedures, and the child should tolerate the surgery well. Hemiepiphysiodesis may also be achieved with the eggshell technique, which will be discussed later.

Hemivertebra Excision
Often there are curves caused by hemivertebrae that produce significant curvature, imbalance, and trunk shift. Lumbosacral hemivertebrae may cause an additional problem of pelvic obliquity and a functional leg-length discrepancy. Correction by the usual methods requires long fusion. A component of kyphosis may also make the usual forms of correction less than ideal. In these situations, excision of the offending hemivertebra may afford excellent correction and often permits fusing of fewer levels than with traditional methods. Most indications for this technique are relative except for the lumbosacral hemivertebra, which presents the only absolute indication for hemivertebral excision.

The hemivertebra that is most easily resected is one that is fully segmented. This allows easy determination of the vertebral body at surgery and allows a more reliable prediction of the correction that can be obtained. Theoretically, a completely unsegmented hemivertebra would not be expected to cause much progression, and it would not be necessary to remove it. However, if it has caused significant imbalance or trunk shift, removing such a vertebra would have the same effect as a spinal osteotomy. Lumbosacral hemivertebrae ought to be excised early to avoid progressive thoracolumbar compensatory curves and to avoid worsening pelvic obliquity.

Hemivertebra excision is most appropriate for hemivertebrae located from the thoracolumbar junc-

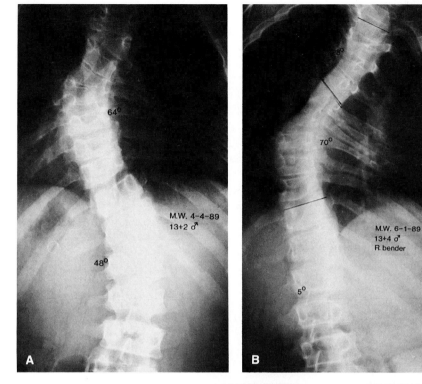

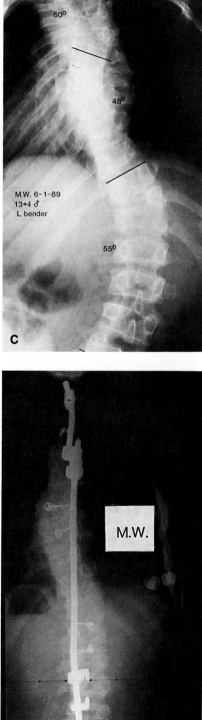

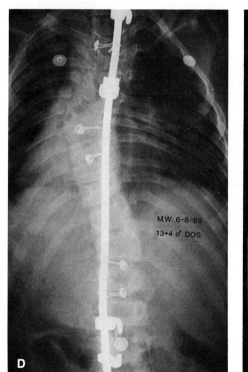

FIG. 15–8. **A.** A 13-year-old boy with congenital scoliosis with an increasing congenital curve and lower compensatory curve. **B,C.** Bending films show the relative flexibility of each curve. **D.** Postoperative anterior-posterior roentgenogram showing the instrumentation in place. **E.** This patient fell down an entire flight of steps 2 weeks after his surgery and displaced the upper hook of his instrumentation system, which at reoperation was found to be a fracture of the lamina. Using a domino on the Cotrel–Dubousset rod, a shorter rod and another hook that went one level above the fractured lamina was attached to the previously inserted rod without having to change the entire instrumentation.

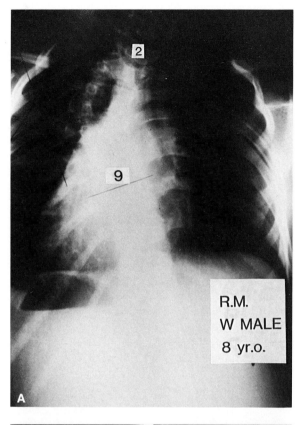

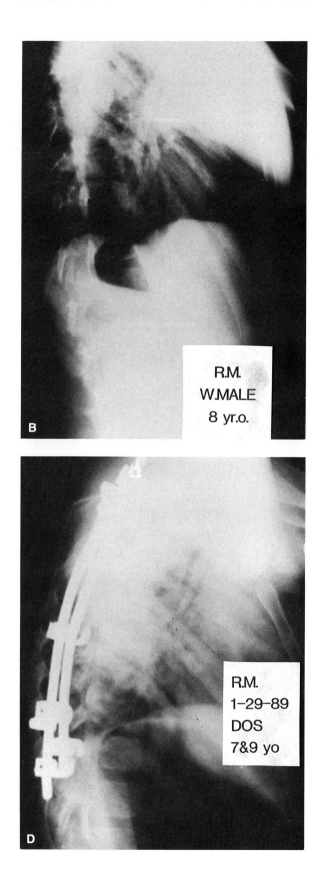

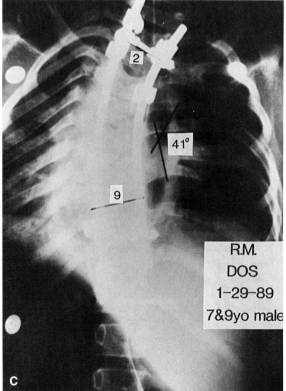

FIG. 15–9.

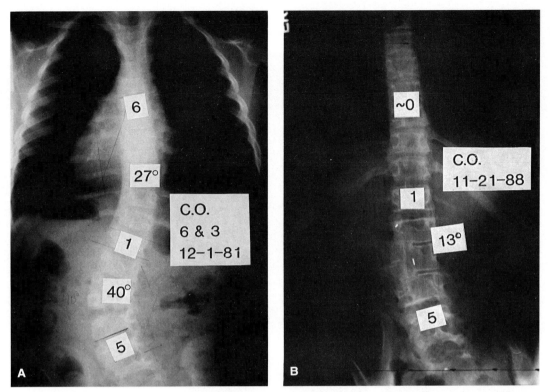

FIG. 15–10. **A.** Preoperative posterior-anterior standing roentgenogram of a 6 + 3-year-old boy with congenital scoliosis. **B.** Seven years later, there has been a marked improvement in his congenital curve and in the upper compensatory curve after anterior and posterior hemi-epiphysiodesis.

tion distally. Excisions in the lumbar spine are safer than in the thoracic. The excision has two effects—control of progression and correction. Preoperative tomography or MRI to define the anatomy is important. Intraoperative localization of the bone to be removed by x-ray films is also important, because counting the vertebrae in the wound may not be reliable in congenital scoliosis.

Hemivertebra excision can be done by the direct approach or the eggshell technique.[14] The eggshell technique offers the advantage of a one-stage, one-approach operation whose major effect is to eliminate the growth potential of the offending hemivertebra. It also can offer some immediate correction when used with internal fixation or a cast. Although many physicians use no internal fixation or external immobilization with the eggshell technique, my colleagues and I have routinely used both. We feel that, although

growth potential may be eliminated, there is not always predictable, immediate correction obtained with this method. However, it does effect a hemi-epiphysiodesis when combined with a convex posterior fusion at the same time.

The eggshell technique should be used with C-arm control. It can be tedious, because it requires patience to avoid trouble. Heinig, who popularized the technique, teaches that the hemilamina should be left in place until the vertebral body resection is completed (C. Heinig, personal communication). This helps protect the dural tube because the curette can safely be levered on this bone. I agree with this. Because experience with this procedure is fairly recent, longer follow-up is required to confirm whether this technique is reliable and efficacious (Figs. 15-11 and 15-12).

Although hemivertebra excision was reported by

(text continues on page 380)

◀ **FIG. 15–9.** **A.** Preoperative posterior-anterior radiograph of Type I congenital scoliosis that was shown to be progressive in an 8-year-old boy. **B.** Preoperative lateral view. **C.** Postoperative anterior-posterior view of the Cotrel–Dubousset instrumentation in place. **D.** Postoperative lateral view showing the instrumentation in place.

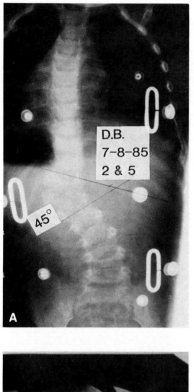

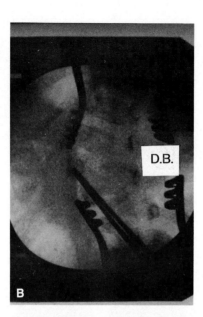

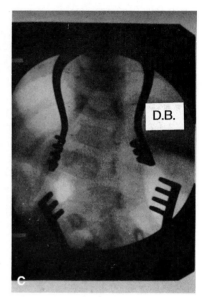

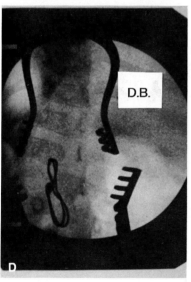

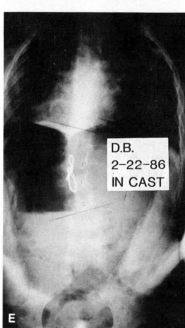

FIG. 15–11. A. A 2 + 5-year-old boy with congenital scoliosis secondary to failure of formation. Preoperative posterior-anterior standing radiograph. **B.** Intra-operative localization of the pedicle of the hemivertebra using the C-arm. **C.** C-arm image after the hemivertebra was removed by the eggshell technique. **D.** C-arm image after correction using a sublaminar wire. **E.** Postoperative standing posterior-anterior radiograph in cast.

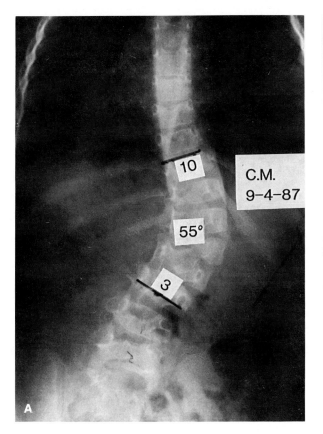

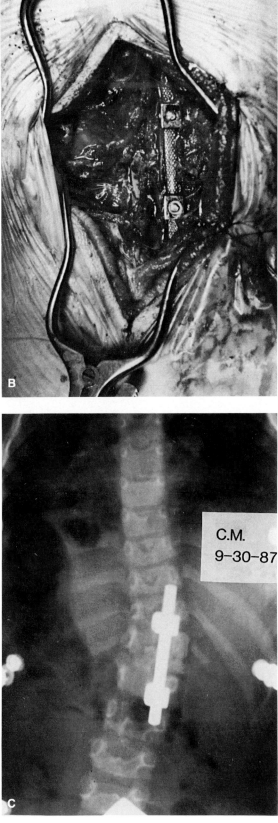

FIG. 15–12. **A.** A young girl with congenital scoliosis secondary to a thoracolumbar hemivertebra. Preoperative posterior-anterior standing radiograph of the spine. **B.** Intraoperative view of posterior instrumentation using pediatric Cotrel–Dubousset instrumentation. **C.** Postoperative standing posterior-anterior radiograph showing instrumentation in place and acute correction of the curve.

Compere many years ago, formal hemivertebra excision was popularized by Leatherman and Dickson.[8, 17] Their technique allows direct visualization of the hemivertebra and complete vertebrectomy without the blind maneuvers of the eggshell procedure. Although originally described as a two-stage procedure, anterior and posterior components can be done together, and there are some advantages to that approach. Particularly in young children, the blood loss should be minimal. For a simultaneous procedure, the patient should be positioned on his or her side and the back, abdomen, flank, and chest should be draped widely, so that adequate exposures can be done anteriorly and posteriorly (see Color Plate 7). Even lumbosacral hemivertebrae can usually be exposed through a flank extraperitoneal approach.

Once the ascending lumbar vein is isolated, ligated, and divided, the iliac vessels can usually be mobilized to visualize the lumbosacral junction. The hemivertebra are then resected back to the pedicle and the posterior longitudinal ligament. At this point, the posterior approach should be made. After the subperiosteal exposure has been completed out to the tips of the transverse processes, the two exposures can be connected. The nerve root at the level of excision should be identified and protected. Completion of the excision can then be performed. Some epidural and bone bleeding are to be expected and can be controlled with gelfoam, bone wax, and bipolar cautery.

One of the major problems is the fixation needed to close the space created by the excision. In my experience, this has been especially difficult in young patients because their bone is small and soft and cannot usually accommodate adult anterior fixation devices, like the Zielke or Dwyer. However, in the larger child or in the adult, these devices may work well. In the young child nonstandard kinds of fixation, such as vertebral body screws passed through a plate or coupled with a twisted wire, can be used anteriorly. Posteriorly, a sublaminar wire or pediatric Cotrel–Dubousset compression system can help hold the wedge-shaped space together (Fig. 15-13). Older and larger children can be managed by standard instrumentation constructs.

The instrumentation may not hold, especially in small children or in those with soft bone, and the use of a pantaloon spica cast incorporating a distal femoral pin in the femur on the high side of the pelvis and a turnbuckle can restore balance and afford correction. Even if internal fixation is used in the young child, the use of a pantaloon spica for 2 or 3 months is probably warranted to ensure adequate initiation of the fusion. This is particularly true when excising lumbosacral hemivertebrae. If a lumbosacral hemivertebrae has stimulated a structural thoracolumbar curve to compensate for it, prolonged use of bracing may be necessary to control that curve. It is important to treat lumbosacral hemivertebrae early to prevent large structural compensatory curves from forming.

The technique of hemivertebrae excision is exacting and should be attempted only by those with the requisite training and experience to do this kind of surgery. Moreover, because the type of fixation needed cannot always be predicted preoperatively, a wide range of instrumentation should be available in the operating room. Evaluation of the spinal canal should be done by myelography or MRI, and spinal cord monitoring with or without the wake-up test should be done during surgery.[22, 33] Fortunately, my colleagues and I have not had any major or permanent neurologic deficits caused by these techniques.

Salvage/Reconstruction

The previous sections outlined methods of controlling or correcting congenital curves while patients are young and before curves are severe. However, some patients present who have had no prior treatment (Fig. 15-14) or who have had prior treatment that has failed or did not give an optimal result. In these situations, corrective surgery becomes more complicated; although it usually cannot correct the curve greatly, it may help with symptoms and achieve better overall balance of the spine. The indications for this surgery are continued progression of the curvature, pain, or neurologic deficits and for the correction of severe cosmetic or functional deformities (Figs. 15-15 and 15-16). This last category points out that, even though fusion in situ may achieve curve control, a grotesque deformity that is cosmetically displeasing and functionally problematic may persist.

Surgery consists of osteotomies, hemivertebrae excision, decompressions, repair of pseudarthrosis, and extension of fusions. Care must be taken in recommending these procedures because they may not produce the expected cosmetic results. Procedures like osteotomies may be associated with a significant threat of neurologic complications.

Newer instrumentation may help in these situations. The Cotrel–Dubousset dominoes and axial connectors (Stuart, Greensburg, PA), as well as the Texas

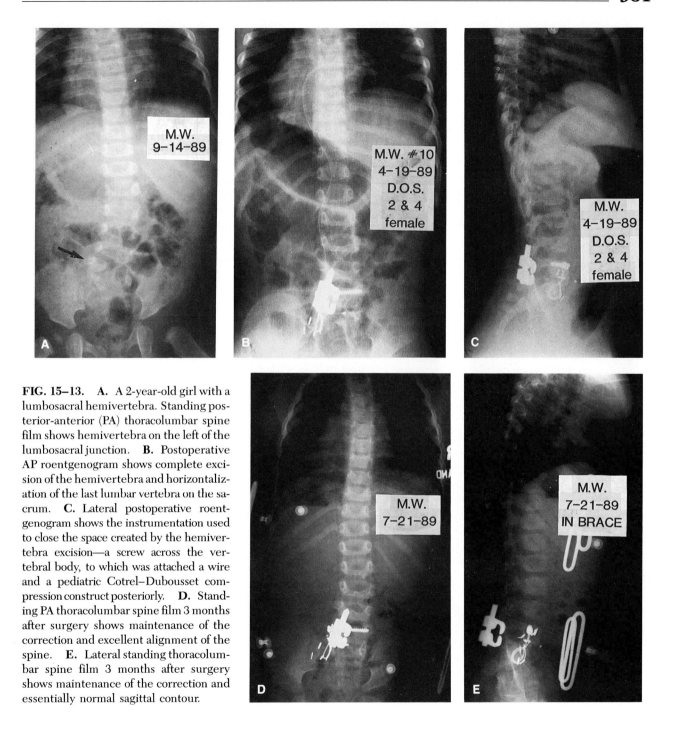

FIG. 15–13. **A.** A 2-year-old girl with a lumbosacral hemivertebra. Standing posterior-anterior (PA) thoracolumbar spine film shows hemivertebra on the left of the lumbosacral junction. **B.** Postoperative AP roentgenogram shows complete excision of the hemivertebra and horizontalization of the last lumbar vertebra on the sacrum. **C.** Lateral postoperative roentgenogram shows the instrumentation used to close the space created by the hemivertebra excision—a screw across the vertebral body, to which was attached a wire and a pediatric Cotrel–Dubousset compression construct posteriorly. **D.** Standing PA thoracolumbar spine film 3 months after surgery shows maintenance of the correction and excellent alignment of the spine. **E.** Lateral standing thoracolumbar spine film 3 months after surgery shows maintenance of the correction and essentially normal sagittal contour.

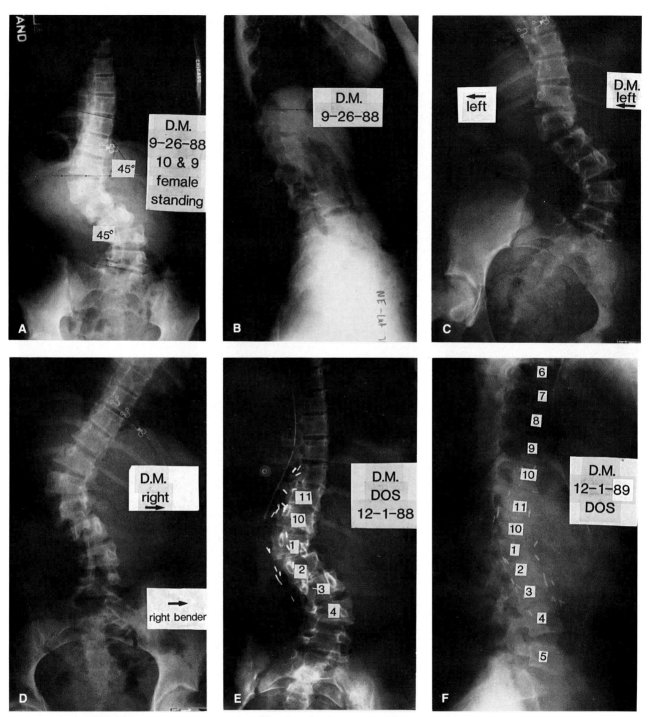

FIG. 15–14. A. A 10 + 9-year-old girl with an apparent congenital scoliosis with wedging of the L4 vertebra and abnormal left pedicle with severe trunk decompensation. Posterior-anterior standing thoracolumbar spine film showing the wedging of L4 and decompensation of the trunk to the left. **B.** Lateral standing thoracolumbar spine roentgenogram showing loss of the normal sagittal contour. **C,D.** Left and right supine forced-bending roentgenograms show the flexibility of the curves. **E,F.** Postoperative anterior-posterior and lateral roentgenograms after anterior release, discectomy, and bone grafting. **G,H.** Postoperative roentgenograms after the final stage, consisting of posterior fusion and Cotrel–Dubousset instrumentation, showing good alignment in the coronal plane and restoration of the sagittal contour.

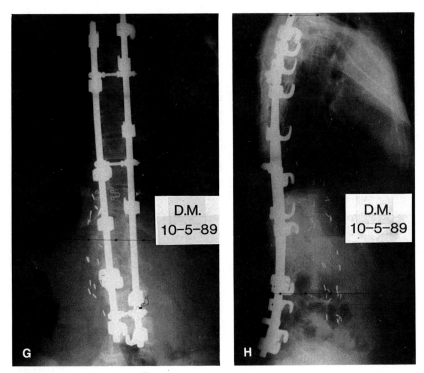

FIG. 15–14.   (*continued*)

Scottish Rite Crosslink system (Danek, Memphis, TN), are very useful for extending existing instrumentation and repairing pseudarthrosis with broken instrumentation. The Cotrel–Dubousset instrumentation is useful as replacement instrumentation if the previous instruments cannot be salvaged and have to be removed. If instrumentation cannot be used, methods such as turnbuckle casts are used to achieve a satisfactory result. Spinal cord monitoring and the wake-up test should be used with these procedures.[22, 33] An appropriate preoperative workup is required to rule out intraspinal abnormalities.

Author's Preferred Treatment

This chapter has reviewed various surgical treatments for congenital scoliosis. Some are more complicated than others, and some offer correction immediately or gradually. The surgeon may feel more comfortable with one procedure than another. All of these factors enter into treatment decisions.

In situ fusions are not 100% effective in curve control. In very young children, a concomitant anterior spinal fusion may be necessary. The addition of the anterior spinal fusion helps to avoid the crankshaft phenomenon. In situ fusions are appropriate in areas where curve correction and surgical exposure are problematic, such as at the cervicothoracic junction. In situ posterior fusions alone are not appropriate for severe curves, especially those with kyphosis, because they neither control the curve nor achieve correction of severe deformity, the magnitude of which may in itself cause functional impairment. In situ fusions should extend across the entire curve and be performed bilaterally with sufficient bone graft to insure a solid arthrodesis.

Anterior-posterior hemiepiphysiodesis is the treatment of choice for mild to moderate curves expected to progress and caused by hemivertebrae. Excellent results have been obtained by doing formal anterior and posterior hemiepiphysiodesis. Convex arthrodeses, anterior alone or posterior alone, cannot achieve curve control or gradually decrease curve magnitude. Gradual curve improvement is the beauty of a well done anterior and posterior hemiepiphysiodesis. The anterior and posterior procedures can be done together. Whether doing this hemiepiphysiodesis by means of the eggshell technique will give comparable results is

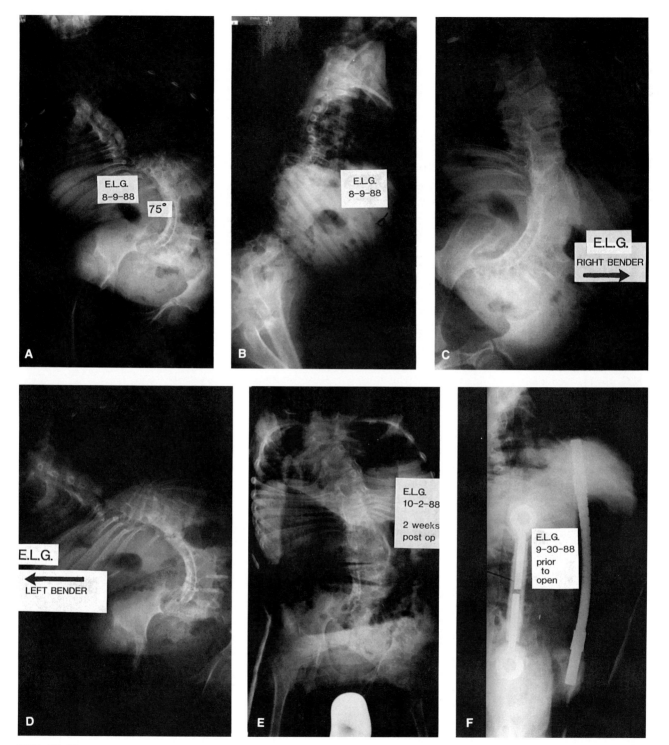

FIG. 15–15.

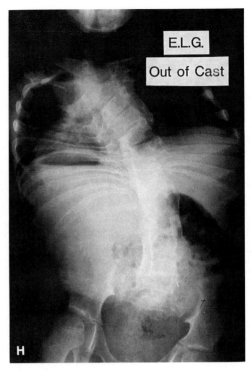

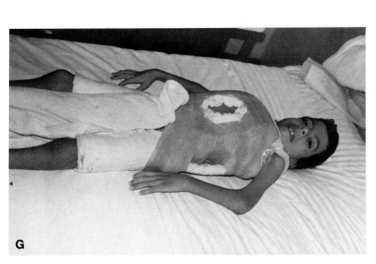

FIG. 15–15. **A.** A 10-year-old boy with congenital scoliosis secondary to failure of segmentation of the lumbar spine who underwent in situ fusion as a young child. Curve control was obtained, but the functional and cosmetic results were poor. Standing posterior-anterior thoracolumbar spine film shows severe trunk decompensation to the left and the left hemipelvis up under the left costal margin. **B.** Lateral standing thoracolumbar spine film showing the sagittal alignment of the spine. **C,D.** Right and left supine forced-bending roentgenograms showing the relative stiffness of even the unfused area of the spine. **E,F.** Anterior-posterior and lateral roentgenograms of the thoracolumbar spine in a pantaloon spica cast with a turnbuckle, after simultaneous anterior and posterior wedge resection of the fusion mass. This child's bone was too soft to be able to use instrumentation to effect correction and stabilization. Attempts at using several different types of instrumentation failed intraoperatively, and the patient was then placed in a cast for gradual correction with the turnbuckle. **G.** Photograph of the patient in his turnbuckle pantaloon cast. **H.** Standing anterior-posterior thoracolumbar spine roentgenogram after cast removal with apparent solid fusion and nice correction.

not yet clear, but it may be an alternative technique to achieve the same result.

Hemivertebra excision should be done when there is a significant deformity that needs correction, not just for curve control or when correction cannot be adequately achieved by other means. This is especially true for lumbosacral hemivertebrae causing pelvic obliquity and significant thoracolumbar compensatory curvatures. Hemivertebra excision should not routinely be done in the thoracic spine owing to the neurologic risk. Formal anterior and posterior pro-

cedures offer the most reliable method of accomplishing this closing wedge osteotomy. However, the eggshell procedure can also be used.

Posterior fusion with instrumentation is indicated in the older child and adult with a moderate to severe curve without significant kyphosis, for which the goal is modest correction and curve control. If the associated kyphosis is significant, preliminary or secondary anterior spinal fusion may be needed to insure a solid fusion.

Instrumentation can be used in any of the pro-

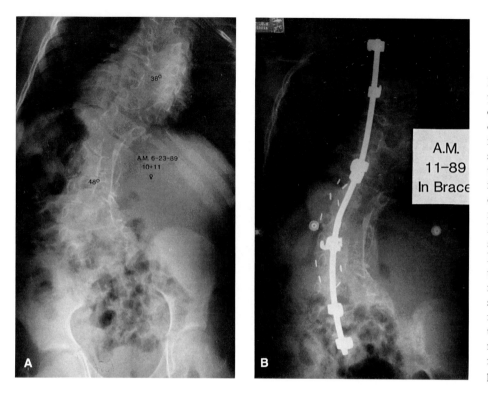

FIG. 15–16. **A.** A 10 + 11-year-old girl with progressive, congenital scoliosis whose myelogram and MRI were seen in Fig. 15-5. She underwent staged anterior and posterior osteotomies with excision of the intraspinal bony spur at the time of her posterior surgery. Anterior-posterior standing thoracolumbar spine roentgenogram showing the congenital anomalies and the decompensation of the spine. **B.** Standing posterior-anterior thoracolumbar spine film showing improvement in the overall alignment of the spine and a well-healed spinal fusion. This patient remained neurologically intact postoperatively.

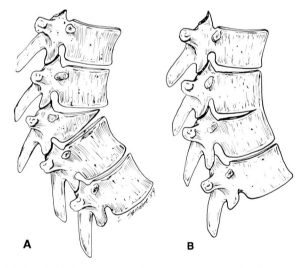

FIG. 15–17. Classification of congenital kyphosis. **A.** Type I, failure of formation. **B.** Type II, failure of segmentation.

cedures mentioned to stabilize the spine as the fusion heals, but its use introduces all its potential problems. The advantages and disadvantages should be considered carefully.

If these procedures are applied before curves become severe, there should be less need for complicated salvage or reconstructive procedures in the future.

CONGENITAL KYPHOSIS

Congenital kyphosis can be classified as Type I (failure of formation) or Type II (failure of segmentation) (Fig. 15-17). The two types are very different. Most notably, neurologic deficit in Type II kyphosis is practically unheard of, even if the deformity is large.[24] Many of these patients have multiple areas of involvement with only a few open disc spaces remaining mobile between long segments of fused vertebrae. The amount of unsegmented disc space determines the amount of progression or the loss of longitudinal growth of the spine. Patients with Type I deformities are more likely to have

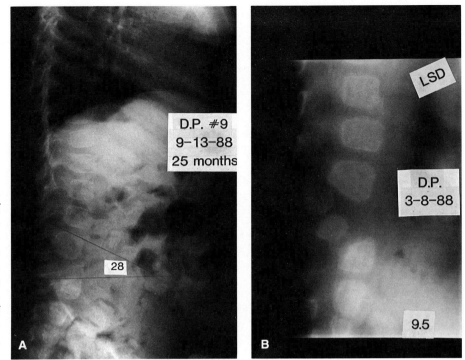

FIG. 15–18. **A.** A 25-month-old boy with Type I failure of formation defect causing a congenital kyphosis in the lower lumbar spine. Standing lateral thoracolumbar spine roentgenogram showing the congenital kyphosis and the vertebral anomalies. **B.** Lateral tomogram of the same patient, better delineating the anatomy of the congenital abnormality.

more progression, and they are at risk for neurologic deficits caused by their curves and vertebral anomalies.[6, 19, 27, 41, 34, 40]

Congenital kyphosis is the most common spinal deformity that produces spinal cord compromise. The patients in whom this occurs tend to be males in their second decade of life, and the problem occurs most often in the thoracic spine. The duration of the neurologic deficit does not necessarily correlate with the result of treatment.[19] In Type I and Type II deformities, increasing kyphosis causes an increase in the compensatory lumbar lordosis, especially if the curve is low thoracic, thoracolumbar, or upper lumbar. In the long run, degenerative disease of the lumbosacral spine may cause more problems than the kyphosis itself, with symptoms of back pain and nerve root compression.

Clinical and Radiologic Evaluation

A workup and evaluation similar to that for congenital scoliosis should be performed for each congenital kyphosis patient. Genitourinary abnormalities, Klippel-Feil syndrome, and intraspinal abnormalities should be sought. Particular attention should be given to the patient's neurologic examination. Signs of myelopathy (i.e, hyperreflexia, clonus, positive Babinski signs) and a history of weakness and difficulty walking should be noted. Patients with spinal cord compression often complain that they have difficulty walking, particularly going up stairs and advancing their legs, yet their muscle testing appears to be relatively normal. Despite this apparent contradiction, the surgeon should be alert for spinal cord compression caused by the spinal deformity.

All of these patients should have renal ultrasonography and cervical spine films. An evaluation of the spinal canal in patients who have neurologic abnormalities or in whom surgical correction is contemplated should also be done. In patients with pure kyphosis, MRI may be very helpful in evaluating the spinal canal. Myelography, however, may be required in some of these patients who also have associated scoliosis. Tomograms may better define the pathologic anatomy and may assist in surgical planning (Fig. 15-18).

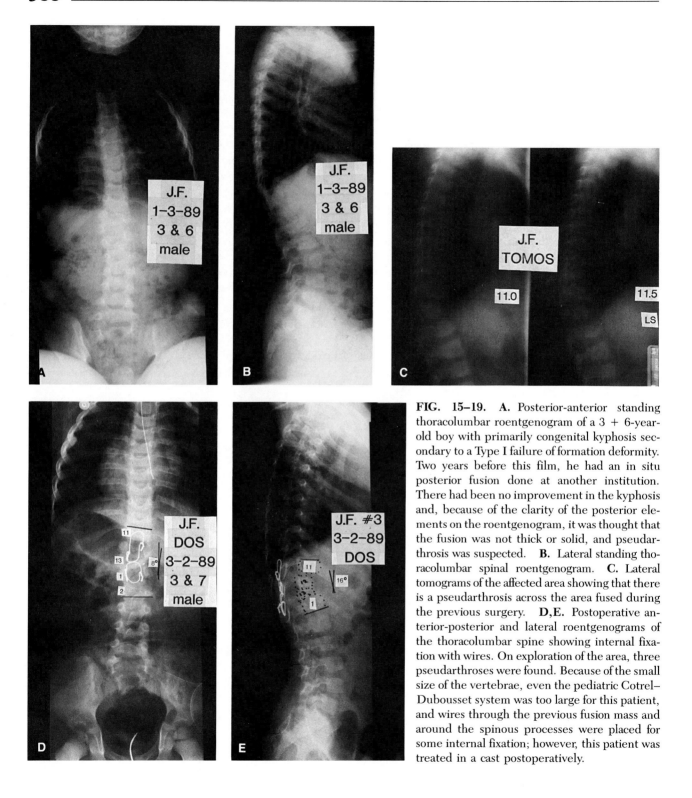

FIG. 15–19. **A.** Posterior-anterior standing thoracolumbar roentgenogram of a 3 + 6-year-old boy with primarily congenital kyphosis secondary to a Type I failure of formation deformity. Two years before this film, he had an in situ posterior fusion done at another institution. There had been no improvement in the kyphosis and, because of the clarity of the posterior elements on the roentgenogram, it was thought that the fusion was not thick or solid, and pseudarthrosis was suspected. **B.** Lateral standing thoracolumbar spinal roentgenogram. **C.** Lateral tomograms of the affected area showing that there is a pseudarthrosis across the area fused during the previous surgery. **D,E.** Postoperative anterior-posterior and lateral roentgenograms of the thoracolumbar spine showing internal fixation with wires. On exploration of the area, three pseudarthroses were found. Because of the small size of the vertebrae, even the pediatric Cotrel–Dubousset system was too large for this patient, and wires through the previous fusion mass and around the spinous processes were placed for some internal fixation; however, this patient was treated in a cast postoperatively.

Careful follow-up with physical examinations is mandatory, especially for patients with Type I deformities, so that early recognition of spinal cord compression can be accomplished.

Treatment

Standard Treatments

Bracing is not a definitive or effective form of treating either type of congenital kyphosis. If there is some flexibility within, above, and below the congenital abnormality, bracing tends to straighten the overall alignment of the spine, but the differential growth pattern characteristic of congenital spinal deformities cannot really be altered by bracing. Without treatment and reduction in the size of the curve, rather rigid compensatory lordoses develop above and below the apex of the kyphotic segment. Therefore, early surgery for both types of deformities is indicated.

In general, kyphosis less than 75° in children younger than 5 years of age responds well to a thick, solid posterior spinal fusion over the congenital segments and extending at least one level above and below.[34] This acts as a hemiepiphysiodesis and allows spontaneous correction to a moderate degree in addition to stabilizing the curve. This effect is more likely to occur with Type I deformities. If this opportunity is lost, more complicated methods are required to ensure correction and a solid fusion.

Type I deformities have an increased incidence of neurologic deficit. The treatment of these curves depends on whether neurologic deficit exists. Some of these patients present so late that their deformities cannot realistically be corrected to any semblance of normal; spinal cord decompression or stabilization of the curve then becomes the primary goal. In patients with Type I deformities who do not have neurologic deficits and have curves less than 75° and in patients younger than 5 years of age, a posterior spinal fusion should be done with prolonged external support to insure solid, rigid fusion. Instrumentation may or may not be used. With this technique, the continuation of anterior growth with the posterior tethering from the fusion mass should theoretically allow some amount of spontaneous correction (Fig. 15-19).

When patients present later with larger deformities, decision making is more difficult. The amount of correction that is obtained depends on the configuration and flexibility of the curve, but anterior interbody or strut grafting followed by posterior fusion and instru-

mentation can offer a significant amount of correction for some of these curves (Figs. 15-20 and 15-21). Some curves, however, are so large and angular that the usual methods of kyphosis correction cannot work, and stabilization is the primary goal. In these patients an anterior strut graft is needed, followed by posterior fusion; posterior fusions alone do not work. The anterior strut construct should be positioned for support in the weight-bearing line of the spine. A hyperextension lateral roentgenogram of the spine is helpful in determining the position and the length of the strut that is needed. In addition, multiple struts may be needed to help support the kyphosis and prevent it from collapsing further. The struts can be vascularized or not and can be autograft or allograft. There has been success in using all of these constructs. However, Bradford and colleagues, using nonvascularized struts, found that 5 of 9 of them placed more than 4 cm from the spine subsequently fractured.[5] Vascularized rib has been shown to incorporate and hypertrophy quickly and may offer an advantage over nonvascularized strut grafts that need to be some distance from the spine.[3] The limiting factor with them, however, is the length of the vascular pedicle.

The use of anterior instrumentation, such as the Kostuik device, may add stability to the construct, but the accurate positioning of the strut grafts, in my opinion, is more important than using instrumentation anteriorly in these patients.[16] When posterior fusion is added, instrumentation may or may not be used, but particularly with Type I deformities, distraction instrumentation increases the risk of neurologic injury from the surgery.[34]

If the patient presents with a severe Type I deformity with neurologic deficit, the appropriate treatment is decompression of the spinal cord and spinal arthrodesis. Decompression allows the spinal cord to fall free of the surrounding bony ring without any pressure above or below the apex of the kyphosis.[5,15] This can be accomplished by realignment of the spine (i.e., correction of the deformity) or direct decompression. In patients with neurologic deficit and kyphosis, Lonstein found that the best results occurred in those who had realignment and correction without exposing the spinal canal.[19] However, this group of patients had flexible curves and mild paraparesis. He found that laminectomy gave poor results in the treatment of the neurologic deficit associated with kyphosis.

However, in those with very severe rigid kyphoses,

(text continues on page 393)

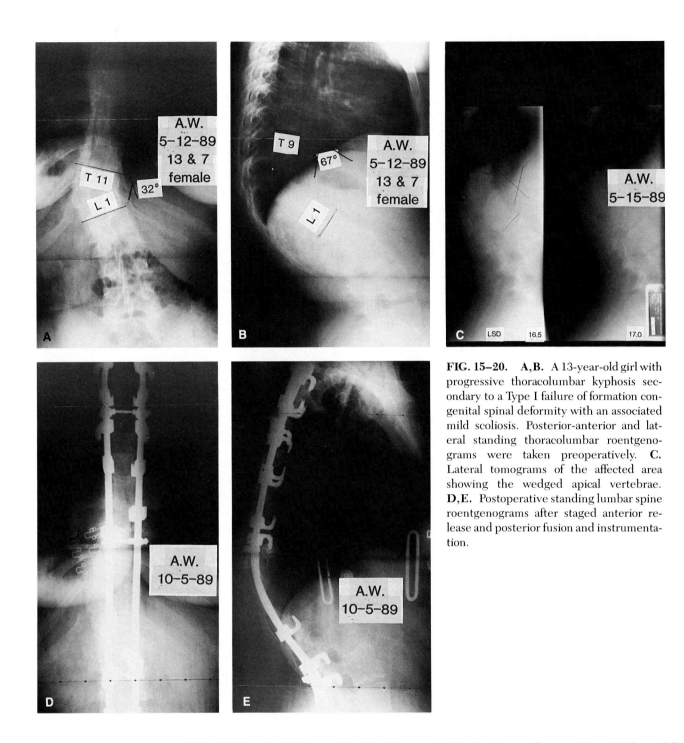

FIG. 15–20.   A,B. A 13-year-old girl with progressive thoracolumbar kyphosis secondary to a Type I failure of formation congenital spinal deformity with an associated mild scoliosis. Posterior-anterior and lateral standing thoracolumbar roentgenograms were taken preoperatively. C. Lateral tomograms of the affected area showing the wedged apical vertebrae. D,E. Postoperative standing lumbar spine roentgenograms after staged anterior release and posterior fusion and instrumentation.

FIG. 15–21.   A. A 10-year-old girl with congenital kyphosis secondary to a Type I failure of formation deformity. Preoperative clinical radiograph of the patient shows the gibbus in the thoracolumbar area.   B,C. Posterior-anterior and lateral standing roentgenograms of the spine showing the marked kyphosis and scoliosis secondary to the congenital anomalies.   D. Lateral roentgenogram after instillation of metrizamide for myelogram showing marked kyphosis and difficulty that the contrast agent had to pass in this area; this patient was neurologically normal preoperatively.   E,F. Standing thoracolumbar roentgenograms after anterior discectomy, interbody and strut graft fusion with autogenous fibula, and posterior fusion with Luque instrumentation. The patient had mild, transient weakness in her quadriceps bilaterally, which resolved within 6 weeks after surgery.

CONCLUSIONS

Caring for congenital spinal deformities requires both a good knowledge of the natural history of the process and experience. The guidelines set forth in this chapter should help the surgeon care for most situations, but nothing works 100% of the time. Even after all the right things have been done for a patient, the result may not be exactly as predicted. The effects of growth are the most important factors. Careful follow-up of these patients until skeletal maturity is necessary. Patients and parents should know at the outset that although the goal is to control the curve with one surgical intervention, others may be needed.

The standards of treatment for congenital spinal deformities have evolved during this century, and some ideas that once fell into disrepute are now being used routinely. Some of the old principles and beliefs about treatment have been abrogated by the results of long-term reviews. The surgeon's thinking must reflect this evolution. Newer procedures, although more complicated and perhaps somewhat riskier, may provide more pleasing results in selected patients than the standard methods of treatment, such as in situ fusion. Only long-term follow-up of treated patients will show—perhaps to the consternation of the surgeon—whether the surgical treatment was truly effective. The unfortunate fact is that nothing can destroy a surgeon's confidence like follow-up.

References

1. Albanese SA, Coren AB, Weinstein MP, et al: Ultrasonography for urinary tract evaluation in patients with congenital spine anomalies. Clin Orthop 228:302, 1988
2. Bassett GS, Bunnell WP, MacEwen GD: Treatment of idiopathic scoliosis with the Wilmington brace: results in patients with a 20–39 degree curve. J Bone Joint Surg 68:602, 1986
3. Bradford DS: Anterior vascularized pedicle bone grafting for treatment of kyphosis. Spine 5:318, 1980
4. Bradford DS: Partial epiphyseal arrest and supplementary fixation for progressive correction of congenital spinal deformity. J Bone Joint Surg [Am] 64:610, 1962
5. Bradford DS, Ganjarian S, Antonious D, et al: Anterior strut grafting for the treatment of kyphosis. J Bone Joint Surg [Am] 64:680, 1982
6. Bradford DS, Lonstein JE, Ogilvie JW, Winter RB (eds): Moe's Textbook of Scoliosis and Other Spinal Deformities, 2nd ed. Philadelphia, WB Saunders, 1987
7. Chou SN: The treatment of paralysis associated with kyphosis: Role of anterior decompression. Clin Orthop 128: 149, 1977
8. Compere EL: Excision of hemivertebrae for correction of congenital scoliosis. J Bone Joint Surg 14:555, 1932
9. Dubousset J: Congenital kyphoses. In Bradford DS, Hensinger RN (eds): The Pediatric Spine. New York, Thieme, 1985
10. Dubousset J, Herring JA, Shufflebarger H: The crankshaft phenomenon. J Pediatr Orthop 9:541, 1989
11. Gillespie R, Faithful DK, Roth A, Hall JE: Intraspinal anomalies in congenital scoliosis. Clin Orthop 93:103, 1973
12. Hall JE: Congenital scoliosis. In Bradford DS, Kensinger RN (eds): The Pediatric Spine. New York, Thieme, 1985
13. Hall JE, Herndon WA, Levine CR: Surgical treatment of congenital scoliosis with or without Harrington instrumentation. J Bone Joint Surg [Am] 63:608, 1981
14. Hodgson AR, Stock FE: Anterior spine fusion. Br J Surg 48:172, 1960
15. Kaneda K: Spinal cord compression secondary to spinal deformity. In Bradford DS, Hensinger RN (eds): The Pediatric Spine. New York, Thieme, 1985
16. Kostuik JP: Anterior Kostuik-Harrington distraction system. Orthopaedics 11:1379, 1988
17. Leatherman KD, Dickson RA: Two-stage correction surgery for congenital deformities of the spine. J Bone Joint Surg [Br] 61:324, 1979
18. Letts RM, Bobechko WP: Fusion of scoliotic spines in young children: Effect on progression and growth. Proceedings and reports of the Canadian Orthopaedic Assn. J Bone Joint Surg [Br] 56:589, 1974
19. Lonstein JE, Winter RB, Moe JH, et al: Neurologic deficits secondary to spinal deformity: A review of the literature and report of 43 cases. Spine 5:331, 1980
20. Lonstein JE, Winter RB: Milwaukee brace treatment of adolescent idiopathic scoliosis: Review of 939 patients. Presented at Spine Research Society meeting, Baltimore, MD, September, 1988
21. Lonstein JE, Winter RB: Milwaukee brace treatment of juvenile idiopathic scoliosis. Presented at Spine Research Society meeting, Baltimore, MD, September, 1988
22. Lubicky JP, Spadaro JA, Yuan HA, et al: Variability of somatosensory cortical evoked potential monitoring during spinal surgery. Spine 14:790, 1989
23. MacEwen GD, Winter RB, Hardy J: Evaluation of kidney anomalies in congenital scoliosis. J Bone Joint Surg [Am] 54:1451, 1972
24. Mayfield JK, Winter RB, Bradford DS, Moe JH: Congenital kyphosis due to defects in anterior segmentation. J Bone Joint Surg [Am] 62:129, 1980
25. McCarroll HR, Costen W: Attempted treatment of scoliosis by unilateral vertebral epiphyseal arrest. J Bone Joint Surg [Am] 42:965, 1960
26. Millis MD, Hall JE: Transiliac lengthening of the lower extremity. J Bone Joint Surg [Am] 61:1182, 1979
27. Morin B, Potras B, Duhaime M, et al: Congenital ky-

phosis by segmentation defect: Etiology and pathogenic studies. J Pediatr Orthop 5:309, 1985

28. O'Donnell CS, Bunnell WP, Betz RR, et al: Electrical stimulation in the treatment of idiopathic scoliosis. Clin Orthop 229:107, 1988

29. Rechles LN, Peterson HA, Bianco AJ, Weedman WH: The association of scoliosis and congenital heart defects. J Bone Joint Surg [Am] 57:449, 1975

30. Roth A, Rosenthal R, Hall JE, Migel M: Scoliosis and congenital heart disease. Clin Orthop 93:95, 1973

31. Sullivan JA, Davidson R, Renshaw TS, et al: Further evaluation of the scolitron treatment of idiopathic adolescent scoliosis. Spine 11:903, 1986

32. Terek R, Wehner J, Lubicky JP: The crankshaft phenomenon in congenital scoliosis. J Pediatr Orthop (in press)

33. Vauzelle C, Stagnara P, Jouvinroux P: Functional monitoring of spinal cord activity during spinal surgery. Clin Orthop 93:173, 1973

34. Winter RB: Congenital Deformities of the Spine. New York, Thieme-Stratton, 1983

35. Winter RB: Convex anterior and posterior hemarthrosis in young children with progressive congenital scoliosis. J Pediatr Orthop 1:361, 1981

36. Winter RB: Scoliosis and spinal growth. Orthop Rev 6:17, 1977

37. Winter RB: The effect of early fusion on spine growth. In Zorab PA (ed): Scoliosis and Spinal Growth. Edinburgh, Churchill Livingstone, 1971

38. Winter RB, Moe JH, Eilers VE: Congenital scoliosis: A study of 234 patients treated and untreated. J Bone Joint Surg [Am] 50:1, 1968

39. Winter RB, Moe, JH, Lonstein JE: The incidence of Klippel-Feil syndrome in patients with congenital scoliosis and kyphosis. Spine 9:363, 1984

40. Winter RB, Moe JH, Lonstein JE: Surgical treatment of congenital kyphosis: A review of 94 patients age 5 years or older with 2 years of more follow-up in 77 patients. Spine 10:224, 1985

41. Winter RB, Moe JH, Wang JF: Congenital kyphosis. J Bone Joint Surg [Am] 55:223, 1973

42. Winter RB, Moe JH: The results of spinal arthrodesis for congenital spinal deformities in patients younger than 5 years old. J Bone Joint Surg [Am] 64:419, 1982

43. Wynne-Davies R: Congenital vertebral anomalies: Etiology and relationship to spina bifida cystica. J Med Gen 12:280, 1975

TETHERED SPINAL CORD

JAMES E. SHOOK

Embryologically the spinal cord terminates in the coccygeal region of the vertebral column. Between the 11-mm and 30-mm stages, the greater part of the coccygeal cord undergoes a process of dedifferentiation. The most cephalic part of this region persists as the ventricularis terminalis; the more caudal part develops into a fibrous strand, the filum terminale.[22] Disproportionate growth rates between the spinal cord and the vertebral column result in an ascent of the spinal cord. The most rapid ascent is before the 17th week of life, when the cord ends opposite L4. The conus reaches the mature adult level (L1–L2) approximately 2 months after a full-term gestation.[4]

Spinal dysraphic states are caused by aberrations in the development of the neural-vertebral axis.[16] These present as a continuum of structural and physiologic defects, including open neural tube defects, lipomas, lipomeningoceles, diastematomyelia, a thickened filum terminale, dermal sinuses, fibrous bands, and abberant nerve roots.[13, 14]

These dysraphic states may prevent normal ascent of the spinal cord to its adult level or may result in loss of normal movements of the spinal cord in flexion and extension, both of which lead to spinal cord "traction" or "tethering."[2, 3, 8] Spinal cord traction produces neural ischemia and cellular dysfunction caused by an alteration in subcellular oxidative metabolism. It is seen clinically as a failure in the development or function of the musculoskeletal, neurologic, or urologic systems.[28]

Open neural tube defects, including meningoceles and myelomeningoceles, are frequently associated with a low-lying spinal cord, disorganized dysfunctional nerve roots, and neurologic dysfunction.[16] Early closure techniques that minimize scar formation have been advocated to avoid spinal cord traction with growth. Spinal cord traction caused by perineural cicatrix formation is occasionally associated with a rapidly progressive scoliosis, foot deformity, or urologic dysfunction and is seen most frequently during periods of rapid growth.[2, 3]

Spinal lipomas and lipomeningoceles are accumulations of normal fat that are frequently associated with developmental abnormalities in the neural vertebral axis.[5, 21] The lipomas may be extraspinal and communicate through posterior defects in the neural arches with a thickened fibrotic filum terminale or with a low-lying conus medullaris. These lipomas may be extradural or intradural. Spinal cord traction may occur because of attachment to these lipomatous lesions during periods of rapid growth or because of hypomobility of the conus medullaris or cauda equina during normal flexion and extension movements of the spine. With weight gain, the lipomatous mass may increase in size and cause cord compression and dysfunction.[5]

Diastematomyelia is a longitudinal bifurcation in the spinal cord with an interposed midline septum. The septum may be osseous, cartilagenous, or fibrous. Diastematomyelia is seen in 4.9% of individuals with congenital scoliosis, and 60% of them have a congenital scoliosis.[12, 27] A diastematomyelia may be asymptomatic or may occur with progressive scoliosis, foot deformity, or urologic dysfunction.[19]

The filum terminale forms from the most caudal end of the embryonic spinal cord. It normally floats free in the cerebrospinal fluid, is not under tension, is less tham 2 mm in diameter, and merges imperceptibly with the conus medullaris. If the filum terminale is developmentally short, fibrotic, or infiltrated with fat, it "tethers" the conus medullaris, preventing the normal ascent of the spinal cord during embryologic development. It may also limit normal movement of the conus medullaris during spinal flexion and extension. This pathologic traction on the conus medullaris may lead to progressive dysfunction of the terminal end of the spinal cord, manifested as musculoskeletal, neurologic, or urologic dysfunction.[15, 18]

Epidermoids, dermoids, and dermal sinuses are heterotopic formations composed of elements of the skin. They are hamartomatous rather than true neoplasms. Epidermoids are composed of the epidermal layers of the skin. Dermoids contain all layers of the skin—epithelial and mesenchymal—and accessory cutaneous organs, such as hair follicles and sebaceous glands. Dermal sinuses are tubular formations that may have the histologic characteristics of epidermoids, dermoids, or both, but that are always directly connected with the skin. Spinal cord traction and dysfunction may be associated with any of these hamartomatous conditions because of direct attachment to the skin through a defect in the posterior neural arches or because of fibrous thickening of the filum terminale associated with one of these lesions.[2, 3, 17]

Spinal cord traction is associated with progressive dysfunction of the musculoskeletal, neurologic, and urologic systems. Musculoskeletal dysfunction is seen as a progressive scoliosis, foot deformity (i.e., clubfoot or cavovarus foot), unstable hip, or limb-length dis-

crepancy.[13, 14, 25, 26] Urologic dysfunction manifests as urgency, frequency, incontinence, progressive vesicoureteral reflux, hydronephrosis, and renal insufficiency.[1] Neurologic dysfunction is revealed by gait disturbance, trophic ulcers of the feet, and pain.[19]

The diagnosis of a tethered spinal cord depends on one's being alert to the possibility. Every patient with a foot or lower-extremity deformity, urologic complaints, or gait disturbance should have a spinal examination. If there is a cutaneous lesion overlying the spine (e.g., hypertrichosis, nevus, dimple, or sinus) or a spinal deformity, a tethered spinal cord should be suspected.[13, 14]

Radiographic evaluation is indicated in patients with suspected spinal cord tethering. Radiographic abnormalities suggestive of cord tethering include spina bifida occulta, congenital vertebral abnormalities (e.g., failure of formation, failure of segmentation, sacral dysgenesis), increased interpedicular distance, and bony spicules (i.e., an osseous diastematomyelia).[13, 14, 19]

If a spinal deformity, extremity deformity, or gait disturbance is associated with an abnormality on plain vertebral x-ray films, cord imaging is indicated. Cord imaging is also indicated for patients without abnormal findings on x-ray films if tethered cord is suspected. In the newborn, incomplete fusion of the posterior neural arches is common and provides a window for sonographic evaluation of the spinal cord; this is a relatively inexpensive screening procedure for spinal dysraphic states.[20] Myelography has been useful in cord imaging (Fig. 15-24).

Criteria for a low-lying cord include a conus below the L2–L3 disc and a thickened filum terminale (i.e., with a diameter greater than 2 mm).[9] Computed tomographic (CT) evaluation of the spinal cord has been useful in the evaluation of patients with suspected spinal cord tethering (Fig. 15-25).[10] Magnetic resonance imaging (MRI) has also been very effective (Fig. 15-26).[23]

Overt or occult urologic dysfunction is common in patients with spinal cord tethering. There is frequently dysynergy between the vesical musculature and the urethral sphincter, causing hypertrophy of the bladder, progressive vesicoureteral reflux, hydronephrosis, and progressive renal insufficiency.[2, 3] It has been suggested that all patients with documented spinal cord tethering should have a urologic evaluation, consisting of a renal ultrasound and a voiding cystourethrogram to rule out hydronephrosis and vesicoureteral reflux.[1]

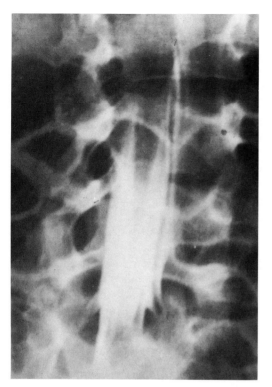

FIG. 15–24. Myelogram showing thickened filum terminale with conus at L4.

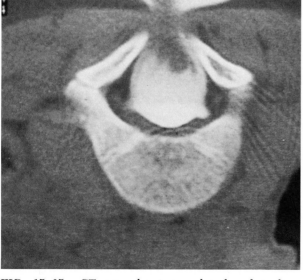

FIG. 15–25. CT scan showing cord tethered to lipomeningocele through neural arch defect.

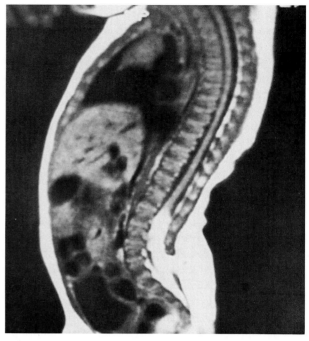

FIG. 15–26. MRI showing cord tethered to lipoma through posterior neural arch defect.

The treatment of symptomatic spinal cord tethering is surgical and includes release of a tight filum terminale, resection of a diastematomyelia, and resection of sacral lipoma.[7] For some patients, cord release improves progressive musculoskeletal, neurologic, or urologic dysfunction.[11, 13, 14] In most patients, however, a halt in progressive dysfunction is the rule.[2, 3, 6, 21, 24, 25]

References

1. Al-Mefty O, Kandzari S, Fox JL: Neurogenic bladder and the tethered spinal cord syndrome. J Urol 122:112, 1979
2. Anderson FM: Occult spinal dysraphism: Diagnosis and management. J Pediatr 73:163, 1968
3. Anderson FM: Occult spinal dysraphism: A series of 73 cases. Pediatrics 55:826, 1975
4. Barson AJ: The vertebral level of termination of the spinal cord during normal and abnormal development. J Anat 106:489, 1970
5. Bassett RC: The neurological deficit associated with lipomas of the cauda equina. Ann Surg 131:109, 1950
6. Bruce DA, Schut L: Spinal lipomas in infancy and childhood. Childs Brain 5:192, 1979
7. Fitz DR, Harwood-Nash DC: The tethered conus. Am J Roent Rad Ther Nucl Med 125:515, 1975

8. Garaceau GJ: The filum terminale syndrome. J Bone Joint Surg [Am] 35:711, 1953
9. Gryspeerdt GL: Myelographic assessment of occult forms of spinal dysraphism. Acta Radiol [Diag] (Stockh) 1:702, 1963
10. Hammerschiag SB, Wolpert SM, Carter BL: Computed tomography of the spinal canal. Radiology 121:361, 1976
11. Hoffman HJ, Hendrick EB, Humphries RP: The tethered spinal cord: Its protean manifestations, diagnosis and surgical correction. Child's Brain 2:145, 1976
12. Hood RW, Risebrough EJ, Nehme kA, et al: Diastematomyelia and structural spinal deformities. J Bone Joint Surg [Am] 62:520, 1980
13. James CCM, Lassman LP: Spinal dysraphism: An orthopedic syndrome in children accompanying occult forms. Arch Dis Child 35:315, 1960
14. James CCM, Lassman LP: Spinal dysraphism: The diagnosis and treatment of progressive lesions in spina bifida occulta. J Bone Joint Surg [Br] 44:828, 1962
15. Jones PH, Love JG: Tight filum terminale. Arch Surg 73:556, 1956
16. Lichtenstein BW: "Spinal dysraphism," spina bifida and myelodysplasia. Arch Neurol Psychiatry 44:792, 1940
17. List CF: Intraspinal epidermoids, dermoids, and dermal sinuses. Surg Gynecol Obstet 73:525, 1941
18. Love JG, Daily DD, Harris LE: Tight filum terminale. JAMA 176:115, 1961
19. McMaster MJ: Occult intraspinal anomalies and congenital scoliosis. J Bone Joint Surg [Am] 66:588, 1984
20. Nadich TP, McLone DG, Shkolnik A, Fernbach SK: Sonographic evaluation of caudal spine anomalies in children. AJNR 4:661, 1983
21. Rogers HM, Long DM, Chou SN, French LA: Lipomas of the spinal cord and cauda equina. J Neurosurg 34:349, 1971
22. Streeter GL: Factors involved in the formation of the filum terminale. Am J Anat 93:1, 1919
23. Szalay EA, Roach JW, Smith H, et al: Magnetic resonance imaging of the spinal cord in spinal dysraphisms. J Pediatr Orthop 7:541, 1987
24. Thomas JE, Miller RH: Lipomatous tumors of the spinal canal. A study of their clinical range. Mayo Clin Proc 48:393, 1973
25. Till K: Spinal dysraphism. J Bone Joint Surg [Br] 51:415, 1969
26. Wilkinson JA: Occult spinal dysraphism in established congenital dislocation to the hip. J Bone Joint Surg [Br] 70:744, 1988
27. Winter RB, Haven JJ, Moe JH, Lagaard SM: Diastematomyelia and congenital spine deformities. J Bone Joint Surg [Am] 56:27, 1974
28. Yamada S, Zinke DE, Sanders D: Pathophysiology of the "tethered cord syndrome." J Neurosurg 54:494, 1981

CHAPTER
16

Spinal Dysraphism

H. Dennis Mollman
Bruce A. Kaufman
Tae Sung Park

CHIARI MALFORMATION, TETHERED CORD, MYELOMENINGOCELE CLOSURE, DIASTEMATOMYELIA, NEURENTERIC CYSTS, AND CONGENITAL DERMAL SINUS

H. DENNIS MOLLMAN

Two percent of live births have major congenital anomalies, and 60% of these anomalies involve the central nervous system (CNS).[34] More than half of CNS malformations are due to abnormal development and closing of the neural tube and its neighboring tissues along the posterior midline of the body. These malformations are grouped under the heading of "cranial and spinal dysraphism." Dysraphism (Greek: *raphe*, seam) describes the defective fusion of parts that normally unite.[45] The term has been extended to encompass all forms of anomalous development of tissue associated with various malformations, regardless of whether malfusion has occurred.

Spinal dysraphism may have permanent adverse consequences for the patient and family. The patient is deprived of independence, physical poise, and intelligence. The defects and their effects range from mild to severe. Despite pessimism about CNS malformations, correction of a defect before irreparable damage in a developing child can be very rewarding.

Neural tube development occurs in three phases: neurulation (days 18–28), canalization of the tail bud (days 28–40), and regression (day 41 through fetal life). The neural tube closes between days 26 and 28. Dysraphic abnormalities are the result of abnormal neurulation.[30] During week 9 of gestation, the vertebral body and spinal cord segments are at the same level. During regression, there is ascension of the spinal cord in the spinal canal with development of the cauda equina and filum terminale. The conus is at the level of the L4 vertebral body by week 18. By term, the conus lies adjacent to the L3 vertebral body, and by 2 months postpartum, it lies at the L1–L2 vertebral level.

Neural tube abnormalities have a poorly understood genetic background. There is no obvious hereditary predisposition to the development of dysraphism in offspring, but the risk of a mother of a dysraphic child having a second child with any form of dysraphism is 3 to 5%. This 3 to 5% risk also applies to children of a mother who has any form of dysraphism. The severity of the malformation is determined by the mechanisms of teratogenesis and the gestational age at the time of occurrence. The incidence of neural tube malformations in the United States and Canada is between 1 and 2 in 1000 births.

This chapter covers several forms of spinal dysraphism: Chiari II malformation, tethered cord, myelomeningocele closure, diastematomyelia, neurenteric cysts, and spinal dermal sinuses. Syringomyelia is discussed in conjunction with the Chiari malformations. Many of the other disease states listed in Table 16-1 are discussed elsewhere in this text.

CHIARI II MALFORMATION

The anatomical description of this brainstem and cerebellar anomaly was first presented by Cleland in 1883.[7] Four types of malformations found in hydrocephalic specimens with spina bifida were described by Chiari in 1891 and 1896 (Table 16-2).[4-6] In 1907, Schwalbe and Gredig, Arnold's laboratory assistants, reviewed the brain anomalies associated with spina bifida and applied Arnold's name to the malformation already described by Chiari.[39] In this chapter, the malformation is referred to as a Chiari malformation, and only the Chiari Type II malformation, seen in dysraphic states, is discussed here. Type I is seen in adults and is treated in the same way as Type II. The Chiari III and IV malformations are seen in stillbirths and are of pathologic interest only.

Six major theories of altered embryogenesis have been proposed to explain the development of the Chiari malformation: the traction theory, Gardner's hemodynamic theory, the overgrowth hypothesis, neuroschisis theory, arrested development theory, and Williams's differential pressure theory.[14] Each describes mechanisms that account for caudal displacement of the brainstem and cerebellar tissue into and through the foramen magnum. Although a combination of Gardner's and Williams's theories is appealing because it can account for the altered anatomy and the associated syringomyelia, there is no conclusive data confirming any of these theories.

A Chiari II malformation occurs in 90% of patients with myelomeningocele. Hydrocephalus, either obstructive or communicating, is present in more than

TABLE 16-1. Classification of Cranial and Spinal Dysraphism

Spina Bifida Aperta

Myeloschisis
Myelomeningocele
Hemimyelomeningocele
Syringomyelomeningocele
Spinal meningocele

Chiari Malformation

Dandy-Walker Malformation

Cranium Bifidum

Cranial meningocele
Encephalomeningocele

Occult Cranial Dysraphism

Cranial dermal sinus

Occult Spinal Dysraphism

Spinal dermal sinus
Tethered cord syndrome
Lumbosacral lipoma
Diastematomyelia
Neurenteric cyst
Combined anterior and posterior spina bifida
Anterior sacral meningocele
Occult intrasacral meningocele

Nondysraphic Malformations

Perineural (Tarlov) cyst
Spinal extradural cyst
Nondysraphic spinal meningocele
Caudal regression syndrome
Sacrococcygeal teratoma

90% of these patients. Obstructive hydrocephalus occurs if there is occlusion of the aqueduct of Sylvius, caused by pressure on the brainstem by the caudally displaced cerebellar tissue or from elongation and narrowing of the aqueduct of Sylvius due to the altered brainstem anatomy. Communicating hydrocephalus, if present, is due to obliteration of the basal subarachnoid cisterns, which in the normal state allow for cerebrospinal fluid (CSF) circulation around the brainstem. The altered anatomy of the cerebellum and brainstem illustrated in Figure 16-1 includes tectal breaking (*diamond*), elongated brainstem, medullary kink (*arrow*), and caudal displacement of the vermis.

Diagnosis requires an alert physician treating dysraphic patients, recognition of the signs and symptoms, and appropriate radiographic imaging. The clinical

TABLE 16-2. Types of Chiari Malformations

Type I	Type II (Infant)	Type III	Type IV
Cerebellar tonsils extend into upper cervical canal	Cerebellar vermis is hypoplastic; tonsils elongated, extend into the cervical canal	Entire cerebellum displaced into cervical canal	Hypoplastic cerebellum
No brainstem abnormality	Elongated IV ventricle		
	Choroid plexus and medulla displaced into cervical canal		
	Dorsal protuberance of medulla and cervical spinal cord		
	May have associated syringomyelia		

signs and symptoms associated with a Chiari II malformation vary with the age of the patient at the time of presentation and are summarized in Table 16-3.[35]

Most infants show improvement or plateauing of the symptoms during the first year of life. During the first 2 years, apneic spells remain the leading cause of death of children being treated for dysraphism. Many of the symptoms seen in the adolescent Chiari II mimic those of syringomyelia or hydromyelia, which produce spinal cord or brainstem dysfunction by cystic dilation of the cord or brainstem. Decreased pain and temperature sensations with preserved proprioception and light touch (i.e., suspended sensory loss) can produce painless injuries and Charcot joints. The symptom complex, even if mild at the time of diagnosis, virtually always progresses and requires surgery.

Cystic dilatations of the spinal cord or brainstem that occur in association with Chiari malformations are hydromyelia, which is dilation of the central canal that is lined with ependymal cells, and syringomyelia, if the cyst involves the cord parenchyma. Hydromyelia and syringomyelia can occur independently or simultaneously. Syringomyelia is probably caused by rupture of a hydromyelic cyst into the cord parenchyma. The extent of cyst formation ranges from very mild and focal to that involving dilatation of the entire central canal from the obex to the conus medullaris (Fig. 16-2). Syringomyelia and hydromyelia are classified as com-

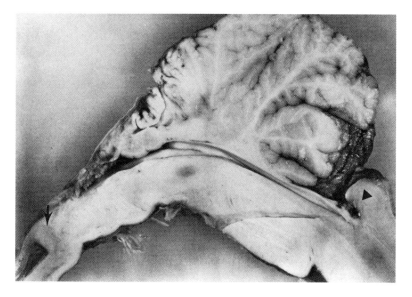

FIG. 16–1. Sagittal section of a brainstem with a Chiari II malformation. Notice: tectal breaking (*diamond*), elongated brainstem, medullary kink (*arrow*), and caudal displacement of the vermis. (With permission from McAdoms AJ: The Arnold-Chiari malformation: Pathology and developmental considerations. In McLaurin RL (ed): Myelomeningocele, p 197. New York, Grune & Stratton, 1977)

TABLE 16-3. Chiari II Signs and Symptoms

Infancy

Inspiratory stridor (X nerve paresis)
Apnea spells
Weak gag reflex
Nystagmus
Fixed retrocollis
Weak cry
Upper extremity weakness, exaggerated deep tendon reflexes,
    increased tone
Peripheral facial paresis

Childhood

Nystagmus
Quadraparesis or upper extremity weakness, exaggerated
    deep tendon reflexes, increased tone
Mirror movements
Ataxia, truncal or extremity
Recurrent aspiration pneumonias
Weak cough
Gastroesophageal reflux

Adolescence

Spastic weakness of upper or lower extremities
Suspsended sensory loss
Hand or upper extremity weakness
Truncal ataxia
XII nerve paresis
Scoliosis

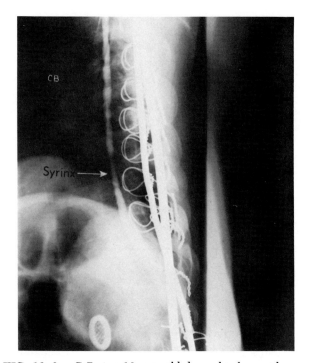

FIG. 16–2.   C.B. is a 16-year-old dysraphic boy with progressive loss of hand function. During attempted myelography, a holocord syringomyelic cavity was injected. Notice the characteristic pattern of alternating dilations and constrictions of the cavity (goose neck appearance).

municating or noncommunicating, depending on communication with the obex. It is thought that all the cysts associated with Chiari II malformations are initially in communication with the obex. With evolution of the cyst, this communication may be lost (Fig. 16-3).

The signs and symptoms of syringomyelia or hydromyelia are due to destruction of the central portion of the spinal cord or brainstem, where the crossing spinothalamic pathways are located. Major clinical signs are suspended or dissociated sensory loss and atrophy and weakness of the upper extremities. Atrophy is most severe in the intrinsic muscles of the hand. If the brainstem is involved, lower cranial nerve dysfunction occurs, producing dysphonia, altered gag reflex, and dysphagia.

Radiographic evaluation should include cervical spine films in flexion and extension, magnetic resonance imaging (MRI) of the head and complete spinal axis, and computed tomography (CT) of the head and craniocervical junction for bone detail. In patients with scoliosis to the degree that MRI is inadequate for de-

tection of a syrinx, myelography may be necessary. Angiography has been replaced by MRI and CT scanning for the detection of caudal migration of the cerebellar tonsils (Fig. 16-4). The cervical spine radiographic evaluation is necessary to detect abnormal movement or anatomy at the craniocervical junction. Other anomalies may coexist with the Chiari II malformation: basilar impression, platybasia, occipitalization of the atlas, atlantoaxial instability, and Klippel-Feil anomalies. MRI scanning defines the anatomy of the brainstem, the extent of caudal migration of the cerebellar tonsils or vermis, and the size of the ventricular system. Spinal MRI can detect the presence of syringomyelia or hydromyelia.

Surgery is indicated for all Chiari II patients who are reasonable surgical candidates and have symptoms referable to the malformation. The first step in treating a Chiari II malformation is to ensure that the hydrocephalic patient has a functioning ventricular shunt.[13] There is often marked improvement in symptoms after placement of a shunt. Even with a shunt, most patients

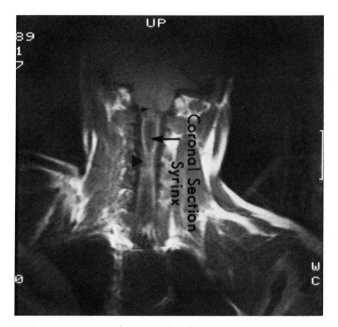

FIG. 16–3. Coronal section of a Chiari II malformation with a cervical syrinx, illustrating how the connection with the obex (*small diamond*) may regress because of segmental constriction (*large diamond*) of the syrinx cavity. The rostral cavity remains in communication with the obex, but the caudal cavity does not.

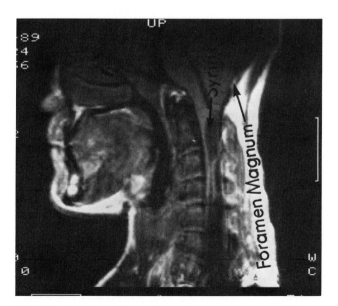

FIG. 16–4. Sagittal spinal MRI demonstrating caudal migration of the cerebellar tonsils below the level of the foramen magnum. Notice associated syrinx.

remain symptomatic and require further surgery. Surgery involves a posterior fossa exploration and cervical laminectomy down to the distal extension of the caudally displaced brainstem and cerebellum.

The patient's position is prone on chest rolls, with the head in a skeletal fixation device. The prone position is chosen for several reasons: the patients are children; there is often displacement of the transverse sinus caudally, increasing the risk of injury to the sinus and resultant air embolism; and caudally displaced cerebellar tissue is more easily manipulated if the caudal gravitational pull is eliminated. A midline incision extends from the inion down to the spinous process at the level of the most caudally displaced cerebellar tissue. It is usually not necessary to extend the incision to expose a more caudal syrinx cavity. A suboccipital craniectomy and cervical laminectomy is carried out. At the C1 level there is often a thick extradural band. Care must be taken in removing the C1 arch to avoid any compression of the underlying neural structures. The dura is then opened in midline. Extreme caution is required to identify the dural sinuses, which are often displaced caudally. The fibrous band frequently present at the C1 level is transected when the dura is opened.

The surgical microscope should be used for the intradural portion of the surgery. Several options exist for the intradural procedure, including placing a dural patch graft with no other manipulation, plugging the obex, resecting the displaced cerebellar tissue that is atrophic, performing a myelotomy into an existing syrinx, and placing a stent into the foramen of Magendie.[2, 16, 36, 38, 47] The necessary manipulation remains a point of controversy. I follow the recommendation of Oakes.[35] Subarachnoid adhesions are taken down, and if a syrinx is accessible without further laminectomy, a myelotomy is performed and a stent placed in the syrinx, draining it to the subarachnoid space. A stent is placed into the foramen of Magendie. A generous elliptical dural patch graft is placed to enlarge the subarachnoid space, allowing room for the caudally displaced cerebellar tonsils and brainstem.

In a patient who has a syrinx distal to the craniocervical exposure and continued neurologic deterioration postoperatively, a laminectomy at the appropriate level over the syrinx and establishment of a syringosubarachnoid or syringoperitoneal shunt may be beneficial. For a few patients, terminal ventriculostomy may be helpful if the syrinx extends to the conus medullaris. This is accomplished by truncating the filum terminale and allowing the syrinx to drain into the subarachnoid space.

The surgical outcome is difficult to assess. Long-term follow-up is required due to the slowly progressive nature of the disease. In infant patients with a Chiari II malformation without a syrinx, controversy exists about the efficacy of posterior fossa surgery. This topic remains under investigation, but clearly these children do respond well to ventricular shunting if there is hydrocephalus. Most children or adolescents with a Chiari II without syrinx respond to surgery with the stabilization of symptoms. Much less frequently there will be improvement in neurologic deficits.[20] Patients who present with severe neurologic deficits due to permanent injury to the brainstem and spinal cord show no improvement with surgery, and the only goal is stabilization of symptoms, which is accomplished in most cases.

Chiari II malformations with syringomyelia present a more difficult problem. The natural history of syringomyelia is slow progression, but the actual course may be erratic. Symptoms may be static for 5 to 10 years and then progress. There is often the feeling of improvement postoperatively, but follow-up is required for at least 5 to 10 years. With appropriate follow-up, 20 to 43% of the patients eventually show progression of symptoms.[11, 36] Reoperation, except for revision of a nonfunctioning shunt, has limited value.

Risks of surgery include infection, hemorrhage, CSF fistula, increased neurologic deficits, and respiratory compromise. The rate of infection is 1% for scalp infections and less than 1% for meningitis. Most infections are treatable with minimal morbitiy if identified early. Postoperative hemorrhage is quite rare but is often associated with significant deficits or death. CSF fistula formation is an unusual complication if 4 days of strict flat bed rest is enforced. If it occurs, reoperation and repair of the CSF leak is required. The potential for new neurologic deficits exists, but with modern microsurgical and anesthetic techniques, it is a very unusual occurrence. Nocturnal respiratory depression can be seen transiently after any posterior fossa procedure. Close monitoring of the patient in the intensive care unit is required postoperatively for 24 to 48 hours.

TETHERED CORD

The tethered cord syndrome has previously been known as tethered conus, filum terminale syndrome,

or meningocele manque.[12, 14, 15, 21, 27, 28, 46, 49] The syndrome consists of neurologic deficits in the lower extremities and sphincter dysfunction, with the conus at a lower than normal spinal level. During embryologic regression, the conus ascends in the spinal canal. The adult conus level is normally between the superior border of the L1 and the inferior border of the L2 vertebral bodies.[37] The syndrome is seen in patients with intraspinal lipomas, diastematomyelia, or spina bifida aperta and postoperatively after repair of a myelomeningocele or myeloschisis.[35]

Pathologically, the abnormality includes a short filum terminale and adhesive bands attaching the distal conus or filum to the dura.[1, 9, 21, 27, 28] In the repaired myelomeningocele, the malfused neural tube or placode is attached to the deep fascia or dural remnants at the level of the previous repair. Cutaneous stigmata are present in approximately half the patients, such as a hairy patch, abnormal pigmentation, subcutaneous lipoma, and congenital dermal sinus. The cutaneous lesion rarely connects with the intradural lesion. The bony abnormalities associated with a tethered cord are usually simpler than those seen with other dysraphic states. Deficits are believed to be the result of microvascular insufficiency within the spinal cord caused by intermittent stress applied to the tethered cord during flexion and extension movements.[48]

Diagnosis of a tethered cord is made between the ages of 11 and 20 years in 42% of the cases, between birth and 5 years in 31%, between 6 and 10 years in 21%, and over 21 years in 6%.[1, 9, 15, 28, 32, 37] The high rate of presentation during adolescence has been attributed to the growth spurt, causing tension on the spinal cord. No conclusive studies have shown a relation between the growth rate and time of onset of symptoms. The signs and symptoms of a tethered cord are presented in Table 16-4. Most symptoms begin in infancy but are often not detected until childhood or

TABLE 16-4.   Signs and Symptoms of a Tethered Cord

Sign or Symptom	Frequency
Gait abnormality, short limb, muscle atrophy, ankle abnormality	93%
Sensory deficit, absent ankle reflex	70%
Bladder dysfunction	40%
Spinal deformity	29%

adolescence. Virtually all patients complain of muscular, low-back pain.

Plain roentgenograms of the spine may show widened interpedicular distances, spina bifida, spinal deformity, and hemivertebra. Spinal MRI is the best method for diagnosing a tethered cord (Figs. 16-5 and 16-6). As with the Chiari malformations, myelography with CT scanning may be needed if there is severe curvature preventing adequate MRI studies.

Surgical technique varies considerably with the complexity of the tethering structures and with the neurologic status of the patient. In the simplest form, a thickened filum terminale is exposed through a one- or two-level laminectomy, and the filum is transected. The next level of complexity consists of fibrous bands and adhesions of the conus to the dura. In a patient with minimal neurologic deficits and intact sphincter function, the goal is to release the tether without risking loss of neurologic function. The exposure requires a laminectomy of at least two levels and often more. The laminectomies are centered over the expected level of the tether. A dural opening is made. If the site of attachment to the dura is visible, the dural opening is made adjacent to this site. The surgical microscope is used to dissect the adhesions and fibrous bands, each being taken down sharply. The filum should again be identified and transected. The most complex surgery is the release of a tether that has occurred after repair of a myelomeningocele, in which the malfused neural tube is tethered to the deep fascia or dural remnants over a large area. Functioning nerve rootlets may be entan-

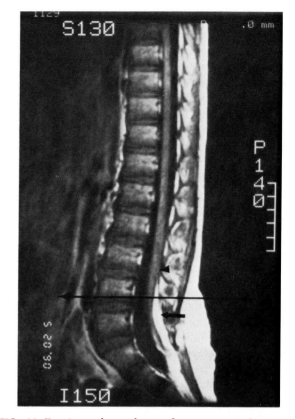

FIG. 16–5. Sagittal spinal MRI demonstrating dorsal migration of a low-lying conus (*diamond*, L4 level) and tethering to a subcutaneous lipoma (*arrow*). The *double-headed arrow* indicates the level of the axial section shown in Fig. 16–6.

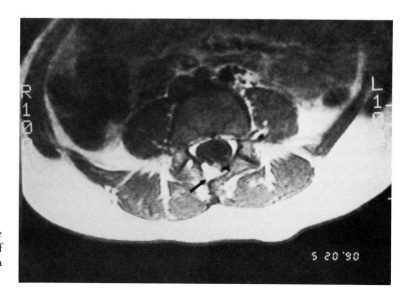

FIG. 16–6. Axial spinal MRI at L4 level (see Fig. 16–5) demonstrating dorsal attachment of the conus (*diamond*) to a subcutaneous lipoma (*arrow*).

gled in the adhesion. Again the dictum of producing no further deficits guides the surgery.

A midline incision is made, with the proximal portion of the incision several centimeters above the superior aspect of the previous myelomeningocele defect. The dissection through the tissue layers is performed sharply, developing multiple tissue planes to be used in closing. The spine is usually bifid, and a cautious approach to the bony lateral masses must be taken to avoid plunging into the unprotected spinal canal. I prefer to approach the spinal canal starting at a vertebral level with an intact lamina. The inferior portion of that lamina is removed and the dura identified. Dissection can then be directed caudally following the extradural plane. It is rare that the dural sac can be dissected through the area of the myelomeningocele repair without entering the sac. In this area, the dura usually blends into the deep fascia, and a plane may need to be developed in order to provide tissue for closure of the sac.

All intradural dissecting should be done with the surgical microscope. The placode is sharply dissected away from its attachment to the scar and subcutaneous tissues. Arachnoid adhesions and fibrous bands are likewise taken down. Often nerve roots will be under tension, extending from the placode to caudal dural exit sites, and contribute to the tethering. These roots can be stimulated to see if there is muscle contraction or increase in bladder tension. A battery-powered nerve stimulator is used to stimulate the root. Muscle contraction in the legs or an increase in the cystomanometer pressure indicates a functioning nerve root. In children with no bowel or bladder function and complete motor and sensory level above the operative level, these roots can be transected. On the other hand, if the patient has sphincter function and motor or sensory function below the operative level, extreme caution must be exercised before dividing any nerve roots.

In patients with myelomeningocele, release of the tethered cord is only considered when a scoliosis surgery is planned that will lengthen the spine. At the time of fusion, the cord can be transected and released. It may be necessary to release the cord to prevent chronic trauma to the normal part of the spinal cord during flexion and extension movements.

After the untethering is accomplished, a watertight closure is needed. If a dural sac exists, normal dural closure techniques are used. In the myelomeningocele patient, a pseudodural plane can be developed and undermined. This allows adequate tissue to form a "dural" sac with the released neural tube enclosed. Several layers of permanent suture are placed to ensure a watertight seal. All patients are maintained on strict flat bed rest for 4 postoperative days to prevent the formation of a CSF fistula.

Prognosis is generally good. More than 80% of the patients have improved motor and bladder function. Approximately 33% of the patients with scoliosis have improvement or stabilization of the degree of angulation.[21] The remaining 67% patients require spinal fusion for the scoliosis at a later date. All patients have relief of the low-back pain.

The risks of surgery include local infection (1%), meningitis (<1%), production of new neurologic deficits (rare), and CSF fistula formation (very unusual after 4 days of strict bed rest).

MYELOMENINGOCELE CLOSURE

Tethered cord and myelomeningocele closure are quite similar. Controversy still exists about whether there are children who should not be treated because of the poor chance for anything but rudimentary existence. The major pitfall of no treatment in these severe cases is that about 30% will survive, and they are more impaired because of a lack of treatment. I feel the only question in regard to open neural tube defects is when to close the defect, early or late. If there are other problems making the risk of general anesthesia and surgery unacceptable, then a late closure is warranted and should be performed at 6 weeks. This period allows a clean epithelial scar to form.

Neonates who are suitable candidates for surgery should have the defect closed, ideally in the first 24 hours after birth. Closure after 48 hours carries a significant risk of meningitis and ventriculitis. The goal of treatment is to protect the functioning neural tissue, not to repair the damaged spinal cord. The exposed neural elements in the myelomeningocele are not fully developed and are not repairable.

In the operating room, meticulous attention must be paid to the neonate's body temperature and fluid balance. The ambient room temperature should be elevated, and overhead heating should be employed to minimize heat loss from the neonate. The procedure is done with the patient prone, supported with soft chest rolls and a foam ring to support the head. Magnified vision should be employed.

A circumferential dissection of the placode is performed at the junction between skin and placode. This dissection leads directly to the intradural space. The rostral and caudal dissection is performed last, after the cord is identified. I do not feel that rolling the placode into a tube and suturing it produces any improvement in outcome. Nerve roots that clearly end in the myelomeningocele defect can be transected as well as the filum. All vascular structures should be preserved if possible. The dura is then freed from the lateral walls of the defect, and a dural tube is constructed. If there is not enough dura to make a watertight tube, a dural substitute should be used as a graft. The dura is closed with a 4-0 silk in a running locked fashion.

Skin closure should be in a direction that results in the least amount of tension on the suture line. After widely undermining the skin, the subcutaneous tissues are closed in several layers of absorbable suture. Skin closure is with a monofilament nylon in a simple running fashion, taking care not to compromise the blood supply to the skin edges. Immaculate hemostasis must be obtained before closure. Because of the infection risk, I do not use any drains. In rare instances, there is not adequate tissue to allow closure of the defect. A plastic surgeon should provide an appropriate myocutaneous flap.

The only significant risk of surgery is infection. The child must be followed expectantly, and any question of infection should prompt CSF examination. Despite the fact that the tissues involved are not ideal, the formation of a CSF fistula is unusual.

DIASTEMATOMYELIA

Diastematomyelia denotes an anomaly in which there is separation of a segment of the spinal cord into two hemicords (Greek: diaste, separation; myelia, marrow). The cord malformation itself may be compatible with normal neurologic function and does not require any surgery.[25, 27] Diastematomyelia often occurs with a bony, cartilaginous, or fibrous septum interposed between the two hemicords and is called diastematomyelia with septum (DWS). This can be a surgical problem. The hemicords usually reunite just below the septum. Septa are present in about 50% of diastematomyelia cases, and virtually all cases have a low-lying conus medullaris.[40]

Several theories have been proposed to explain the formation of diastematomyelia. Because of the known association of neurenteric cysts with diastematomyelia, the theory most accepted proposes a persistent accessory neurenteric canal or division of the neural ectoderm by the posterior blastopore into two parts.[40] Neurologic deficits and pain are due to the fixation of the spinal cord by the septum. With physical activity, especially spinal flexion, traction is applied to the spinal cord, causing injury from direct pressure or because of vascular compromise.[17]

DWS occurs 3.5 times more frequently in females than males. The diagnosis of DWS is made on the basis of cutaneous manifestations and recognition of three clinical presentations. The cutaneous lesions include localized hypertrichosis (40%), subcutaneous lipoma, nevoid skin, atretic meningocele, and dermal sinus. The clinical presentations include the orthopedic syndrome (OS) of infants and young children; pain, sphincter dysfunction, and spastic paraparesis without OS in any child; and congenital scoliosis. The OS was coined by James and Lassman to describe a constellation of signs: hemiatrophy and monoparesis of a lower extremity, shortness of the involved lower extremity, ipsilateral absent ankle jerk, decreased sensation in the foot, and pes cavus and clawing of the toes, usually noted in infants or young children younger than 2 years old.[26] The group without OS presents with back and leg pain, weakness of the legs and bowel, and bladder dysfunction, all of which are often exacerbated by physical activity. Scoliosis is present in almost 67% of children with DWS. Detection and removal of the septum before surgical correction of scoliosis is mandatory to prevent postoperative paraplegia.[23]

Radiographic evaluation is best accomplished by iopamidol myelography with CT scanning (Fig. 16-7). Plain spine films may fail to demonstrate a fibrous or cartilaginous septum (Fig. 16-8). In some cases without scoliosis, MRI can give an excellent illustration of the altered anatomy (Fig. 16-9). The vertebral anomalies associated with DWS are listed in Table 16-5.[35] The septum is most often (28 of 37 cases) located between L1 and L4.[17] Thoracic septa are rare, and cervical septa are reported even less frequently.[44]

Surgery is indicated in patients with progressive neurologic deficits or before surgical correction of scoliosis. The treatment of all patients with DWS without symptoms is controversial, and an argument can be made for close follow-up. Because of reports of sudden neurologic deterioration with paraplegia and the finding that most children eventually become symptomatic, I generally recommend surgery on all cases of

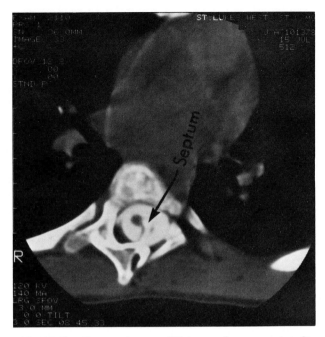

FIG. 16–7. Postmyelogram CT image demonstrating diastematomyelia with bony septum.

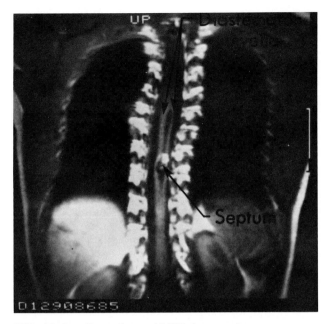

FIG. 16–9. Coronal spinal MRI showing the same patient as in Fig. 16–8. Notice the diastematomyelia (two light gray columns) and the septum.

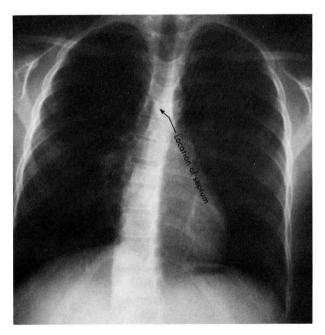

FIG. 16–8. Anterior-posterior thoracic roentgenogram showing the subtle appearance of a septum in DWS on plain radiograms.

TABLE 16-5. Vertebral Anomalies of Diastematomyelia with Septum

Central bony spur
Broadened spinal canal
Spina bifida
Vertical laminar fusion
Fused vertebral bodies
Split vertebral body
Hemivertebral hypoplasia
Fused or deformed spinous processes
Unsegmented bars

DWS in children. Asymptomatic DWS in adults can be followed and the patients physical activity restricted.

The surgical technique was first described by Shillito and Matson.[42] A midline incision is made, excising scar or meningocele. A subperiosteal dissection is performed on the spinous processes and lamina of the malformation and at the adjacent levels directly above and below the malformation. Care must be exercised to prevent plunging through a spina bifida; in certain instances, it is best to dissect in a layer above the periosteum, avoiding any dense fibrous tissue.

The septum is approached from its cephalic aspect. The surgical microscope or magnifying loops should be used. Removal of the septum is accomplished with a small rongeur or drills, working in the gap between the two hemicords. The septum and its dural sheath must be resected down to the posterior border of the vertebral body. The dura usually is divided at the septum and envelops each hemicord. The large blood vessels between the dural sheath and the septum must be coagulated. The hemicords must be freed of any adhesions to the surrounding dura to release the tether.

The ventral dural sheath need not be closed. The dorsal dura is closed in a watertight fashion. Permanent suture material is used to close the fascial, subcutaneous and skin layers. In a majority of cases, the filum is transected through the same exposure and through a separate, single-level laminectomy, if necessary. All patients are kept at strict flat bed rest for 4 postoperative days to avoid potential CSF leakage.

Outcome is good for deficits of recent onset. Weakness improves in muscles that are not severely atrophied in almost all cases. Bladder dysfunction improves in almost all cases. Pain always is relieved. Foot deformities require orthopedic follow-up and often need correction. Follow-up is required to detect the rare retethering at the surgical site.[18]

The risks of surgery are the same as those discussed in the previous sections. The major risk is a local skin infection in about 1% of cases. CSF fistula and the production of new neurologic deficits are both rare complications.

NEURENTERIC CYSTS

Neurenteric cysts are the result of a teratogenic process in which endodermal tissue herniates dorsally through the mesoderm into the spinal canal ventral to the neural plaque.[3, 8, 10, 19, 22, 24, 29, 31, 41, 43] The resultant communication between the yolk sac (future gut) and the amniotic cavity allows the development of intramedullary or intradural, extramedullary neurenteric cysts. Gut malformations frequently are associated with the spinal cysts. These include enteric cysts, enteric diverticula, and mediastinal cysts. Neurenteric cysts occur most commonly in the cervical and conus levels.

These cysts produce symptoms typical for slowly

expanding intraspinal lesions: quadraparesis, central cord syndrome, hemiparesis, and paraparesis. Local back pain, radicular pain, and meningismus are the most common symptoms. Recurrent bouts of meningitis, especially with gram-negative bacteria, should prompt appropriate radiographic testing. The diagnosis is best made with MRI. Most patients present during the first decade.

Treatment is surgical. The approach depends on the complexity of the abnormality. In some cases, the spinal and prevertebral components can be approached simultaneously, but others require separate surgical procedures for each component. The intraspinal resection can usually be accomplished by a posterolateral approach, although certain thoracic lesions require a thoracotomy. Complete resection is not always possible, and simple drainage of the cyst with partial resection of the sac produces good results. Most patients have marked improvement of neurologic function unless there were preoperative, long-standing fixed deficits.

CONGENITAL DERMAL SINUS

Congenital dermal sinuses are lined by stratified squamous epithelium and are located in the midline from the nasion to the coccyx. The most frequent locations are lumbosacral and occipital. This section discusses only the spinal location.

Dermal sinuses result from abnormal midline fusion occurring during week 4 of gestation. They are found with other types of dysraphism, but alone, they are usually not associated with other CNS abnormalities. The sinus may go just beneath the skin or may extend to the central canal of the spinal cord. There is often an associated extradural or intradural dermoid cyst. The lumbosacral lesion can extend rostrally to the conus. Sacral dimples very rarely communicate with the subarachnoid space.[33]

The usual mode of presentation is infection, either meningitis or epidural abscess. Close examination of the midline dermis is required to detect the sinus tract, unless associated signs of infection make the area of the sinus more prominent. Typical cutaneous stigmata of dysraphism are often present, including hypertrichosis and abnormal pigmentation.

Radiographic diagnosis is best made with spinal MRI. Alternatively, iopamidol myelography with CT scanning provides excellent imaging of the malformation. Injection of radiographic contrast material into the sinus tract is not a useful technique and risks introducing bacteria into the spinal canal.

The goal of surgery is complete excision of the sinus tract and associated cysts. Standard laminectomy techniques are employed, with exposure from the cutaneous opening of the sinus to the conus, if needed. The use of the surgical microscope is recommended for removal of tissue around nerve roots or the conus. Good surgical judgement is required to prevent neurologic deficits when attempting total excision of a lesion near the conus. It is sometimes necessary to leave a residual capsule and treat the capsule with laser coagulation to prevent recurrence.[33] Outcome is usually quite good.

The risks of infection and CSF fistula are as described in preceding sections. New neurologic deficits involving bowel and bladder dysfunction can be avoided only if surgery is very conservative in attempting to obtain a complete excision of the capsule.

References

1. Anderson FM: Occult spinal dysraphism: Diagnosis and management. J Pediatr 73:163, 1968
2. Barnett HJM, Foster JB, Hudgson P: Syringomyelia. Philadelphia, WB Saunders, 1973
3. Bently JFR, Smith JR: Developmental posterior enteric remnants and spinal malformations: The split notochord syndrome. Arch Dis Child 35:76, 1960
4. Carmel PW, Markesbery WR: Early descriptions of Arnold-Chiari Malformation: The contribution of John Cleland. J Neurosurg 37:543, 1972
5. Chiari H: Uber veranderungen des kleinhirns, des pons und der medulla oblongata infolge von congenitaler hydrocephalie des grosshirns. Denschr Akad Wiss Wien 63:71, 1896
6. Chiari H: Uber veranderungen des kleinhirns infolge von hydrocephalie des grosshirns. Deutsch Med Wochenschr 17:1172, 1891
7. Cleland J: Contribution to the study of spina bifida, encephalocele, and anencephalus. J Anat Physiol 17:257, 1983
8. Cohen J, Sledge CB: Diastematomyelia: An embryological interpretation with report of a case. Am J Dis Child 100:257, 1960
9. Craig WM, Mulder DW: Late neurologic symptoms of spinal bifida occulta: Report of a case. Mayo Clin Proc 31:98, 1956
10. Dorsey JF, Tabrisky J: Intraspinal and mediastinal foregut cyst compressing the spinal cord. Report of a case. J Neurosurg 24:562, 1966
11. Faulhauer K, Loew K: The surgical treatment of syringomyelia: Long-term results. Acta Neurochir (Wein) 44:215, 1978
12. Fitz CR, Harwood-Nash DC: The tethered conus. AJR 125:515, 1975
13. Fitzsimmons JS: Laryngeal stridor and respiratory obstruction associated with myelomeningocele. Dev Med Child Neurol 15:533, 1973
14. French BN: Midline fusion defects and defects of formation. In Youmans JR (ed): Neurological Surgery. Philadelphia, WB Saunders, 1982
15. Garceau GJ: The filum terminale syndrome (the cord traction syndrome). J Bone Joint Surg [Am] 35:711, 1953
16. Gardner WJ: Hydrodynamic mechanism of syringomyelia: Its relation to myelocele. J Neurol Neurosurg Psychiatry 28:247, 1965
17. Guthkelch AN: Diastematomyelia with median septum. Brain 97:729, 1974
18. Guthkelch AN, Hoffman GT: Tethered spinal cord in association with diastematomyelia. Surg Neurol 15:352, 1981
19. Harriman DGF: An intraspinal enterogenous cyst. J Path Bact 75:413, 1958
20. Hoffman HJ, Hendrick EB, Humphreys RP: Manifestations and management of Arnold-Chiari malformations in patients with myelomeningocele. Childs Brain 1:255, 1975
21. Hoffman HJ, Hendrick EB, Humphreys RP: The tethered spinal cord: Its protean manifestations, diagnosis and surgical correction. Childs Brain 2:145, 1976
22. Holcomb GW, Matson DD: Thoracic neurenteric cyst. Surgery 35:115, 1954
23. Hood RW, Riseborough EJ, Nehme AM, et al: Diastematomyelia and structural spinal deformities. J Bone Joint Surg [Am] 62:520, 1980
24. Jackson FE: Neurenteric cysts. Report of case of neurenteric cyst with associated chronic meningitis and hydrocephalus. J Neurosurg 18:678, 1961
25. James CCM, Lassman LP: Diastematomyelia and the tight filum terminale. J Neurol Sci 10:193, 1970
26. James CCM, Lassman LP: Spina Bifida Occulta: Orthopaedic, Radiological and Neurosurgical Aspects. New York, Grune & Stratton, 1981
27. James CCM, Lassman LP: Spinal Dysraphism. Spinal Bifida Occulta. London, Butterworth, 1972
28. Jones PH, Love JG: Tight filum terminale. Arch Surg 73:556, 1956
29. Laha RK, Huestis WS: Intraspinal enterogenous cyst: Delayed appearance following mediastinal cyst resection. Surg Neurol 3:67, 1975
30. Lemire RJ: Embryology of the central nervous system. In Davis JA, Dobbing J (eds): Scientific Foundations of Pediatrics. London, William Heinemann Medical Books, 1974
31. Levin P, Antin SP: Intraspinal neurenteric cyst in the cervical area. Neurology 14:727, 1964
32. Love JG, Daly DD, Harris LE: Tight filum terminale. Report of condition in three siblings. JAMA 176:31, 1961
33. McComb JG: Congenital dermal sinus. In Wilkins RH, Rengachary SS (eds): Neurosurgery, vol. 3, p 2081. New York, McGraw-Hill, 1985

34. Murphy DP: The etiology of congenital malformations in light of biological statistics. Am J Obstet Gynecol 34:890, 1973
35. Oakes JW: Chiari malformations, hydromyelia, syringomyelia. In Wilkins RH, Rengachary SS (eds): Neurosurgery, vol 3. New York, McGraw-Hill, 1985
36. Paul KS, Lye RH, Strang FA, Dutton J: Arnold-Chiari malformation: Review of 71 cases. J Neurosurg 58:183, 1983
37. Reiman AF, Anson BJ: Vertebral level of termination of the spinal cord with report of a case of sacral cord. Anat Rec 88:127, 1944
38. Rhoton AL: Microsurgery of Arnold-Chiari malformation in adults with and without hydromyelia. J Neurosurg 45:473, 1976
39. Schwalbe E, Gredig M: Uberent wicklungstorungen des kleinshirns and halmarks bei spina bifida (Arnold'sche und Chiarische mibbildung). Beitr Path Anat 40:132, 1907
40. Scott G, Musgrave MA, Harwood-Nash DC, et al: Diastematomyelia in children: Metrizamide and CT metrizamide myelography. AJR 135:1225, 1980
41. Scoville WB, Manlapaz JS, Otis RD, Cabieses F: Intraspinal enterogenous cyst. J Neurosurg 20:704, 1963
42. Shillito J, Matson DD: An Atlas of Pediatric Neurosurgical Operations, pp 484–487. Philadelphia, WB Saunders, 1982
43. Silvernail WI Jr, Brown RB: Intramedullary enterogenous cyst. Case report. J Neurosurg 36:235, 1972
44. Simpson RK, Rose JE: Cervical diastematomyelia: Report of a case and review of a rare congenital anomaly. Arch Neurol 44:331, 1987
45. Stedman's Medical Dictionary. Baltimore, Williams & Wilkins, 1976
46. Till K: Spinal dysraphism. A study of congenital malformations of the lower back. J Bone Joint Surg [Br] 51:415, 1969
47. Williams B: A critical appraisal of posterior fossa surgery for communicating syringomyelia. Brain 101:223, 1978
48. Yamada S, Zinke DE, Sander D: Pathophysiology of "tethered cord syndrome." J Neurosurg 54:494, 1981
49. Yarhon D, Beaty RA: Tethering of the conus medullaris within the sacrum. J Neurol Neurosurg Psychiatry 29:244, 1966

SPINAL DYSRAPHISM

BRUCE A. KAUFMAN

TAE SUNG PARK

The term *spinal dysraphism* encompasses a large number of congenital spine and spinal cord defects. These defects involve the imperfect development of the neuropore during embryogenesis and the subsequent maldevelopment of the adjacent bone and mesenchymal structures. They are the most common birth defects seen by neurosurgeons, and, with their sequelae, they affect more children than traumatic paraplegia and muscular dystrophy.[1]

Although the primary lesions are within the spinal portion of the central nervous system, their presenting manifestations and sequelae are frequently more pervasive, affecting the brain, spine, extremities, bowel, and bladder. The more severe types have been described as being the most complex developmental defects compatible with life.[2] Thus, the care of these patients requires consideration of both the symptoms and the primary cause, not only on presentation, but during the lifelong follow-up they require.

DEFINITIONS

The terminology of spinal dysraphism can be quite confusing, and the classifications vary among authors.

Spinal dysraphism describes the overall group of defects that result from the maldevelopment of the ectodermal, mesodermal, and neuroectodermal tissues in the region of the spine and spinal cord. *Myeloschisis* refers to the cleavage of the spinal cord; it may be complete or partial, ventral or dorsal. *Rachischisis* describes the extreme condition in which complete failure of neural tube closure has occurred and the entire brain and spinal cord are exposed to the external environment; this defect is not compatible with survival.

Spina bifida cystica typically refers to the meningoceles and myelomeningoceles; *spina bifida aperta* has been used to categorize the subgroup of defects that are open or exposed.[3] *Spina bifida occulta* in the strictest definition refers only to those spinal abnormalities identified on plain radiographs. These typically involve a failure of posterior arch fusion at one or more levels, usually in the lower lumbosacral region. The phrase *occult spinal dysraphism* is a better term for these entities, such as diastematomyelia, tight filum terminale, dorsal dermal sinus, and spinal lipoma; previously, these conditions would have been classified as *spina bifida occulta* (see later discussion under "Closed Dysraphic States").

The classification used by Naidich and McLone is straightforward and more pertinent to the evaluation and treatment of these patients (Table 16-6).[4] Those lesions with an absence of skin covering the defect, such as the classic myelomeningocele, form one group.

TABLE 16-6. Classification of Spina Bifida Lesions

Absent Skin Covering	Intact Skin Covering
Myelomeningocele	Lipomas of the spinal cord
	Lipomyelomeningocele
Myelocele	Intradural lipoma
	Dermal sinus
	Diastematomyelia
	Anterior meningocele
	Tight filum terminale
	Myelocystocele

They may have some degree of myeloschisis, posterior spina bifida, and protrusion and exposure of all or some of the neural elements. In the other group, skin completely covers the lesions. This group includes the dorsal dermal sinus, diastematomyelia, spinal lipoma, anterior sacral meningocele, and tight filum terminale. These may also have some degree of myeloschisis and spina bifida, but no neural elements are exposed.

HISTORY

The open lesions (myelocele, myelomeningocele) and their associated hydrocephalus were known to Hippocrates, Aristotle, and other ancient physicians.[5, 6] By the 19th century, physicians had associated the open spinal dysraphic state with concurrent paraplegia. Crude attempts were made to surgically correct the lesions, quite unsuccessfully.[7–9] In the early 20th century, surgical techniques had progressed to allow the closure of open defects without the immediate perioperative mortality that was usually due to infection.[10] The untreated hydrocephalus, however, ruined most of the survivors.

Effective treatment of the hydrocephalus with shunting began in the 1950s.[11] Only then did a large proportion of the myelomeningocele patients receive aggressive care. As they survived, however, many continued to suffer from significant physical and mental disabilities, which at the time were difficult or impossible to treat. They developed deformity of their affected extremities and severe scoliosis. Shunt infections and malfunctions left many more with decreased intelligence, and urinary tract dysfunction was a major source of late morbidity and mortality.[3, 12]

From this experience, it was suggested that only the "best" patients be selected for treatment.[13] An extensive debate ensued over the relative merits and the ethics of selection versus nonselection for treatment.[14] In 1986, McLone reviewed the largest series of unselected and aggressively treated patients and compared them with a group of highly selected patients who had been treated.[13, 15–18] When comparing factors that included social continence, renal function, ambulation, mortality, and intelligence, he found that the aggressively treated but unselected patient populations had better function than the selected groups.

It has become clear that the aggressive treatment of all but the moribund patients can allow many of them to lead productive lives. As described in later sections, sequelae that were previously thought to be inevitable are continuing to be identified as correctable.

EPIDEMIOLOGY

The incidence and epidemiology of the open forms of spinal dysraphism are studied the most frequently. In the North American continent, the incidence of myelomeningocele is approximately 1 per 1000 live births.[19–22] A geographic variation is seen, with some regions having a more frequent incidence. Ireland has 4 or 5 cases per 1000 live births. In other regions, a gradient exists; across the United States the frequency increases going west to east, and across the British Isles it increases in a southeast to northwest direction.[23–25] Ethnicity also is involved to some degree. Population studies of Celtic immigrants in Boston have shown an incidence that remains higher than the surrounding population.[26] Black and Asian populations tend to have a lower incidence than the white population.[24] Interestingly, the overall incidence has been declining for the past 15 years.[19, 27, 28]

Based on these geographic and cultural variations, extensive searches for etiologic factors or agents have been undertaken, with the overall conclusion that this disease has heterogeneous causes.[29] Attempts to determine factors related to the season, maternal age, or parity have been unsuccessful.[19, 30–32] Renwick theorized that an agent in potatoes caused the increased incidence in the Irish population, but subsequent evaluations and trials failed to support this theory.[33–35] Drugs, infections, and nutritional deficiency states also have been explored as potential etiologic agents. For the most part, no conclusive evidence for these suggested teratogens has been found.[36–46] The anticonvulsant valproic acid, however, has been associated with neural tube defects in the children of some women on the medication.[47] Recently, the use of periconceptual vitamin supplementation—folic acid in particular—has been suggested to prevent neural tube defects.[48, 49] No clear evidence, however, indicates that this therapy is effective; most of the studies have been relatively small, nonrandomized, and retrospective and did not control for maternal and ethnic factors or suffered from poor subject compliance.[2, 36, 49–54]

Genetic factors do seem to have a role in some cases.[55, 56] The risk of one child having spinal dysraphism is estimated at 0.1% to 0.2%; however, with one affected sibling, the risk of a second affected child increases to 2% to 5%, and the risk of a third affected child increases again to 10% to 15%.[22, 57, 58] These occurrences do not fit a mendelian pattern of transmission. Other genetic mechanisms of transmission, such as an X-linked recessive gene, a dominant gene with variable penetrance, or polygenic transmission, have been suggested to explain this tendency to recur within families.[59–61]

Spina bifida occulta is much more prevalent than the open forms. Estimates of its frequency have come from recent reviews of spinal radiographs taken for reasons unrelated to the spine or nervous system. In the "normal" population, 17% to 30% have been found with a spinal defect.[62, 63] It is seen more commonly in males, and most frequently at the L5 or S1 level. By itself, this ubiquitous finding is of no clinical significance. However, finding a significant underlying dysraphic state is much more likely when spina bifida occulta is associated with subtle neurologic symptoms or with cutaneous abnormalities, such as hypertrichosis, dimples, sinus tracts, or capillary hemangiomas, in the same area.

NORMAL EMBRYOLOGY

The lesions of spina bifida are all aberrations of the normal development of the spine and spinal cord. A review of normal spinal embryologic development provides a better understanding of the origin of these defects. It also helps to define the abnormal anatomic relationships observed on diagnostic studies and at surgery. Only a brief review of the pertinent embryology is presented here.

By embryonic stage 7 (approximately days 16–17), the embryo is trilaminar, composed of the endoderm adjacent to the yolk sac, the ectoderm adjacent to the

amnion, and the mesoderm between. The endoderm ultimately develops into the gut structures, the mesoderm into the musculature and skeleton, and the ectoderm into the skin and nervous system. As the mesoderm proliferates, cells condense in the midline, extending from the primitive node (Henson's node) to the prochordal plate (Fig. 16-10). This thickening of cells is called the *notochordal process*.

The primitive pit, starting at Henson's node, deepens and extends through the notochordal process, forming a hollow tube (Fig. 16-11). Along its ventral surface, the notochordal tube fuses with the endoderm, and multiple areas of endodermal cell breakdown occur, allowing a temporary communication of the yolk sac and amnion through what is called the neurenteric canal. This process is called the *intercalation* of the notochordal plate (Fig. 16-12). The notochordal plate then reforms into a solid cylinder, the true notochord, and allows the endoderm to reestablish its continuity. This process is called the *excalation* of the notochord (Fig. 16-13).

With the development of the notochord, the process of *neurulation*, or neural tube formation, begins (stages 8 to 12, days 18 to 27). The underlying notochord causes the ectoderm rostral to Henson's node to differentiate into the neural plate. The cells of the neural plate proliferate and heap up on each side of a developing longitudinal groove to form the neural folds on each side of the neural groove. Laterally, the neural

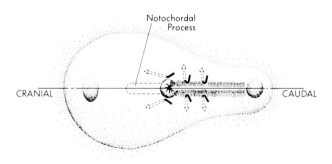

FIG. 16–10. Formation of the trilaminar embryo. The stage 7 embryo viewed from the ectodermal side. The mesoderm forms from cells that condense in the midline and invaginate between the ectodermal and endodermal layers (*curved arrows*). A thickening of cells in the midline, rostral to the primitive node, forms the notochordal process. (Redrawn from Moore KL: The Developing Human: Clinically Oriented Embryology, 2nd ed, p 46. Philadelphia, WB Saunders, 1970)

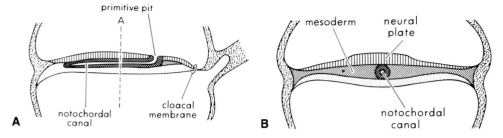

FIG. 16–11. Formation of the notochordal process. **A.** Midsagittal section of the notochordal canal within the notochordal process. The canal extends from the primitive pit throughout the length of the notochordal process. **B.** A representative axial section taken at level A in part A. The relationship of the notochordal canal within the mesoderm and between the endodermal and ectodermal layers is seen. The ectoderm adjacent to the notochordal process is the neural plate, precursor of the neuroectoderm. (Redrawn from Moore KL: The Developing Human: Clinically Oriented Embryology, 2nd ed, p 49. Philadelphia, WB Saunders, 1970)

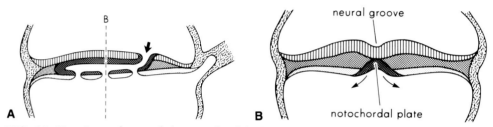

FIG. 16–12. Intercalation of the notochordal plate. **A.** Midsagittal section with areas of endodermal breakdown. Fusion of the notochordal tube with the endoderm occurs. A temporary communication, the neurenteric canal, is established between the amnion and yolk sac (*arrow*). **B.** Axial section at level B in part A. The notochordal tube has fused with the endoderm and is evaginating in the process of intercalation, forming the notochordal plate. (Redrawn from Moore KL: The Developing Human: Clinically Oriented Embryology, 2nd ed, p 50. Philadelphia, WB Saunders, 1970)

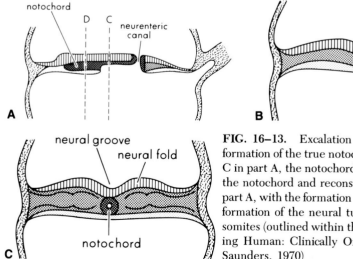

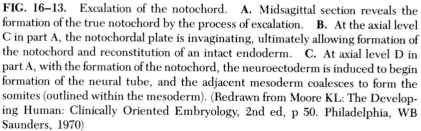

FIG. 16–13. Excalation of the notochord. **A.** Midsagittal section reveals the formation of the true notochord by the process of excalation. **B.** At the axial level C in part A, the notochordal plate is invaginating, ultimately allowing formation of the notochord and reconstitution of an intact endoderm. **C.** At axial level D in part A, with the formation of the notochord, the neuroectoderm is induced to begin formation of the neural tube, and the adjacent mesoderm coalesces to form the somites (outlined within the mesoderm). (Redrawn from Moore KL: The Developing Human: Clinically Oriented Embryology, 2nd ed, p 50. Philadelphia, WB Saunders, 1970)

plate is in continuity with the ectoderm from which it derived (Fig. 16-14).

Concurrently, the notochord has induced the paraxial mesoderm to thicken and form longitudinal columns. These cell masses condense and segregate into paired segments called *somites*. When finally formed, there are approximately 42 to 44 pairs, consisting of 4 occipital, 8 cervical, 12 thoracic, 5 lumbar, 5 sacral, and 8 to 10 coccygeal segments. Ultimately, the first occipital and the caudalmost 5 to 7 coccygeal segments regress.[64]

As the neural folds grow, they meet and fuse in the midline to form the neural tube (stage 10, day 22–23) (Fig. 16-15). Closure occurs at each level at approximately the same time as each somite pair is formed. The first portion of the neural tube to form occurs at the third to fourth somite, the future site of the craniovertebral junction. Closure then progresses caudally and rostrally as additional somites form. The most rostral portion of the tube closes at stage 11 (day 24–25), with

final closure at the posterior neuropore (caudal end) at the level of the future L1 or L2 vertebral body (stage 12, day 26–27). The lower portion of the spinal cord forms by a separate process called *canalization.*

As the neural tube folds and fuses into a tube, the superficial ectoderm disconnects from the neural tube (disjunction), then fuses in the midline, dorsal to the tube. This process reconstitutes a continuous ectoderm (the future skin). The mesenchyme migrates from the sides into a position between the neural tube and ectoderm and ultimately forms the meninges, neural arches, and paraspinal muscles.

In the process of canalization, the distal spinal cord forms after neurulation is complete. The caudal cell mass forms from the aggregation of undifferentiated cells, the remnants of the notochord, and the caudal end of the neural tube. This structure is adjacent to the developing hindgut and mesonephros. Vacuoles form within the caudal cell mass, begin to coalesce, and ultimately connect with the central canal of the formed spinal cord more rostrally.

Along this distal canal, the cells differentiate toward glia. The most cephalic portion becomes the conus medullaris. The remainder involutes, by a process called *retrogressive differentiation,* to form the filum terminale. At the time the conus medullaris is formed, it is located at approximately the second or third coccygeal level. The spinal cord does not involute further, but the spinal column grows at a relatively faster rate than the spinal cord, resulting in the apparent "ascension" of the conus to the L2–L3 level at birth.[65]

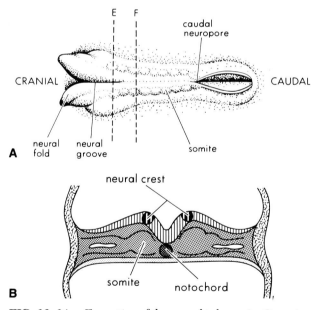

FIG. 16–14. Formation of the neural tube. **A.** Overview of the embryo from the ectodermal surface. As the somites form on each side of the neural groove, the neural tube is induced to form, extending in both the rostral and caudal directions simultaneously. **B.** Axial section representative of level E in part A. The neural folds move medially, with eventual fusion of the neural crest cell mass dorsal to the neural tube, and reformation of the ectodermal layer most dorsally. (Redrawn from Moore KL: The Developing Human: Clinically Oriented Embryology, 2nd ed, p 52. Philadelphia, WB Saunders, 1970)

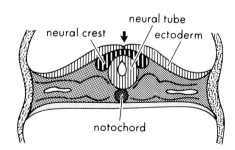

FIG. 16–15. Neural tube. Axial section through the developing neural tube corresponding to level F in Figure 16–14A. The neural tube has formed at this level. The ectoderm has separated from the neural crest cells and is about to fuse in the midline (*arrow*), reconstituting an intact layer. (Redrawn from Moore KL: The Developing Human: Clinically Oriented Embryology, 2nd ed, p 328. Philadelphia, WB Saunders, 1970)

OPEN DYSRAPHIC STATES

Some forms of spinal dysraphism appear to be related to the formation of the neural tube (neurulation defects), whereas others are related to events after neurulation (so-called postneurulation defects). Neurulation defects include abnormal development due to failure of neural tube closure, abnormal disjunction of the neural plate and ectoderm, and abnormal mesenchymal migration. The most common form of neurulation defect gives rise to the myelomeningocele.

Myelomeningocele

Embryology

This malformation of the neural tube may be the result of a primary failure of neural tube closure, with the neural folds failing to roll up and fuse, or it may be due to a secondary reopening of the closed neural tube from rupture of an expanding central canal.[66–70] Experimental evidence supports both theories.[71, 72] The best evidence supports the failure of the tube to close primarily, with the neural plate remaining flat until birth. The development of the associated Chiari malformation has been suggested to occur later in gestation.[73]

When the tube fails to close, the superficial ectoderm remains attached and lateral to the flat neuroectoderm. The mesenchyme and somites cannot migrate medially, and they form the bony, cartilaginous, and muscular elements laterally. The laminae appear bifid, and the structures that form are essentially everted (Fig. 16-16).

At the level of the defect, a number of contiguous vertebrae are affected. The pedicles and laminae have developed laterally and appear rotated outward.[4] The transverse processes are directed anteriorly. This process, however, effectively decreases the anterior-posterior (AP) dimension of the canal. If the laminae have rotated far enough, the AP dimension of the canal can be reduced to zero. The transverse diameter of the canal is usually the greatest and the AP diameter the least at the level of the greatest displacement of the lamina. In some cases of extensive pedicle rotation, the paraspinal muscles develop anterior to the midcoronal plane of the spine. In this position, they become flexors of the spine and can cause or aggravate a kyphosis, particularly when they occur at the upper lumbar or lower thoracic level.

Presentation

The prenatal diagnosis of myelomeningocele has increased markedly with the more routine use of screening tests, such as alpha-fetoprotein determinations, amniocentesis, and ultrasound examinations. This diagnosis allows not only for a more thorough education of the expectant parents but also for preparation of definitive care at the time of delivery.

Myelomeningoceles not diagnosed prenatally are apparent at birth. The goals of evaluation and treatment are to assess the general health of the baby; to identify associated problems, particularly those that potentially preclude early operative closure of the defect; to protect and preserve neural function; and to close the defect and prevent infection. Routine, although somewhat more extensive, neonatal care is be-

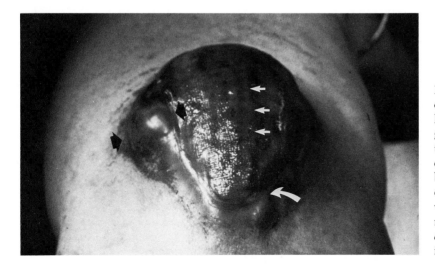

FIG. 16–16. Lumbar myelomeningocele. In this preoperative photograph of a lumbar myelomeningocele, the midline groove is discernible (*white arrows*), but the superior opening to the central canal is out of view. The membranous connection between the placode and the skin edges is easily seen (between *black arrows*) and is of variable width. Epithelialization up to the neural placode is seen at one point (*curved arrow*). (Courtesy of Dr. Keith Rich, Washington University, St. Louis)

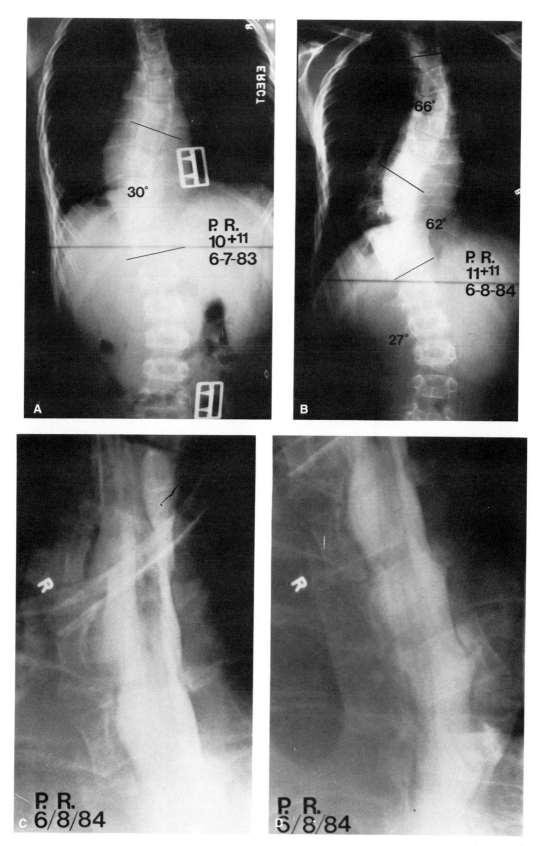

(continued)

451

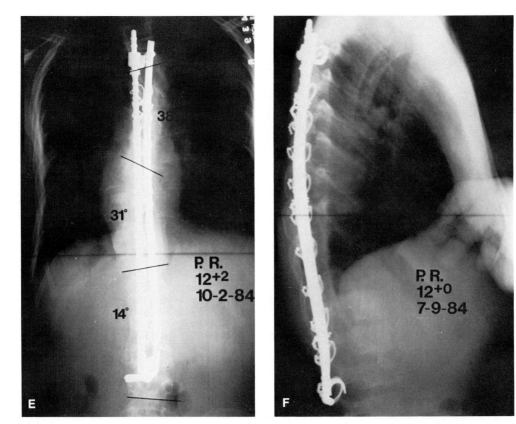

FIG. 17–3. (*continued*)

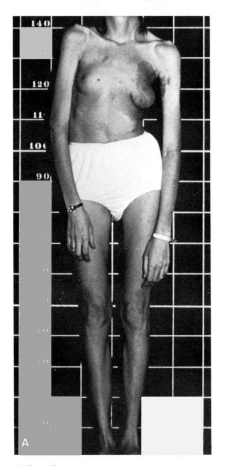

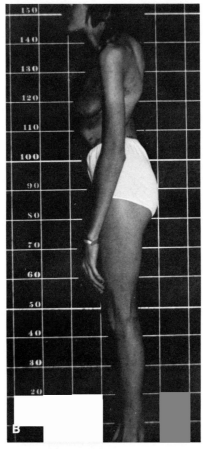

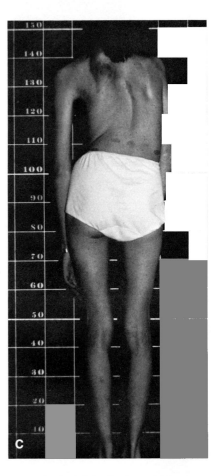

FIG. 17–4.

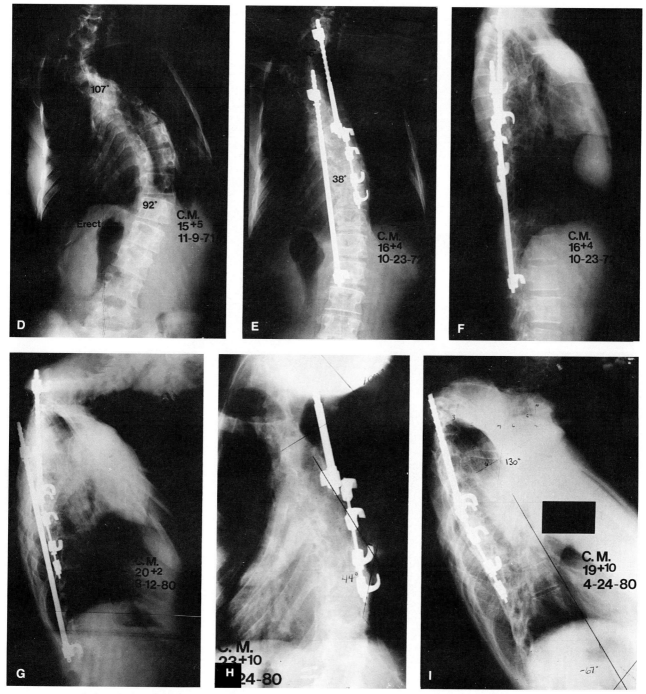

FIG. 17–4. Patient with progressive deformity above the solid fusion. **A–C.** Preoperative clinical photographs. **D.** Erect preoperative anterior-posterior films of first operation showing a curve of 107°. **E, F.** Postoperative Harrington instrumentation and fusion showing correction to 56° and minimal kyphosis. **G.** Note the patient's hook cutting out at the top of the fusion; progressive kyphosis is developing above fusion. **H, I.** Tip of rod removed, allowing further kyphotic progression. Kyphosis is 130° and scoliosis increased to 100°.

(continued)

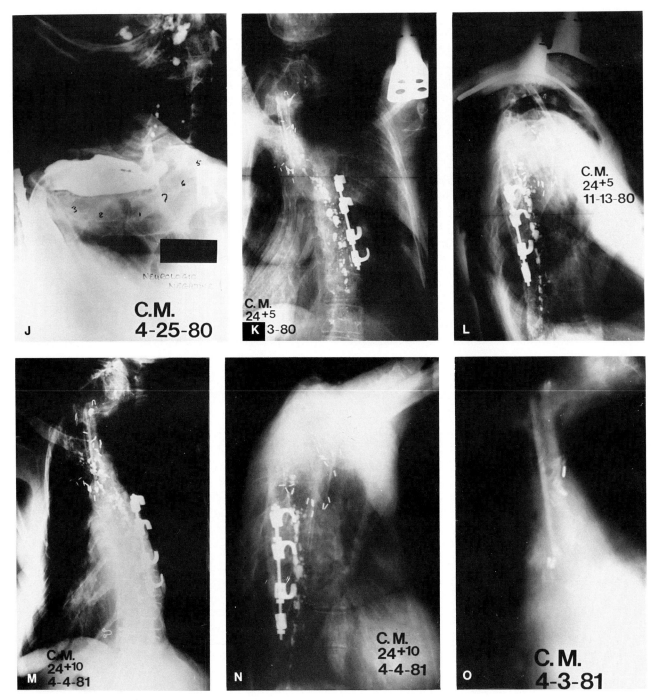

FIG. 17–4. *(continued)* **J–L.** Myelogram shows marked bony constriction and cord compression. Patient underwent posterior osteotomy and anterior cord decompression and strut graft with subsequent paralysis. She was maintained in a halo cast after surgery. **M–O.** Paralysis has resolved, and the patient has solidified anterior and posterior fusion, as confirmed by tomograms.

Results have not been universally satisfactory with these combined procedures. Hsu, in reviewing 5 of 13 patients who had an angular kyphosis and underwent anterior and posterior spinal fusion, noted that none of the 5 did well. One had a pseudarthrosis, and the other 4 had progressive kyphosis despite a solid fusion.[21] Together with other authors, Hsu has attributed some of these failures to poorly done anterior surgery.

To be satisfactory, the anterior graft should be contiguous to all the vertebral body levels it is attempting to fuse and should extend through all of the dysplastic vertebrae anteriorly, ideally to a level segment above and below. Too short a graft allows progressive kyphosis or scoliosis above or below. If soft tissue surrounds the graft, there is a high risk of poor incorporation or graft resorption. Many authors have pointed out the difficulty of placing such a graft at the apex of the acutely angulated curve, emphasizing the need for relatively early operative treatment to obtain optimal results.

In addition to the technical problems of graft placement and instrumentation, several authors have pointed to the increased bleeding that occurs because of plexiform venous abnormalities and increased vascularity of neurofibromatous tissue. Autologous and cell-saver salvaging of blood intraoperatively is mandatory.[21, 31]

Most authors have demonstrated improved correction and decreased risk of progression following fusion when instrumentation is used. Winter reported correction from 69 to 36° with Harrington rod instrumentation, and from 64 to 48° without instrumentation.[50] Chaglassian reported that 5 patients treated with posterior spinal fusion alone (without rods) had an average of 28° of progression postoperatively.[7]

Instrumentation is sometimes difficult owing to the severity of the deformity, osteoporotic bone, or both. Winter has advocated the use of segmental instrumentation, such as segmental wires, to accomplish satisfactory segmental control of these curves. As newer instrumentation techniques are developed, such as Cotrel–Dubousset instrumentation (Fig. 17-5), the use of segmental wires or a simple Harrington construct may become outmoded.[47]

POSTOPERATIVE CARE

Postoperatively all patients with neurofibromatosis who have undergone surgery on the spine should be immobilized in a cast or a brace. Immobilization should be continued until there is strong radiographic evidence of fusion on anterior-posterior, lateral, and oblique x-ray films. If there is any doubt that a solid fusion has occurred, reexploration and reinforcement of the fusion with autologous bone graft should be considered. After the fusion is solid, the patient should be followed at yearly intervals, because neurofibromata can erode into what was previously a solid fusion mass, creating a pseudarthrosis and an increasing deformity.

Decompressive laminectomy has been performed in the past to remove intraspinal tumors. If this approach is indicated, it must be combined with a posterior spinal fusion, preferably with instrumentation. If decompressive laminectomy is performed alone, there may be a temporary neurologic improvement. However, if the spine is further destabilized and deformity increases, the neurologic status will deteriorate further.[50]

If the neurologic abnormalities are caused by the angular deformity of the spine, laminectomy is contraindicated. An anterior decompression and strut grafting followed by a posterior spinal fusion with instrumentation is the appropriate approach in most cases. A posterior spinal fusion alone does not adequately address the problem and has been associated with continued curve and neurologic deterioration and an unacceptable pseudarthrosis rate.[5, 21, 50]

CERVICAL SPINE DEFORMITIES

Deformities of the cervical spine can present as either lordotic or kyphotic. Klose, in 1926, was the first to report such a case in association with neurofibromatosis.[27] Since then, reference to the cervical spine and neurofibromatosis in the literature has been very sparse. In 1962, Heard reported 5 cases of severe cervical kyphosis. Three patients had neurologic compromise, and 2 had no signs or symptoms referable to their severe deformity.[18] More recently, Yong-Hing, in reviewing 34 scoliotic patients, found that 44% had cervical lesions. He noted a significant association with other spinal deformities. Cervical abnormalities seemed to be increased in patients with short kyphotic thoracic or thoracolumbar curves greater than 65°. Interestingly, many of his patients were asymptomatic, perhaps indicating why the cervical spine in neurofibromatosis has not been closely evaluated.[51]

Many of these patients present to the orthopedist

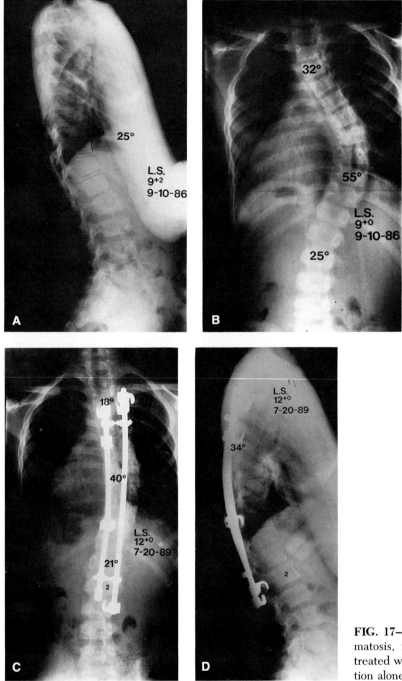

FIG. 17–5. A 10 + 5-year-old boy with neurofibromatosis, nondysplastic curve, and minimal kyphosis, treated with posterior Cotrel–Dubousset instrumentation alone.

after an evaluation of a cervical mass that is to be excised by another surgical service. Usually a cervical spine x-ray film showing multiple abnormalities has already been obtained. Adkins and Ratvich reported that 19 (22%) of 85 patients with neurofibromatosis presented with complaints of head or neck masses. Other presenting signs and symptoms have been dysphagia, torticollis, and neurologic deficits.[1]

Treatment of these deformities depends on their progression and neurologic status. If either deteriorates, posterior fusion is necessary. If the anterior vertebral bodies are severely dysplastic, a strut graft may be necessary. If cord compression occurs anteriorly, decompression is indicated. A halo vest may be needed postoperatively.

Complete cervical dislocation has been reported twice.[38, 42] One case was poorly documented, and the other responded well to halo traction, followed by application of a halo-thoracic jacket. Two cases of spontaneous thoracic dislocation have also been reported.[38, 43]

SPONDYLOLISTHESIS

Spondylolisthesis secondary to neurofibromatosis has been reported in only 11 cases. This is a much lower incidence than occurs in the general population. Winter's well-documented case report in 1981 reinforces the concept that this is an insidiously progressive disease that will gradually intensify the deformity.[48] In his case, the spondylolisthesis developed slowly and progressively over 6 years, with the dystrophic changes of elongated pedicles, vertebral body scalloping, and foraminal enlargement all progressing. A large meningocele sac was discovered in the workup.

INTRATHORACIC MENINGOCELE AND DUMB-BELL LESIONS

Intrathoracic meningoceles are found rarely in neurofibromatosis. There are fewer than 50 cases reported, the first by Pohl in 1933.[35] The best imaging modality that can be used for this diagnosis is a high-volume, complete myelogram. As MRI techniques improve, myelography may be replaced.

Deformity of the pedicles and widening of the intervertebral foramina may be caused by the saccular dilatation of the dura (dural ectasia) or by the presence of dumb-bell tumors (intraspinal neurofibromata). The

preoperative myelogram helps to avoid intraoperative problems during anterior surgery.

References

1. Adkins JC, Ratvich MD: The operative management of von Recklinghausen's neurofibromatosis in children, with special reference to lesions of the head and neck. Surgery 82:343, 1977
2. Biot B, Fauchet R, Robert JM, Stagnara P: Les lesions vertebrales de la neurofibromatose. Rev Chir Orthop 60:607, 1974
3. Brooks B, Lehman EP: The bone changes in Recklinghausen's neurofibromatosis. Surg Gynecol Obstet 38:587, 1924
4. Brasfield RD, Das Gupta TK: Von Recklinghausen's disease: A clinicopathological study. Ann Surg 175:86, 1972
5. Calvert PT, Edgar MA, Webb PJ: Scoliosis in neurofibromatosis. The natural history with and without operation. J Bone Joint Surg [Br] 71:246, 1989
6. Casman J: Scoliose dans des cas de dysplasie fibreuse des os et de neurofibromatose. Acta Orthop Belg 90:252, 1959
7. Chaglassian JH, Riseborough EJ, Hall JL: Neurofibromatous scoliosis: Natural history and results of treatment in thirty-seven cases. J Bone Joint Surg [Am] 58:695, 1976
8. Crawford AH Jr, Bagamery N: Osseous manifestations of neurofibromatosis in childhood. J Pediatr Orthop 6:72, 1986
9. Crawford AH Jr: Neurofibromatosis in children. Acta Orthop Scand Suppl 218:1, 1986
10. Crowe FW, Schull WJ, Neel JU: In A Clinical, Pathological and Genetic Study of Multiple Neurofibromatosis. Springfield, IL, Charles C Thomas, 1956
11. Curtis BH, Fischer RL, Butterfield WL, Saunders FP: Neurofibromatosis with paraplegia. J Bone Joint Surg [Am] 51:843, 1969
12. Dickson RA: Thoracic lordoscoliosis in neurofibromatosis treatment by a Harrington rod with sublaminar wiring [letter]. J Bone Joint Surg [Am] 67:822, 1985
13. DiSimone RE, Berman AT, Schwentker EP: The orthopedic manifestations of neurofibromatosis. A clinical experience and review of the literature. Clin Orthop 230:277, 1988
14. Fauchet J, Gounot C, Gouyet P, et al: Problemes poses par certaines formes de scoliose dans la neurofibromatose de Recklinghausen. Rev Chir Orthop 54:239, 1968
15. Flood BM, Butt WP, Dickson RA: Rib penetration of the intervertebral foraminae in neurofibromatosis. Spine 11:172, 1986
16. Gould EP: The bone changes occurring in von Recklinghausen's disease. Q J Med 11:221, 1918
17. Hagelstam L: Deformite de la collone dans la multiple neurofibromatose. Acta Chir Scand 39:169, 1948
18. Heard CE, Holt JF, Naylor B: Cervical vertebral defor-

mity in von Recklinghausen's disease of the nervous system. J Bone Joint Surg [Br] 44:880, 1962

19. Holt JF: Neurofibromatosis in children. AJR 130:615, 1928
20. Hosoi K: Multiple neurofibromatosis (von Recklinghausen's disease) with special reference to malignant transformation. Arch Surg 22:258, 1931
21. Hsu LCS, Lee PC, Leong JCY: Dystrophic spinal deformities in neurofibromatosis, treatment by anterior and posterior fusion. J Bone Joint Surg [Br] 66:495, 1984
22. Hunt JC, Pugh DG: Skeletal lesions in neurofibromatosis. Radiology 76:1, 1961
23. Isu T, Miyasaka K, Abe H, et al: Atlantoaxial dislocation associated with neurofibromatosis. Report of 3 cases. J Neurosurg 58:45, 1983
24. James JIP: Kyphoscoliosis. J Bone Joint Surg [Br] 37:414, 1955
25. Kerr JG: Scoliosis with paraplegia. J Bone Joint Surg [Am] 35:769 1953
26. Kessel AWL: Intrathoracic meningocele, spinal deformity and multiple neurofibromatosis. J Bone Joint Surg [Br] 33:87, 1951
27. Klose J: Recklinghausensche Neurofibromatose mit schwerer Deformierung der Halswirbelsaule. Klin Wochenschr 5:817, 1926
28. Kornberg M, Dupuy TE: Thoracic vertebral erosion secondary to an intrathoracic meningocele in a patient with neurofibromatosis. Report of 3 cases. J Neurosurg 58:45, 1983
29. Laws JW, Pallis C: Spinal deformities in neurofibromatosis. J Bone Joint Surg [Br] 45:674, 1963
30. Lonstein JE, Winter RB, Moe JH, et al: Neurologic deficits secondary to spinal deformity. Spine 5:331, 1980
31. McCarroll HR: Clinical manifestations of congenital neurofibromatosis. J Bone Joint Surg [Am] 32:601, 1950
32. Meslet PAF: Contribution a l'etude des nevromes plexiformes. These de Bordeaux No. 6, 1982
33. Miller A: Neurofibromatosis with reference to skeletal changes, compressive myelitis and malignant degeneration. Arch Surg 32:109, 1936
34. Phillipat TM: Scoliose grave et neurofibromatose infantile. Acta Neurol Psychiat 4:384, 1962
35. Pohl R: Meningokele im Brustraum unter dem Bilde eines intrathorakalen Rundschattens. Roentgenpraxis 5:747, 1933
36. Preiser SA, Davenport CB: Multiple neurofibromatosis (von Recklinghausen's disease) and its inheritance. Am J Med Sci 156:507, 1918

37. Rezaian SM: The incidence of scoliosis due to neurofibromatosis. Acta Orthop Scand 47:534, 1976
38. Rockower S, McKay D, Nason S: Dislocation of the spine in neurofibromatosis. A report of two cases. J Bone Joint Surg [Am] 64:1240, 1982
39. Saville PD, Nassim JR, Stevenson RH, et al: Osteomalacia in von Recklinghausen's neurofibromatosis: Metabolic study of a case. Br Med J 1:1311, 1955
40. Savini R, Parisini P, Cervellati S, et al: Surgical treatment of vertebral deformities in neurofibromatosis. Ital J Orthop Traumatol 9:13, 1983
41. Savini R, Vincenzi G: Le deformita del rachinde nella neurofibromatosi. Studio clinicoradiografico di 46 casi. Ital J Orthop Traumatol 2:37, 1976
42. Scott JC: Scoliosis and neurofibromatosis. J Bone Joint Surg [Br] 47:240, 1965
43. Stone JW, Bridwell KH, Shackelford GD, Abramson CL: Dural ectasia associated with spontaneous dislocation of the upper part of the thoracic spine in neurofibromatosis. A case report and review of the literature. J Bone Joint Surg [Am] 69:1079, 1987
44. Veliskakis KP, Wilson PD, Levine DB: Neurofibromatosis and scoliosis. Significance of the short angular spinal curve. J Bone Joint Surg [Am] 52:833, 1970
45. Weiss RA: Curvature of the spine in von Recklinghausen's disease. Arch Dermatol Syph 3:144, 1921
46. Winter RB, Edwards WC: Case report—neurofibromatosis with lumbosacral spondylolisthesis. J Pediatr Orthop 1:91, 1981
47. Winter RB: Thoracic lordoscoliosis in neurofibromatosis: Treatment by a Harrington rod with sublaminar wiring. Report of two cases. J Bone Joint Surg [Am] 66:1102, 1984
48. Winter RB, Lonstein JE, Anderson M: Neurofibromatosis hyperkyphosis: A review of 33 patients with kyphosis of 80 degrees or greater. J Spinal Disorders 1:39, 1988
49. Winter RB, Swayze C: Severe neurofibromatosis kyphoscoliosis in a Jehovah's Witness. Anterior and posterior spinal fusion without blood transfusion. Spine 8:39, 1983
50. Winter RB, Moe JH, Bradford S, et al: Spine deformity in neurofibromatosis. J Bone Joint Surg [Am] 61:677, 1979
51. Yong-Hing K, Kalamchi A, MacEwen GD: Cervical spine abnormalities in neurofibromatosis. J Bone Joint Surg [Am] 61:695, 1979

SPINAL DEFORMITY ASSOCIATED WITH MARFAN'S SYNDROME

DAVID H. DONALDSON

Spinal deformities associated with Marfan's syndrome include scoliosis, kyphosis, and lumbar spondylolisthesis (Fig. 17-6).

The incidence of associated scoliosis is between 34 and 73%.[3, 5, 7, 8, 10, 14] Robins found that of 65 patients with Marfan's syndrome, 35 had scoliosis.[10] Fahey reported 45 patients with scoliosis among 132 patients with Marfan's syndrome.[5] Orcutt and DeWald stated that scoliosis occurred in 73% of their patients with Marfan's.[8]

According to most reports, scoliosis occurs more frequently in infantile and juvenile patients than in adolescents. Robins and colleagues reported that 44% of the patients in their study had juvenile or infantile scoliosis. Scoliosis began at less than 3 years of age for 4 patients, between 4 and 10 years of age for 8 patients, and after 10 years of age for 13 patients.[10] Sliman reported that among 16 patients, 9 developed scoliosis during their juvenile years and 6 developed scoliosis during infancy.[12]

Although females with Marfan's syndrome have a higher incidence of scoliosis than males, the rate is less than among patients with idiopathic adolescent scoliosis. In one series, 23 of the patients with scoliosis were female, and 11 patients were male.[10] Birch reported 10 females among 14 patients with scoliosis associated with Marfan's syndrome.[2]

Hyperkyphosis occurs much less frequently in Marfan's syndrome than scoliosis. Robins and colleagues found that kyphosis occurred in only 1 patient in their series.[10] Birch reported 4 patients with thoracolumbar kyphosis; 2 of them also had scoliosis. Two patients had true thoracic kyphosis.[2] Severe kyphosis can be a significant problem, as indicated in Figure 17-7.

The incidence of spondylolisthesis associated with Marfan's syndrome is unknown. Only four cases of severe Grade IV spondylolisthesis associated with painful scoliosis and cauda equina tension symptoms have been reported.[11, 13, 15] Isolated cases of Grade I deformity have also been reported.[7]

Reports concerning the severity of scoliosis in patients with Marfan's syndrome vary.[3–6, 14] Among Fahey's 45 Marfan's patients with scoliosis, none was serious enough to treat.[5] Wilner also reported that none of his 18 patients had scoliosis severe enough to treat.[14] In contrast, two studies reported that scoliosis associated with Marfan's syndrome can be quite severe.[4, 6] In Daudon's report of 21 patients with scoliosis, 66% of the curves had magnitudes ranging from 50 to 150°.[4]

Scoliosis associated with Marfan's syndrome is more structural than adolescent idiopathic scoliosis, according to Daudon, who writes that 60% of his patients with scoliosis did not correct on side-bending x-ray films.[4] In the series reported by Robins, only 36% correction was noted on bending films among curves averaging 72°.[10]

Scoliosis associated with Marfan's syndrome becomes painful in many patients. Robins stated that 74% of patients with scoliosis had back pain, and Moe noted that 5 of 18 of his patients with scoliosis experienced pain.[7, 10]

Chest deformities like pectus excavatum and decreased anterior-posterior chest diameter add to the problems of scoliosis and decreased pulmonary function.

NATURAL HISTORY

Few reports are available describing the natural history of scoliosis associated with Marfan's syndrome.[7, 10] Daudon studied 9 patients for whom longitudinal follow-up was available. The curves of all of these patients progressed, with the greatest progression occurring during adolescence. The curves of males progressed an average of 7.2° per year; the curves of females progressed an average of 5.8° per year.[4] Although documented progression is lacking in most series, the reports of severe deformities in a significant number of patients tend to corroborate the impression that scoliosis associated with Marfan's syndrome is a progressive deformity.

RADIOGRAPHIC FEATURES

The vertebral bodies of patients with Marfan's syndrome are typically elongated. This produces an exag-

(text continues on page 462)

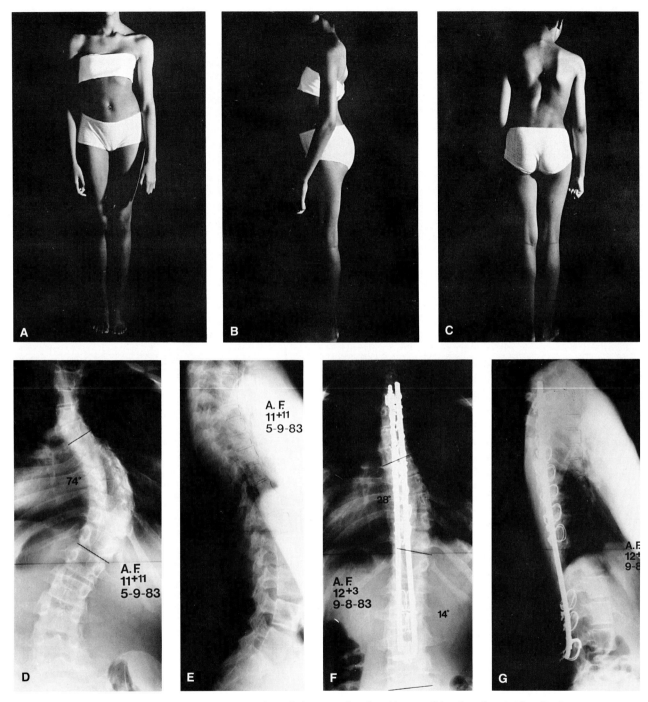

FIG. 17–6. A–C. Preoperative clinical photographs of an 11-year-old girl with a rigid scoliosis secondary to Marfan's syndrome. The side view illustrates significant lumbar lordosis. **D, E.** Anterior-posterior and lateral roentgenograms of the patient with a rigid 74° curvature. **F, G.** Postoperative roentgenograms indicating significant correction of this fairly rigid deformity with segmental instrumentation and Harrington–Luque technique.

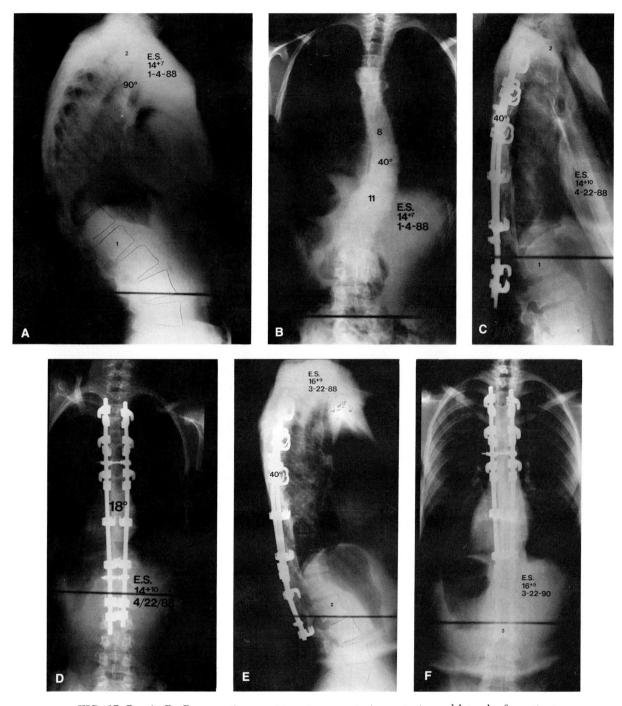

FIG. 17–7.   A, B. Preoperative roentgenograms, anterior-posterior and lateral, of a patient with a kyphosis of 90° and a scoliosis of 40°.   **C, D.** Postoperative roentgenograms of the same patient with significant correction of the scoliosis to 18° and significant correction of the kyphosis to 40°. Unfortunately, the correction was extended to L1 distally and has fallen off at the L1 to L2 level. The lesson is that the instrumentation must extend distally to intersect the sagittal vertical line dropped from C7. This patient should have been fused to L2 or L3.   **E, F.** Indicated extension of the fusion distally with instrumentation to L2 and satisfactory appearance of the spine.

geration of the normal concave posterior surface.[14] Widening of the canal in the lumbar region can also be observed. The curve patterns in scoliosis associated with Marfan's syndrome are similar to those occurring in idiopathic scoliosis. However, frequencies of these curve patterns differ.[3, 10] Unlike idiopathic scoliosis, the prevalence of double-major right thoracic, left lumbar curves has been reported to be greater than the prevalence of single, right thoracic curves in Marfan's (Fig. 17-8).[2, 10]

TREATMENT

Nonsurgical Treatment

The results of brace treatment for scoliosis in Marfan's syndrome have been poor. According to Robins, progression occurred among all 5 patients treated by cast or underarm orthosis. Fourteen patients were treated by Milwaukee brace wear. Only 6 patients who corrected to 30° or less in the brace were maintained by its use; 5 of these patients had progression of the curve after brace treatment was discontinued. Brace failures were attributed to curve severity and rigidity.[10] Birch indicated that brace treatment was successful in only 1 of 9 patients.[2] Success in this patient was thought to be largely due to skeletal maturity. Eight patients demonstrated progression, requiring spinal fusion.

Indications for Surgery

Surgical treatment of Marfan's syndrome has been recommended for patients who develop curvature of 45° to 50° or who have had significant progression despite brace wear.[2, 4, 10] It has been suggested that these patients do not require treatment because many die of cardiovascular disease at an early age. McKusick, in 1972, reported an average life span of 32 years among the patients he studied.[6] However, owing to recent advances in cardiovascular surgery, these individuals will probably have a relatively normal life span; for that reason, surgical treatment for progressive scoliosis should not be withheld.

A significant number of patients with scoliosis associated with Marfan's require surgical treatment for curve progression and pain. In the series reported by Robins and colleagues, 40% of their patients required

fusion, which was usually performed in late adolescence.[10]

Preoperative Evaluation

Operative candidates should have a thorough assessment of their cardiovascular status, because valvular insufficiencies with or without dissecting aortic aneurysms are contraindications to surgery.

These conditions can often be treated before any surgical treatment of the spine. Ophthalmologic evaluation should determine the presence or absence of ectopia lentis. An anesthesiologist familiar with Marfan's syndrome should be available, because special problems related to respiratory function (e.g., emphysema and spontaneous pneumothorax) have been reported.

Surgical Techniques

Posterior spinal fusion with instrumentation is the recommended treatment for scoliosis associated with Marfan's. Robins reported the results of 14 patients treated by posterior spinal fusion, in which 11 were instrumented with Harrington rod instrumentation. Correction of 41%, with an average loss of 7°, was obtained.[10] Birch reported correction of 31%, from an average scoliosis of 55 to 38°.[2]

Thoracic lordosis is a relatively common finding in patients with Marfan's syndrome. Sagittal-plane balance is necessary to correct this situation. The Cotrel–Dubouset instrumentation seems to be an effective way to handle this problem. Segmental instrumentation is also useful in creating a more normal degree of kyphosis. One goal of treatment is to provide a more normal anterior-posterior diameter, since this is frequently quite narrow. The technique of instrumentation and fusion levels are the same as those used for idiopathic scoliosis patients. Bending x-ray films are useful in selecting fusion levels and hook sites.

Amis and Herring reported a case of facet dislocation and disc-space disruption caused by overzealous correction with a Harrington rod.[1] This complication was secondary to increased ligamentous laxity, which occurs in patients with Marfan's syndrome.

Severe spondylolisthesis associated with Marfan's syndrome can be successfully treated with surgery, as described by Winter in his report of 2 cases of Marfan's

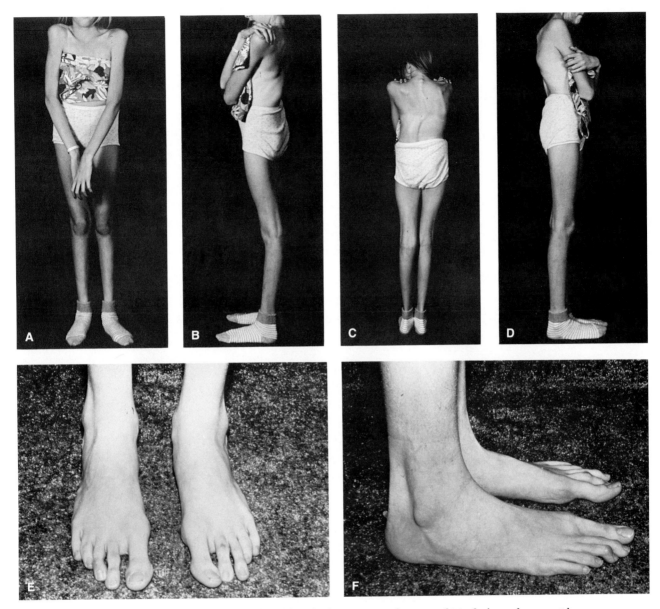

FIG. 17–8. **A–D.** A 9-year-old child with characteristic features of Marfan's syndrome with pronounced right thoracic, left lumbar scoliosis and a very narrow anterior-posterior chest diameter. **E–F.** Clinical photographs indicating the characteristic elongated feet (12 AAAA).

(continued)

syndrome with severe spondylolisthesis and neurologic involvement. He suggested a causal relationship between the severe displacement and Marfan's syndrome. Both patients had successful treatment, one with an in situ fusion and the other with decompression of the nerve roots and decompression with an anterior-posterior fusion.[15] Taylor similarly has reported a Grade IV spondylolisthesis treated successfully with an in situ fusion.[13]

(text continues on page 466)

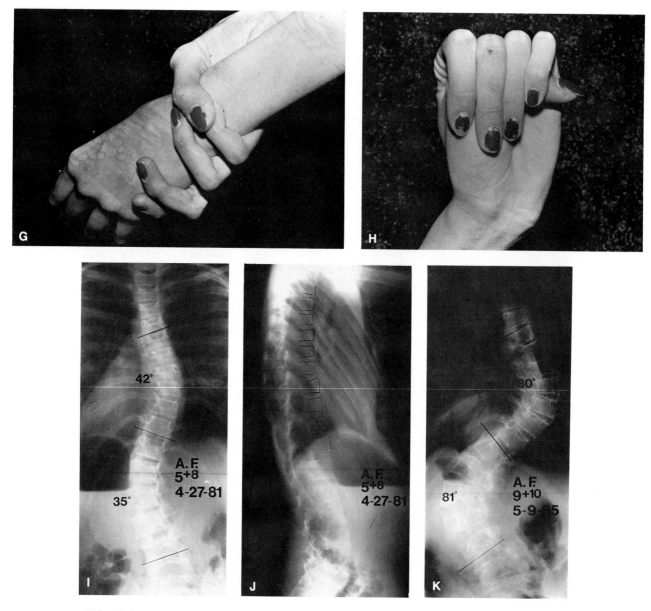

FIG. 17–8. (*continued*) **G, H.** Clinical photographs indicating arachnodactyly, as indicated by overlapping of the thumb and fifth finger, and a positive Steinberg thumb sign. **I–L.** Roentgenograms taken at age 5, indicating a significant curvature, which progressed rapidly to 80° in spite of TLSO brace treatment. **M, N.** Roentgenograms taken 4 years after surgery, indicating fairly satisfactory maintenance of the instrumented spine with Harrington–Luque segmental instrumentation and contouring of the rods. **O–Q.** Postoperative photographs 4½ years after surgical stabilization of the spine, with marked improvement over the preoperative clinical photographs.

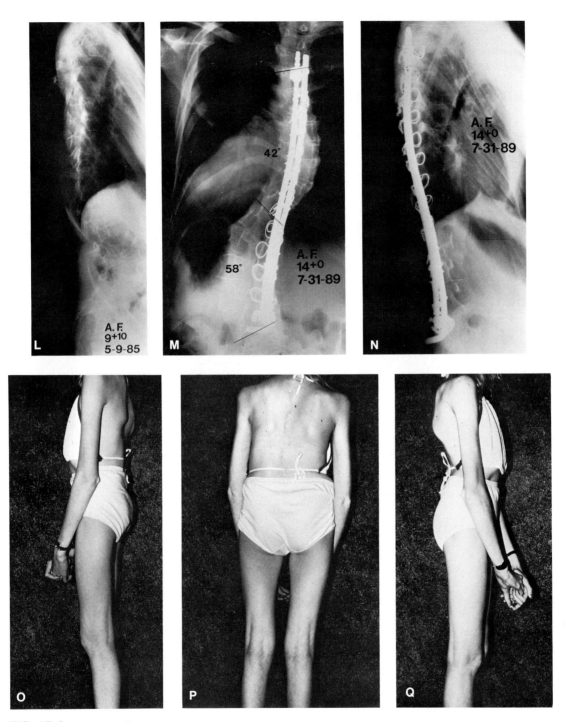

FIG. 17–8. (*continued*)

Complications

Pseudarthroses have occurred frequently among these patients. Robins has reported pseudarthrosis in 5 of 14 patients, requiring additional bone graft.[10] Birch reported only 3 cases of solid fusions among 9 patients in whom a posterior spinal fusion alone was performed.[2] Four patients required a total of 19 revisions for multiple pseudarthroses. Treatment was complicated in all 4 patients by the development of kyphotic deformities. A combined anterior and posterior fusion should be carried out in patients who develop a kyphosis secondary to pseudarthrosis. Two of the 9 patients undergoing a posterior spinal fusion lost 20° of correction, but no reoperation was performed. In patients who have a kyphosis associated with scoliosis, a combined anterior and posterior spinal fusion with instrumentation should be carried out. Birch pointed out, however, that not all adolescent cases of kyphosis progress to require surgery.[2]

References

1. Amis J, Herring JA: Iatrogenic kyphosis: A complication of Harrington instrumentation in Marfan's syndrome. J Bone Joint Surg [Am] 66:460, 1984
2. Birch JG, Herring JA: Spinal deformity in Marfan syndrome. J Pediatr Orthop 7:546, 1987
3. Brenton DP, Dow CJ: Homocystinuria and Marfan's syndrome. J Bone Joint Surg [Br] 54:227, 1972
4. Daudon DP: Contribution a l'étude du syndrome de Marfan: Les deviations vertébrales de ce syndrome propos de 21 observations du centre de Massues. Ph.D. Thesis, Lyon, France 1972
5. Fahey JJ: Muscular and skeletal change in arachnodactyly. Arch Surg 39:741, 1939
6. McKusick VA: Heritable Disorders of Connective Tissue. St. Louis, CV Mosby, 1972
7. Moe JH, Winter RB: Scoliosis in Marfan's syndrome. J Bone Joint Surg [Am] 51:204, 1969
8. Orcutt FV, DeWald RL: The special problems which the Marfan syndrome introduces to scoliosis. J Bone Joint Surg [Am] 56:1763, 1974
9. Pyeritz RE, McKusick VA: The Marfan syndrome: Diagnosis and management. N Engl J Med 300:772, 1979
10. Robins PR, Winter RB, Moe JH: Scoliosis in patients with Marfan's syndrome. J Bone Joint Surg [Am] 57:358, 1975
11. Savini R, Cervellati S, Beroaldo E: Spinal deformities in Marfan's syndrome. Ital J Orthop Traumatol 6:19, 1980
12. Sliman N: A propos de 16 cas de scoliosis-Marfan. Tunis Med 2:93, 1971
13. Taylor LJ: Severe spondylolisthesis and scoliosis in association with Marfan's syndrome. Clin Orthop 221:207, 1987
14. Wilner HI, Finby N: Skeletal manifestations in the Marfan syndrome. JAMA 187:490, 1964
15. Winter RB: Severe spondylolisthesis in Marfan's syndrome: Report of 2 cases. J Pediatr Orthop 2:51, 1982

SPINAL PROBLEMS IN DWARFS

MICHAEL R. MOORE

Spinal abnormalities are commonly associated with dwarfism. Because the underlying pathology in skeletal dysplasias involves abnormal bone development and structure, it is not surprising that spinal abnormalities producing progressive deformity or neurologic sequelae are frequently observed.

Because of the relative rarity of many dwarfing conditions and the variety of phenotypic expressions of these disorders, guidelines for the treatment of spinal disorders in particular dwarfing syndromes are lacking. In discussing spinal disorders in dwarfs, most authors have focused on specific dwarfing syndromes and reviewed the spinal problems found in the small number of cases of the particular syndromes.[10, 12, 33] However, when dwarfs are considered as a group, a limited number of significant spinal problems are identified. Many of the specific spinal disorders, such as atlantoaxial instability, thoracolumbar kyphosis, or scoliosis, are found in many dwarfing syndromes. Table 17-1 lists the spinal problems reported for some dwarfing conditions.

The discussion in this subchapter focuses on the spinal problems and their treatment, rather than on the particular dwarfing conditions.

ATLANTOAXIAL INSTABILITY AND ODONTOID HYPOPLASIA

Atlantoaxial instability, with or without associated odontoid hypoplasia, is associated with several dwarfing conditions (Table 17-1). Odontoid hypoplasia is usually associated with some degree of atlantoaxial instability and produces myelopathy in approximately 50% of cases.[31]

TABLE 17-1. Dwarfing Syndromes and Associated Spinal Problems*

Syndrome	Atlanto-Axial Instability	Odontoid Hypoplasia	Occipitocervical Anomaly	Cervical Kyphosis	Thoracolumbar Kyphosis	Scoliosis	Spinal Stenosis	Spondylolysis Spondylolisthesis
Achondroplasia			49, 54, 4, 33, 37, 40, 44		4, 10, 21, 29, 48, 50, 53	4, 20, 29, 39, 51	4, 10, 20, 21, 29, 34, 36, 40, 41, 43, 48	
Pseudoachondroplasia	31, 32	20, 31, 32				7, 20, 32		
Chondrodysplasia punctata	8	8, 10				10, 45, 46, 47		
Spondyloepiphyseal dysplasia	32, 15	10, 20, 31, 32			15, 52	10, 16, 20, 39		
Metatrophic dwarfism	10, 20	20			10	10, 20, 42	32	
Diastrophic dwarfism				9, 25, 26, 30	9	2, 7, 9, 20, 25, 26, 39		
Kniest's dysplasia		20				20, 42		
Multiple epiphyseal dysplasia		20				3, 20, 24		
Pyknodysostosis						19, 28		19 (cervical)
Dyggve-Melchior-Clausen syndrome		28			10, 22	18, 28, 47		
Mucopolysaccharidoses	6, 10, 20, 22, 31, 32, 34	34, 31, 10, 20, 22				10, 20, 32, 38		
Spondylometaphyseal dysplasia	10, 20, 28, 31	20, 31				10, 20		
Camptomelic dysplasia	27			14		14		14 (lumbar)

*Numbers are reference numbers at the end of this subchapter for published studies.

There is an early, universal association of symptomatic atlantoaxial instability with Morquio syndrome.[11, 31, 32] In his review of 18 patients with Morquio syndrome, Kopits found atlantoaxial instability in all patients and noted that signs of cervical compression usually become apparent by age 6. The most common presenting symptom was reduced exercise tolerance, followed by progressive upper motor neuron signs. Because of the universal occurrence of atlantoaxial instability in patients with Morquio syndrome and the fact that neurologic losses did not usually recover after surgery, Kopits recommended that surgery be performed as soon as any signs of myelopathy were identified.[32] Lipson also recommended early posterior cervical fusion in patients with Morquio syndrome to avoid catastrophic and unrecoverable neurologic loss.[34] In an earlier review, Kopits recommended posterior atlantoaxial fusion, but he later mentioned posterior occipitocervical fusion.[31, 32] Because occiput–C1 instability in Morquio syndrome has not been reported, fusion of the C1–C2 complex is the indicated procedure.

In other dwarfing conditions, atlantoaxial instability is less common. In Bethem's review of 12 patients with spondyloepiphyseal dysplasia, only 2 patients had odontoid hypoplasia, and neither patient had demonstrable instability or neurologic deficit. In the same review, Bethem found 2 of 4 patients with metatrophic dwarfism who had atlantoaxial instability that required fusion. In both cases, fusion was performed from the occiput to C3, although the reason for the inclusion of the occiput was not clear.[10] Kopits reported performing occipitocervical fusion on 1 of 31 patients with pseudoachondroplasia.[32] Bethem also reported atlantoaxial instability in 1 of 2 patients with metaphyseal chondrodysplasia who required fusion because of 5 mm of subluxation.[10]

Summary

Atlantoaxial instability and odontoid hypoplasia are frequently associated with dwarfing conditions, and evaluation of any patient presenting with a dwarfing condition should include an evaluation of the upper cervical spine. Instability does not always accompany a hypoplastic odontoid, and progression to cervical cord compression is not inevitable, with the exception of the Morquio syndrome. Surgical treatment consists of posterior atlantoaxial fusion, sometimes extended to the occiput.

OCCIPITOCERVICAL JUNCTION PROBLEMS

Symptomatic abnormalities of the occipitocervical junction have not been frequently reported in association with dwarfing conditions. Bailey found that most adult achondroplastic dwarfs had mild symptoms of neurologic disturbance.[4] He attributed some of these to constriction of the foramen magnum. Hancock and Phillips reported 2 achondroplastic dwarfs with basilar impression, one of whom also had narrowing of the foramen magnum. This patient underwent a suboccipital decompression, was quadriplegic postoperatively, and died on the fifth postoperative day.[21]

Occipitalization of the first cervical vertebra has also been associated with achondroplasia.[44] Yamada and colleagues reported 6 achondroplastic infants with respiratory problems and quadriparesis due to a small foramen magnum. All 6 patients were treated with suboccipital craniectomy, and all demonstrated significant neurologic improvement.[54] Luyendijk also reported significant postoperative neurologic recovery in a 15-year-old girl with a similar problem.[37] Yamada and colleagues speculated that an unrecognized stenosis of the foramen magnum might account for the increased infant mortality in achondroplastic dwarfs.[54]

Summary

Narrowing of the foramen magnum and basilar impression is increasingly recognized in patients with achondroplastic dwarfism. From the limited reports available, it appears that surgery is effective in restoring neurologic function if deficits exist. Evaluation of neurologic deficit in an achondroplastic dwarf must include imaging studies of the foramen magnum and occipitocervical junction. The role of prophylactic surgery for stenosis at this level has not been studied. Determination of the level of constriction and appropriate decompression with bony stabilization have been associated with good results.

CERVICAL KYPHOSIS

Cervical kyphosis occurs in diastrophic dwarfism.[10, 25, 26, 30] The deformity has been catastrophic in some cases; in others, it has resolved spontaneously or responded to treatment with a Milwaukee brace. Descriptions of surgical treatment are rare, but treatment has been reported with anterior strut grafting and fusion, followed by posterior fusion.[25] Deaths have been reported in untreated cases, warranting a fairly aggressive surgical approach.[30] Cervical kyphosis up to 150° has been reported in camptomelic dysplasia, and surgery has been associated with complications of neurologic loss, wound infection, pseudarthrosis, graft absorption, and progression of deformity.[14]

THORACOLUMBAR KYPHOSIS

Thoracolumbar kyphosis is common in achondroplasia (Figs. 17-9 and 17-10) but has also been observed in spondyloepiphyseal dysplasia, metatrophic and diastrophic dwarfism, and in the Hurler, Morquio, and Maroteaux-Lamy syndromes (see Table 17-1). Although a mild thoracolumbar kyphosis is a common finding in achondroplasia, it is usually neither a progressive nor a severe problem.[32, 53] Bethem reported 2 patients with metatrophic dwarfism who had thoracolumbar kyphosis in association with other complex spinal deformities.[10] Other authors have not reported this deformity in metatrophic dwarfism.[28, 42] Bethem reported 2 patients with diastrophic dwarfism who had thoracolumbar kyphosis, although Herring did not mention this finding in his series of 8 patients with diastrophic dwarfism.[9, 25]

The effectiveness of bracing in the treatment of mild thoracolumbar kyphosis is not clear. Because most of these deformities are nonprogressive in achondroplastic dwarfs, bracing may appear to be more effective than it actually is. Bethem treated 2 patients with Milwaukee braces and reported that 1 patient's kyphosis was reduced from 48 to 5° in 18 months. A second patient, whose kyphosis measured 67° at age 3, wore a Milwaukee brace for 9.5 years and did not show progression.[10] Whether the bracing had any impact on the natural history is impossible to determine.

Some patients with thoracolumbar kyphosis exhibit curve progression and develop neurologic symptoms.[5, 10, 22, 39] Such neurologic manifestations are most common in achondroplasia because of the associated spinal stenosis. Laminectomy for this condition has predictably poor results, and surgical treatment must include anterior decompression and strut grafting.[10, 22, 23] Depending on the stability achieved by the anterior approach, posterior instrumentation and fu-

sion can be considered. As in the treatment of other types of kyphosis, a fusion of adequate length must be carried out to achieve adequate correction and prevent progression above or below the fused segments.

Summary

Thoracolumbar kyphosis is associated with several dwarfing conditions, most noticeably achondroplasia. In most instances, this is a nonprogressive condition. Bracing may be effective in preventing progression. When progression leads to neurologic compromise, surgery is indicated to reduce deformity and relieve spinal cord compression. The appropriate surgical plan must include anterior decompression and strut grafting. A fusion of adequate length can minimize the tendency for progression after fusion.

SCOLIOSIS

Scoliosis, together with thoracolumbar kyphosis, is one of the most commonly reported spinal problems associated with dwarfing conditions (see Table 17-1). As in all forms of scoliosis, the clinical concerns are curve progression leading to cardiopulmonary compromise or an increasingly severe cosmetic problem. Because of the limited number of patients reported with scoliosis in any particular dwarfing condition, it is difficult to extract useful information.

Although many dwarfing conditions have radiographically abnormal vertebrae, scoliosis is due to specific congenital anomalies, such as hemivertebra or failure of segmentation, in a limited number of syndromes, such as Conradi's form of chondrodysplasia punctata, some subgroups of multiple epiphyseal dysplasia, and camptomelic dysplasia.[3, 14, 20] Scoliosis associated with specific congenital verebral anomalies should be treated in the same manner as other congenital scolioses, with early surgical intervention to prevent relentless progression. A convex hemiepiphysiodesis and arthrodesis can be considered as treatment for scoliotic deformities, although this approach has not been reported in dwarfs.[13, 49]

The surgical indications for treatment of scoliosis in dwarfing conditions are somewhat broader than for a typical idiopathic scoliosis because of the practical difficulties with bracing in dwarfs. The weight of a brace is a significant consideration, because it may amount to up

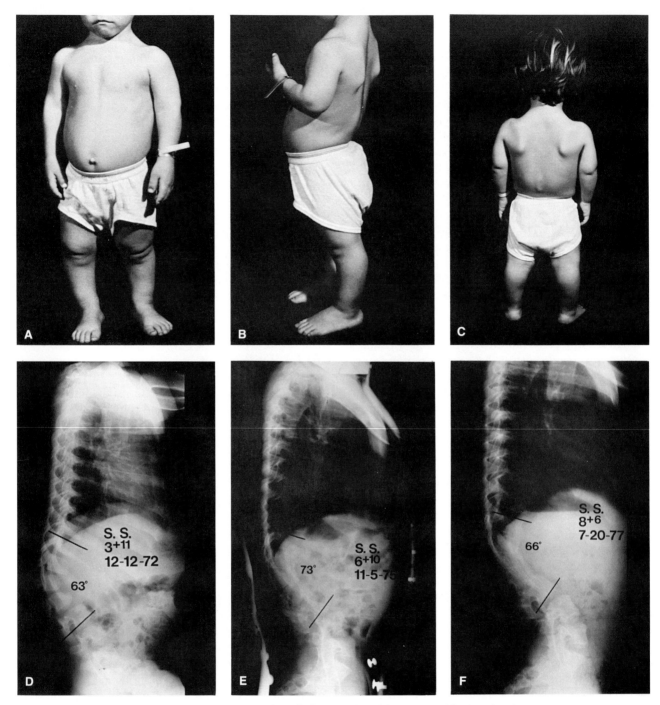

FIG. 17–9. A–C. Postoperative clinical photographs of this 4-year-old achondroplastic dwarf demonstrating the pronounced gibbus deformity in the lumbar area and the other characteristic features of achondroplasia. **D.** Preoperative lateral roentgenogram demonstrating the 63° kyphos in the lumbar area of the spine. **E.** Lateral roentgenogram demonstrates a 73° curve 1 year after an anterior spine fusion with strut grafting, followed by a posterior spine fusion in situ. The patient is being maintained in a TLSO jacket. **F.** Lateral x-ray film of the thoracolumbar spine, demonstrating slight progression of the kyphos, in spite of a solidly healed fusion 3 years after surgery. **G, H.** Anterior-posterior and lateral roentgenograms demonstrating continued and progressive deformity of the lumbar kyphos. Although this patient was ambulatory and without symptoms, one must be skeptical of the length of the fusion because the kyphosis progressed despite a successful fusion both anteriorly and posteriorly.

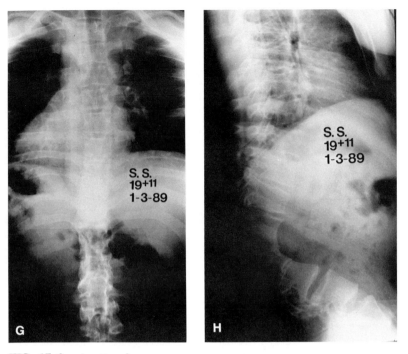

FIG. 17–9. *(continued)*

to 10% of a dwarf's body weight. In addition, the disproportion of limb length to trunk size exaggerates the problems imposed by the lack of spinal flexibility in a brace and makes activities of daily living and personal hygiene extremely difficult.[3] The frequent association of dwarfing conditions and cervical spine problems also makes Milwaukee brace treatment less attractive. No studies exist that demonstrate conclusively that brace treatment modifies the natural history of scoliosis in dwarfing conditions.

Although scoliosis is common in dwarfing conditions, it is usually mild and slowly progressive.[20] In his review of 47 achondroplastic dwarfs, Bailey found a mild scoliosis (less than 20°) in 25 patients and a moderate curve (20–45°) in 7 patients.[4] No patients required surgery. Diamond, reporting on four generations of a family with spondyloepiphyseal dysplasia tarda, noted that only 3 of 31 patients had scoliosis serious enough to be treated with spinal fusion.[16] Although scoliosis is often associated with mucopolysaccharidosis, the pronounced deformity is more frequently kyphosis. In Bethem's series, only 10 of 18 patients with mucopolysaccharidosis had any measurable scoliosis, and the largest curve was 38°. Some patients were treated

with bracing, although this had minimal impact. No patients in Bethem's series were treated surgically.[10]

Severe scoliotic deformities are consistently reported in diastrophic and metatrophic dwarfism (Fig. 17-11). Herring reported 7 patients with diastrophic dwarfism, 5 of whom had scolioses ranging from 20 to 80°. Three patients had been followed long enough to observe significant progression. Two patients treated with Harrington instrumentation and posterior spinal fusion had satisfactory correction.[25] Bethem found scoliosis in 9 of 9 patients with diastrophic dwarfism. All patients over the age of 8 years showed significant progression to curvatures as high as 135°. Surgery was recommended for significant progression, although some difficulties with instrumentation have been encountered owing to fragile bone.[9] Kopits considers scoliosis to be a constant feature of diastrophic dwarfism and recommends early posterior spinal fusion alone, because growth after the age of 10 is minimal.[32]

Metatrophic dwarfs are also reported to have significant scoliosis, although few detailed reports have been published.[10, 20, 42] Bethem reported on 4 patients with metatrophic dwarfism, 2 of whom had severe scoliosis.

(text continues on page 474)

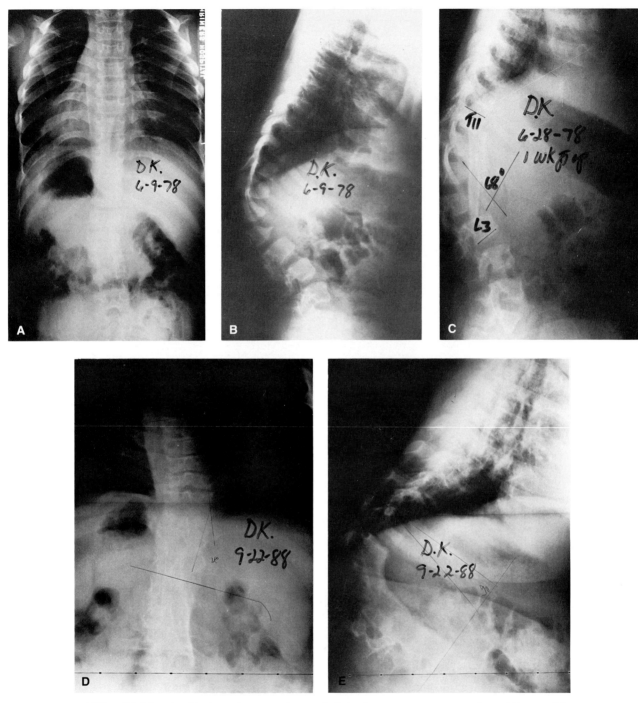

FIG. 17–10. **A, B.** Anterior-posterior and lateral roentgenograms of a 4.5-year-old achondroplastic illustrate a 90° kyphos in the thoracolumbar area. **C.** Lateral roentgenogram demonstrating a 68° kyphosis after an anterior strut grafting. **D, E.** Anterior-posterior and lateral roentgenograms of the same patient 10 years after surgery, demonstrating the pronounced progression of the deformity despite a solidly healed anterior spinal fusion. This case illustrates the difficulty in making decisions about fusion of this particular deformity in achondroplastics. It is apparent that a 360° fusion must be carried out to prevent progression. One must also consider a more lengthy fusion to keep the deformity from progressing as the patient continues to grow. Resolution of the kyphosis has also been reported in patients with severe kyphos at a young age.

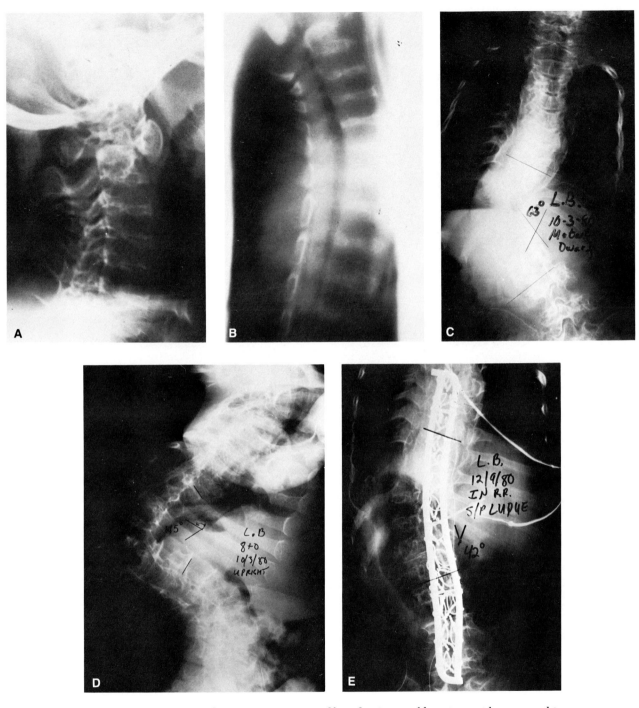

FIG. 17–11. **A.** Lateral postoperative x-ray film of a 6-year-old patient with metatrophic dwarfism with atlantoaxial instability of the cervical spine. This patient presented with quadriparesis. **B.** Lateral roentgenogram of the air myelogram indicating a block at the C2 level. **C, D.** Anterior-posterior and lateral roentgenograms of the same patient with metatrophic dwarfism with pronounced kyphoscoliosis. **E, F.** Postoperative spinal fusion after segmental instrumentation with Luque instruments, with excellent correction of the deformity.

(continued)

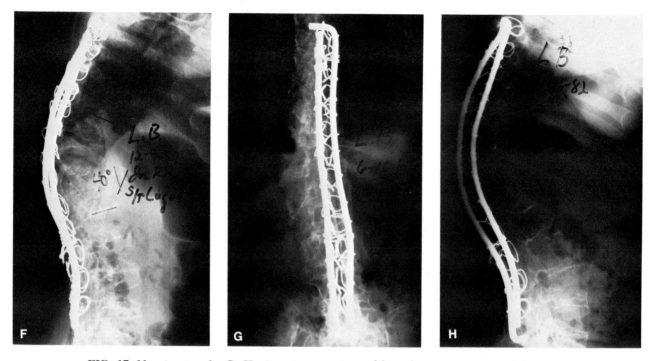

FIG. 17–11. *(continued)* **G, H.** Anterior-posterior and lateral roentgenograms of the same patient 2 years after surgery demonstrating maintenance of the curve. The patient was asymptomatic and normal neurologically.

Both of these patients were treated with halo-femoral traction, followed by posterior spinal fusion without instrumentation. One patient developed pseudarthrosis, and the other died 1 year later during intubation for an unrelated surgical procedure.

Coscia reported 8 patients with camptomelic dyplasia, 7 of whom had a scoliotic curve averaging 63°.[14] Treatment ranged from bracing to posterior fusion without instrumentation to subcutaneous Harrington rods to sublaminar wiring. Significant complications were identified (i.e., cervical kyphosis), yet these authors recommended an aggressive approach to the treatment of spinal deformity in these patients, with their final recommendation being anterior and posterior fusion followed by casting.

Summary

Scoliosis is frequently associated with dwarfing conditions, although in most syndromes it is not severe or rapidly progressive. The value of bracing in moderate curves is unknown. Patients with diastrophic dwarfism or metatrophic dwarfism show early progression to severe curves, and early surgical intervention is indicated. Congenital curves occurring in dwarfs should be treated in a similar fashion to congenital curves in nondwarfs. All dwarfs need to be evaluated for scoliosis and followed for progression.

SPINAL STENOSIS

Spinal stenosis is a consistent feature of achondroplasia (Fig. 17-12).[4, 10, 29, 32, 36, 43, 51] The narrowed interpediculate distance that is a constant radiographic feature of achondroplasia is not a reliable index to the degree of spinal stenosis, because the stenoses are due more to the short pedicles, high laminar angle, and the resultant decreased anteroposterior diameter.[29, 35, 48, 51] However, some authors have identified a relation be-

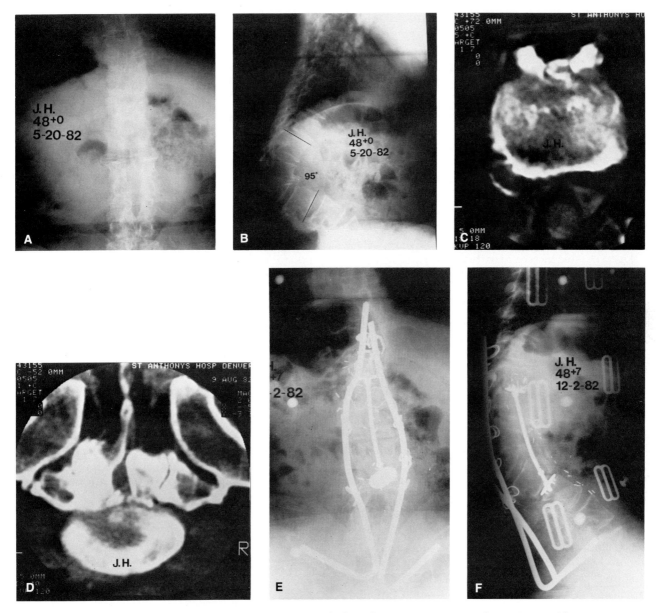

FIG. 17–12. A, B. Anterior-posterior and lateral roentgenograms of a 48-year-old achondroplastic with progressive paraparesis after a decompressive laminectomy for spinal stenosis. **C.** A cross-section of a contrast myelogram at the apex of deformity indicating the very short pedicles and attenuated spinal canal. **D.** A CT scan indicating cross-sectional area of the spinal canal with severe stenosis, which is characteristic of achondroplastic patients. **E, F.** Anterior-posterior and lateral roentgenograms after anterior decompression of the spinal canal and an anterior corrective device and fusion, followed by segmental instrumentation posteriorly. Multiple revisions were subsequently necessary. Despite adequate and extensive anterior decompression, this patient failed to regain neurologic function, a situation that sometimes occurs in achondroplastic patients with spinal stenosis.

tween interpediculate distance in the existence of neurologic symptoms. Wynne-Davies and colleagues reported that if the ratio of the interpediculate distance at L1 to that at L4 was greater than 1.3 and there was a persistent thoracolumbar kyphosis, the risk of neurologic sequelae was increased.[51] Kahanovitz and colleagues reported that an L1 interpediculate distance of less than 20 mm or an L5 interpediculate distance of less than 16 mm was associated with symptoms of spinal stenosis.[29]

The preexisting spinal canal stenosis makes the achondroplastic dwarf particularly prone to serious neurologic complications associated with disc herniation, degenerative arthroses, and kyphotic deformity. Schreiber and Rosenthal reported 2 patients who developed paraplegia secondary to disc herniation superimposed on the characteristically narrowed spinal canal.[43] Both patients had significant neurologic improvement after laminectomy and discectomy. Several authors have noted the increased likelihood of symptoms when stenosis is associated with kyphosis.[21, 29, 39, 51] Kahanovitz and colleagues reported that thoracolumbar kyphosis was identified with increasing frequency in groups of patients with intensifying severity of stenosis symptoms.[29] Vogl and Osborne were able to observe pathologic changes in the lower spinal cord produced by hypertrophic arthrosis of the facet joints that reduced the size of an already congenitally narrowed canal.[48]

Achondroplastic dwarfs presenting with symptoms of spinal claudication without objective neurologic deficit have been reported to improve with a brief period of rest alone.[29] Patients presenting with paraparesis or a cauda equina syndrome required canal decompression and evaluation for the presence of a herniated nucleus pulposus. Bethem and coworkers recommended that fusion accompany a posterior decompression, although Kopits stated that this was not necessary, provided that the facets were not damaged in the decompression.[10, 32] The plan for treatment of a patient presenting with significant symptoms must also include evaluation of the sagittal-plane deformity. If kyphosis is associated with stenosis and neurologic deficit, the anterior compression resulting from the deformity must be ameliorated. Lutter and colleagues, in their series of patients with spinal stenosis and mild kyphosis, found that after laminectomy 2 patients were unchanged, 2 were worse, and 2 were slightly improved but not normal. Laminectomy alone in the treatment of combined ste-

nosis and kyphosis produces poor results, and anterior decompression and strut grafting should be considered.[10, 22, 23]

Early treatment of spinal stenosis in patients with achondroplasia has been recommended by several authors.[1, 10, 17] Bethem reported on 6 patients with paraparesis, for 6 weeks to 2 years, who were treated with laminectomy. No patient showed neurologic improvement. This suggests that surgical treatment should be pursued before the development of neurologic deficit or as soon as possible after its onset.

Summary

Lumbar spinal stenosis is common in achondroplasia and requires decompressive laminectomies when symptoms do not respond to conservative measures or when objective neurologic deficit is present or imminent. The need for fusion at the time of decompression is controversial, but it is probably unnecessary unless the integrity of the facet joints is compromised. If kyphosis accompanies stenosis, the approach must be one of anterior decompression and strut grafting.

SPONDYLOLYSIS AND SPONDYLOLISTHESIS

Spondylolysis and spondylolisthesis have been mentioned in association with pyknodysostosis and camptomelic dysplasia.[14, 19] No specific guidelines for treatment of this condition in these syndromes have been advanced.

References

1. Alexander E: Significance of the small lumbar spinal canal: Cauda equina compression syndromes due to spondylosis. Part 5. Achondroplasia. J Neurosurg 31: 513, 1969
2. Amuso SJ: Diastrophic dwarfism. J Bone Joint Surg [Am] 50:113, 1968
3. Bailey JA: Disproportionate Short Stature; Diagnosis and Treatment. Philadelphia, WB Saunders, 1973
4. Bailey JA: Orthopaedic aspects of achondroplasia. J Bone Joint Surg [Am] 52:1285, 1970
5. Beighton P, Bathfield CA: Gibbal achondroplasia. J Bone Joint Surg [Br] 63:328, 1981
6. Beighton P, Craig J: Atlantoaxial subluxation in the Morquio syndrome: Report of a case. J Bone Joint Surg [Br] 55:478, 1973

7. Beighton P: Orthopaedic problems in dwarfism. J Bone Joint Surg [Br] 62:116, 1980

8. Bethem D: Os odontoideum in chondrodysplasia calcificans congenita. A case report. J Bone Joint Surg [Am] 64:1385, 1982

9. Bethem D, Winter RB, Lutter L: Disorders of the spine in diastrophic dwarfism. J Bone Joint Surg [Am] 62:529, 1980

10. Bethem D, Winter R, Lutter L, et al: Spinal disorders of dwarfism. Review of the literature and report of 80 cases. J Bone Joint Surg [Am] 63:1412, 1981

11. Blaw ME, Langer LO: Spinal cord compression in Morquio-Brailsford disease. J Pediatr 74:593, 1969

12. Bradford DS, Lonstein JE, Ogilvie JW, Winter RB: Moe's Textbook of Scoliosis and Other Spinal Deformities, 2nd ed. Philadelphia, WB Saunders, 1987

13. Bradford DS: Partial epiphyseal arrest and supplemental fixation for progressive correction of congenital spinal deformity. J Bone Joint Surg [Am] 64:610, 1982

14. Coscia MF, Bassett GS, Bowen JR, et al: Spinal abnormalities in camptomelic dysplasia. J Pediatr Orthop 9:6, 1989

15. Diamond LS: Management of inherited disorders of the skeleton. Instr Course Lect 25:107, 1976

16. Diamond LS: A family study of spondyloepiphyseal dysplasia. J Bone Joint Surg [Am] 52:1587, 1970

17. DuVoisin RC, Yahr MD: Compressive spinal cord and root syndromes in achondroplastic dwarfs. Neurology 12:202, 1961

18. Dyggve HU, Melchior JC, Clausen J: Morquio–Ullrich's disease. An inborn error of metabolism? Arch Dis Child 3F:525, 1962

19. Elmore SM: Pyknodysostosis: A review. J Bone Joint Surg [Am] 49:153, 1967

20. Goldberg MJ: Orthopedic aspects of bone dysplasias. Orthop Clin North Am 7:445, 1976

21. Hancock DO, Phillips DG: Spinal compression in achondroplasia. Paraplegia 3:23, 1965

22. Hensinger RN: Kyphosis secondary to skeletal dysplasias and metabolic disease. Clin Orthop 128:113, 1977

23. Herring JA: Kyphosis in an achondroplastic dwarf. J Pediatr Orthop 3:250, 1983

24. Herring JA: Rapidly progressive scoliosis in multiple epiphyseal dysplasia. J Bone Joint Surg [Am] 58:703, 1976

25. Herring JA: The spinal disorders in diastrophic dwarfism. J Bone Joint Surg [Am] 60:177, 1978

26. Hollister DW, Lachman RS: Diastrophic dwarfism. Clin Orthop 114:61, 1976

27. Holmes JC, Hall JE: Fusion for instability and potential instability of the cervical spine in children and adolescents. Orthop Clin North Am 9:923, 1978

28. Jones KL: Smith's Recognizable Patterns of Human Malformation, 4th ed. Philadelphia, WB Saunders, 1988

29. Kahanovitz N, Rimoin D, Sillence DO: The clinical spectrum of lumbar spine disease in achondroplasia. Spine 7:137, 1982

30. Kash IJ, Sane SM, Samaha FJ, Briwer J: Cervical cord compression in diastrophic dwarfism. J Pediatr 84:862, 1974

31. Kopits SE, Perovic MN, McKusick VA, et al: Congenital atlantoaxial dislocations in various forms of dwarfism. J Bone Joint Surg [Am] 54:1349, 1972

32. Kopits SE: Orthopaedic complications of dwarfism. Clin Orthop 114:153, 1976

33. Leatherman KD, Dickson RA: The Management of Spinal Deformities. London, Wright, 1988

34. Lipson SJ: Dysplasia of the odontoid process in Morquio's syndrome causing quadriparesis. J Bone Joint Surg [Am] 59:340, 1977

35. Lutter LD, Lonstein JE, Winter RB, Langer LO: Anatomy of the achondroplastic lumbar canal. Clin Orthop 126:139, 1977

36. Lutter LD, Langer LO: Neurological symptoms in achondroplastic dwarfs—surgical treatment. J Bone Joint Surg [Am] 59:87, 1977

37. Luyendijk W, Matricali B, Thomeer RTWM: Basilar impression in an achondroplastic dwarf: Causative role in tetraparesis. Acta Neurochir 41:243, 1978

38. Melzak J: Spinal deformities with paraplegia in two sisters with Morquio-Brailsford syndrome. Paraplegia 6:246, 1969

39. Nelson MA: Orthopaedic aspects of the chondrodystrophies. The dwarf and his orthopaedic problems. Ann Royal Coll Surg Engl 47:185, 1970

40. Nelson MA: Spinal stenosis in achondroplasia. Proc Royal Soc Med 65:18, 1972

41. Nelson MA: Spinal stenosis in achondroplasia. J Bone Joint Surg [Am] 52:1285, 1970

42. Rimoin DC, Siggens DC, Lachman RS, Silberberg R: Metatrophic dwarfism, the Kneist syndrome, and the pseudo-achondroplastic dyplasias. Clin Orthop 114:70, 1976

43. Schreiber F, Rosenthal H: Paraplegia from ruptured lumbar discs in achondroplastic dwarfs. J Neurosurg 9:648, 1952

44. Scott CI: Achondroplastic and hypochondroplastic dwarfism. Clin Orthop 114:18, 1976

45. Selakovitch WG, White JW: Chondrodystrophia calcicans-congenita: Report of a case. J Bone Joint Surg [Am] 37:1271, 1955

46. Spranger J: The epiphyseal dysplasias. Clin Orthop 114:46, 1976

47. Spranger J, Maroteaux P, Der Kaloustian VM: The Dyggve-Melchior-Clausen syndrome. Radiology 114:415, 1975

48. Vogl A, Osborne RL: Lesions of the spinal cord (transverse myelopathy) in achondroplasia. Arch Neurol Psychiatry 61:644, 1949

49. Winter RB, Lonstein JE, Denis F, Sta-Ana de la Rosa H: Convex growth arrest for progressive congenital scoliosis due to hemivertebrae. J Pediatr Orthop 8:633, 1988

50. Winter RB, Hall JE: Kyphosis in childhood and adolescence. Spine 3:285, 1978

51. Wynne-Davies R, Walsh WK, Gormley B: Achondroplasia and hypochondroplasia: Clinical variations and spinal stenosis. J Bone Joint Surg [Br] 63:508, 1981

52. Wynne-Davies R, Hall C, Ansell BM: Spondyloepiphyseal dysplasia tarda with progressive arthropathy. A "new" disorder of autosomal recessive inheritance. J Bone Joint Surg [Br] 64:442, 1982

53. Wynne-Davies R, Hall CM, Apley AG: Atlas of Skeletal Dysplasias, 3rd ed. Edinburgh, Churchill Livingstone, 1985

54. Yamada H, Nakamura S, Kageyama N: Neurological manifestations of pediatric achondroplasia. J Neurosurg 54:49, 1981

SPINAL DEFORMITY AFTER LAMINECTOMY

DAVID H. DONALDSON

Many reports describe spinal deformities after laminectomy for resection of spinal cord tumor, decompression of spinal cord injury, spondylosis, cervical disc disease, and syringomyelia (Fig. 17-13).[3, 9, 10, 15, 33]

Spinal deformity occurs most frequently in the cervicothoracic spine, followed by the thoracic spine, and rarely, in the lumbar spine. Kyphosis is the most commonly reported deformity.[14] Scoliosis occurs occasionally.[9] Atlantoaxial rotary subluxation has also been reported in conjunction with kyphosis after laminectomy.[34]

The reported frequency of deformities after laminectomy varies. Sim observed that only 21 patients developed swan-neck deformity among 673 patients for whom laminectomy was performed.[29] However, this was a mixed group of patients that included partial and complete laminectomies. Mikawa reported that 23 (36%) of 64 patients developed a change in curve type after multiple laminectomies. Nine (14%) of 64 patients developed frank deformity.[20] Lonstein has speculated that the incidence is approximately 49%, based on a review of several series.[14]

The frequency of spinal deformity after laminectomy is higher in children than in adults. Matson found that as many as 80% of children undergoing laminectomy for tumor required orthotic treatment or operation.[17] In Lonstein's series of patients younger than 20 years, all 32 developed deformity after laminectomy. Twenty-six developed kyphosis, with an average curve magnitude of 82°.[15] Yasuoka reported that, among 58 patients who underwent laminectomy, only patients younger than 15 years developed deformity.[38] Sim noted that 5 (14%) of 35 patients between the ages of 13 and 18 years developed spinal deformity.[29] This was compared with 21 (< 3%) of 673 patients who developed swan-neck deformity in the older age group. Haft, Ransohoff, and Carter reported 10 of 17 children who developed kyphoscoliosis; however, only 1 required fusion.[10]

ETIOLOGIC CONSIDERATIONS

Spinal deformity after laminectomy has been largely attributed to the imbalance created by resection of bone and ligamentous structures.[35] The extent of resection performed at each level, the number of levels performed, and the location of levels performed appear to be significant factors in the development of spinal deformity. Callahan reported that 7 of 13 patients who had laminectomy performed at only one or two levels developed significant deformity.[2] Fraser reported severe spinal deformity in patients with an average age of 4 years at the time of diagnosis.[9] Patients with an average age of 10 years at the time of diagnosis had no deformity. Cervical deformity did not correlate with the age of diagnosis in this series. These authors speculated that deformity was due to the extent of resection at any one level. Sim wrote that spinal deformity usually followed bilateral laminectomy.[29] However, he described one case of deformity after unilateral resection at C5, C6, and C7. He recommended preservation of articular processes if possible.

Lonstein noticed a positive correlation between the extent of laminectomy and the location of the apex.[14] He found that the apex typically was located at the level in which the articular processes had been removed. Mikawa observed that patients developed a sharp angular kyphosis if the facets were completely removed, but a rounded kyphosis developed when the facets were preserved.[20] Fraser stated that the higher the level of laminectomy, the greater the likelihood of deformity.[9] The extent of laminectomy did not correlate with deformity in their series.

Spinal deformity after laminectomy occurs more often in children than in adults. Some authors have attributed the increased frequency to greater ligamentous laxity in young patients.[3, 33] Fielding thinks that the more horizontal orientation of the facets in a child's

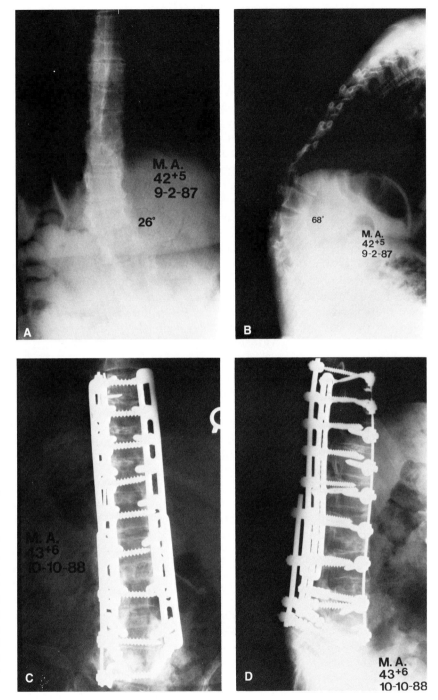

FIG. 17–13. **A, B.** Anterior-posterior roentgenograms that demonstrate the deformity resulting from extensive laminectomies done for the purpose of rhizotomies. The patient had wide-open laminectomies posteriorly, which required pedicle fixation of the spine for solid stabilization. An anterior fusion with a Zielke device was also carried out. **C, D.** Anterior-posterior and lateral roentgenograms demonstrating the extensive instrumentation used in this patient. With Steffee plates inserted in the pedicles posteriorly and the Zielke instrumentation done anteriorly, this patient was solidly healed at 1 year after surgery.

spine may allow greater subluxation and translation of vertebrae.[7]

Patients with muscle imbalance secondary to paralysis are at greater risk of developing spinal deformity after laminectomy, with younger patients having the greatest risk. In Morgan's series of 186 patients with spinal cord injury at 18 years of age or younger, 86 patients had undergone laminectomy. Thirty-six of the 86 patients developed kyphosis, and 16 developed kyphoscoliosis. Kyphosis, which most often developed in the cervical and thoracic spine, ranged from 10 to 110°, averaging 41°. Patients who had not undergone laminectomy more commonly developed scoliosis.[21] Among Malcolm's group of patients who had undergone laminectomy after spinal injury, patients with a thoracic-level injury had an average increase in kyphosis of 15° over patients who had not had laminectomy.[16] Patients with thoracolumbar-level injuries had an average increase of 13°, and patients with a lumbar-level injury had an average increase of 11°. Yasuoka reported that patients with paralysis developed kyphosis at the laminectomy site, with scoliosis and pelvic obliquity below that area.[37] Fraser documented severe scoliosis in 2 patients and mild scoliosis in 2 others after thoracic laminectomy.[9] Paraplegia also occurred in the severe cases.

Natelson describes development of kyphosis in 3 patients who underwent laminectomy and facetectomy for lumbar spinal stenosis.[22] This deformity was attributed to progression of compression fractures unrecognized at the time of surgery.

Patients receiving irradiation to the spine have an increased risk of developing spinal deformity, especially if laminectomy has also been performed.

NATURAL HISTORY

Development and progression of spinal deformity after laminectomy is not reported uniformly. According to Mikawa, spinal deformity in 2 juvenile patients developed soon after laminectomy, and fusion was required to avoid neurologic complications.[20] Winter tells of the case of a 20-month-old child who underwent extensive laminectomy; 3 years later, he developed paraplegia secondary to progressive kyphosis.[36] Kyphosis after laminectomy is invariably progressive, with the greatest progression occurring during the adolescent growth spurt.[20] Of Mayfield's 7 patients who developed

progressive kyphosis after thoracolumbar spinal cord injuries, a kyphosis progression of 5° per year among 4 patients who had prior laminectomies was compared with an average of 1° per year among 3 patients in whom laminectomies were not performed. Kyphosis progressed more rapidly in the thoracolumbar than thoracic spine injuries after laminectomy. Spinal deformity occurred more frequently in the postadolescent group when laminectomy was performed. Patients in the preadolescent group developed significant paralytic deformity with or without laminectomy.

TREATMENT

Conservative measures, primarily bracing, have been attempted to prevent spinal deformity after extensive laminectomy. Although Sim noted that bracing has been effective in preventing the development of kyphosis after laminectomy, my experience does not support this. He has also reported spontaneous fusion after a prolonged period of bracing. Wearing orthoses has been recommended to decrease symptoms of nerve irritation after laminectomy.[29] Bracing must be applied at the first signs of deformity.[14]

In patients with an existing deformity, correction can rarely be obtained by brace wear. Rather, a goal should be to control the deformity until the patient is mature enough to undergo fusion.

Several surgical treatments have been recommended as more definitive methods of preventing deformity after laminectomy. These methods include various fusion techniques and reconstructive procedures. Many physicians have recommended fusion combined with laminectomy.[3, 13, 29] Callahan suggested using posterolateral cervical facet fusion to stabilize the spine after laminectomy to prevent progressive deformity.[2] He reported the results of 52 patients in whom solid fusion occurred in 50 at a mean period of 6.5 months. He recommended fusion for children, young adults, patients with injury to the intervertebral ligaments, and those who had had foramenotomy or extensive resection of articular processes performed. Mikawa states that adults do not usually become unstable after laminectomy.[20] In his series, no patient demonstrated greater than 3.5 mm of displacement after laminectomy during follow-up. Southwick reported 63 patients who had undergone posterior facet fusion after laminectomy with corticocancellous bone grafts. All patients fused; however, 2 required revision surgery. Several patients developed kyphosis below their fusion at the cervicothoracic junction. Fraser also experienced displacement above the anterior fusion.[9] Southwick cited immediate stability and lack of interference with decompression as advantages to this technique.[31]

Other surgeons have argued against posterior cervical fusion at the time of laminectomy because of increased blood loss and possible damage to the exposed cord. These authors, although also recommending fusion if instability occurs after laminectomy, advocated anterior fusion. Earlier consolidation and lack of future problems, if further decompression is needed, were cited as advantages to anterior spinal fusion. Sim recommended that the fusion extend the full length of the laminectomy to prevent progressive deformity below.[29] Smith and Robinson suggested that anterior fusion be performed before wide laminectomy.[30] Critics of anterior spinal fusion pointed out the lack of immediate stability provided by these grafts. For this reason, the use of plaster jackets, halo vests, or traction has been recommended for support until fusion takes place.

Several authors have advocated replacement of the posterior cervical laminae and attached ligaments as a method to prevent deformity.[24] Various modifications of this laminoplasty procedure have been described, but all remove the laminae and attached ligaments as a single structure after bilateral osteotomy. The laminae are then replaced and sutured into position.

Surgical Treatment of the Cervical Spine

Correction of an existing cervical deformity has not achieved normal alignment in most cases. Sim reported complete correction in 4 patients, partial correction in 7, and no correction in 9 after anterior release and fusion.[29] Correction achieved the best results for mild deformity. Preoperative traction has not been particularly effective in reducing deformity.[3, 29] Francis recommended preoperative traction followed by anterior release and strut graft with iliac or fibular graft if the deformity is secondary to deficient posterior elements alone.[8] Rigid halo immobilization is maintained for 3 to 4 months. Good results were achieved with this technique. A number of physicians have reported that, as the length of anterior fusion increases, the complications increase also.[1, 4, 30]

Contoured loop fixation with sublaminar wiring through burr holes in the occiput to C3, C4, and C5 has been effective in controlling craniocervical instability.

Indications for Surgery

Children and adults who demonstrate steady progression of deformity should be considered for fusion. This is particularly true for children with growth potential who have progressed despite adequate bracing (Fig. 17-14). Considerable variables exist in these individuals, especially with respect to neurologic function, the presence of pelvic obliquity, and scoliosis. Aggressive treatment is warranted because unacceptable deformity can occur quite rapidly and neurologic risk is high.

Surgical Treatment of the Thoracolumbar Spine

The major problem confronted in deformity after extensive laminectomy is the lack of posterior elements. There is minimal bone surface available posteriorly to accept graft. Attempts to fuse posteriorly alone have resulted in a high pseudarthrosis rate (57%). My recommended treatment is a combined anterior and posterior fusion, with some form of instrumentation. In patients with pure kyphosis, strut grafting anteriorly with rib graft obtained during the transthoracic approach or a fibular graft allows fusion on the compression side of the spine. It can provide considerable correction. The discs should be completely cleaned of soft tissue, and endplates should be exposed to fresh cancellous bone. Additional bone obtained locally from the vertebral bodies or from the ilium should be packed into the open disc space.

If laminectomy in the upper thoracic area is associated with a significant scoliosis below, anterior instrumentation using a Zielke or Dwyer device should be considered. This is particularly useful in paralytic curves. All patients should have a posterior fusion in addition. Instrumentation should be used if possible. If the laminectomy is extensive, the defect may be crossed with posterior instrumentation. An attempt to provide segmental fixation with wire loops around the transverse processes or remaining laminae can be useful in most cases. In the thoracolumbar area, fixation with a pedicle system provides good fixation. In neuro-

(text continues on page 484)

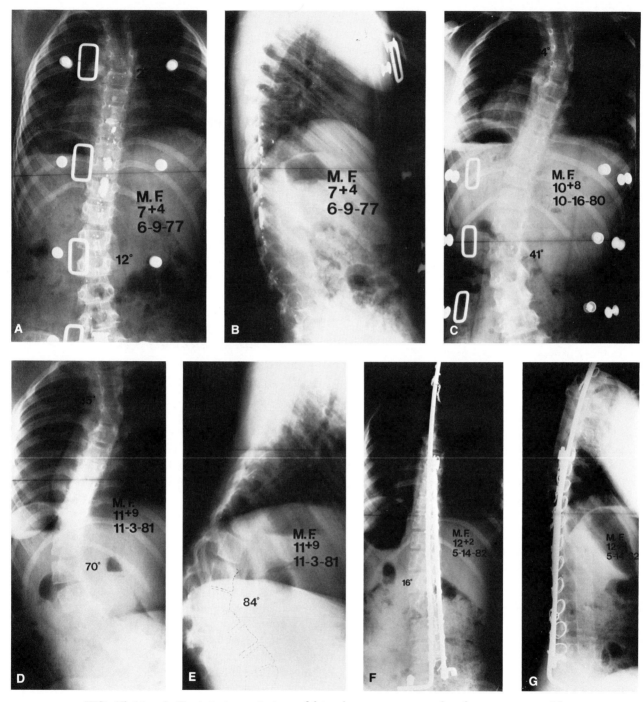

FIG. 17–14. **A, B.** Anterior-posterior and lateral roentgenograms that demonstrate a mild scoliosis being maintained in a TLSO jacket. This 7-year-old child had sustained a fracture and complete spinal cord injury at T5 to T6 at age 6. Extensive upper thoracic laminectomy was carried out at the time of the injury. **C.** Anterior-posterior roentgenogram indicates the significant progression of the deformity despite TLSO treatment. **D, E.** Anterior-posterior and lateral roentgenograms of the spine at age 11 indicates pronounced progression in the anterior-posterior and sagittal planes. This was associated with pronounced pelvic obliquity. **F, G.** Anterior-posterior and lateral roentgenograms indicate the excellent correction of the spine after segmental instrumentation to the pelvis. **H, I.** Anterior-posterior and lateral roentgenograms indicate reinstrumentation after pseudarthrosis and collapse of the spine at the mid-thoracic and lumbosacral junction.

(*continued*)

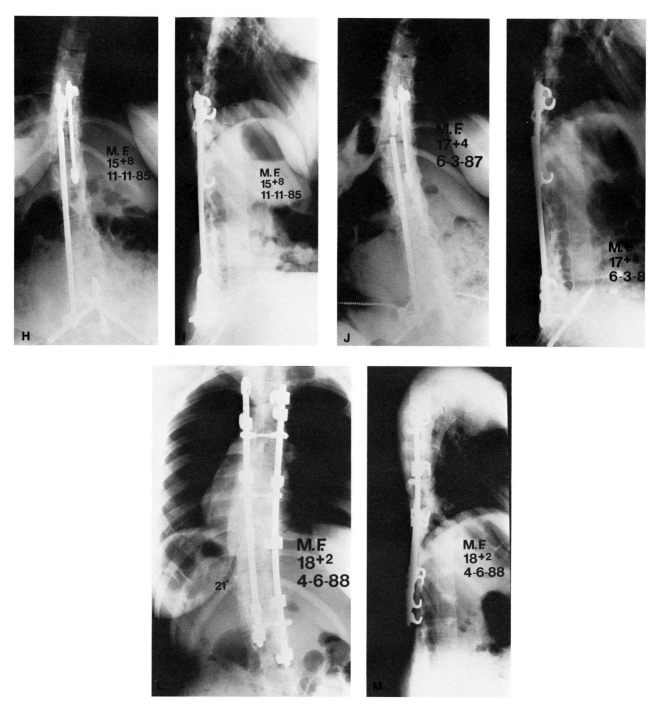

FIG. 17–14. *(continued)* **J, K.** Anterior-posterior and lateral roentgenograms indicate further progression of the curve and fracture of the Harrington rod, indicating a pseudarthrosis at the superior portion. **L, M.** Spine with reinstrumentation using Cotrel–Dubousset instrumentation and an anterior spinal fusion to obtain a solid spinal fusion. The patient recovered quite satisfactorily, despite multiple operative procedures.

This case indicates the severe progression that can occur in a child injured at an early age and the difficulties in obtaining a solid fusion in a child with laminectomy and spinal cord injury. This patient should have been considered originally for an anterior fusion at the time of the original instrumentation.

logically normal individuals, however, I am reluctant to use pedicle screws in the thoracic area. For significant pelvic obliquity in individuals with a paralytic curve, fusion must be done to the pelvis.

One must be aware of the midline defect and avoid risk to the spinal canal. This can be done with a midline incision, but with lateral exposure of the bony structures and the edge of the laminectomy defect. The dura does not need to be dissected free of adherent tissue. A high fusion rate can be expected after the combined anterior-posterior approach; however, patients must be protected for at least 6 months in a well-fitted TLSO jacket or cast.

References

1. Bailey RW, Badgley CE: Stabilization of the cervical spine by anterior fusion. J Bone Joint Surg [Am] 42:565, 1960
2. Callahan RA, Johnson RM, Margolis RN, et al: Cervical facet fusion for control of instability after laminectomy. J Bone Joint Surg [Am] 59:991, 1977
3. Cattell HS, Clark GL Jr: Cervical kyphosis and instability after multiple laminectomies in children. J Bone Joint Surg [Am] 49:713, 1967
4. Cloward RB: The anterior approach for ruptured cervical discs. J Neurosurg 15:602, 1958
5. Dubousset J, Guillaumat J, Mechin JF: Paper presented to Neurosurgical Congress of Infants, Versailles, 1970. In Rongerie J (ed): Les Compressions Medullaires Non-traumatiques de l'Enfant. Paris, Masson, 1973
6. Fager CA: Results of adequate posterior decompression in the relief of spondylotic cervical myelopathy. J Neurosurg 38:684, 1973
7. Fielding JW, Hawkins RJ: Roentgenographic diagnosis of the injured neck. Instr Course Lect 25:149, 1976
8. Francis WR, Noble DP: Treatment of kyphosis in children. Spine 13:883, 1988
9. Fraser RD, Paterson DC, Simpson DA: Orthopaedic aspects of spinal tumors in children. J Bone Joint Surg [Br] 59:143, 1977
10. Haft H, Ransohoff J, Carter S: Spinal cord tumors in children. Pediatrics 23:1152, 1959
11. Hirabayashi K, Watanabe K, Wakano K, et al: Expansive open-door laminoplasty for cervical spinal stenotic myelopathy. Spine 8:693, 1983
12. Jenkins DHR: Extensive cervical laminectomy. Long-term results. Br J Surg 60:852, 1977
13. Johnston CE II: Post-laminectomy kyphoscoliosis after surgical treatment for spinal cord astrocytoma. Orthopedics 9:587, 1986
14. Lonstein JE: Post-laminectomy kyphosis. Clin Orthop 128:93, 1977
15. Lonstein JE, Winter RB, Moe JH, et al: Post-laminectomy spinal deformity. J Bone Joint Surg [Am] 58:727, 1976
16. Malcolm BW, Bradford DS, Winter RB, Chou SN: Post-traumatic kyphosis. J Bone Joint Surg [Am] 63:891, 1981
17. Matson DD: Neurosurgery of Infancy and Childhood, 2nd ed. Springfield, IL, Charles C Thomas, 1969
18. Mayfield FH: Cervical spondylosis: A comparison of the anterior and posterior approaches. Clin Neurosurg 13:181, 1966
19. Mayfield JK, Erkkila JC, Winter RB: Spine deformity subsequent to acquired childhood spinal cord injury. J Bone Joint Surg [Am] 63:1401, 1981
20. Mikawa Y, Shikata J, Zamamuro T: Spinal deformity and instability after multilevel cervical laminectomy. Spine 12:6, 1987
21. Morgan R Jr, Brown JC, Bonnett C: The effect of laminectomy on the pediatric spinal cord patient. J Bone Joint Surg [Am] 56:1767, 1974
22. Natelson SE: The injudicious laminectomy. Spine 11:966, 1986
23. Panjabi MM, White AA III, Johnson RM: Cervical spine mechanics as a function of transection of components. J Biomech 8:327, 1975
24. Raimondi AJ, Gutierrez FA, DiRocco C: Laminectomy and total reconstruction of the posterior spinal arch for spinal canal surgery in childhood. J Neurosurg 45:555, 1976
25. Ransford AO, Crockard HA, Pozo JL, et al: Craniocervical instability treated by contoured loop fixation. J Bone Joint Surg [Br] 68:173, 1986
26. Robinson RA, Southwick WO: Indications and techniques for early stabilization of the neck in some fracture dislocations of the cervical spine. South Med J 53:565, 1950
27. Rogers L: The surgical treatment of cervical spondylotic myelopathy. Mobilisation of the complete cervical cord into an enlarged canal. J Bone Joint Surg [Br] 43, 1961
28. Scoville WB: Cervical spondylosis treated by bilateral facetectomy and laminectomy. J Neurosurg 18:423, 1961
29. Sim FH, Svien HJ, Bickel WH, et al: Swan neck deformity after extensive cervical laminectomy. A review of twenty-one cases. J Bone Joint Surg [Am] 56:564, 1974
30. Smith GW, Robinson RA: The treatment of certain cervical spine disorders by anterior removal of the intervertebral disc and interbody fusion. J Bone Joint Surg [Am] 40:607, 1958
31. Southwick WO, Johnson RM, Callahan RA, et al: Cervical laminectomy and facet fusion—fifteen years' experience. J Bone Joint Surg [Br] 59:121, 1977
32. Stauffer ES, Kelly EG: Fracture-dislocations of the cervical spine: Instability and recurrent deformity after treatment by anterior interbody fusion. J Bone Joint Surg [Am] 59:45, 1977
33. Tachdjian MO, Matson DD: Orthopaedic aspects of intraspinal tumors in infants and children. J Bone Joint Surg [Am] 47:223, 1965
34. Taddonio RF, King AG: Atlanto-axial rotatory fixation after decompressive laminectomy. A case report. Spine 7:540, 1982
35. White AA III, Johnson RM, Panjabi MM, Southwick WO: Biomechanical analysis of clinical stability in the cervical spine. Clin Orthop 109:85, 1975

36. Winter RB, McBride GG: Severe postlaminectomy kyphosis. Treatment by total vertebrectomy (plus late recurrence of childhood spinal cord astrocytoma). Spine 9:690, 1984

37. Yasuoka S, Peterson HA, Laws ER Jr, MacCarty CS: Pathogenesis and prophylaxis of postlaminectomy deformity of the spine after multiple level laminectomy: Difference between children and adults. Neurosurgery 9:145, 1981

38. Yasuoka S, Peterson HA, MacCarty CS: Incidence of spinal column deformity after multilevel laminectomy in children and adults. J Neurosurg 57:441, 1982

SCOLIOSIS SECONDARY TO RADIATION

DAVID H. DONALDSON

Arkin first reported radiation-induced scoliosis in an 8-year-old patient treated at 19 months of age with 9600 rad for Wilms' tumor.[1] Other authors have reported spinal deformity in patients receiving irradiation to the spine for childhood malignancy.[9, 15, 16, 19, 21, 24, 27] This occurs most often in the treatment of neuroblastoma, Wilms' tumor, and medulloblastoma—the three most common neonatal and childhood malignancies—although deformity following irradiation of intra-abdominal tumor and benign hemangioma has also been reported.[7–10, 15, 19, 21, 24, 26, 27]

Spinal deformity appears to be related to the inhibitory effect of radiation on bone growth.[2, 4, 6, 10, 12, 22] Growth inhibition occurs primarily at the vertebral physeal plate, which has been described by Bick and Capel as the region responsible for longitudinal growth.[6] Soft tissue fibrosis and contracture produced by radiation exposure also contribute to spinal deformity by their tethering effects.[24, 27]

Arkin and Engel have demonstrated that growth inhibition is inversely proportional to the age at the time of irradiation and directly proportional to the radiation dose.[2, 10] Hinkel, Barr, and Reidy found that more than 600 rad produce growth retardation and that complete inhibition of growth occurred with doses of more than 1200 rad.[4, 12, 22] Rubin reported that maximal damage was caused by 1200 to 3000 rad and that 5000 rad caused bone necrosis.[26]

Curve pattern and magnitude are related to radiation dosage.[15, 19, 23, 24, 28] Mayfield reported a mean dose of 2281 rad (range, 73–6250 rad) in 20 patients with curves less than 20°, and a mean dose of 3588 rad (range, 2138–4988 rad) in 8 patients with curves greater than 20°.[19] Mayfield and Riseborough demonstrated that little or no skeletal abnormality developed after less than 1000 rad administered to skeletally immature patients. Patients with deformities of less than 25° had a mean dose of 3159 rad, and patients with curves greater than 25° had received a mean dose of 3608 rad.[24]

It is generally held that patients developing kyphosis have received more radiation than those who develop scoliosis. In a review of patients treated for neuroblastoma, the patients developing kyphosis had received a mean dose of 3746 rad (range, 1821–6250 rad), compared with a mean dose of 3588 rad for patients developing scoliosis curves larger than 25°.[19] Patients developing both kyphosis and scoliosis had received the largest amounts of radiation—a mean dose of 4032 rad (range, 2688–6250 rad).[19] The kyphosis associated with scoliosis was usually more severe than kyphosis occurring alone.[19, 24] New cobalt 60 and linear accelerators providing equivalent tumor dose with decreased bone resorption may lower the incidence of spinal deformity.

In addition to patient age and radiation dose, the symmetry of irradiation fields may be important in the development of skeletal deformity.[2, 10, 15, 19, 21, 23, 24, 26, 28] Arkin first produced scoliosis by asymmetric irradiation of the spine.[3] Mayfield reported that asymmetric irradiation was responsible for more frequent and severe deformity.[19] He reported that 71% of patients with asymmetric irradiation developed scoliosis, but only 50% with midline irradiation developed scoliosis. Only 1 of 6 patients with a curve greater than 30° had midline irradiation. Despite attempts to produce symmetric radiation fields, some investigators have pointed out that rapid fall-off of radiation peripherally still allows asymmetry of radiation.[26] Neuhauser proposed that the entire width of the vertebral body should be included in the radiation field to avoid asymmetry of growth.[21] Inclusion of the entire vertebral body is still thought to be important in reducing growth asymmetry.

Spinal deformity may also develop due to involvement of bone by tumor, because of paralysis after spinal cord injury, or after decompressive laminectomy. Mayfield reported that the most severe scoliosis and ky-

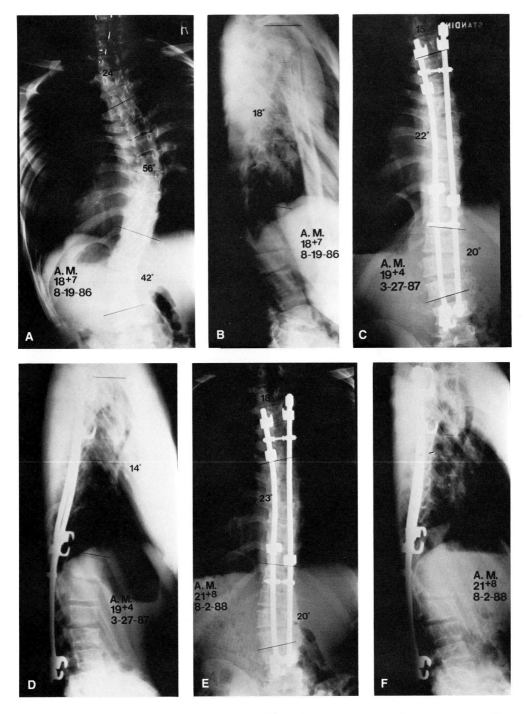

FIG. 17–15. A, B. The anterior-posterior and lateral roentgenograms show an 18-year-old patient who had a Wilms' tumor irradiated at age 1. The patient developed progressive scoliosis and thoracolumbar kyphosis. **C.** Anterior-posterior roentgenogram 1 month after with Cotrel–Dubousset instrumentation shows excellent anterior-posterior alignment. **D.** Postoperative film shows that the patient had only minimal correction of his lumbar kyphosis. An anterior fusion with strut grafting would improve the sagittal plane alignment significantly. **E, F.** The anterior-posterior and lateral roentgenograms demonstrate a solidly healed fusion at 2½ years after surgery. Although the patient was completely asymptomatic, with no pain in the lumbar area, an ideal correction of the sagittal plane curvature was not obtained.

phosis was due to epidural spread with deformity secondary to laminectomy and paraplegia.[19]

INCIDENCE

The reported frequency of spinal deformity after irradiation of childhood malignancies varies considerably, but most survivors will develop some degree of abnormality.[9, 19, 24] Rubin reported that 9 of 10 patients surviving more than 2 years after irradiation for Wilms', neuroblastoma, or medulloblastoma had scoliosis.[25] Katzman and Waugh followed 15 of 51 survivors with Wilms' tumor and 13 of 46 patients with neuroblastoma.[2, 14, 15] Of the 28 survivors, 20 (71%) developed scoliosis. Vaeth found only mild scoliosis in 12 patients surviving Wilms' tumor.[27] Riseborough, reporting 81 patients with Wilms' tumor, noted the development of spinal deformity in 59.[24] Scoliosis was present in 38, kyphoscoliosis in 19, and kyphosis in 2. Mayfield stated that, of 74 patients treated for neuroblastoma, 56 (74%) developed spinal abnormalities after an average follow-up of 12.9 years.[19] Scoliosis was present in 50%, kyphosis in 16%, and kyphoscoliosis in 9% of the patients.

RADIOGRAPHIC FEATURES

Neuhauser first described the radiographic changes apparent after irradiation of the spine.[21] These changes include horizontal growth arrest lines (producing an os within an os appearance), endplate irregularity with scalloping, loss of vertebral height, and asymmetric or symmetric failure of vertebral body development, producing gross contour abnormalities.[15, 21, 24] Anterior narrowing or a biconvex oval configuration are the most common contour abnormalities. Riseborough reported that failure of vertebral body development (75%) and endplate irregularity (68%) were the most common abnormalities.[24] He found that radiographic alterations, usually growth arrest lines, may be apparent as early as 6 months after irradiation.[24]

Irradiation of the spine may produce pure scoliosis, kyphosis, or kyphoscoliosis (Fig. 17-15). Kyphosis most commonly develops at the thoracolumbar junction. Mayfield reported 6 (67%) of 9 patients developed kyphosis within this region.[19] The mean kyphosis of these patients was 39° (range, 13–61°).

Right and left scoliotic curves occur equally.[24] The association between curve direction and irradiation may depend on tumor location.[15] Riseborough found that the concavity of thoracolumbar curves developed on the irradiated side in patients treated for Wilms' tumor. He speculated that this might be related to consistent tumor location. In contrast, no correlation was observed in patients treated for neuroblastoma. Mayfield, in a review of patients irradiated for neuroblastoma, also found that the side of irradiation did not correlate with the curve pattern.[19]

NATURAL HISTORY

Reports concerning the likelihood of progression of radiation-induced scoliosis have varied.[26] Katzman reported that scoliosis is usually not progressive.[15] Similarly, Neuhauser observed little progression of scoliosis with growth.[21] In contrast, Mayfield reported that the incidence and severity of scoliosis were related to the length of follow-up.[19] These findings were related to a significant increase in scoliosis during the adolescent growth period.[19, 24] Of 30 prepubertal patients, 12 (40%) had scoliosis, and only 13% of prepubertal patients had scoliosis curves greater than 20°. In contrast, of 13 skeletally mature patients, 46% had curves greater than 20° at skeletal maturity. Overall, 40% of prepubertal patients and 85% of postpubertal patients had developed scoliosis at long-term follow-up. Riseborough reported no scoliosis greater than 20° in patients less than 10 years old.[24] A number of reports of minimal progression lack follow-up through the adolescent period.[26]

Despite the frequency of radiation-induced scoliotic deformity, most curves remain small and do not need treatment. Riseborough speculated that only 12% of patients treated with radiation for Wilms' tumor would have required treatment for their scoliosis by today's standards.[24] Mayfield believed that only 11% of patients treated with radiation for neuroblastoma would have required treatment by today's standards.[9, 20]

Mayfield reported that most kyphotic deformities develop before puberty, with progression during the adolescent growth spurt, similar to scoliosis. The rate of progression, however, is slightly greater—approximately 3° per year.[19] Kyphosis has been reported to progress after skeletal maturity.[23] Severe kyphosis is more often associated with scoliosis greater than 25°.

Kyphosis accounts for the majority of patients referred for treatment.[18] In one series, 95% of patients referred for treatment of postradiation spinal deformity had kyphosis. The actual number of patients requiring fusion is small, however. Mayfield speculated that 9% of patients treated for neuroblastoma and 6% of patients treated for Wilms' tumor would have required fusion for kyphosis by current standards.

TREATMENT

Few reports are available in the literature on conservative treatment of irradiation-induced scoliosis and kyphoscoliosis. Riseborough reported that brace treatment of these patients was poor.[23, 24] He noted that even small curves become rigid at an early age. Mayfield, in a review of 44 patients seen at the Twin Cities Scoliosis Center, reported the results of 16 patients treated by bracing.[18] Twelve patients were treated in a Milwaukee brace and 4 in an underarm brace. Patients were followed for an average of 2.4 years from a mean age of 12.5 years. Fifty percent of the patients improved or maintained their prebrace curve magnitude; the other 50% progressed to a point requiring surgery. Progression was greatest in curves exhibiting a thoracolumbar kyphosis.[18]

Indications for Surgery

The indications for surgical treatment of radiation-induced scoliosis and kyphoscoliosis include thoracolumbar kyphosis greater than 40 to 50° and scoliosis greater than 40°.[16, 18, 23] Patients demonstrating progression despite brace treatment are also candidates for surgical treatment. Procrastination in treating a steadily progressing curve is not indicated.

Patients presenting with radiation-induced spinal abnormalities may have any curve pattern, although those requiring surgical treatment most commonly have kyphoscoliosis. Obtaining satisfactory correction and solid fusions in this patient population is difficult.[24] Of 8 patients who were surgically treated by Riseborough, 3 developed pseudarthroses. King and Stowe linked 13 patients treated surgically for spinal deformity after radiation with 8 kyphotic and 5 scoliotic deformities.[16] Ten pseudarthroses developed in these patients, requiring 28 fusion procedures.

Kyphosis and prior laminectomy often inhibit obtaining solid fusions in these patients (Fig. 17-16). King

and Stowe reported 8 patients with kyphosis treated by posterior spinal fusion with casting.[16] Six patients' curves progressed whether prior laminectomy had been performed or not. Riseborough had 3 patients with pseudarthroses in 8 patients treated with posterior spinal fusion and Harrington rod instrumentation.[24] The 3 patients were members of a group of 5 patients who had kyphoscoliotic deformities. Repeat fusion was unsuccessful in all except 1 patient with only 18° of curvature. The 2 remaining patients were successfully treated by anterior interbody fusion. Given the results of these studies, kyphosis should be treated by combined anterior and posterior fusion.[16, 18, 24] Flexible kyphotic curves may be treated by interbody fusion. Rigid kyphotic curves should be treated by disc excision and strut grafting.

Combined anterior and posterior spinal fusion may not result in a solid fusion in patients treated by prior laminectomy. King and Stowe reported 7 patients treated for spinal deformity after radiation for neuroblastoma.[16] Five patients had laminectomies at an early age. The spinal deformities included five kyphotic curves, one scoliosis, and one lumbar hyperlordosis. An average of 2.7 fusions per patient were required to obtain a solid fusion. Seven anterior pseudarthroses were observed in this group.

Comparison of surgical results among patients in which prior laminectomy was not performed have not indicated significantly improved results. Mayfield reported patients who had no laminectomy procedures.[12, 18] Fourteen of the 21 patients required surgery. Of these patients, 71% required reoperation. The majority of these curves were kyphotic.

Surgical Technique

The choice of surgical instrumentation should be governed somewhat by the degree of kyphosis present. At this time, it is appropriate to use segmental instrumentation, and I have used the Cotrel–Dubousset technique. Other types of fixation, as illustrated in Figure 17-17, can be successfully used. A circumferential fusion with anterior strut graft or anterior interbody fusion should be strongly considered for patients with a kyphos of greater than 40° in the lumbar area. Anterior instrumentation is rarely indicated because of the unpredictable nature of the irradiated anterior bone stock. The fusion area should be selected in the same way as idiopathic curves. A large quantity of cancellous bone should be used from a nonirradiated iliac site.

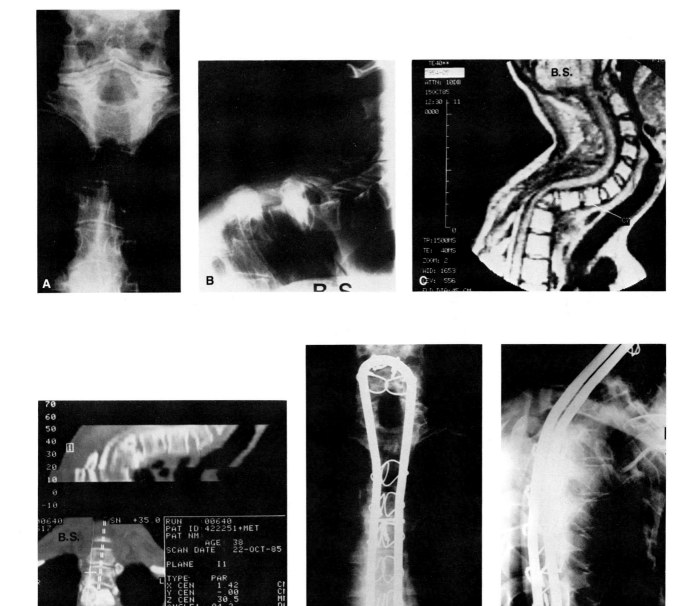

FIG. 17–16. A, B. The anterior-posterior and lateral roentgenograms of the cervicothoracic area after an extensive thoracic laminectomy was carried out for non-Hodgkin's lymphoma demonstrate a severe kyphos at T1 to T2 that permitted an end-on view of the cervical spinal canal.   **C.** MRI study demonstrating the severity of the deformity and the compromise of the spinal canal.   **D.** A CT scan with contrast demonstrates the route of the spinal cord as it runs over the kyphotic deformity. Despite an 80° kyphos, the patient had normal neurologic function, but the progressive deformity was associated with pain.   **E, F.** Anterior-posterior and lateral radiographs demonstrate a surgical approach. The patient had an anterior strut graft carried out through an axillary approach to the upper thoracic spine, followed by posterior stabilization with Luque ring and segmental wiring of the remaining cervical lamina. Although normal sagittal plane alignment was not restored, the patient had significant improvement of her deformity, and a solid fusion was obtained.

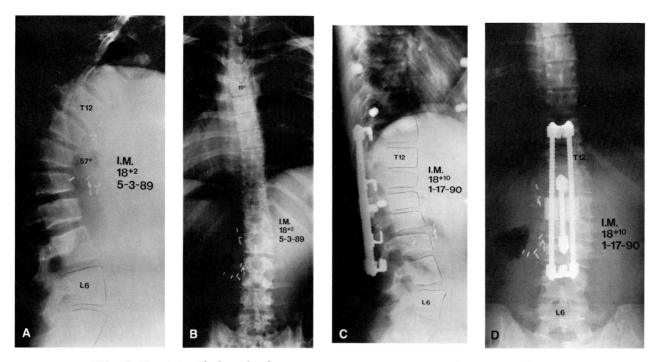

FIG. 17–17. **A, B.** The lateral and anterior-posterior roentgenograms of an 18-year-old patient with a history of Wilms' tumor in infancy who had radiation and an anterior resection. The roentgenograms illustrate a significant lumbar kyphosis of 57° and a mild scoliosis. **C, D.** The postoperative films show a posterior fusion using Edwards instrumentation to reverse the severe kyphosis. The procedure was preceded by anterior releases and interbody fusions.

Severe scarring may be encountered in the retroperitoneal space during the anterior approach, making the exposure difficult.

Complications

Complications after spinal fusion for radiation-induced deformity have included pseudarthrosis, an increased infection rate, and paralysis.[16, 19, 23, 24] The high rate of pseudarthrosis has been attributed to poor bone quality, decreased bone vascularity, and skeletal immaturity, as well as prior kyphosis and laminectomy.[23] The increased incidence of infection has been attributed to the poor vascularity and quality of overlying skin caused by radiation damage.[23, 27] Paralysis has been associated with an underlying predisposition of radiation-induced myelopathy.[16] Berg and Lindgren observed a time-dose relationship between radiation and associated myelopathy due to vascular compromise.[5]

Postoperative Care

In addition to combined anterior and posterior fusion, many authors recommend reoperation at 6 months for supplementary bone grafting of the fusion mass.[18] Prolonged casting or bracing for a period extending as long as 12 months has also been recommended.[16, 18] A plastic TLSO jacket is indicated until a healed fusion is obtained.

References

1. Arkin AM, Pack GT, Ransohoff NS, Simon N: Radiation-induced scoliosis. J Bone Joint Surg [Am] 32:401, 1950
2. Arkin AM, Simon N: Radiation scoliosis. J Bone Joint Surg [Am] 32:396, 1950
3. Arkin A, Simon N, Siffert R: Asymmetrical suppression of vertebral epiphyseal growth with ionizing radiation. Proc Soc Exper Biol Med 69:171, 1948
4. Barr JS, Lingley JR, Gall EA: The effect of Roentgen irradiation on epiphyseal growth. I. Experimental studies upon the albino rat. AJR 49:104, 1943
5. Berg NO, Lindgren M: Time-dose relationship and morphology of delayed radiation lesions of the brain in rabbits. Acta Radiol 167:1, 1958
6. Bick EM, Capel JW: Longitudinal growth of the human osteogeny. J Bone Joint Surg [Am] 32:803, 1950
7. Bodian M: Neuroblastoma. Pediatr Clin North Am 6:449, 1959

8. Dargeon HW: Neuroblastoma. J Pediatr 61:456, 1962
9. Donaldson WF, Wissinger HA: Axial skeletal changes after tumor dose radiation therapy. J Bone Joint Surg [Am] 49:1469, 1967
10. Engel D: Experiments on the production of spinal deformities by radium. AJR 42:217, 1939
11. Godwin-Austen RB, Howell DA, Worthington B: Observations on radiation myelopathy. Brain 98:557, 1940
12. Hinkel CL: The effect of irradiation upon the composition and vascularity of growing rat bones. AJR 50:516, 1943
13. Hinkel CL: The effect of Roentgen rays upon the growing long bones of albino rats. I. Quantitative studies of the growth limitations following irradiation. AJR 47:439, 1942
14. Hinkel CL: The effect of Roentgen rays upon the growing long bones of albino rats. II. Histopathological changes involving endochondral growth centers. AJR 49:321, 1943
15. Katzman H, Waugh T, Berndon W: Skeletal changes after irradiation of childhood tumors. J Bone Joint Surg [Am] 51:825, 1969
16. King J, Stowe S: Results of spinal fusion for radiationscoliosis. Spine 7:574, 1982
17. Kun LE: Post-irradiation myelopathy in children. Am Neurol 5:106, 1979
18. Mayfield JK: Postradiation spinal deformity. Orthop Clin North Am 10:829, 1979
19. Mayfield JK, Riseborough EJ, Jaffe N, Nehme AM: Spinal deformity in children treated for neuroblastoma. J Bone Joint Surg [Am] 63:183, 1981
20. Mayfield JK, Sundberg SB, Moe JH: Post-radiation spinal deformity: Results of treatment. Paper presented at the meeting of the American Academy of Orthopaedic Surgeons, Atlanta, GA, February 10, 1980
21. Neuhauser EBD, Wittenborg MN, Berman CZ, Cohen J: Irradiation effects of Roentgen therapy on the growing spine. Radiology 59:637, 1952
22. Reidy JA, Lingley JR, Gall EA, Barr JS: The effect of Roentgen irradiation on epiphyseal growth. II. Experimental studies upon the dog. J Bone Joint Surg 29:853, 1947
23. Riseborough EJ: Irradiation-induced kyphosis. Clin Orthop 128:101, 1977
24. Riseborough EJ, Grabias SL, Burton RI, Jaffe N: Skeletal alterations after irradiation for Wilms' tumor. J Bone Joint Surg [Am] 58:526, 1976
25. Rubin P, Andrews JR, Swarm R, Gump H: Radiation-induced dysplasias of bone. AJR 82:206, 1959
26. Rubin P, Duthie RB, Young LW: The significance of scoliosis in postirradiated Wilms' tumor and neuroblastoma. Radiology 79:539, 1962
27. Vaeth JM, Levitt SH, Jones MD, Holtfreter C: Effects of radiation therapy in survivors of Wilms' tumor. Radiology 79:560, 1962
28. Whitehouse WM, Lampe I: Osseous damage in irradiation of renal tumors in infancy and childhood. AJR 70:721, 1953

SPINAL DEFORMITY ASSOCIATED WITH OSTEOGENESIS IMPERFECTA

DAVID H. DONALDSON

Patients with osteogenesis imperfecta (Fig. 17-18) have abnormal collagen production resulting in defective bone and connective tissue. The precise cause is unknown, but it has been speculated that spinal deformity may be related to fractures through defective bone with collapse, ligamentous laxity, damaged growth plate, and disc abnormality.

INCIDENCE

Spinal abnormalities associated with osteogenesis imperfecta have been reported in the cervical, thoracic, and lumbar regions. The most commonly associated abnormality reported is scoliosis. Reported frequencies of scoliosis associated with osteogenesis imperfecta range from 25 to 71%.[3–6, 10, 16]

The frequency of scoliosis increases with patient age. Benson reported that 26% of patients between 1 and 5 years of age exhibited scoliosis. In contrast, 80% of patients older than 12 years demonstrated scoliosis.[2] Moorefield reported a 50% incidence of scoliosis among 31 adults followed for more than 10 years.[12]

The incidence of scoliosis also appears to be related to the severity of osteogenesis imperfecta. Several authors have reported the frequency of scoliosis associated with mild disease to be approximately 10%.[1, 6, 8] Bauze reported that 16 of 17 severely involved patients had scoliosis.[1]

Classification schemes do not necessarily correlate with the severity of bony involvement.[6, 10] As a result, prediction of scoliosis based on these classification systems has not been accurate. Hanscom developed a classification system that correlates with the degree of bony involvement and the likelihood of developing spinal abnormality.[8] Patients are grouped into categories A through E. Patients with type A disease have mild, bony abnormalities with normal vertebral contours. Patients with type B disease have biconcave vertebrae and no acetabular protrusion. Type C deformity has a trefoil pelvis, thin, long bones that are

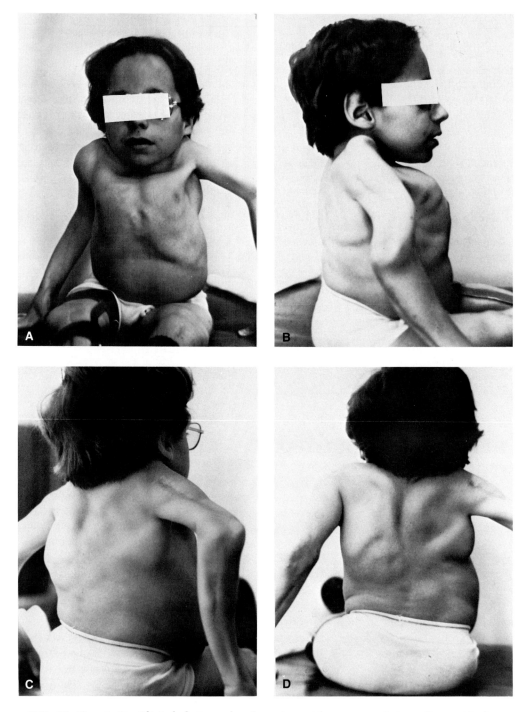

FIG. 17–18. A–D. Clinical photographs of a patient with osteogenesis imperfecta with characteristic upper extremity deformities, a relatively flat back without pronounced rotational changes, and pectus carinatum with an extremely short trunk.

bowed, and a characteristic acetabular protrusion, which develops at approximately 8 to 10 years of age. Patients with type D deformity have pelvic findings similar to type C and develop cystic changes in the metaphyses and epiphyses of the femur and tibia at 3 to 5 years of age. Patients with type E deformity demonstrate the most severe changes, with lack of cortex on long bones usually evident by 2 to 3 years of age. The incidence of scoliosis increases from groups A through E. Scoliosis occurred in 46% of the patients in type A, but all patients in types C and D had developed scoliosis by adolescence.

Thoracic lordosis and hyperkyphosis have also been reported. Lumbosacral spondylolysis has been reported with the appearance of elongated pedicles secondary to microfractures.[13]

Cervical abnormalities associated with osteogenesis imperfecta include isolated cases of fracture of the odontoid and C2, as well as spondyloptosis at the cervicothoracic junction and cervical kyphosis.[10, 11, 15, 18]

NATURAL HISTORY

Several physicians have reported progression of spinal deformity in patients with osteogenesis imperfecta.[2, 9, 12, 14] Both kyphosis and scoliosis may be progressive. Benson reported a higher percentage of progressive scoliosis among patients with severe osteogenesis imperfecta and patients older than 8 years.[2] Norimatsu reported rapid curve progression after 5 years of age among patients with severe deformity and after 50° of scoliosis had been reached. He also reported curve progression after physeal closure of the lower extremities in some cases.[14]

TREATMENT

Bracing has been recommended for scoliosis demonstrating curve progression greater than 20°. The results of brace treatment for scoliosis depended on the severity of the curve and the severity of the osteogenesis imperfecta. Hanscom reported successful correction in patients with minimal deformity.[8] Poor results were obtained in patients with severe deformity. Patients in types B, C, and D demonstrated minimal correction, with increased curve magnitude after brace treatment. Poor results in bracing of severe deformity have been attributed to vertebral body deformity and ribs too

weak to withstand the pressure of bracing. Production of chest wall deformity with curve progression has been reported.[2, 8, 17] It has been recommended that bracing be continued for 18 months after maturity in curves that are responding to brace treatment. Benson reported 9 patients treated in the Milwaukee brace.[2] He found brace treatment to be ineffective, producing rib deformity in most cases.

Yong-Hing reported 73 patients treated by bracing, most of whom were in a Milwaukee brace.[17] Fifteen patients demonstrated equal or decreased curve magnitude after brace treatment. However, only 2 patients were out of the brace, and 7 patients had been in the brace less than 1 year at the time of this report. The curves of 79% of the 73 patients progressed in the brace. Progression did not appear to be influenced by age or severity, because all but 1 of 23 patients with curves less than 30° progressed. Thirteen of 73 patients developed rib deformity during brace wear. Twenty-nine patients required fusion, although this was not performed in all of the patients. Bracing is usually contraindicated in these patients because severe distortion of their rib cage is far more likely than effective control of spinal deformity.

Several authors have described the surgical treatment of spinal deformity associated with osteogenesis imperfecta.[4, 7, 9, 10, 17] Recommendations for spinal fusion of scoliosis at 35 to 40° have been made. Advocates of early fusion maintain that hook purchase is decreased in the weak bone with increased deformity, which may occur by waiting.[2] Others maintain that fusion should be performed during adolescence because of increased bone mass and strength.[10] Yong-Hing reported 60 patients who had spinal fusions for spinal deformity related to osteogenesis imperfecta. Fifty-five patients underwent posterior spinal fusion, 39 of whom had Harrington rod instrumentation. Four patients underwent anterior spinal fusion, and 1 patient underwent combined anterior and posterior spinal fusion. The average preoperative curve magnitude was 74°; this was corrected to an average of 47°—a 36% correction. Patients with Harrington instrumentation demonstrated a 7% increase in correction over those without. However, complications were much higher in the instrumented group. Forty-five patients were followed more than 18 months. Eight patients demonstrated progression, which was thought to be secondary to bending of the fusion mass and pseudarthrosis in some cases. Two pseudarthroses were noted among 8 patients fused for kyphoscoliosis greater than 60°[17]

(text continues on page 496)

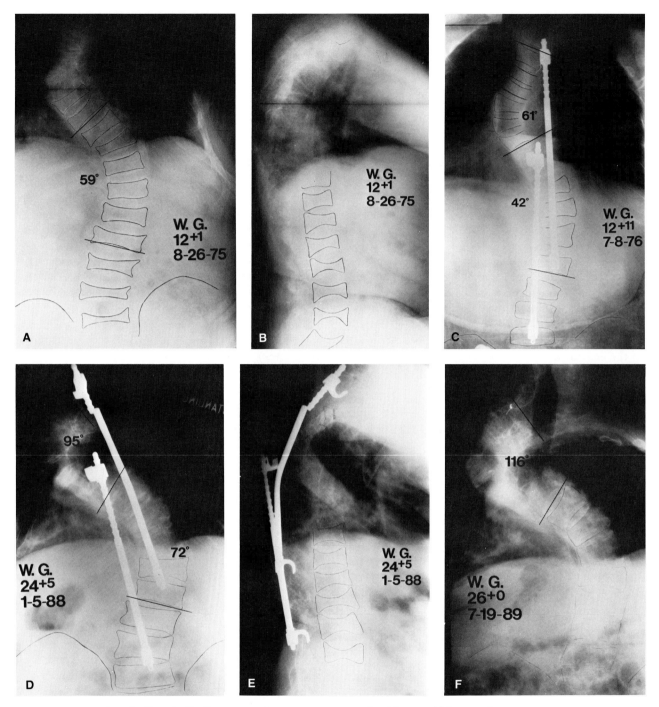

FIG. 17–19. A, B. Preoperative roentgenograms of a 12-year-old boy with severe osteogenesis imperfecta with a 79° left thoracic and 59° right thoracolumbar curvature. He has severe osteopenia with characteristic flattening of the vertebral bodies. **C.** Postoperative anterior-posterior roentgenogram of the patient instrumented with overlapping Harrington rods. This procedure was carried out without methylmethacrylate and obtained good correction of the curvature. **D, E.** Roentgenograms taken 12 years after the original surgery, indicating a fractured Harrington rod and significant progression of the spine deformity. The rods were removed and no evidence of a pseudarthrosis was identified, despite progression of the curvature from 61° to 95°. **F.** A roentgenogram of the same patient, 14 years after his original instrumentation, indicating continued progression of the curvature despite a solid fusion. The patient was relatively asymptomatic and functioned well.

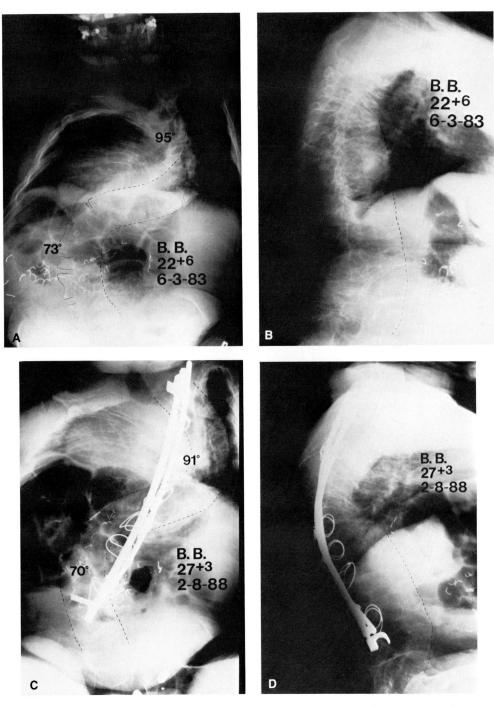

FIG. 17–20. **A, B.** Roentgenograms of an adult osteogenesis imperfecta patient with a pronounced 95° cervicothoracic curve to the right and 73° lumbar curve to the left. Despite instrumentation with some segmental fixation, there was no improvement of curvature. **C, D.** This patient did not, however, increase his curvature 5 years after the instrumentation was carried out. He was essentially free of pain and functioned satisfactorily.

Most authors have recommended that segmental fixation be performed, owing to the poor quality of bone. Attempts at overcorrection of the deformity should also be avoided. Hanscom stated that some of the most severe cases of deformity and bone abnormality may be inoperable.[9] Others have recommended anterior and posterior fusion with methylmethacrylate augmentation as a possible solution to stabilization of severe deformity.[7]

SURGICAL CONSIDERATIONS

Indications for Surgery

Patients should be considered operative candidates when a curve shows significant progression beyond 40 to 50°. This consideration should be made whether a patient has the "mild" or "severe" type of osteogenesis imperfecta. Patients with the mild form of the disease may be treated like patients with idiopathic scoliosis, although the surgeon must be less aggressive about correction and more attentive to the technical aspects of fusion. Procrastination about surgical treatment is discouraged, even in relatively young age groups, because severe progression of these curves is well documented.

Patients with the severe type of osteogenesis imperfecta cannot be treated by nonoperative techniques, and an aggressive attitude toward surgery should be maintained. Allowing a curve to progress to severe levels before surgery creates more difficult technical problems and does not allow increased truncal height. These children can be expected to have short stature with or without surgery.

Preoperative Assessment

The patient's pulmonary status must be evaluated, especially those with severe thoracic curves. Gitelis and colleagues reported a vital capacity of 35% in a child with a thoracic curve of 138°. Although these patients are amazingly resilient, pulmonary consultation and management is an important part of the surgical approach. Preoperative evaluation by an anesthesiologist familiar with the anesthetic problems associated with osteogenesis imperfecta patients is also appropriate. Body temperature control during surgery may be a problem; a thermal mattress should be used during spine procedures.

Surgical Technique

The procedure of choice is posterior fusion with instrumentation. Although the bony structures are quite fragile and heroic measures to gain correction are not indicated, the posterior arch is usually adequate for gentle distraction or fixation. The technique for hook placement does not vary from the standard techniques, although care should be taken to avoid notching or cutting the laminae to be instrumented. No beveled or sharp hooks should be used in the Harrington technique. For example, segmental fixation using the Luque technique or Cotrel–Dubousset instrumentation adds to overall stability, but it is more time consuming. It is desirable to have two experienced spine surgeons involved in the surgical team to decrease operating time. Excessive blood loss during operative exposure requires attention to hemostasis and decreasing the time of surgery. A cell saver is essential, because osteogenesis imperfecta patients are generally too small to contribute autologous blood.

Anterior spinal fusion with instrumentation has been successfully used in severe scoliosis.[7] The technique does not vary from other types of anterior fusion, with the exception of dealing with pronounced osteopenia. Methylmethacrylate used to supplement screw fixation can significantly improve pull-out strength of the staple-screw couple.

Posterior spinal fusion must be carried out with meticulous detail. Each facet must be curetted thoroughly and packed with autologous bone, if available. Bone graft should be obtained from the iliac crest, if possible. Because an inadequate amount of bone is usual, bank bone should be available and liberally used. U-shaped pedicle hooks should be placed around the pedicle, rather than in the pedicle, as is suggested by a standard Harrington technique. Decortication of bony surfaces should be carried out thoroughly to provide additional graft material. Standard-sized instrumentation can be used in most patients, although it is appropriate to have pediatric instruments available. One should not expect to gain a great deal of correction, and any corrective force on the instruments should be to "hold" the spine. Cotrel–Dubousset instrumentation is well suited for this problem, provided no serious effort is made to rotate the spine (Figs. 17-19 to 17-21). The rods must be bent to conform to the contours of the spine in the frontal and sagittal planes.

Methylmethacrylate has been very useful in maintaining and supplementing hook placement, and its

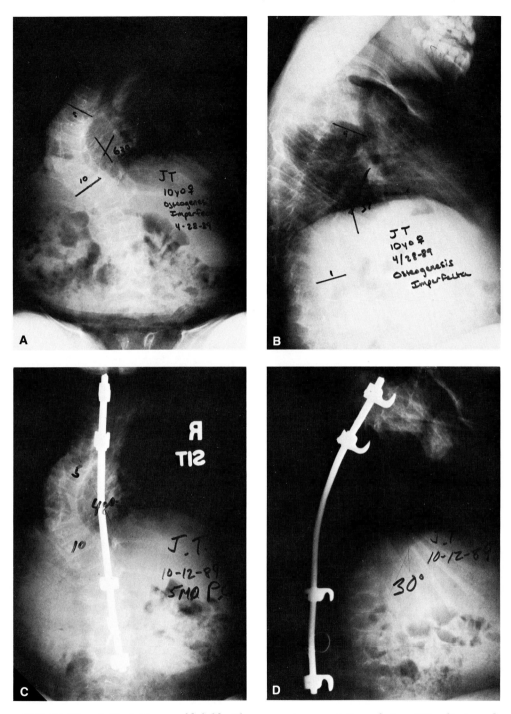

FIG. 17–21.   A, B. A 10-year-old child with severe osteogenesis imperfecta, a 63° scoliosis, and a relatively rigid curvature.   **C, D.** The minimal correction obtained using a single Cotrel–Dubousset rod. Correction was maintained 5 months after surgery, and it appeared that the patient was healing satisfactorily.

use should be considered in most patients. The technique has been described by Benson and Newman.[3] They prefer to leave the spinous process of the adjacent vertebra in place, decorticate the side opposite the hook placement, and graft that opposite side. Methylmethacrylate is then placed around the hook, the lamina, and the spinous process of the vertebra, as well as the vertebrae above and below (Fig. 17-22). This allows adequate surface area for fusion and maximizes the surface area for fixation.

Complications

Problems faced when attempting to obtain a solid fusion in osteogenesis imperfecta are largely related to instrument failure or hook pull-out. These problems can be minimized with careful placement of segmental instrumentation and the use of methylmethacrylate in tenuous hook placement. Although infection has been reported, the incidence is quite small. Blood loss can be very large, representing a large percentage of total blood volume in these small patients.

Postoperative Care

A body jacket is necessary postoperatively and should be maintained for 6 to 9 months if possible. A two-piece plastic TLSO, which allows easy removal for nursing care, is preferable. It should be fitted after the surgery to accommodate any change in body configuration.

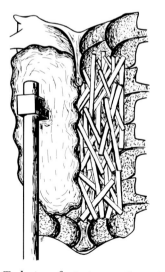

FIG. 17–22. Technique for instrumenting osteogenesis imperfecta with methylmethacrylate.

Acknowledgment

We thank our spine fellows Clay Baynham, M.D., and Michael Moore, M.D., for their research and help in the preparation of this chapter.

References

1. Bauze RJ, Smith R, Francis MJO: A new look at osteogenesis imperfecta: A clinical, radiological, and biochemical study of forty-two patients. J Bone Joint Surg [Br] 57:2, 1975
2. Benson DR, Donaldson DH, Millar EA: The spine in osteogenesis imperfecta. J Bone Joint Surg [Am] 60:925, 1978
3. Benson DR, Newman DC: The spine and surgical treatment in osteogenesis imperfecta. Clin Orthop 159:147, 1981
4. Cristofaro RL, Joek KJ, Bonnett CA, Brown JC: Operative treatment of spinal deformity in osteogenesis imperfecta. Clin Orthop 139:40, 1979
5. Fairbank HAT: Osteogenesis imperfecta and osteogenesis imperfecta cystica. J Bone Joint Surg [Br] 30:164, 1948
6. Falvo KA, Root L, Bullough PG: Osteogenesis imperfecta: Clinical evaluation and management. J Bone Joint Surg [Am] 56:783, 1974
7. Gitelis S, et al: The treatment of severe scoliosis in osteogenesis imperfecta. Clin Orthop 175:56, 1983
8. Hanscom DA, Bloom BA: The spine in osteogenesis imperfecta. Orthop Clin North Am 19:449, 1988
9. Hanscom DA, et al: Spinal deformities in osteogenesis imperfecta—natural history and treatment. Presented at the Minnesota Orthopaedic Society, May 1986
10. King JD, Bobechko WP: Osteogenesis imperfecta. An orthopaedic description and surgical review. J Bone Joint Surg [Br] 53:72, 1971
11. Meyer S, Villarreal M, Ziv I: A three-level fracture of the axis in a patient with osteogenesis imperfecta. Spine 11:505, 1986
12. Moorefield WG, Jr, Miller GR: Aftermath of osteogenesis imperfecta: The disease in adulthood. J Bone Joint Surg [Am] 62:113, 1980
13. Newman PH: The etiology of spondylolisthesis. J Bone Joint Surg [Br] 45:39, 1963
14. Norimatsu H, Mayuzumi T, Takahashi H: The development of the spinal deformities in osteogenesis imperfecta. Clin Orthop 162:20, 1982
15. Rush GA, Burke SW: Hangman's fracture in a patient with osteogenesis imperfecta. J Bone Joint Surg [Am] 66:778, 1984
16. Versfeld GA, Beighton PH, Katz K, Solomon A: Costovertebral anomalies in osteogenesis imperfecta. J Bone Joint Surg [Br] 67:602, 1985
17. Yong-Hing K, MacEwen GD: Scoliosis associated with osteogenesis imperfecta. Results of treatment. J Bone Joint Surg [Br] 64:36, 1982
18. Ziv I, Rang M, Hoffman HJ: Paraplegia in osteogenesis imperfecta. J Bone Joint Surg [Br] 65:184, 1983

PART
IV

DEFORMITY: SAGITTAL PLANE

CHAPTER 18

Kyphosis

Kim W. Hammerberg

■

MORPHOLOGY AND BIOMECHANICS

An understanding of the normal sagittal contour of the spine is a prerequisite to a discussion of the biomechanics of kyphotic deformity. The normal spine is rectilinear in the coronal plane. In the sagittal plane, the spine develops four balanced, undulating curvatures. The cervical spine is lordotic and is usually the least pronounced of the curvatures. The thoracic spine is kyphotic, the curvature extending from T2 to T12. The lumbar region is lordotic, extending from the thoracolumbar junction to the lumbosacral junction. The sacral curvature is kyphotic, beginning at the lumbosacral disc and ending at the coccyx.

The thoracic and sacral curvatures are considered primary because they are present at birth. These kyphotic regions are relatively rigid. The cervical and lumbar lordosis are secondary or compensatory. At birth, the spine demonstrates a long, simple kyphosis from occiput to coccyx. As the infant begins to gain head control, in sitting and crawling, the cervical region reverses its contour to lordosis. After the toddler stands and begins to walk, the lumbar region assumes a lordotic contour.

The compensatory lordosis in the cervical and lumbar regions is necessary to maintain balance in the upright position. Compared with a rectilinear spinal column, a curved spine is more dynamic, allowing greater flexibility and shock absorption. A column with four alternative curvatures is more resilient to stress than a straight column.[39]

In relaxed stance, the spine and pelvis balance on the femoral heads. Obviously, a relationship exists between the attitude of the hips and the sagittal spinal contour. For example, fixed flexion deformity of the hips is compensated by increased lumbar lordosis in a flexible spine. In equipoise, the activity of the back musculature is low. A shift in the center of gravity requires an active counterbalancing muscle force on the opposite side.[72] The natural tendency of the thoracic spine is toward a flexion moment, resulting in increased kyphosis. The lordotic curvature of the lumbar region of the spine permits the dorsal musculature of the back to resist anterior moments.

A broad range of sagittal contours reflects the morphologic latitude of the human species. Stagnara believes that each subject has a unique spinal physiognomy, just as each has a unique facial physiognomy.[63] For purposes of discussion, a normal range of sagittal contours can be defined, but for each patient, the overall balance of the sagittal contour must be assessed on an individual basis. The normal thoracic kyphosis is in the range of 20 to 50°.[6, 23] The most dorsal vertebra is T7, which is also horizontally situated. The thoracic vertebrae superior to the apex are ventrally inclined, and those inferior are dorsally inclined. The normal lumbar lordosis is approximately 40 to 60°.[6, 23, 63, 71] The most ventral vertebra, again horizontally oriented, is L3. The lumbar vertebrae above the apex are dorsally inclined, and those below are ventrally inclined (Fig. 18-1).

A kyphotic deformity is defined as an abnormal dorsal curvature of the spine in the sagittal plane. In the thoracic spine, the curvature can be considered pathologic if it is greater than the upper range of normal, 50 to 55°. In the normally lordotic cervical and lumbar spines, any degree of dorsal curvature represents a kyphotic deformity. A configuration with less than normal lordosis, but with maintenance of some ventral angulation, is called hypolordosis.

In stance, the thoracic kyphosis and lumbar lordosis and the lesser cervical and sacral curvatures are balanced. The weight-bearing line, or sagittal vertical axis, falls from the craniovertebral articulation through the bodies of the cervical vertebrae and anterior to the thoracic spine (see Fig. 18-1). The axis crosses the spinal column at T12 and lies posterior to the lumbar

spine. The axis again crosses the spine at the lumbosacral articulation and is located anterior to the second sacral vertebra. The sagittal vertical axis must be in this orientation for the lateral contours to balance. The concept of the sagittal vertical axis is an important consideration in the realignment of sagittal-plane deformities.

The anterior elements of the spinal column, vertebral body, intervertebral disc, and associated ligaments resist compressive forces. The posterior osteoligamentous structures resist tensile forces.[73] A kyphotic deformity occurs when the spinal column is unable to resist one or both of these forces. Anterior column failure results in the inability of the spine to withstand compression, causing relative shortening of the anterior column. Disruption in the posterior column results in an inability to resist tension and relative lengthening of the posterior column. These deficiencies can be caused by growth disturbances, trauma, tumor, infection, degenerative diseases, or iatrogenic processes. The surgical correction of kyphosis is accomplished by shortening the posterior column and lengthening the anterior column.

SURGICAL CONSIDERATIONS

The treatment of a structural kyphotic deformity is surgical. With the exception of Scheuermann's kyphosis, nonoperative methods are ineffective in providing permanent correction. As a kyphosis progresses, the weight-bearing axis migrates further anterior, increasing the tendency toward progression. A vicious circle is created unless normal sagittal balance can be restored. The pathomechanics of the deformity dictate that, in most situations, both anterior and posterior surgery be performed.

In kyphosis, posterior fusion and instrumentation experience tensile forces. Anterior fusion experiences primarily compressive forces, which Wolff's law indicates is an optimal situation. Many kyphotic deformities are a result of anterior column deficiencies. Correction of the kyphosis lengthens the anterior column. Unless the anterior column deficit is supported, posterior fusion and instrumentation is doomed to failure.

The expectations and specific methods employed to correct the deformity are determined to a large extent by the personality of the kyphosis—that is, its magnitude, angularity, and flexibility. Kyphotic defor-

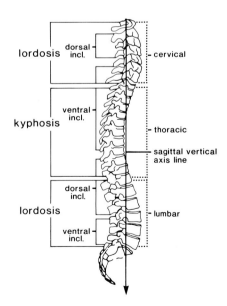

FIG. 18–1. Balance of sagittal contour depends on the sagittal vertical axis. Each vertebra has a unique orientation and spatial relationship to the apical vertebra.

mities can be broadly classified as two types. The first includes deformities with a uniform posterior curvature over many segments of the spine (Fig. 18-2). These curvatures may be flexible or rigid. A flexible kyphosis is one that corrects to within normal range with hyperextension. These curvatures can be corrected initially by posterior instrumentation and then have augmentation of the fusion by anterior inlay or strut graft of the residual kyphosis. The advantage of this method is the strength of a single, solid anterior support. A more rigid kyphosis demands primary anterior release and fusion, followed by posterior instrumentation and fusion. Although a single anterior strut is advantageous, the restoration of a more physiologic sagittal contour is critical. To obtain a balanced spine, the sagittal vertical axis must be properly oriented.

The second type of kyphosis is acute and angular. This type of deformity is usually quite rigid, as seen in post-traumatic, healed Pott's, or congenital kyphosis. A patient with this type of deformity is at a much greater risk for the development of neurologic impairment, especially if the kyphosis is located in the thoracic spine.[38] Often, the objective of surgical intervention in this type of deformity is the protection or decompression of the neural elements. The deformity is stabilized in situ or with minimal correction, in conjunction with anterior spinal cord decompression (Fig. 18-3). Correction of this type of kyphosis can be accomplished, but it is certainly hazardous.[4] The principles of lengthening the anterior column, restoring adequate anterior support, and shortening the posterior column must be followed.

METHODS OF ANTERIOR RECONSTRUCTION

The successful surgical treatment of kyphosis frequently depends on the reconstruction of the anterior column. Without sufficient support in the anterior column, the posterior instrumentation and fusion remain under tension and will fail. A variety of bone grafting techniques and instrumentation are available for the reconstruction of the anterior column.

Fusion Techniques

Anterior spinal fusion can be accomplished by interbody, inlay, or strut grafting techniques.[11, 14] Interbody grafting and inlay grafting are most appropriate for moderate kyphosis in which correction close to a physiologic contour is anticipated. Curvatures that are relatively stiff should first be released anteriorly and grafted by the interbody technique. A more supple kyphosis can be initially corrected by posterior instrumentation and then grafted by an inlay rib technique.

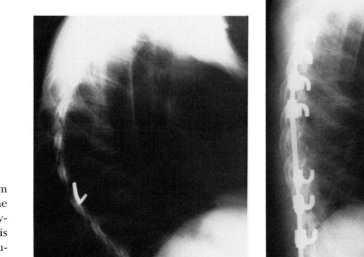

FIG. 18–2. A. Gentle, uniform deformity over many levels of the spine is typical of Scheuermann's kyphosis. **B.** Correction of kyphosis by anterior release and interbody fusion, followed by posterior Harrington compression, instrumentation, and fusion.

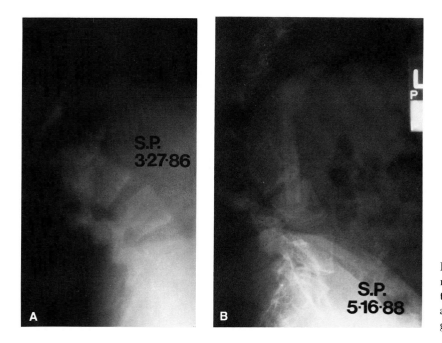

FIG. 18–3. **A.** Acute, angular deformity secondary to healed tuberculosis of the spine. **B.** Residual deformity after anterior decompression and fibular strut graft. Apex of gibbus has been removed.

The rib should be placed as far anterior in the vertebral body as possible to provide maximal resistance to compressive forces.

Alternatives to rib for inlay grafting include autogenous fibula and homogenous rib or fibula. For shorter reconstructions, tricortical ilium can be employed, as well as a variety of allografts including ilium, femoral head, or diaphyseal bone. The best use of these grafts is for the reconstruction of short segmental column defects resulting from trauma, tumor, or infection.

Anterior strut grafting is necessary for rigid angular kyphosis in which significant deformity will persist. The fibula is the preferred graft because of its length and strength, although rib can also be used. The graft must span the entire length of the structural curve. Inadequate length of the strut graft will result in "adding on" to the kyphosis proximally or distally.[64] The graft should be vertical in the coronal and sagittal planes. If a concomitant scoliosis is present, the strut should be in the concavity of the curve.

The spine is exposed through a standard anterior approach. The segmental vessels are identified, isolated, and ligated. A subperiosteal flap is raised, including the periosteum, annulus fibrosus, and anterior longitudinal ligament. Optionally, an osteoperiosteal flap may be elevated with an osteotome. This technique may improve osteogenesis, but it will increase blood loss, which could be prohibitive.

A thorough discectomy is performed at each intervening level between the end vertebrae (Fig. 18-4). A tunnel is created in the end vertebrae to accept the ends of the fibula strut graft. Manual pressure at the apex of the kyphosis produces partial correction and lengthening of the anterior column. The fibula should be cut to 1 to 2 cm longer than the corrected position. Manual pressure is again applied to the gibbus, and the

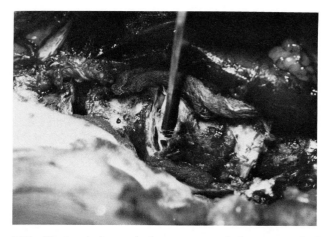

FIG. 18–4. A thorough discectomy, including removal of cartilaginous endplates, is necessary for interbody or inlay fusion. An osteotome is used to excise the endplates (ventral is to the top; cephalad is to the right).

strut graft is impacted into place. The tunnels should be made well anterior in the vertebral body, so that, if subsidence should occur, the ends of the strut graft will rest on the dense subchondral bone of the endplates and not in the spinal canal. Depending on the magnitude and angularity of the kyphosis, several struts of various lengths may be inserted. Morselized rib graft and cancellous bone are packed in the intervertebral spaces and between the gibbus and the strut graft. The periosteal flap serves as a shelf for the cancellous graft deep to the struts at the apex of the kyphosis. The periosteum can usually be closed at the ends of the strut.

Supplementary posterior instrumentation and fusion is necessary to augment the strength of the stabilized segment (Fig. 18-5).[11, 14, 43, 64] Cotrel–Dubousset instrumentation is used; the hook pattern and technique of insertion is similar to that described for Scheuermann's kyphosis. In a thin patient with a severe kyphosis, the Cotrel–Dubousset instrumentation may be prominent, especially over the gibbus. In these circumstances, the small Keene compression system is used.

An autologous fibular strut provides an immediate strong, physiologic, anterior support. However, rib or fibular graft may take up to 2 years to incorporate and undergo revascularization by creeping substitution. The graft is weakest at approximately 6 months postoperatively and is subject to fracture. Bradford reported a 50% failure of strut grafts placed more than 4 cm anterior to the apex.[11] To overcome the problem of strut fracture, several methods have been devised. Vascularized grafts are attractive in that they obviate the need for revascularization of the grafts. The use of a vascularized rib graft for the treatment of a kyphotic deformity was first reported by Rose in 1975.[53] Since then, Bradford has reported extensively on the use of vascularized pedicle rib graft for strut fusion or with allograft as an inlay for segmental defects.[7, 10, 44] The superiority of vascularized rib grafts over non-vascularized grafts has been demonstrated by biologic and mechanical testing.[58]

The technique of vascularized pedicle rib graft has been described in detail.[12] In high thoracic kyphosis, the rib selected for transfer is two to three levels below the apex. The distal end of the rib is rotated up. In lower thoracic kyphosis, the rib chosen is two to three levels above the apex, and the distal end is rotated down.

The patient is positioned for a standard thoracot-

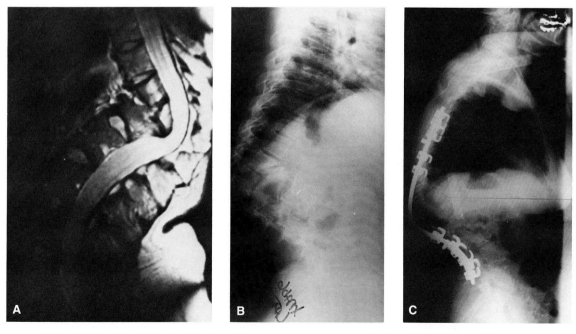

FIG. 18–5. **A.** MRI of Pott's disease demonstrating acute angular kyphosis compromising the spinal canal. **B, C.** Preoperative and postoperative radiographs demonstrate anterior decompression, fibular strut graft, and posterior instrumentation and fusion.

omy. The skin and superficial musculature of the chest are divided in the usual fashion. The periosteum of the rib to be used is not incised and circumferentially elevated; instead, the rib is isolated by cutting the intercostal musculature on either side. Superiorly, the muscle can be cut at its insertion onto the superior edge of the rib. Inferiorly, a cuff of muscle should be left on the rib to prevent injury to the intercostal vessels. The length of rib to be used and the length of the vascular pedicle are dependent on the kyphosis and must be determined on an individual basis. The appropriate length of rib is sectioned from the shaft of the rib, lateral to the angle. Before transection, the periosteum is incised and circumferentially elevated at the points to be cut to prevent injury to the vessels. The proximal portion of the vascular pedicle is mobilized from the costal groove by sharp dissection. The proximal rib, angle, neck, and head are removed. The distal vessels are divided, and vascularity is confirmed by brisk bleeding. The proximal pedicle can be further mobilized, if necessary, by dividing the foraminal branch of the segmental vessel overlying the vertebral body.

The spine is prepared for inlay or strut grafting in the usual fashion. If the rib is to be used as an inlay graft, the periosteum of the upper third of the cephalad edge of the rib is stripped. This edge is then placed deep in the trough to provide bone-to-bone contact. When used as a strut graft, the periosteum is left intact except for 1 to 2 cm at both ends, where the strut is inserted into the end vertebra. The remainder of the fusion is performed in a standard manner as previously described (Fig. 18-6).

Free vascularized fibular strut graft has also been reported for the treatment of kyphosis.[30, 35] The use of a free vascularized fibular strut requires the anastomosis of the nutrient vessels, a procedure not needed for a pedicle rib graft. The advantages of a free fibular graft are greater strength and length of the strut than for a rib. Because the fibula is not restricted by a vascular pedicle, it may be used anywhere in the spinal column, including the cervical and lumbosacral regions.

Anterior Instrumentation

The use of posterior compression instrumentation in the correction and stabilization of kyphotic deformities is well established. The role of anterior distraction instrumentation for the treatment of kyphosis is not as clearly defined. The appeal of anterior fixation is that it may eliminate the necessity of second-stage posterior surgery. However, elongation of the anterior column without shortening and compression of the posterior column may not be a sound mechanical construct. The practical experience of anterior instrumentation for kyphosis as reported in the literature is limited.

In 1978, Pinto described an anterior distractor for the intraoperative correction of angular kyphosis.[49] Analogous to the Harrington outrigger used for scoliosis, this device is temporarily inserted at surgery

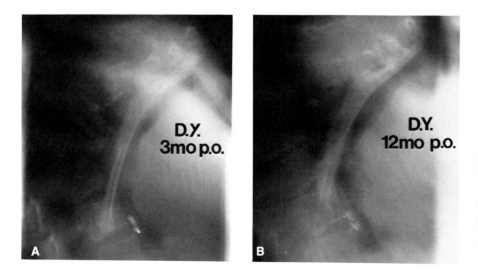

FIG. 18–6. Progressive kyphosis secondary to lymphangiomatosis stabilized by vascular rib strut. **A.** Incorporation of strut ends after 3 months. **B.** At 12 months, the strut has hypertrophied with further dissolution of the spine. (Courtesy of John P. Lubicky, M.D.)

to "take out the slack" in the spine. Strut grafts are then inserted after taking advantage of whatever correctability exists, but not forcing the spine beyond its natural limits. Posterior instrumentation and fusion are still advised because loss of correction and pseudarthrosis would otherwise be likely.

In 1981, Slot reported a new distraction system for the intraoperative correction of kyphosis.[60] Similar to Pinto's device, this system was not designed as an implant. Slot did mention that an anterior implant could be employed to strengthen the bone graft reconstruction. He described a variation of VDS instrumentation using Zielke screws and a solid distraction rod (Fig. 18-7). Micheli reported a similar modification of the Dwyer system at the same time.[45]

Dunn, in 1984, reported on a new anterior implant of his design used in 48 patients.[21] Although designed primarily for the treatment of acute burst fractures, the ability to apply distraction force allowed for its application in the treatment of short-segment kyphosis. However, later reports of failure of the device and vascular catastrophe led to the recall of this device by the manufacturer.[15]

Other devices that have been developed for the stabilization of burst fractures can be applied to short-segment kyphosis.[24, 34] Kostuik reported one of the largest series of patients treated by anterior instrumentation.[36] In his series of 279 patients, 123 patients

were treated for kyphosis of different causes, including Scheuermann's and post-traumatic kyphosis. The instrumentation uses simple standard Harrington instrumentation, heavy compression rods, and collar-end and distraction-end vertebral body screws. Kostuik concluded that this was a reliable and versatile system of anterior fixation. Posterior instrumentation and fusion was rarely necessary in this series.

Interest in the surgical treatment of kyphosis led to the development of a fiber-metal strut.[20] The implant has undergone several design changes and now consists of 3-mm titanium wire mesh sintered to a 6.3-mm solid titanium core. The concept for this implant is similar to porous-coated-surface replacements, and it has been shown to encourage bone ingrowth.[41] The fiber-metal device is available in various lengths and can be used as an inlay or strut. The implant is intended to augment the rib or fibular graft, avoiding the period of structural weakness that occurs before completion of revascularization (Fig. 18-8). The fiber-metal implant does not provide torsional or lateral stability, and posterior instrumentation and fusion are recommended. This device has been employed for anterior reconstruction in 11 patients with benign kyphotic conditions. The average follow-up is 60 months, with a 22-month minimum. One implant fractured and one subsided; neither patient had had posterior stabilization. These implants function as an adjunct to bone

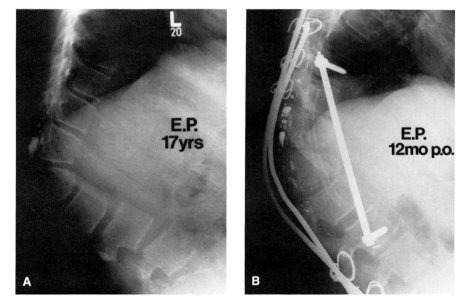

FIG. 18–7. **A.** Progressive kyphosis secondary to extensive laminectomies in a growing child. **B.** Correction and stabilization by anterior VDS rod and inlay rib graft, and posterior stabilization by the Luque technique.

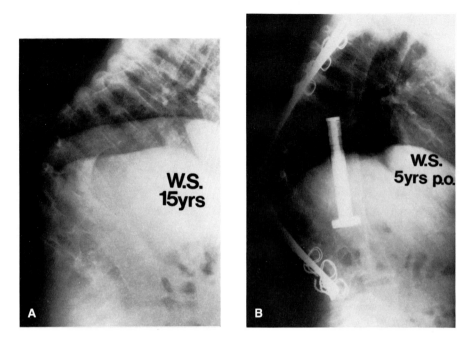

FIG. 18–8. **A.** Progressive congenital kyphosis despite previous anterior fusion. **B.** Stabilization of deformity by fibular strut graft augmented by fiber metal strut yielded a solid fusion.

grafting or as a substitute if autologous graft is unavailable.

SCHEUERMANN'S KYPHOSIS

Scheuermann's kyphosis is the prototype for discussion of the surgical treatment of uniform, round-back deformity. The deformity was first described by Scheuermann in 1921 as resembling Calvé-Perthes disease of the spine. He labeled the kyphosis osteochondritis deformans juvenilis dorsi.[56] Recent studies have demonstrated abnormal cartilage matrix with diminished glycoproteins and a different type of collagen in affected vertebral end plates.[31] Other theories have suggested that juvenile osteoporosis may play a role in the progressive kyphosis.[9, 33]

The cause of Scheuermann's kyphosis remains obscure, but the radiographic characteristics are well described. Sorenson, in 1964, described endplate irregularity, Schmorl's nodes, and wedging of at least 5° of three adjacent vertebrae typical of this process (Fig. 18-9).[61] Bradford classified atypical variants of this process as vertebral body changes without wedging and as increased kyphosis without vertebral body changes.[12] At times, it may be difficult to distinguish milder forms of Scheuermann's kyphosis from postural roundback.[75]

The mechanism of progression in Scheuermann's kyphosis is shortening of the anterior column. The anterior portion of the apophyseal plate is involved, decreasing anterior vertical growth, and with normal posterior growth, wedging of the vertebral bodies occurs.[50] As the kyphosis progresses, increased compressive forces result across the anterior epiphyseal plate, compounding the growth disturbance. Roaf, in 1960, pointed out that once a deformity exists, a vicious circle of aggravated progression is created.[51]

Indications

The natural history of Scheuermann's kyphosis is not as well understood as that of idiopathic scoliosis, and the latitude of physiologic sagittal contours is relatively broad. Consequently, the indications for surgery are not well defined. Progressive kyphosis despite bracing, intractable back pain, neurologic compromise, or significant deformity with little or no growth remaining are indications for surgery.

Bracing has proved effective in the correction of moderate deformities if adequate growth occurs. However, the greater the curvature at the onset of treatment, the greater the residual curvature at the conclusion of treatment and the less favorable final result. Sachs and colleagues, in a review of 120 patients, concluded that an initial kyphosis of more than 74° was

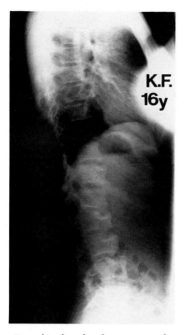

FIG. 18–9. True lumbar kyphosis secondary to Scheuermann's disease. Notice vertebral wedging, endplate irregularity, and Schmorl's nodes. The compensatory thoracic lordosis represents an attempt to maintain sagittal balance.

associated with a higher percentage of unsatisfactory treatment results.[54] Montgomery and Erwin suggested that it may not be justified to brace patients with curvatures greater than 75° if the expected result is in the range of 60°.[47]

Surgery should be considered in a growing child with a kyphosis in the range of 70 to 75°. In a more mature patient, surgery should be considered for curvatures greater than 60 to 65°, because these deformities are cosmetically objectionable, often symptomatic, and may progress during adult life. This is especially true for females, because preexisting juvenile kyphosis may increase the propensity to develop a severe senile kyphosis secondary to osteoporsis.

Literature Review

Before the introduction of Harrington instrumentation, the surgical treatment of Scheuermann's kyphosis was only sporadically reported.[2, 22, 51] Bradford, in 1975, presented the first large series of patients treated with Harrington compression instrumentation.[13] Satisfactory initial correction and pain relief was obtained in all 22 patients. Significant loss of correction

occurred in 16 patients. Other complications included 3 infections, 5 instrumentation failures, 1 deep vein thrombosis, 1 psychotic episode, and 1 superior mesenteric artery syndrome. The complication rate was so high that the procedure was recommended only for disabling pain or spinal cord compression. Anterior release and interbody fusion followed by posterior instrumentation and fusion was suggested for curvatures greater than 70° to reduce loss of correction.

Taylor and associates, in 1979, reported a similar group of 27 patients who underwent Harrington compression instrumentation.[68] This group included both Scheuermann's kyphosis and postural roundback. The proximal and distal hooks were placed under the lamina to reduce pull-out. Fifteen of the patients had a correction loss of 5° or more. Three patients had hook pull-out, 4 had upper gastrointestinal obstruction, 1 had tension pneumothorax, 1 had graft site hematoma, and 1 had ulnar paresthesias.

To overcome the problem of significant loss of correction with a high rate of pseudarthrosis and metal failure, combined anterior and posterior fusion was recommended. Bradford reported 24 patients who underwent anterior release and interbody fusion, intercurrent traction, and posterior instrumentation and fusion.[8] Significant loss of correction was not observed in the instrumented region and only one pseudarthrosis was noted. Herndon and Nerubay reported similar low rates of correction loss and pseudarthrosis after combined fusions.[29, 48] They concluded that traction did not improve the final correction.

Staged surgeries remain a formidable undertaking, as is demonstrated by a high rate of complications. Bradford reported complications of pulmonary embolisms, deep wound infection, persistent pneumothorax, and superior mesenteric artery syndrome.[8] Herndon reported 1 death, 1 deep vein thrombosis, 2 psychotic episodes, and 1 transient lower extremity paresis in only 13 patients.[29]

In 1986, Speck and Chopin reported a series of 59 patients who underwent surgical correction of Scheuermann's kyphosis.[62] Pain was the presenting complaint in 46% of their patients. They recommended posterior surgery alone for skeletally immature patients with a Risser sign, Stage 3 or 4, after a period of preparatory mobilization treatment. Improvement of the vertebral wedging and filling in of the anterior column was anticipated with continued spinal growth. For more mature patients, combined anterior and posterior surgery offered the best results. Loss of correction of more than 10° was noted in 9 patients, primarily due to inadequate length of fusion. The complication rate was modest, including 4 deep infections, 1 transient Brown-Séquard syndrome, and 1 broken rod.

The use of Luque instrumentation has been recently studied (Fig. 18-10). The advantage of this system appeared to be improved maintenance of correction and elimination of postoperative immobilization. A worrisome 16% incidence of "transient hyperesthesia" was reported.[40] A longer follow-up of this technique observed the development of a junctional kyphosis at the superior end of the instrumentation in almost 67% of the cases.[17] This study suggested that Luque instrumentation is a poor construct for the management of Scheuermann's kyphosis.

Another recent development in the surgical treatment of Scheuermann's kyphosis is the use of Cotrel–Dubousset instrumentation. In 1988, Shufflebarger presented a series of 15 patients with an average follow-up of 26 months.[59] Anterior release and interbody fusion was followed by Cotrel–Dubousset instrumentation. The mean preoperative kyphosis of 81° was corrected to a mean 33°, with negligible loss of correction. Although the experience is limited, the versatility of this instrumentation system in hook placement, rod contour, and application of corrective forces represents a significant improvement over other systems.

Alternative methods of correction include anterior distraction instrumentation and multilevel posterior pedicle instrumentation. Further follow-up is needed to substantiate the success of these new techniques.

Preoperative Assessment

The selection of levels to include in the instrumentation is critical. Historically, the loss of correction has been primarily due to inadequate fusion length, either proximal or distal. Theoretically, Cotrel–Dubousset instrumentation should cause less proximal junctional kyphosis because the interspinous ligaments and ligamentum flavum are preserved at the most superior level. In part, the proximal level of instrumentation is determined by the apex of the kyphosis. In patients with a fairly high apex, such as T7 or T8, instrumentation is routinely extended to T1.

A part of this deformity is the compensatory cervical hyperlordosis that results in the characteristic head and neck thrust. The head and neck thrust can be quantified by having the patient stand with his or her back touching a wall and measuring the horizontal distance from the wall to the point of maximal cervical lordosis. This has been referred to as the cervical fleche in the French literature. Extending the instrumentation to T1 has been most effective in reducing the head and neck thrust, which can be an unsightly residual after the correction of a kyphotic deformity (Fig. 18-11). The development of a junctional kyphosis

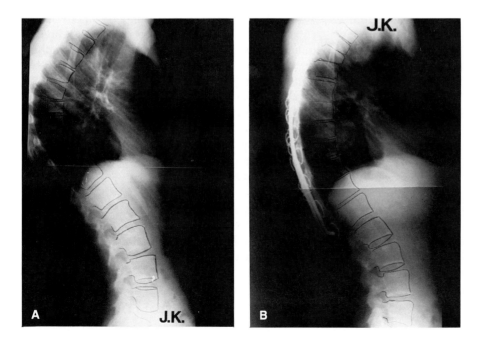

FIG. 18–10. Typical Scheuermann's kyphosis stabilized by anterior release and fusion and by posterior Luque instrumentation and fusion. This technique has a relatively high incidence of neurologic sequelae and may lead to a junctional kyphosis proximally.

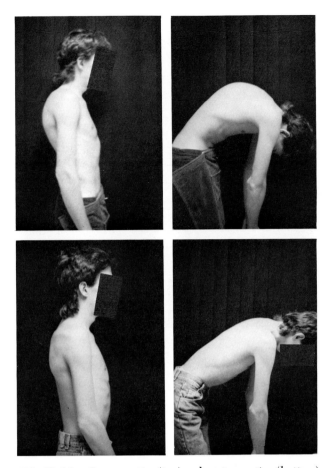

FIG. 18–11. Preoperative (*top*) and postoperative (*bottom*) photographs of patient whose radiographs are in Fig. 18–12. Notice restoration of sagittal alignment and elimination of the head and neck thrust.

at this level is unlikely because the sagittal vertical axis crosses the spinal column and thoracic kyphosis is reversing to cervical lordosis.

Kyphotic deformities with apices in the lower thoracic or thoracolumbar regions do not require as much proximal extension of the instrumentation. However, the instrumentation must extend proximally to include the entire pathologic kyphos and at least one neutral level beyond the curvature. In high deformities, with an apex of T6 or above, this may require instrumentation into the lower cervical region. If the sagittal vertical axis can be restored, the spine should remain balanced.

The distal extent of the instrumentation is determined by evaluating the preoperative standing lateral radiographs and flexion and extension studies. The principles of the sagittal vertical axis and balanced

contour must be kept in mind. In the normal spine, the T11, T12, and L1 section is neutral, and lordosis generally begins at the L1–L2 interspace. The instrumentation should extend the full length of the kyphosis and into the neutral section at the thoracolumbar junction. The standing lateral and hyperextension radiographs must be analyzed to estimate the location of the sagittal vertical axis after correction. The distal extent of the instrumentation is generally two levels distal to the last vertebra in the curve.

Another method for determining the inferior extent of instrumentation is to position the patient supine over a bolster and obtain a hyperextension radiograph that includes the lumbar spine (Fig. 18-12). Instrumentation should be carried distally to the neutral vertebra, which is the vertebra perpendicular to the long axis of the spine. The intervertebral disc space below the instrumentation must be mobile, opening dorsally and ventrally on flexion and extension, to accommodate any compensation that may be necessary. In my experience, the instrumentation should include the initiation of the lordotic curve, generally L2, and sometimes in larger kyphosis L3.

Surgical Technique

Surgical correction of a kyphosis requires both anterior and posterior surgery. To produce a mechanically sound reconstruction, the anterior column must be lengthened and provided adequate support, and the posterior column must be shortened. Currently, this is best achieved by anterior release and interbody fusion, followed by posterior Cotrel–Dubousset instrumentation and fusion.

Anterior release and fusion are performed first. The levels of anterior release are those with the most wedging and least flexibility on hyperextension. This region generally includes seven or eight interspaces centered on the apex of the kyphosis.

The patient is preferably positioned in the right lateral decubitus position with the left side up, unless a concomitant scoliosis exists. Then the spine is best approached on the convexity of the scoliosis. The patient is appropriately padded, and the operating table is flexed to improve access to the spine. A standard thoracotomy is performed with resection of a rib to be used for bone graft. The selected rib corresponds to the most proximal level to be released.

The parietal pleura is incised longitudinally over the spine. If an anterior release, including simple discectomy and interbody fusion is planned, the segmen-

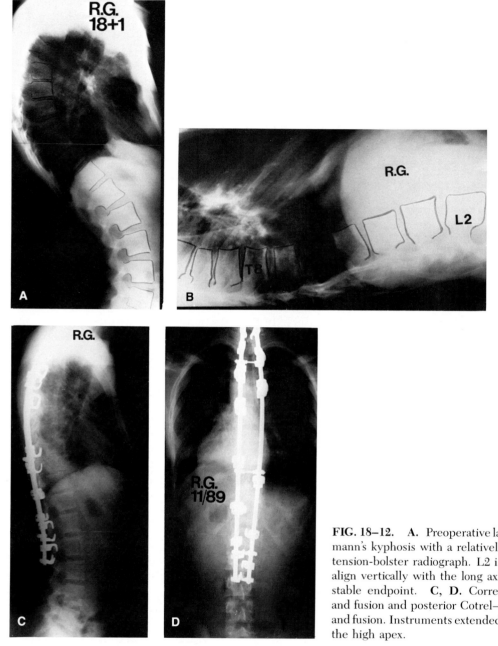

FIG. 18–12. **A.** Preoperative lateral radiograph of Scheuermann's kyphosis with a relatively high apex. **B.** Hyperextension-bolster radiograph. L2 is the first distal vertebra to align vertically with the long axis of the spine, indicating a stable endpoint. **C, D.** Correction after anterior release and fusion and posterior Cotrel–Dubousset instrumentation and fusion. Instruments extended proximally to C7 because of the high apex.

tal vessels may be spared at some or all levels. This may reduce the likelihood of a vascular-related spinal cord injury. In most cases, especially in the more rigid kyphoses, a thorough release of the anterior longitudinal ligament and annulus is necessary and the segmental vessels must be ligated to gain adequate exposure. After a complete discectomy with curettage of the cartilaginous endplates, an interbody fusion using the

morselized rib graft is performed. An alternative is to create a trough and perform an inlay rib graft. The resulting cancellous bone from the trough is used for the interbody fusion. The inlay rib graft does not appear to restrict the correction obtained at the time of posterior instrumentation (Fig. 18-13).

Between the staged surgeries, the patient is encouraged to be mobile. While at bed rest, the patient

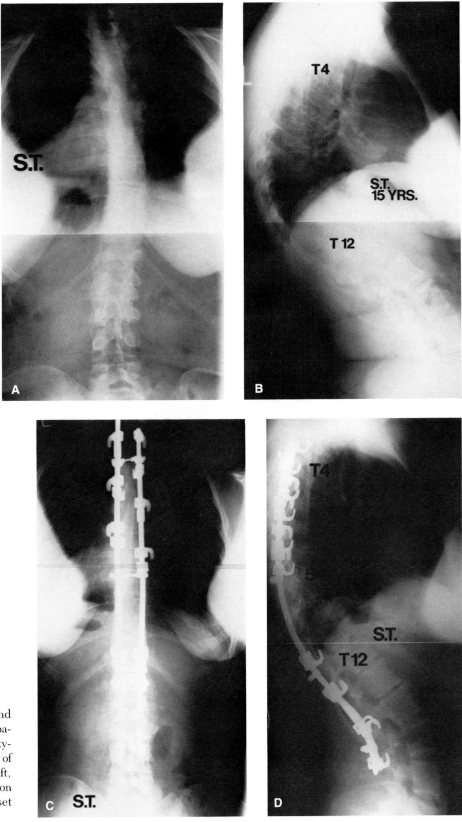

FIG. 18–13. Preoperative and postoperative radiographs of a patient with Scheuermann's kyphosis. The first stage consisted of anterior release and inlay rib graft, which did not restrict correction with posterior Cotrel–Dubousset instrumentation.

can be positioned supine over a blanket roll or bolster to encourage passive correction of the deformity. When more comfortable, after 4 to 5 days, the patient can be sent to physical therapy to work on active extension exercises of the thoracic spine.

The posterior spinal surgery usually follows the first stage by 7 to 10 days. The patient is positioned prone in Gardner-Wells tongs on a Stryker frame. The instrumentation is routinely extended proximally to T1 or, in some cases, C7. Frequently, exposure and instrumentation of the cervicothoracic junction is difficult because it is in the depths of the wound. The tongs help elevate and stabilize the cervicothoracic junction. The Stryker frame facilitates the use of the tongs and may provide some passive correction. Abdominal compression may be partially relieved by blanket rolls placed transversely under the chest and pelvis.

The apex of the kyphosis is determined on the preoperative radiographs. Three sets of hooks above the apex and at least two sets below are mandatory. For the most part, bilateral pediculotransverse claws are avoided because this places excessive stress at one level, and disruption of the posterior elements may occur. The pattern of hook placement is evolving. Currently, a spread pediculosublaminar claw is used proximally between T2 and T1. Closed offset cervical hooks are placed over the cephalad lamina of T1, and closed pedicle hooks are inserted at T2. Two pediculotransverse claws are staggered on each side on the spine above the apex. Staggering the claw constructs disperses the forces at each level and increases segmental fixation. This configuration allows improved placement and contact of bone graft from one level to the adjacent levels.

At least two and preferably three sets of hooks are placed distally to the apex of kyphosis. Open pedicle hooks are usually inserted at the lower thoracic levels. If possible, these hooks are also staggered. Sometimes, in the transitional thoracolumbar junction, infralaminar open thoracic hooks are inserted if pedicle hooks seem ill fitting. The distal terminal hook placement is critical, because hook dislodgment may occur. I prefer a spread claw on one side and a single level sublaminar claw on the opposite. This construct resists the tendency for hook dislodgment, improves contact between the two lower levels for bone graft, and disperses forces. Moreover, compression between the two lower levels initiates lumbar lordosis. The use of thin-blade hooks reduces the amount of metal within the spinal canal at a single level.

The patient is nursed postoperatively on a standard hospital bed. The patient is dangled at bedside on day 2 or 3 after surgery and ambulates soon afterward, as tolerated. Postoperative bracing is not used for most adolescents unless bone quality and fixation is thought to be tenuous. A Milwaukee brace for kyphosis provides the best immobilization. In adults, a molded, bivalve TLSO is often used for patient security. If postoperative immobilization is deemed necessary, a Milwaukee brace is employed.

POST-TRAUMATIC KYPHOSIS

Post-traumatic kyphosis is an angular deformity with increased local kyphosis. It represents a failure of initial fracture treatment, operative or nonoperative, to restore spinal stability. Intrinsic causes of post-traumatic instability are persistent angular deformities of the vertebral bodies or attenuated healing of posterior element disruption.[42] As with other types of kyphosis, the deformity results from loss of anterior column support and lack of posterior column restraint. Fractures predisposed to kyphotic deformity are those with more than 30° of local kyphosis or 30% loss of anterior body height, especially at the thoracolumbar junction.[70] Thoracic compression fractures at two or more adjacent levels have the potential for increasing late deformity (Fig. 18-14).[65] The most malignant form of post-traumatic kyphosis occurs in the unstable fracture treated by laminectomy.

Indications

The delayed development of kyphosis after fracture of the spine may result in a painful deformity, persistent or progressive neurologic compromise, and restricted rehabilitation. The development of a progressive post-traumatic kyphosis should be regarded as an ominous event. As the kyphosis progresses, the sagittal vertical axis moves farther anteriorly, increasing the kyphotic tendency. Once this cycle starts, operative intervention is the only treatment that can halt the process.

The indications for surgical intervention are a progressive deformity, pain, and persistent or progressive neurologic compromise.[5, 25, 74]

Literature Review

Malcolm and colleagues, in 1981, reported the results of 48 patients surgically treated for post-traumatic kyphosis.[43] Pain was noted in 94% of the patients, pro-

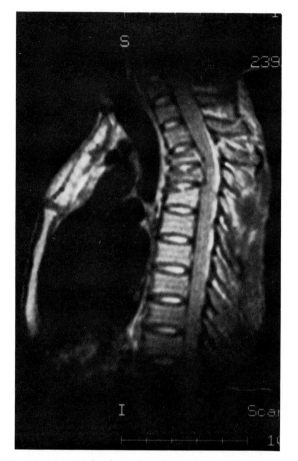

FIG. 18–14. Multiple, contiguous thoracic compression fractures have a high propensity for developing post-traumatic kyphosis. As this MRI scan demonstrates, these injuries also have a high risk of neurologic compromise.

gression of deformity in 46%, and increasing neural deficit in 27%. Anterior surgery alone failed in 6 of 12 patients, but significantly, 50% of these failures had previous laminectomies. Pain relief was significant in 98% of the patients. Of the 14 patients undergoing anterior decompression, 5 were improved, 5 unchanged, and 4 made worse. No patient improved neurologically after posterolateral decompression or repeat laminectomy. Complications included 3 superficial wound infections, one chest wound dehiscence, one persistent pleural effusion, and 1 persistent pneumothorax. They recommend augmenting anterior fusions with posterior instrumentation and fusion to lessen the rate of pseudarthrosis and loss of correction.

Roberson and Whitesides reported a group of 34 patients undergoing surgical treatment for post-trau-

matic kyphosis.[52] Twenty-one patients presented with neurologic symptoms. Only 2 patients had posterior surgery alone. Eighteen patients had anterior decompression and fusion, of whom 17 attained good spinal stability. The lone failure occurred in a patient with compromised posterior stability secondary to a previous laminectomy. No patient was made worse by anterior decompression, 5 were improved, and 13 were unchanged. Postoperative complications were recorded in 24% of the patients, the most significant being death from a pulmonary embolus. The researchers concluded that the treatment of late post-traumatic kyphosis should follow basic biomechanical principles by replacing the aspect of spinal stability that is compromised, whether anterior, posterior, or both.

Kostuik reported the results of anterior stabilization, instrumentation, and decompression for post-traumatic kyphosis.[37] Stable arthrodesis and correction of the deformity was achieved in 36 of 37 patients. The one failure was in a patient with a previous laminectomy. Pain, the presenting complaint of all patients, was reduced in 78%. Anterior decompression improved neurologic function in 3 of 8 patients. Complications included Horner's syndrome, a hemothorax, an incisional post-thoracotomy syndrome, and adult respiratory distress in 3 patients. One patient had a diaphragmatic rupture 2 months after surgery, requiring reconstruction. Kostuik suggested that anterior instrumentation and fusion are sufficient for most cases of post-traumatic kyphosis. Posterior instrumentation and fusion are recommended in cases with previous destabilizing laminectomy.

Preoperative Assessment

A thorough history and physical examination are the cornerstones of the preoperative assessment of a patient with a post-traumatic kyphosis. Special emphasis must be placed on the neurologic examination, looking for subtle deficits. Dynamic bladder function studies may reveal occult sphincter dysfunction.

Radiographic evaluation includes full-length posterior-anterior and lateral radiographs in a weight-bearing position, either sitting or standing. Stability of the kyphosis is demonstrated by flexion-extension lateral radiographs centered on the apex of the deformity. At times, the posterior elements ankylose after trauma, and the lack of motion should be noted. If a concomitant scoliosis exists, side-bending radiographs are helpful in determining flexibility. Tomography may provide the best evaluation of the bony architecture at the apex of the deformity.

In the presence of a neurologic deficit, whether progressive or static, the spinal canal should be imaged to determine the location and extent of canal compromise. Traditionally, this has been accomplished by myelography. Computed tomography (CT) is a great adjunct. Specifically, the axial views are helpful in planning the side of approach if anterior decompression is considered. Recently, magnetic resonance imaging (MRI) has proved successful in evaluating the spinal canal, especially with the gradient-echo techniques that produce CSF myelograms.[3] MRI provides information about possible post-traumatic changes within the spinal cord or cauda equina, including hematomyelia and arachnoiditis. This information clearly influences surgical planning and the prognosis for anterior decompression.

Operative Management

The surgical treatment of post-traumatic kyphosis is determined by the magnitude of deformity, presence of neurologic deficit, stability of the posterior column, and integrity of the anterior column. Reconstruction should follow sound biomechanical principles. Posterior spinal instrumentation and fusion are not sufficient treatment for the correction of a progressive post-traumatic kyphosis. Posterior fusion in the presence of significant residual kyphosis places the bone graft under tension, with the inevitable result of pseudarthrosis. Correction of a kyphosis by posterior instrumentation must create a significant anterior column deficit, which, if unsupported, will again cause tension-side failure.

Patients with a modest local kyphosis of 30 to 40° and a stable posterior column can be treated with anterior surgery alone (Fig. 18-15). Intact posterior elements and ligamentous stability are prerequisites for solitary anterior fusion. If an incomplete or increasing neurologic deficit is present or a significant canal compromise coexists with a progressive kyphosis, anterior decompression is indicated. Autogenous tricortical iliac graft is used for most reconstruction. The graft is slotted into the vertebral bodies above and below the fracture level. The graft is placed anterior in the bodies to maximize anterior support. Iliac graft is preferred over fibula because of faster incorporation of the cancellous bone. The harvesting of a substantial iliac graft is not without its own complications, and

allograft is being used with increasing frequency. Anterior instrumentation is an attractive addition if the device is low-profile and can provide torsional, frontal, and lateral stability.

In patients with local kyphosis greater than 40 to 45°, instability, previous laminectomy, or multilevel anterior column deficits, anterior and posterior surgery are indicated. In patients with instability or sufficient flexibility to correct to a physiologic sagittal contour, posterior instrumentation and fusion may be performed first, followed by anterior fusion (Fig. 18-16). Patients with a more rigid deformity or neurologic compromise are best managed by anterior decompression and fusion, followed by posterior instrumentation and fusion. Short-segment kyphosis in the lumbar spine or at the thoracolumbar junction can be stabilized by posterior pedicle screw fixation to minimize encroachment on the lower lumbar levels. Longer deformities are fixed with Cotrel–Dubousset instrumentation in a compression construct.

The guidelines about when to perform osteotomies to gain correction of a rigid kyphotic deformity are not provided in the literature. Frequently, the goal of surgical intervention in a rigid kyphosis is not correction of the deformity but protection of the neural elements and stabilization of the kyphosis. Several reports infer that the more severe deformities should be treated by anterior release, osteotomies and fusion, and then second-stage posterior instrumentation and fusion.[26, 43, 52] The restoration of a more normal sagittal balance increases the likelihood of fusion and reduces the stress on the instrumentation. Furthermore, it may reduce the development of pain and degenerative changes that frequently occur in the compensatory lumbar hyperlordosis distal to the kyphotic segment. If the cause of neurologic compromise is the angular kyphotic deformity of the canal rather than absolute spinal stenosis, realignment of the spinal canal may relieve the neurologic disability. In other words, decompression is achieved by correction of the deformity.

SENILE KYPHOSIS

At the opposite end of the spectrum from Scheuermann's kyphosis is the development of kyphotic deformity in the elderly. A correlation between increased kyphosis, decreased lordosis, and aging is well established.[46, 66, 69] The pathogenesis of progressive ky-

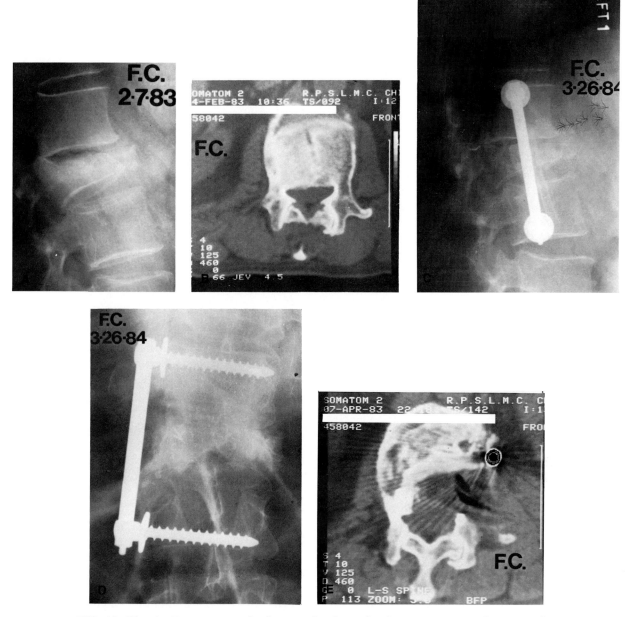

FIG. 18–15. A. Post-traumatic kyphosis at the thoracolumbar junction. **B.** CT scan at the level of injury demonstrates a 50% canal occlusion. **C, D.** Postoperative radiographs after anterior decompression, rib inlay strut graft and VDS instrumentation. **E.** Postoperative CT scan demonstrating decompression, rib graft, and instrumentation.

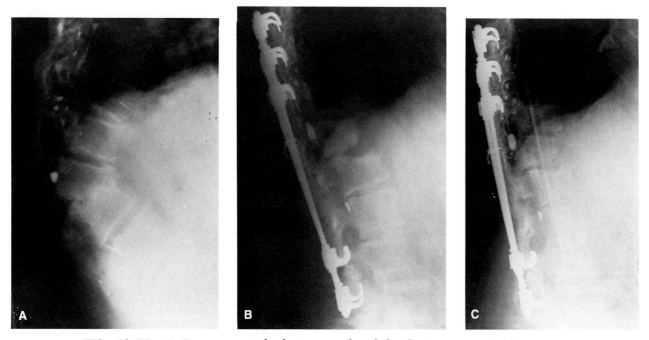

FIG. 18–16. **A.** Post-traumatic kyphosis exacerbated by laminectomy. **B.** Correction achieved by posterior compression instrumentation, taking advantage of the instability. Notice the significant anterior column defect. **C.** Anterior column reconstructed with an inlay fibular graft.

phosis in the elderly includes loss of posterior muscle and ligamentous tone and loss of anterior support by vertebral compression fractures and disc degeneration.[16, 19, 67]

The scope of this problem is growing as our elderly population increases. Clinically significant osteoporosis occurs in approximately 15% of postmenopausal women.[28] As many as 5% of white women have suffered an osteoporotic burst fracture by age 70.[32] These may be conservative estimates, because other reports indicate that as many as 40% of women have at least one compression fracture before they reach age 80.[18] Many of these fractures do not lead to a progressive kyphosis, but they do represent a huge pool of potential problems.

For the most part, the management of kyphosis in the elderly is conservative. These measures include nonsteroidal anti-inflammatory medication, analgesics, and a variety of orthotics, ranging from reinforced support garments to molded-plastic braces. Equally important is the treatment of the underlying metabolic defect. A variety of endocrine abnormalities may contribute to a progressive kyphosis in any age group, and most are amenable to medical treatment. Medical

treatment of the primary metabolic condition may alleviate the need for surgical intervention. Even if surgery is necessary, the treatment of the primary condition allows a more positive intervention (Fig. 18-17).

Indications

The indications for surgical intervention are pain unresponsive to medical management, progressive kyphosis interfering with function, or neurologic impairment. Senile kyphosis is a pathologic situation in a usually compromised patient. The goals of treatment must be appropriately limited to alleviate pain and restore or preserve neurologic function. Correction of the deformity should not be a priority in the surgical treatment of senile kyphosis.

Kyphosis in the elderly may be progressive, primarily owing to a lack of posterior restraint. This may be similar to the senile kyphosis described by Schmorl, in which the anterior column is shortened by disc degeneration and posterior restraint is lost by attrition of muscle and ligaments.[57, 67] For the most part, these curvatures are flexible unless secondary spondylosis has occurred. The deformity is frequently accom-

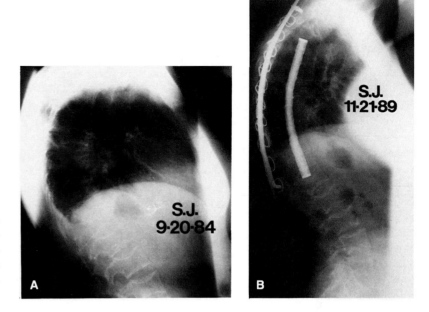

FIG. 18–17. A. Progressive kyphosis secondary to hypophosphatemic osteomalacia treated before surgical intervention. **B.** Stabilization with Luque instrumentation and anterior inlay fiber metal strut.

panied by mechanical pain in the compensatory cervical hyperlordosis and by fatigue pain in the lumbar hypolordosis. A physiologic contour can be restored by posterior instrumentation and fusion (Fig. 18-18).

Kyphosis may also develop due to deficits in the anterior column from osteoporotic fractures. The kyphosis may be due to a senile burst fracture, causing an acute local kyphosis. These pathologic fractures have a previously unrecognized high risk of neurologic complications.[1, 27, 55] The kyphosis may be a uniform rounding as a result of multiple thoracic wedge compression fractures. This deformity may also produce neurologic

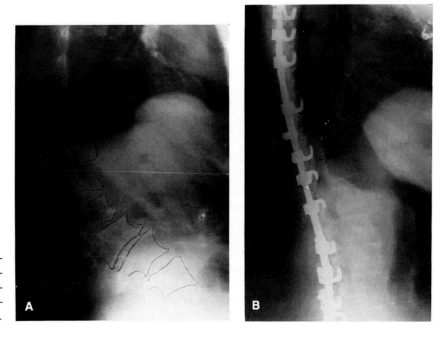

FIG. 18–18. A. Senile kyphosis secondary to attrition of posterior ligamentous structures and anterior disc degeneration. **B.** Realignment with Cotrel–Dubousset instrumentation and fusion.

compromise, depending on the degree of vertebral compression and kyphosis.

Surgical Technique

Bradford recommended that these deformities be stabilized by posterior instrumentation and fusion.[12] Anterior surgery is reserved for those patients with neurologic compromise necessitating anterior decompression. Little is to be gained by anterior release in an attempt to correct the kyphosis, and it exposes an elderly patient to the risks of an additional major surgery.

The senile burst fracture is associated with a relatively high risk of neurologic compromise. This demands anterior decompression. Even without neurologic compromise, the segmental anterior column deficit that characterizes this injury often requires anterior reconstruction to stabilize the local kyphosis. Anterior reconstruction is accomplished by the use of allograft. Autograft can be used, but because of the generalized osteoporosis, it usually does not have sufficient strength to provide the necessary structural support. Methylmethacrylate alone or in conjunction with internal fixation can provide immediate stability. The long-term efficacy of such constructs is questionable because of the disproportionate strength between the

fixation and the host bone. Subsidence of the construct and fracture above or below the fixation are likely.

An alternate method of decompression of the neural elements is by the transpedicular technique. Although this technique does not allow as direct a decompression as the anterior approach, significant decompression can be achieved. This technique is particularly useful in patients with multiple fractures requiring lengthy posterior instrumentation or multiple levels of cord compression or for those who cannot tolerate anterior surgery. The vertebral body is approached through the pedicle on the side of maximal compromise as determined by preoperative CT scans. As much of the lamina as possible should be preserved to minimize instability. The pedicle is followed to its junction with the dorsolateral vertebral body. After the floor of the canal and the ventral aspect of the dural sac are identified, the soft osteoporotic bone is removed with straight and reverse-angle curettes. After completion of the decompression, the spine is stabilized by posterior instrumentation. The spine is stabilized in the "collapsed" position, because correction or elongation of the spine would increase the anterior column deficiency (Fig. 18-19).

My current treatment for the typical osteoporotic kyphosis is posterior Cotrel–Dubousset instrumentation and cancellous allograft fusion. Because the actual

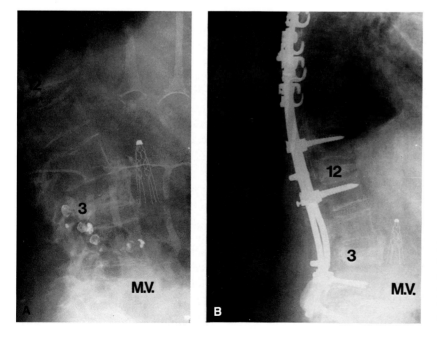

FIG. 18–19. A. Osteoporotic fractures causing increased local kyphosis and canal compromise at T12 and L3. **B.** Transpedicular decompression at T12 and L3 with stabilization by a hybrid screw-hook Cotrel–Dubousset construct.

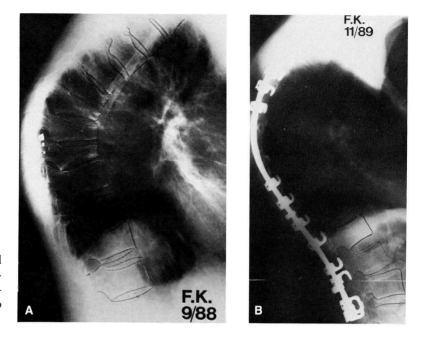

FIG. 18–20. **A.** Typical, uniform, round back deformity caused by multiple compression fractures. **B.** Stabilization by a Cotrel–Dubousset compression construct similar to that used for Scheuermann's kyphosis.

healing and quality of the fusion are dubious, fixation is maximized. The instrumentation is extended proximally and distally of the kyphosis to limit adding on by further compression fractures. Usually the instrumentation is carried to T1 proximally (Fig. 18-20).

The hook placement is similar to that described for Scheuermann's kyphosis, with some modifications. Although the posterior elements are surprisingly strong despite the generalized osteoporosis, the transverse processes do not offer much fixation. Thoracic hooks are placed sublaminar. At T1, cervical hooks are used bilaterally and are placed sublaminar. At the other thoracic levels, bilateral placement of hooks is avoided to minimize canal encroachment and to disperse stresses. The rods are contoured to the spine to avoid preloading the instrumentation, decreasing the likelihood of pull-out. The procedure is essentially an in situ stabilization. Without lengthening the anterior column, the need for anterior surgery is diminished.

Postoperatively, the patient is nursed on a standard hospital bed. The patient is encouraged to sit up and stand at bedside on the first postoperative day, because the problems of prolonged bedrest in the elderly are well known. A molded TLSO is fabricated and worn while out of bed for 6 months. The use of the brace is as much for the patient's security as for protection of the instrumentation.

SUMMARY

The techniques of the surgical correction of kyphosis continue to evolve. The use of autologous bone graft is biologic and a well-proven technique. Vascularized autologous bone grafts provide an even more physiologic method to reconstruct the anterior spinal column. A vascularized graft promotes more rapid incorporation and will hypertrophy under stress, but it does demand a higher degree of technical skill. Allograft bone offers an alternative if autogenous bone is not available or is of poor quality. Anterior instrumentation for the stabilization of kyphosis is appealing. Correction of the deformity and placement of the bone graft under compression can be accomplished in one surgery. The early success of some of these systems is promising, and further development and refinement is anticipated.

The indications for operative intervention in Scheuermann's kyphosis are intractable pain, progressive deformity, and neurologic impairment. The indications for surgical intervention in females may be set at a lower limit because of their predisposition toward kyphotic deformity secondary to osteoporosis. Anterior and posterior spinal surgery is advocated. The first stage includes anterior release to accommodate lengthening of the anterior column and interbody or inlay graft to provide support. The second stage consists of posterior fusion and instrumentation in a compression construct to shorten the posterior column. The entire length of the kyphosis must be stabilized to prevent adding on to the deformity.

Post-traumatic kyphosis is a result of failure of the initial fracture management. The best treatment is its prevention by appropriate early fracture care. The sequelae of post-traumatic kyphosis are the development of a progressive, painful deformity and the risk of neurologic compromise. Laminectomy, without stabilization, has no role in fracture management. Anterior decompression can produce significant neurologic recovery in some cases, even if performed quite late. Reconstruction of post-traumatic kyphosis must follow biomechanical principles. Anterior fusion is appropriate for mild deformities with posterior stability. Anterior and posterior surgery are required for the more severe or unstable deformity.

The surgical treatment of senile kyphosis should be regarded as a salvage procedure. The indications for intervention are intractable pain and neurologic compromise. The goals of surgery are the in situ stabilization of pathologic fractures and the decompression of the neural structures. Of course, the optimal treatment of osteoporotic kyphosis is prevention through appropriate exercise, nutrition, and hormonal replacement.

A better understanding of the biomechanics of the kyphotic deformity has led to a more rational approach to its surgical correction. The basic principles of elongating the anterior column, providing adequate anterior support, and shortening the posterior column must be observed. The sagittal vertical axis provides a guide to the restoration of a physiologic sagittal balance. The importance of maintaining a normal sagittal contour is now being recognized in the correction of frontal-plane deformities as well. Despite these advances, the surgical correction of kyphotic deformity remains a challenge.

References

1. Arciero RA, Leung KYK, Pierce JH: Spontaneous unstable burst fracture of the thoracolumbar spine in osteoporosis. Spine 14:114, 1989
2. Berg A: Contribution to the technique in fusion operations on the spine. Acta Orthop Scand 17:1, 1948
3. Berns DH, Blaser SI, Modic MT: Magnetic resonance imaging of the spine. Clin Orthop 244:78, 1989
4. Bjerkreim I, Magnoaes B, Semb G: Surgical treatment of severe angular kyphosis. Acta Orthop Scand 53:913, 1982
5. Bohlman HH: Late progressive paralysis and pain after fractures of the thoracolumbar spine. J Bone Joint Surg [Am] 58A:728, 1976
6. Bradford DS: Kyphosis [editorial]. Clin Orthop 128:2, 1977
7. Bradford DS: Anterior vascular pedicle bond grafting for the treatment of kyphosis. Spine 5:318,1980
8. Bradford DS, Ahmed KB, Moe JH, et al: The surgical management of patients with Scheuermann's disease. A review of twenty-four cases managed by combined anterior and posterior spine fusion. J Bone Joint Surg [Am] 62:705, 1980
9. Bradford DS, Brown DM, Moe JH, et al: Scheuermann's kyphosis: A form of osteoporosis. Clin Orthop 118:10, 1976
10. Bradford DS, Daher YH: Vascularized rib grafts for stabilization of kyphosis. J Bone Joint Surg [Br] 68:357, 1986
11. Bradford DS, Ganjavian S, Antonious D, et al: Anterior strut grafting for the treatment of kyphosis. J Bone Joint Surg [Am] 64:680, 1982
12. Bradford DS, Lonstein JE, Ogilvie JW, Winter RB: Scoliosis and Other Spinal Deformities, 2nd ed. Philadelphia, WB Saunders, 1987
13. Bradford DS, Moe JH, Montalvo FJ, Winter RB: Scheuermann's kyphosis: Results of surgical treatment by posterior spine arthrodesis in twenty-two patients. J Bone Joint Surg [Am] 57:439, 1975
14. Bradford DS, Winter RB, Lonstein JE, Moe JH: Techniques of anterior spinal surgery for the management of kyphosis. Clin Orthop 128:129, 1977
15. Brown LP, Bridwell KH, Holt RT, Jennings J: Aortic erosions and lacerations associated with the Dunn anterior spinal instrumentation. Orthop Trans 10:16, 1986
16. Chow RK, Harrison JE: Relationship of kyphosis to physical fitness and bone mass on post-menopausal women. Am J Phys Med 66:219, 1987
17. Coscia MF, Bradford DS, Ogilvie JW: Scheuermann's kyphosis: Results in 19 cases treated by spinal arthrodesis and L-rod instrumentation. Orthop Trans 12:255, 1988
18. Cummings SR: Epidemiology of osteoporotic fractures. In Genaut HK (ed): Osteoporosis Update 1987, p 7. San Francisco, Radiology Research and Education Foundation, 1987
19. Desmet AA, Robinson RG, Johnson BE, et al: Spinal compression fractures in osteoporotic women: Patterns and relationships to hyperkyphosis. Radiology 166:497, 1988
20. DeWald RL, Shook JE, Rodts MF: Fiber-metal struts for spinal kyphotic afflictions. Orthop Trans 8:152, 1984
21. Dunn HK: Anterior stabilization of thoracolumbar injuries. Clin Orthop 189:116, 1984
22. Fergusson AB: The etiology of preadolescent kyphosis. J Bone Joint Surg [Am] 38:149, 1956
23. Fon GT, Pitt MJ, Theis AC Jr: Thoracic kyphosis: Range in normal subjects. AJR 134:979, 1980

24. Gardner A, Wozniak AP, Logroscino C: The use of an anterior spinal distractor in the treatment of kyphotic deformity and post-traumatic instability. Orthop Trans 11:95, 1987

25. Gillet P, Jodoin A: Post-traumatic chronic kyphosis: A report of 13 cases. J Bone Joint Surg [Br] 68:853, 1986

26. Gurr KR, McAfee PC: Cotrel–Dubousset instrumentation in adults: A preliminary report. Spine 13:510, 1988

27. Hammerberg KW, DeWald RL: Senile burst fracture: A complication of osteoporosis. Orthop Trans 13:97, 1989

28. Healey JH, Lane JM: Structural scoliosis in osteoporotic women. Clin Orthop 195:216, 1985

29. Herndon WA, Emans JB, Micheli LJ, Hall JF: Combined anterior and posterior fusion for Scheuermann's kyphosis. Spine 6:125, 1981

30. Hubbard LF, Herndon JH, Buouanno AR: Free vascularized fibula transfer for stabilization of the thoracolumbar spine. A case report. Spine 10:891, 1985

31. Ippolito E, Ponseti IV: Juvenile kyphosis. Histological and histochemical studies. J Bone Joint Surg [Am] 63:175, 1981

32. Jensen GF, Christiansen C, Boesen J, et al: Epidemiology of postmenopausal spinal and long bone fractures: A unifying approach to postmenopausal osteoporosis. Clin Orthop 166:75, 1982

33. Jones ET, Hensinger RN: Spinal deformity in idiopathic juvenile osteoporosis. Spine 6:1, 1981

34. Kaneda K, Kuniyoshi A, Fujiya M: Burst fractures with neurologic deficits of the thoracolumbar spine: Results of anterior decompression and stabilization with anterior instrumentation. Spine 9:788, 1984

35. Kaneda K, Kurakami C, Minami A: Free vascularized fibular strut graft in the treatment of kyphosis. Spine 13:1273, 1988

36. Kostuik JP: Anterior Kostuik-Harrington distraction systems. Orthopedics 11:1379, 1985

37. Kostuik JP, Matsusai H: Anterior stabilization, instrumentation, and decompression for post-traumatic kyphosis. Spine 14:379, 1989

38. Lonstein JE, Winter RB, Moe JH, et al: Neurologic deficits secondary to spinal deformity: A review of the literature and report of 43 cases. Spine 5:331, 1980

39. Louis R: Surgery of the Spine. Surgical Anatomy and Operative Approaches, p 50. Berlin, Springer-Verlag, 1983

40. Lowe TG: Double L-rod instrumentation in the treatment of severe kyphosis secondary to Scheuermann's disease. Spine 12:336, 1987

41. Lubicky JR, Fredrickson BE, Yuan HA, Froehling A: Sintered fibermetal implants: An experimental evaluation. Orthop Trans 8:152, 1984

42. Malcolm BW: Spinal deformity secondary to spinal injury. Orthop Clin North Am 10:943, 1979

43. Malcolm BW, Bradford DS, Winter RB, Chou SN: Post-traumatic kyphosis: A review of forty-eight surgically treated patients. J Bone Joint Surg [Am] 63:891, 1981

44. McBride GG, Bradford DS: Vertebral body replacement with femoral neck allograft and vascularized rib strut graft: A technique for treatment of post-traumatic kyphosis with neurologic deficit. Spine 8:406, 1983

45. Micheli LJ, Yost J, Hall JE: Indications for solid rod Dwyer instrumentation. Orthop Trans 6:29, 1982

46. Milne JS, Lander IJ: Age effects in kyphosis and lordosis in adults. Ann Hum Biol 1:327, 1974

47. Montgomery SP, Erwin WE: Scheuermann's kyphosis—long-term results of Milwaukee brace treatment. Spine 6:5, 1981

48. Nerubay J, Katznelson A: Dual approach in the surgical treatment of juvenile kyphosis. Spine 22:101, 1986

49. Pinto WC, Avanzi O, Winter RB: An anterior distraction for the intraoperative correction of angular kyphosis. Spine 3:309, 1978

50. Riseborough EJ, Herndon JH: Scoliosis and Other Deformities of the Axial Skeleton. Boston, Little, Brown, 1975

51. Roaf R: Vertebral growth and its mechanical control. J Bone Joint Surg [Br] 42:40, 1960

52. Roberson JR, Whitesides TE: Surgical reconstruction of late post-traumatic thoracolumbar kyphosis. Spine 10:307, 1985

53. Rose GK, Owen R, Sanderson JM: Transposition of rib with blood supply for the stabilization of spinal kyphos. J Bone Joint Surg [Br] 57:112, 1975

54. Sachs B, Bradford DS, Winter RB, et al: Scheuermann's kyphosis: Follow-up of Milwaukee-brace treatment. J Bone Joint Surg [Am] 69:50, 1987

55. Salomon C, Chopin D, Benoist M: Spinal cord compression: An exceptional complication of spinal osteoporosis. Spine 13:222, 1988

56. Scheuermann HW: Kyphosis dorsalis juvenilis. Z Orthop Chir 41:305, 1921

57. Schmorl Gl, Junghauns H: The Human Spine in Health and Disease, p 354. New York, Grune & Stratton, 1971

58. Shaffer JW, Davy DT, Field GA: The superiority of vascularized compared to nonvascularized rib grafts in spine surgery shown by biological and physical methods. Spine 13:1150, 1988

59. Shufflebarger HL: Cotrel–Dubousset instrumentation for Scheuermann's kyphosis. Orthop Trans 13:90, 1989

60. Slot GH: A new distraction system for the correction of kyphosis using the anterior approach. Orthop Trans 6:29, 1982

61. Sorenson KH: Scheuermann's Juvenile Kyphosis. Copenhagen, Munksgaard, 1964

62. Speck GR, Chopin DC: The surgical treatment of Scheuermann's kyphosis. Spine 68:189, 1986

63. Stagnara P, DeMauroy JC, Drau G, et al: Reciprocal angulation of vertebral bodies in a sagittal plane: Approach to references for the evaluation of kyphosis and lordosis. Spine 7:335, 1982

64. Streitz W, Brown JC, Bonnett CA: Anterior fibular strut grafting in the treatment of kyphosis. Clin Orthop 128:140, 1977

65. Sutherland CJ, Miller F, Wang GJ: Early progressive kyphosis after compression fractures. Two case reports and a series of "stable" thoracolumbar compression fractures. Clin Orthop 173:216, 1983

66. Suzuke N: Studies on posture of healthy Japanese adults: A classification of postures and their relation to changes in different age groups. J Jpn Orthop Assoc 52:471, 1978

67. Takemitsu Y, Harada Y, Iwahara T, et al: Lumbar degenerative kyphosis: Clinical, radiological and epidemiological studies. Spine 13:1317, 1988
68. Taylor TC, Wenger DR, Stephen J, et al: Surgical management of thoracic kyphosis in adolescents. J Bone Joint Surg [Am] 61:496, 1979
69. Thevnon A, Pollez B, Cantegrit F, et al: Relationship between kyphosis, scoliosis, and osteoporosis in the elderly population. Spine 12:744, 1987
70. Tupper JW, Gunn DR: Factors influencing stability of spine fractures. Orthop Trans 1:132, 1977
71. Voutsinas SA, MacEwen GD: Sagittal profiles of the spine. Clin Orthop 210:235, 1986
72. White AA, Panjabi MM: Clinical Biomechanics of the Spine, p 4. Philadelphia, JB Lippincott, 1978
73. White AA, Panjabi MM, Thomas CL. The clinical biomechanics of kyphotic deformities. Clin Orthop 128:8, 1977
74. Whitesides TE: Traumatic kyphosis of the thoracolumbar spine. Clin Orthop 128:78, 1977
75. Winter RB, Hall JE: Kyphosis in childhood and adolescence. Spine 3:285, 1978

CHAPTER

19

∎∎∎

Ankylosing Spondylitis

Kim W. Hammerberg
Hans-Joachim Hehne
Klaus Zielke

∎

ANKYLOSING SPONDYLITIS

KIM W. HAMMERBERG

Ankylosing spondylitis is a chronic inflammatory disease that affects the axial skeleton, causing pain and progressive stiffness. Ankylosing spondylitis is a member of a group of rheumatoid diseases called seronegative spondyloarthropathies.[10] Other members of this group include spondylitis associated with colitis, psoriasis, and Reiter's syndrome.[11, 12] Ankylosing spondylitis has been referred to as Marie-Strümpell disease or Von Bechterew arthritis in the European literature. Past reports have called it rheumatoid spondylitis, pelvospondylitis ossificans, and spondylitis ankylopoietica. Owing to the propensity for spinal fractures and the development of spinal deformity, ankylosing spondylitis is the spondyloarthropathy that most frequently requires the attention of the spinal surgeon.

The prevalence of ankylosing spondylitis is estimated to be 0.5 to 1.0 per 1000 in the white male population.[18, 38] The prevalence in white females is almost equal to males, greater than previously thought. The course of the disease is generally more severe in males.

PATHOGENESIS

Ankylosing spondylitis is associated with the histocompatibility antigen HLA-B27. Histocompatibility testing has identified the HLA-B27 antigen in 88 to 96% of patients with ankylosing spondylitis.[7, 54] This antigen is found in only 7% of the general white population. The HLA-B27 antigen is uncommon in blacks, which accounts for the lower prevalence of this disease among them.[4]

HLA-B27 is inherited in a mendelian fashion. Studies of the prevalence of ankylosing spondylitis in families and racial groups clearly indicate that heredity is a factor in disease pathogenesis.[64] However, ankylosing spondylitis is seen in patients without the HLA-B27 antigen, suggesting that other factors, perhaps environmental, are also necessary for the development of the disease.

The HLA-B27 antigen appears to be a common denominator with the other seronegative spondyloarthropathies. The HLA-B27 antigen may distinguish a group of individuals whose immune response to an infectious agent predisposes them to the development of a spondyloarthropathy through the phenomenon of molecular mimicry.

In patients with ankylosing spondylitis, a direct connection between positive fecal cultures for *Klebsiella pneumoniae* and disease activity has been demonstrated.[25] *Klebsiella pneumoniae* shares a sequence of six consecutive amino acids with the HLA-B27 antigen.[56] Antibodies raised against a peptide derived from HLA-B27 cross-reacted with a peptide derived from *Klebsiella* and vice versa. Although not yet substantiated, this response suggests that, through molecular mimicry, an immune reaction stimulated by the invading organism could be redirected against the host tissue. In fact, these antibodies have reacted with articular tissue from HLA-B27–positive patients with ankylosing spondylitis.[57, 69]

PATHOLOGY

The progressive inflammatory changes seen in ankylosing spondylitis primarily involve the articulations of the spine and frequently the hip and shoulder. Less commonly, the peripheral joints are affected; on occasion, the eye and heart are involved.

The earliest histopathologic changes occur in the sacroiliac joints. Lone sacroiliitis is uncommon, and progression up the spine is a function of disease duration. Skip lesions rarely occur, but they are more likely to occur in women.[15]

The diarthrodial joints of the spine and peripheral joints exhibit a synovitis that resembles rheumatoid arthritis. Proliferation of the synovium is accompanied by focal accumulation of lymphoid and plasma cells. Pannus formation produces cartilage destruction and bony erosions. Ultimately, these changes are followed by a reparative phase, causing fibrous and bony ankylosis.

The sequence of events in cartilaginous joints, synchondroses, is somewhat different. These joints include the intervertebral disc, symphysis pubis, manubriosternal, and the sacroiliac joint. Initially, chronic inflammatory cells are localized to the subchondral bone on either side of the joint. The radiographic changes at this time are manifested by periarticular osteopenia.[22] Second, the articular cartilage is destroyed by osteoclasts and replaced by exuberant granulation tissue. The corresponding radiographs

show extensive erosion and destruction of the joint space. The late stage of the disease consists of ossification and complete obliteration of the joint. The pattern of new bone formation varies considerably from patient to patient. Radiographs demonstrate sclerotic bone of early healing and later normal density bone after remodelling.

The primary site of inflammation is at the junction of fibrous and bone tissue, such as the bony insertion of a tendon or ligament.[3] The resulting enthesitis leads to bone erosion and eventual ossification of these structures. In the spine, the enthesitis occurs at the insertion of the annulus fibrosus on the vertebral body. The erosive phase of the inflammation at this site gives the vertebra a square appearance on radiographs (Fig. 19-1). Ossification of the annulus fibrosus produces the syndesmophytes and eventually the "bamboo spine" picture typical of ankylosing spondylitis (Fig. 19-2). Surprisingly, the anterior longitudinal ligament remains free of ossification.

Cardiac involvement may occur in ankylosing spondylitis. Specifically, focal necrosis at the root of the aorta producing dilatation of the aortic ring causes aortic insufficiency. Fibrosis may invade the membranous septum and the atrioventricular bundle, causing conduction defects. Other nonskeletal sites of involvement include the anterior uvea, kidney, and lung.

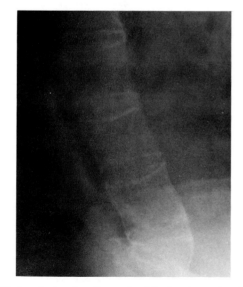

FIG. 19–1. Lateral radiograph of the lumbar spine demonstrating the early changes of ankylosing spondylitis. Notice squarish corners of the vertebral bodies and fine bridging syndesmophytes.

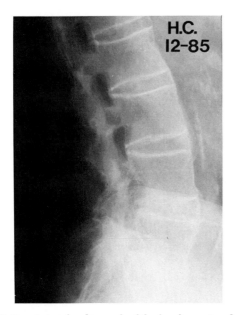

FIG. 19–2. Lateral radiograph of the lumbar spine demonstrating well-developed syndesmophytes secondary to ossification of the annulus fibrosus. Also notice ossification of the posterior ligamentous structures.

CLINICAL MANIFESTATIONS

The onset of symptoms from ankylosing spondylitis typically occurs between the ages of 15 and 50 years.[59] A subgroup of patients with the onset of symptoms who were younger than 16 years has been identified as having juvenile-onset ankylosing spondylitis. There seems to be few differences in overall outcome between juvenile-onset and adult-onset ankylosing spondylitis other than a greater disposition toward hip involvement in the juvenile type.[16]

The insidious onset of low back pain usually heralds the onset of symptoms. The pain is associated with stiffness and may be referred to the buttocks or posterior thighs. The complaints are episodic, with varying intensity and duration. As the disease becomes more established, the patient frequently notices increased pain and stiffness in the morning. Also, the patient notices ascension of the discomfort up the spine to include the thoracic cage and shoulders. Peripheral joints may be stiff and tender, especially at the entheses. After the spine is ankylosed, the majority of symptoms resolve. The inflammatory process appears to quiesce by the time the patient reaches the late fourth or fifth decade.[20]

A late, but fortunately rare, manifestation of ankylosing spondylitis is a cauda equina syndrome. Patients with quiescent disease may present acutely with lower extremity numbness and weakness, impotence, and incontinence. Myelography demonstrates multiple arachnoid cysts. The pathogenesis is not understood.[27, 50, 52] Another serious neurologic manifestation of ankylosing spondylitis is spontaneous atlantoaxial subluxation; this has been reported in both juvenile and adult-onset disease.[58, 66]

Nonskeletal manifestations of the disease include acute anterior uveitis, uremia secondary to renal amyloidosis, and pulmonary fibrosis. Aortic insufficiency and conduction defects characterize cardiac involvement. These conditions may contribute to the cause of death in up to 10% of ankylosing spondylitis patients.[13, 22]

DIAGNOSIS

Physical Examination

The patient with advanced ankylosing spondylitis is easily identified by his or her stooped posture and rigid, kyphotic spine. In the upright position, increased thoracic kyphosis is observed with loss of the normal lumbar lordosis. As the disease progresses, the loss of normal sagittal contour becomes more pronounced, with the development of a general hyperkyphosis (Fig. 19-3).

Motion of the lumbar spine is demonstrated by the Schober test. The Schober test is performed by marking the lumbosacral junction and midline points 10 cm above and 5 cm below it. The patient then bends forward maximally. Normal lumbar motion increases the distance between these two points by at least 5 cm. Costovertebral joint involvement is demonstrated by measuring chest expansion at the nipple line. In normal young men, chest expansion of at least 5 cm is expected.

Motion at the hips should be a standard part of the examination. Fixed flexion deformities of the hip are common in ankylosing spondylitis. The hip deformities must be included in the assessment of the overall trunk deformity. Correction of severe hip flexion deformities by arthroplasty can allow enough compensation of trunk balance that the spinal deformity will not require realignment.

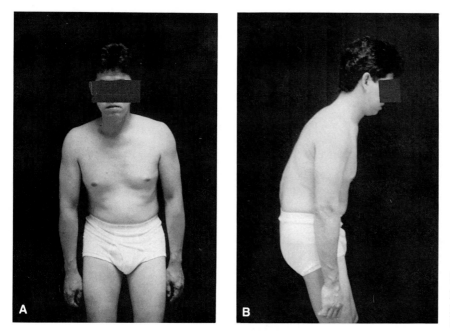

FIG. 19–3. Generalized rigid kyphosis of the entire spine. Stooped posture is compensated by flexion at hips and knees.

Early in the disease, physical findings may be minimal and nonspecific because of the variable penetrance and expression of the disease. The enthesopathy can be elicited as tenderness to direct palpation over the heels, greater trochanters, iliac crests, spinous processes, and costosternal joints. Sacroiliac involvement can be demonstrated by provocative maneuvers, such as Gaenslen's test, that stress the sacroiliac joint. The test is performed with the patient supine with one buttock extending over the edge of the table. Both hips are maximally flexed, and the ipsilateral leg is slowly extended over the edge of the table, hyperextending the hip. A positive test results in the reproduction of sacroiliac pain.

Laboratory Evaluation

The erythrocyte sedimentation rate (ESR) is elevated in approximately 80% of ankylosing spondylitis patients. The ESR may be normal despite inflammation that appears to be quite active. The ESR does not accurately reflect fluctuations of disease activity in the same patient. Serum creatinine phosphokinase is frequently elevated and may be a more sensitive and specific indicator of disease activity.[14,45]

The cerebral spinal fluid may demonstrate a mild to moderate elevation of protein. Peripheral joint fluid analysis reveals a moderate neutrophilic leukocytosis.

The rheumatoid factor is invariably negative, even in active peripheral joint disease. Testing for the HLA-B27 antigen is positive in approximately 90% of white patients with ankylosing spondylitis. A negative rheumatoid factor and a positive HLA-B27 strongly suggest ankylosing spondylitis in a patient with suspicious symptoms but without confirmatory radiographic findings.

Radiography

Early in the course of the disease radiographic findings may be minimal, and radionucleotide scanning may prove more useful. Technetium 99 bone scan can demonstrate the sacroiliitis before radiographic changes.[51]

The radiographic changes of well-established ankylosing spondylitis are diagnostic. The earliest changes are visible at the sacroiliac joint. These changes occur in three distinct phases, the first characterized by subchondral or periarticular osteopenia. As the inflammation advances, erosion and loss of the articular space is noted. The healing phase is denoted by subchondral sclerosis that increases until new bone formation bridges, then obliterates, the joint.[48]

An early radiographic change in the spine is squaring of the anterior corners of the thoracic and lumbar vertebrae. Vertebral osteoporosis frequently accompanies the loss of normal endplate concavity.[29]

Paravertebral ossification is manifested by syndesmophyte formation. This ossification occurs within the substance of the annulus fibrosus and forms a bony bridge between the involved vertebra. Early the syndesmophytes are fine and well demarcated; in later stages, they give rise to the typical bamboo spine appearance.

The posterior spinal structures are also included in the disease process, including the capsules of the zygapophyseal joints, the interspinous and supraspinous ligaments, and the ligamentum flavum. Advanced involvement of these structures can give the spine a "trolley track" appearance on radiographs (Fig. 19-4).

The upper cervical spine may paradoxically demonstrate hypermobility in ankylosing spondylitis. Perhaps as a result of the extensive ankylosis of the subaxial spine, atlantoaxial instability has been observed.[5]

Radiographic changes in peripheral joints are also noted in ankylosing spondylitis. The changes are osteopenia, erosion, and ossification consistent with inflammation and later healing at the common sites of entheseopathy. The hip joints may be more selectively involved in the process than the other peripheral joints. The hips may undergo severe erosive changes and ossification resulting in complete ankylosis. Total hip arthroplasty is eventually required by a large percentage of patients with ankylosing spondylitis (Fig. 19-5).[17]

MEDICAL MANAGEMENT

Approximately 10 to 20% of HLA-B27−positive patients develop ankylosing spondylitis.[18] The prognosis for an individual patient is difficult to predict; however, most patients with ankylosing spondylitis have a good prognosis for a productive life, despite intermittent pain.

Nonsteroidal anti-inflammatory medication is the main modality in the treatment of the discomfort associated with ankylosing spondylitis. Unlike rheumatoid arthritis, gold and penicillamine have no role in the management of ankylosing spondylitis. The most effective medication appears to be phenylbutazone. Indomethacin is almost as effective and is the drug of choice because of its lesser toxicity. Aspirin does not appear to be beneficial in the management of ankylosing spondylitis.[26]

In part, the purpose of medication is to enable the patient to participate in a regular, regimented exercise program. The spine and hip involvement produces increased thoracolumbar kyphosis and fixed flexion deformities. A postural exercise program is designed to maintain extension of the spine and hips. Stretching exercises can increase and maintain hip motion in ankylosing spondylitis if performed conscientiously.[9, 46] The patient must adopt an overall lifestyle conducive to proper spinal alignment and normal activity.

SURGICAL TREATMENT

Most patients with ankylosing spondylitis do not require surgical intervention. Spinal surgery, if necessary, is indicated in two situations: the correction of fixed flexion deformities of the spinal column, and the stabilization of spine fractures and their sequela, spondylodiscitis, which are relatively frequent occurrences in ankylosing spondylitis. In fact, the proclivity of the spine to suffer fractures in ankylosing spondylitis may be a primary factor in the subsequent development of flexion deformities.

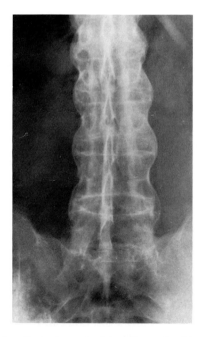

FIG. 19–4. Posterior-anterior radiograph of lumbar spine demonstrating advanced ankylosis and typical bamboo spine picture. Ankylosis of posterior structures gives rise to trolley track appearance and complete obliteration of the sacroiliac joints.

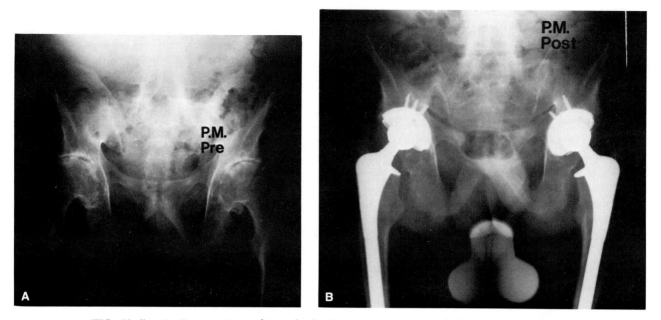

FIG. 19–5.   **A.** Preoperative radiograph of pelvis in patient with ankylosing spondylitis and marked hip involvement.   **B.** Postoperative radiograph after bilateral total hip replacements.

Fixed Flexion Deformities

Surgical Indications

The indications for the correction of a fixed flexion deformity of the spine are relative. The primary indications are the magnitude of deformity and the functional limitations it produces. For many patients, the chief complaint at presentation is the inability to look straight ahead. The kyphotic deformity restricts daily activities like interpersonal communication and driving because of a fixed, inadequate line of view. These indications, of course, are balanced by the patient's age, general health, and willingness to accept the risks and rigors of major spinal surgery.

Preoperative Assessment

The preoperative assessment of an ankylosing spondylitis patient for corrective surgery must be directed at determining the primary site of the deformity. The assessment should also evaluate associated conditions that could complicate or alter the surgical decision.

The kyphotic spinal deformity is frequently accompanied by an associated fixed flexion deformity of the hips. In a few instances, correction of the hip deformity by arthroplasty allows sufficient motion to compensate for the residual trunk deformity. In most cases, the hip ankylosis should be addressed before correcting the

spinal deformity. Unless the hips can be fully extended in the upright position, the sagittal vertical axis will remain well anterior of the spinal column. This unbalanced posture makes any posterior fixation and healing tenuous at best. The chin–brow vertical angle is a means of quantifying the clinical deformity (Fig. 19-6). The goal of surgery is to restore a horizontal gaze. Standing posterior-anterior and lateral radiographs of the entire spine are useful for assessing the overall deformity. Tomography may be helpful to image the cervicothoracic junction. Spot radiographs of the lumbar spine may demonstrate levels of incomplete or "soft" ankylosis, which may be preferable sites for osteotomy.

The most significant correction of a fixed kyphotic deformity can be achieved by osteotomy at the site of the major deformity. The chin-on-chest deformity obviously demands osteotomy at the base of the cervical spine.

Patients with thoracolumbar kyphosis fall into two main categories. The first group consists of patients with a significant thoracic kyphosis and a fairly normal cervical and lumbar lordosis. This group requires correction at the site of the major deformity, the thoracic spine, by multiple posterior osteotomies. The second group of patients demonstrates a generalized kyphosis of the entire thoracolumbar spine, with loss of lumbar

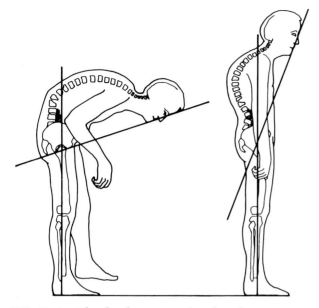

FIG. 19–6. The chin-brow vertical angle is the intersection of a line drawn from the chin to the brow and a vertical line. The angle corresponds to the correction needed to restore a horizontal line of vision. (With permission of Simmons EH: Surgery of the spine in ankylosing spondylitis and rheumatoid arthritis. In Chapman MW (ed): Operative Orthopedics, vol 3, p 2087. Philadelphia, JB Lippincott, 1988)

lordosis. In this group, spinal alignment can be corrected by a compensatory osteotomy in the lumbar spine. This can obviate the need for multiple osteotomies at the spinal cord level. The most important goal is to restore a physiologic sagittal vertical axis.

Isolated kyphosis of the lumbar spine is best managed by lumbar osteotomy. At any level, overcorrection must be avoided because of the lack of compensatory motion. The overall deformity may be so severe that osteotomy at more than one region of the spine is necessary. In these instances, the cervical osteotomy should be performed first.

Lumbar Osteotomy

Smith-Peterson and colleagues, in 1945, described a technique of posterior osteotomy for the correction of a fixed flexion deformity of the spine.[63] The report details the surgical technique employed in 6 cases. The osteotomies were V-shaped, performed at one or more levels, and closed by forced hyperextension. The levels on radiographs that demonstrated the least anterior ossification were selected for osteotomy. Often overlooked, this report included a case of multilevel thoracic osteotomies.

A year later, LaChappelle advocated a two-stage procedure for the correction of this deformity.[35] The first stage consisted of a posterior laminectomy under local anesthesia; the second stage, performed 2 weeks later, was an anterior-opening wedge osteotomy and fusion.

Further modification and refinements in surgical technique have been reported by many authors. Herbert recommended a one- or two-stage procedure, depending on the amount of correction achieved at the posterior osteotomy and osteoclasis.[31, 32]

In 1969, Law reported a series of 120 lumbar osteotomies. These were performed after the Smith-Peterson technique with the patient in the prone or lateral position. The objectives included restoration of erect posture, relief of rib encroachment on the abdomen, and improvement in diaphragmatic excursion. He indicated that thoracic osteotomy is possible, but it is much more difficult because the fused costotransverse joints and the smaller spinal canal allow for less correction.[36, 37]

Law recognized the advantage of internal fixation of the osteotomy in maintaining correction and permitting earlier mobilization of the patient. Other large series attest to the benefit of internal fixation.[43, 60]

Thomasen described a combined laminectomy and posterior decancellation of the L2 vertebral body.[65] It is similar to a procedure described by Scudese and Calabro 20 years earlier.[55] The operation shortens the vertebral column, avoiding stretch of the anterior neurovascular structures, a problem recognized by Adam in 1952.[1]

Zielke recommended multilevel osteotomy and pedicle screw fixation.[30, 47] Realignment over multiple levels, in theory, should restore a more physiologic sagittal contour. My experience is similar to that of McMaster, who noted that, despite multilevel osteotomies, the majority of the correction almost invariably occurred at one level.[44] Multilevel osteotomies increase the likelihood of pseudarthrosis and risk the potential complications involved in the osteotomies themselves.

Surgical Technique. Our technique of lumbar osteotomy is a modification of the Smith-Peterson operation. Surgery is performed in the prone position under general endotracheal anesthesia. Before surgery, the patient can be tried on the Relton-Hall frame. At the same time, the wake-up test is rehearsed. Alternatives to the frame include blanket rolls or foam rubber cushions placed transversely across the chest and abdomen. In cases of extreme deformity, the patient is placed in a lateral decubitus position. An awake, fiberoptic intubation is performed before general anesthesia is induced (Fig. 19-7). Somatosensory evoked potentials are employed for monitoring. The patient is carefully rolled on the frame to minimize risk of cervical fracture. The frame is elongated as much as possible, and the legs are elevated on cushions to facilitate the forced lordotic osteoclasis.

The lumbar spine is exposed through a midline longitudinal skin incision. The paraspinal musculature is stripped subperiosteally to the tips of the transverse processes. A single osteotomy is performed, usually at the L3–L4 interspace. The L2–L3 interspace may be used if radiographs demonstrate a soft ankylosis at this level.

The osteotomy is performed as described by Smith-Peterson. The amount of bone to be removed is determined by the brow–chin vertical angle. The patient's occupation must be considered; for example, a desk worker might be better off with a little less correction than the neutral position. The apex of the wedge is centered on the annulus of the L3–L4 disc and the base over the L3–L4 interspace. Care must be taken to free the dura from the undersurface of the lamina. The dura frequently adheres to the ligamentum flavum at its insertion under the posterior arch. The lamina must be undercut to avoid impingement on the cauda

equina with closure of the osteotomy. Similarly, the pedicles may be partially or completely removed to avoid nerve root entrapment.

Before completion of the osteotomy, hook sites are prepared for the Cotrel–Dubousset instrumentation above and below the osteotomy (Fig. 19-8). Harrington compression instrumentation has been used but does not provide for claw fixation or transverse linkage. Luque instrumentation does not provide the necessary compressive forces, and the passage of sublaminar wires is hazardous because of the frequent dural adhesions.

The osteotomy is closed by firm manual pressure (Fig. 19-9). The anterior structures give way suddenly with a soft snap; Urist describes the sensation "as the sound of breaking a branch from a green tree."[68] If the osteoclasis is complete, the correction is maintained after release of manual pressure. The instrumentation is inserted and secured. The wake-up test is performed to assure the preservation of normal neurologic function. An autologous bone graft is harvested from the ilium and applied to the decorticated lumbar spine. Cancellous allograft bone is often used to supplement the autologous graft because it is frequently rather meager. The wound is closed over a drain in a routine fashion.

In most instances, the disc space opens widely in the front, creating a substantial anterior column defect (Fig. 19-10). A tendency toward a flexion deformity

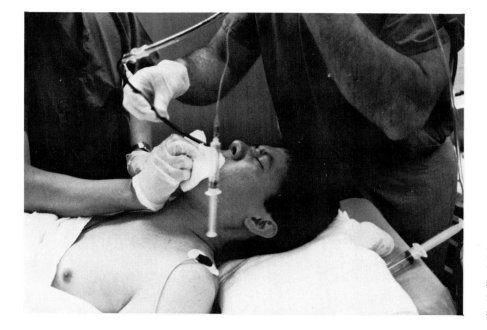

FIG. 19–7. Fiberoptic intubation is routine in patients with ankylosing spondylitis to minimize manipulation of the cervical spine.

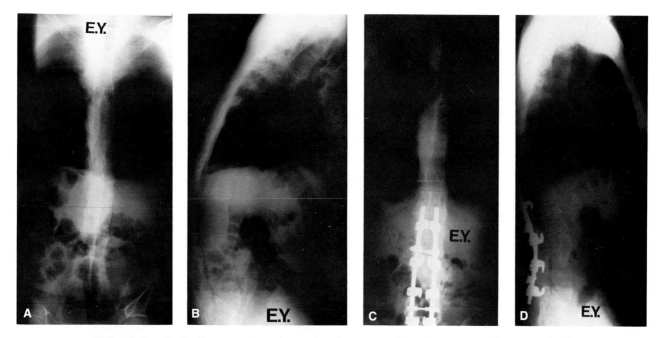

FIG. 19–8. **A, B.** Preoperative radiographs of patient in Fig. 19–3. Notice the generalized ankylosis and kyphosis of the entire spine. **C, D.** Postoperative radiographs after one-level posterior osteotomy and fusion and one-level anterior fusion with an allograft ilium. Sagittal vertical axis has been restored.

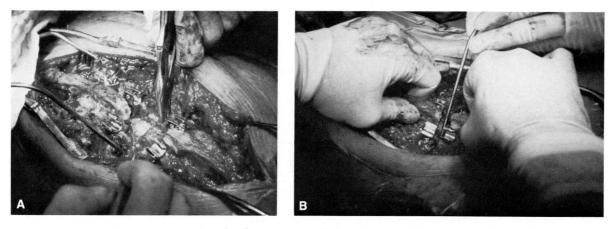

FIG. 19–9. **A.** Preparation of wide osteotomy of L3 to L4 (cephalad is to the left). Bone has been undercut to avoid impingement of cauda equina with closure. Instrumentation sites have already been prepared. **B.** Osteotomy during forced manual osteoclasis. Notice approximation of the hooks.

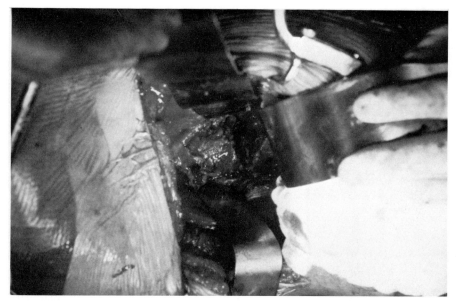

FIG. 19–10. Anterior column defect produced by posterior osteotomy in Fig. 19–8 (ventral is superior, dorsal is inferior, and cephalad is to the right).

persists even though the sagittal vertical axis is shifted posterior to the osteotomy. The bone in ankylosing spondylitis is osteoporotic, offering a less than optimal bone–implant interface. A one-level anterior interbody fusion offers greater stability and improved healing with minimal increase in operative morbidity. The anterior procedure is generally done as a second stage under the same anesthesia (Fig. 19-11).

The patient is nursed postoperatively on a standard hospital bed. Ambulation is encouraged on the second day after surgery. A molded TLSO is fabricated to be worn when out of bed, usually for 6 to 7 months until the fusion is solid.

Thoracic Osteotomy

Simmons indicated that primary thoracic kyphosis can be classified into two groups.[60] In one group, the kyphotic deformity is somewhat flexible, perhaps owing to incomplete anterior ossification or soft ankylosis. The other group consists of patients with rigid primary thoracic deformities.

In the first group with a relatively soft primary thoracic kyphosis, the deformity may correct with gradual halo-gravity traction. After traction satisfactorily realigns the spine, posterior fixation with compression instrumentation and fusion can be performed. If necessary, multiple posterior osteotomies can be done to augment correction by shortening the posterior column. Posterior surgery is not sufficient because of the magnitude of the original deformity and the underlying softness or deficiency of the anterior col-

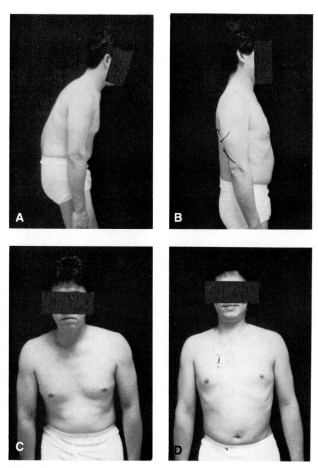

FIG. 19–11. Preoperative and postoperative photographs of patient in Figs. 19–8 and 19–9. Full extension at the hips and a horizontal line of vision have been restored.

umn. The anterior column must be strengthened by inlay and strut grafts.

In the second group of patients with a rigid primary thoracic kyphosis, halo-gravity traction does little. The treatment plan for these patients is similar to that for patients with rigid Scheuermann's kyphosis. Multilevel anterior osteotomy, disc resection, and interbody fusion through the major portion of the kyphosis is the first step. Anterior instrumentation plays no role in this disease because of the extensive posterior ankylosis.

The benefit of intercurrent halo-gravity traction is dubious because of the posterior ankylosis. The second-stage posterior procedure requires multilevel posterior osteotomies, posterior fixation, and autologous bone graft. Cotrel–Dubousset instrumentation, as in Scheuermann's kyphosis, is very effective in correcting and maintaining the deformity. Because the osteoporosis associated with ankylosing spondylitis produces brittle bone, extremes of correction should not be sought to avoid failure at the bone–implant interface.

Correction of the thoracic kyphosis at one level is not advised. The thoracic spinal canal is relatively small, with narrow limits of tolerance. The vascularity of the mid-thoracic spine is the watershed area as described by Dommisse.[23, 24] Because of the costotransverse joint ankylosis, the potential movement at one interspace is quite limited. As Simmons points out, the correction at each level is minimal, yet over multiple levels, a satisfactory cumulative correction can be achieved.

Cervical Osteotomy

The successful correction of a cervical kyphosis was reported by Mason, Cozen, and Adelstein in 1953.[42] A posterior osteotomy was performed distal to C7, and correction was achieved through gradual traction. Urist, in 1958, described a successful correction of a cervical kyphosis by posterior osteotomy and gradual correction in an adjustable brace.[68] Urist recommended that the procedure be performed on a patient under local anesthesia in the sitting position. He emphasized that the optimal site for a cervical osteotomy was between C7 and T1. At this interspace the spinal canal is relatively wide, and the vertebral arteries have not yet entered the foramen transversorum. The seventh and eighth cervical roots are fairly mobile, and if a spinal cord injury was incurred, the upper brachial plexus could be preserved.

Tomography is helpful in the preoperative assessment of these patients. Some cervical kyphoses are

secondary to occult fractures and can be corrected by gradual traction. Tomography can also help assess the degree of anterior ankylosis (Fig. 19-12). In some patients with relatively soft ankylosis, gradual traction can obtain sufficient correction to eliminate the need for posterior osteotomy. If realignment is obtained, it can be maintained by a posterior fusion and halo-vest immobilization.

Simmons reported extensively on osteotomy of the cervical spine in ankylosing spondylitis. In 1982, he summarized 15 years' experience with 67 osteotomies of the spine in 66 patients.[60–62] He developed a technique that satisfactorily corrected the deformity with minimal risk.

Surgical Technique. The technique that follows is essentially that of Simmons and has previously been described in detail.[60–62] A halo cast is applied several days before the procedure. The operation is done with the patient in the sitting position with 9 lb of overhead traction. The patient is awake and alert, not intubated, and local anesthesia is employed.

A posterior midline longitudinal incision is made over the cervicothoracic junction. Deep infiltration of additional local anesthesia is used as necessary. The spine is exposed from approximately C5 to T1. The entire posterior elements of C7 are removed, as well as

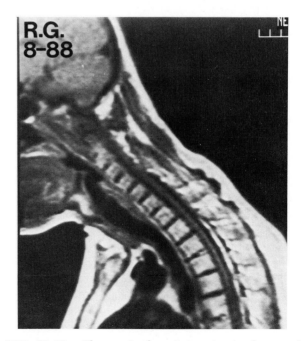

FIG. 19–12. The cervicothoracic junction is often poorly imaged by conventional radiographic techniques, but MRI can be helpful in assessing the deformity.

the caudal half of C6 and the cephalad half of T1. The osteotomy is continued laterally through the facets and lateral masses, out the neural foramen of the eighth cervical nerve (Fig. 19-13).

The amount of bone resection is decided by the difference between the brow–chin line and the vertical angle. The apex of the wedge osteotomy is at the posterior longitudinal ligament, and the base is centered over the lamina of C7 (Fig. 19-14). The amount of bone resected is usually 1.5 to 2.25 cm. At times, the inferior portion of the C7 pedicles and the superior portion of the C8 pedicles must be resected to prevent a pincher effect on the C8 nerve root on closure of the osteotomy. The laminotomies of C6 and C8 should be ovate and undercut to avoid impingement on the cervical cord.

Before the osteoclasis, the deep muscle sutures are placed but not tied, and the drain is placed. The patient is given 100% oxygen for 10 to 15 minutes, and just before the fracture is administered halothane. The neck is extended, fracturing the anterior structures, by the surgeon grasping the halo through the drapes and pulling the head backwards. The osteotomy is closed until the lateral masses appose. An ungowned assistant

stabilizes the head while 100% oxygen is again administered, and normal neurologic function is confirmed. The resected bone is placed laterally and the deep sutures are tied. The remainder of the closure is routine.

After closure, the surgeon can make final adjustments to the head position and stabilize it by attaching the cast uprights to the halo. The patient ambulates to a Circ-o-lectric bed for postoperative management.

At our institution, this procedure has been performed with modification. The patient is fitted with a halo 1 or 2 days before the operation. The halo application is performed in the operating room under local anesthesia and serves as a dress rehearsal for the actual procedure. The patient helps position himself on the operating table in a sitting position comfortable for both him and the surgeon. A molded polyethylene vest with adjustable uprights is used instead of a cast.

The operation is performed on a standard operating table preflexed to a sitting position. The halo uprights are loosely connected to the halo to provide stability during the procedure. Although verbal communication with the patient is beneficial, we feel that the maintenance of an airway is paramount. The patient

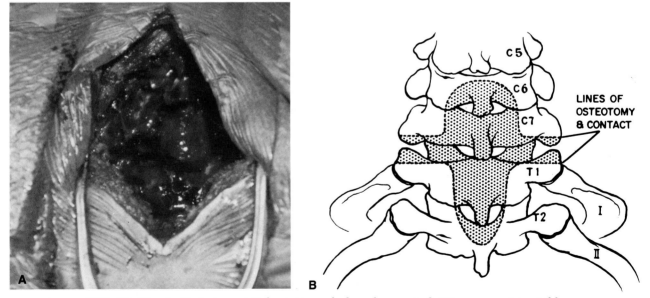

FIG. 19–13. **A.** Posterior cervical osteotomy before closure. Left C8 nerve root is visible exiting the canal. Lamina must be generously resected and undercut. Pedicles can be resected to avoid root entrapment. **B.** Illustration demonstrating ovate osteotomy extending through the lateral masses. (With permission from Urist MR: Osteotomy of the cervical spine. Report of a case of ankylosing rheumatoid spondylitis. J Bone Joint Surg [Am] 40:833, 1958)

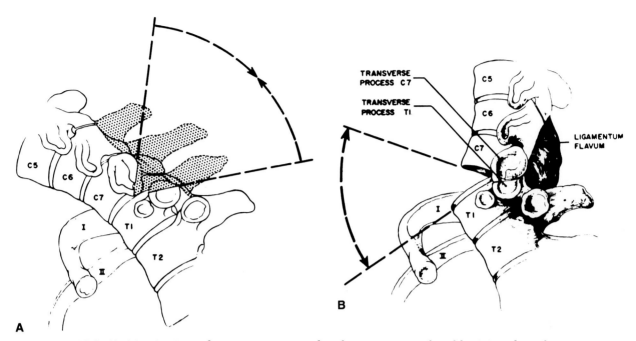

FIG. 19–14. **A.** Apex of osteotomy is centered on the posterior annulus of the C7–T1 disc. The base overlies the C7–T1 interspace. **B.** The osteotomy is closed until contact is obtained between the transverse processes and lateral masses. Care must be taken not to allow translation of C7 on T1. (With permission from Urist MR: Osteotomy of the cervical spine. Report of a case of ankylosing rheumatoid spondylitis. J Bone Joint Surg [Am] 40: 833, 1958)

undergoes an awake fiberoptic endotracheal intubation. This technique is also used for cases of cervical instability, such as fractures and rheumatoid arthritis.

Local anesthestic is employed. Sedation is maintained by a methotrexital sodium infusion. This drug is a rapid, ultrashort-acting barbituate that allows an almost immediate and repeatable wake-up test. Before surgery the patient is taught an elaborate wake-up test to demonstrate intact function of all four extremities. Somatosensory evoked potentials are also used.

The exposure and osteotomy are the same as described by Simmons. The osteoclasis is performed gently; the anterior spine does not crack but seems to give way. Care must be taken to tilt C7 backwards on T1 and not to allow anterior translation. The position is secured by tightening the halo attachments (Fig. 19-15). Bone graft is placed laterally to avoid midline pressure, and the wound is closed routinely over a drain.

After surgery, the patient is transferred to a standard hospital bed. The patient is ambulated the day after surgery. Surprisingly, these patients complain of little postoperative pain. They are often ready for home discharge 7 to 10 days after surgery (Fig. 19-16).

The halo vest is generally maintained for 3 months, followed by a rigid collar for an additional 3 months. Tomograms are obtained approximately 2.5 months after surgery. If healing of the posterior fusion is questionable or if filling of the anterior defect is delayed, an anterior keystone type cervical fusion is performed. The halo vest is maintained until healing is confirmed by tomography (Fig. 19-17).

Internal fixation of the osteotomy provides greater stability, but this advantage is outweighed by several drawbacks. If the deformity is overcorrected or the eighth nerve is entrapped, the head and neck position can be adjusted to reach a neutral position. If incomplete correction is achieved, the patient can be sedated at a later time and further extension achieved by adjusting the halo-vest uprights. Lateral tomography should be obtained before secondary adjustments to evaluate possible anterior translation of C7 on T1. If

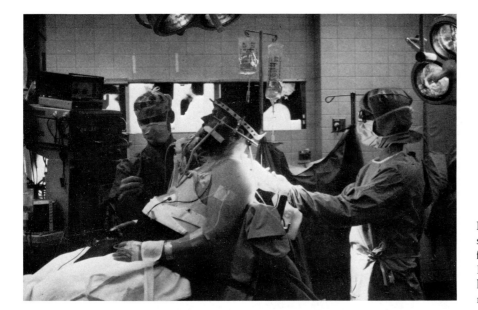

FIG. 19–15. Patient at conclusion of operation. Position is comfortable for patient and surgeon. Extension osteotomy is secured by locking halo-vest uprights in corrected position.

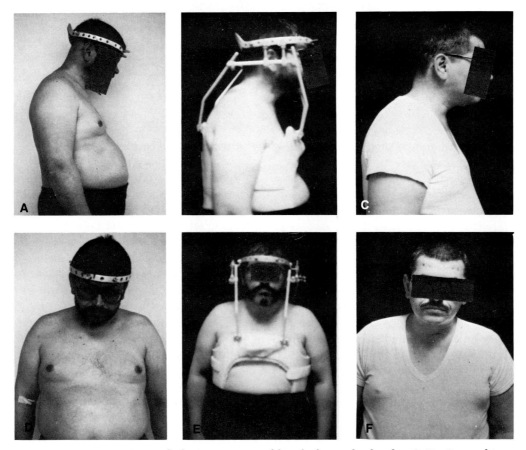

FIG. 19–16.   A, B. Patient before surgery is unable to look straight ahead.   **C, D.** Secured in halo vest. Ambulatory and discharged to home on day 5. Notice change in position of halo.   **E, F.** After anterior keystone fusion, the patient is again able to drive and shave without difficulty.

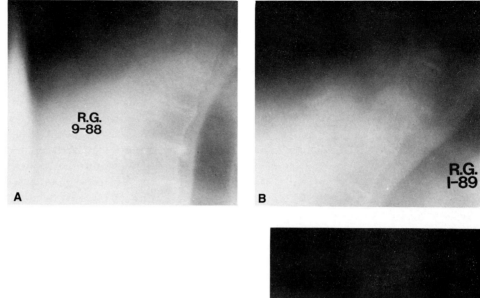

FIG. 19–17. **A.** Lateral tomographs of patient in Fig. 19–16. **B.** Two months after surgery, the anterior healing was questionable. Therefore, an anterior keystone fusion was performed. Notice slight anterior translation of C7 on T1. This must be guarded against during manipulation. **C.** Solid anterior fusion obtained with iliac graft.

significant translation is present, a compromised correction should be accepted. A safer approach to achieve a horizontal gaze may be to perform a compensatory lumbar osteotomy at a later date.

Complications

The complication rate after spinal osteotomy for fixed flexion deformities of the spine has been significant. The mortality rate has been reported as 8 to 10% and the rate of neurologic injury as high as 30%.[43, 60] Herbert and Law both reported an 8% mortality rate.[32, 37] In Herbert's and Law's experiences, approximately half of the deaths were the sequelae of spinal cord injury, such as pneumonia and perforation of gastric ulcers. Law reported 1 patient with cauda equina syndrome and 3 with lumbar root palsies in 120 cases of lumbar

osteotomy. These series include cervical, thoracic, and lumbar osteotomies, and they represent evolutionary experiences in surgical and anesthetic techniques.

Simmons reported a 4% mortality rate.[60] In this series, the causes of death were pulmonary embolism, myocardial infarction, and perforation of a peptic ulcer. He experienced no major neurologic catastrophies but did report 4 cases of C8 root deficits. Camargo and associates reported a series of 66 lumbar osteotomies with no significant neurologic complications.[19] Postoperative ileus, nausea, vomiting, and urinary retention were the most common problems. One patient died 9 days after surgery because of a ruptured aorta. This complication is rare, but it has been reported by others.[39, 71]

Recurrence of the deformity and nonunion of the

osteotomy are often complementary. Their incidence can be reduced by internal fixation of the posterior osteotomy and immediate grafting of the anterior column deficit.

Neurologic injuries appear to be less frequent in more recent series, perhaps owing to improved neurologic monitoring and earlier intervention before end-stage deformity is reached. Advances in patient selection, anesthetic techniques, and postoperative care should decrease the medical complications as well.

Fractures

The spine in ankylosing spondylitis is at high risk for the development of fractures, even after trivial trauma

(Fig. 19-18).[28, 67] These fractures are described by some authors as stress fractures, by others as compression fractures.[33, 34] They are pathologic fractures secondary to the generalized osteoporosis and ossification of the spinal ligaments. The spine cannot absorb the energy of an injury because of the loss of normal resilience.

The mid-cervical spine is the most frequent site of fracture, followed by the thoracolumbar junction.[53, 70, 72] The physician must be alert because these injuries may follow minimal trauma. Demonstration of these fractures radiographically may be difficult owing to the osteopenia and associated deformities. Tomography can often be helpful in demonstrating occult fractures (Fig. 19-19). Following more significant trauma, multiple spine fractures may occur.

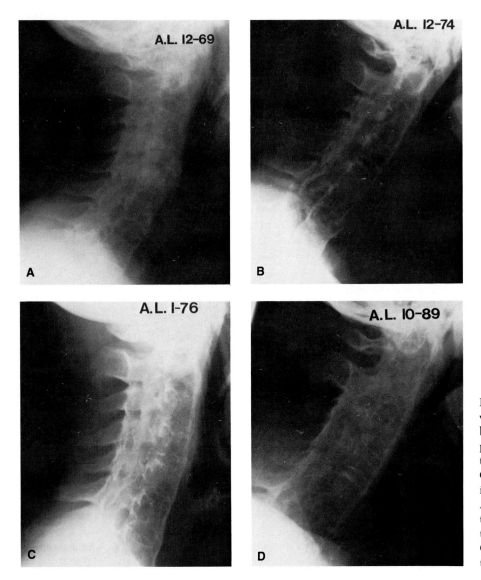

FIG. 19–18. **A.** A.L. in 1969 with fracture at C4 to C5, treated by benign neglect. **B.** Same patient in 1974 with fracture at C6 to C7, treated with halo cast. **C.** A.L. in 1976; notice remodeling of anterior column. **D.** A.L. in 1989 with neck pain after trivial trauma. Suspicion and interruption of ossified ligaments at C6 to C7 revealed another fracture.

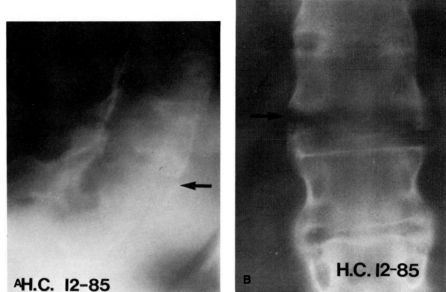

FIG. 19–19. A slip on ice resulted in a double fracture for H.C. **A.** Tomographs demonstrated a fracture at C7 to T1. **B.** A fracture at T12 to L1 was also recognized.

The fractured spine in advanced ankylosing spondylitis can be extremely unstable. Ossification of both anterior and posterior ligamentous structures creates a rigid ring. Fracture of one column of the spine cannot occur alone. Thus, a three-column injury is sustained, resulting in an extremely unstable injury. The most benign-appearing fractures can displace with tragic consequences.

Fractures of the spine are often accompanied by neurologic injury. Wade and colleagues reported a spinal cord injury rate after thoracolumbar fractures in ankylosing spondylitis patients that was twice the rate in the normal population.[70] Hunter and Dobo reported a 75% incidence of neurologic injury in spondylitic spine fractures.[34]

Unrecognized or untreated spine fractures contribute to the development of the typical flexion deformity. Simmons reported that, in a group of patients undergoing surgery for fixed flexion deformities of the cervical spine, 36% recalled a traumatic event.[60] Bailey also observed that a traumatic event, although trivial, often preceded the development of the chin-on-chest deformity.[2]

Chronic, nonunited fractures are also responsible for the development of spondylodiscitis. This phenomenon was once thought to represent a localized expression of the inflammatory process. Most authors now regard spondylodiscitis as a pseudarthrosis resulting from the instability of a chronic nonunion.[21, 73] Wu and coworkers examined the histology of these lesions and found that they were most compatible with a pseudarthrosis (Fig. 19-20).

Epidural bleeding after an acute spinal fracture is commonplace. In ankylosing spondylitis, this scenario can cause an expanding hematoma confined within a rigid tube. Sudden neurologic deterioration should suggest this possibility or the acute displacement of the fracture. This instance may be one of the few indications for laminectomy in trauma surgery, but it must be accompanied by stabilization with instrumentation.

Cervical Fractures

Cervical fractures in ankylosing spondylitis have a high risk of neurologic injury and fatality. Bohlman reported 8 ankylosing spondylitis patients.[6] All had neurologic injury and 5 died. In another series of 20 patients, Woodruff and Dewing reported 9 deaths.[72] The neurologic complications may be delayed, emphasizing the need for prompt intervention.[8]

Cervical fractures with no or little displacement, a fairly normal sagittal contour of the neck, and no neurologic injury should be managed emergently in halo traction on a Stryker frame. The possibility of acute displacement of the fracture must be guarded against. The patient can later, electively, be transferred to a halo vest and mobilized. At times, concomitant thoracolumbar deformity prevents positioning on a standard Stryker frame; the patient is then placed immediately

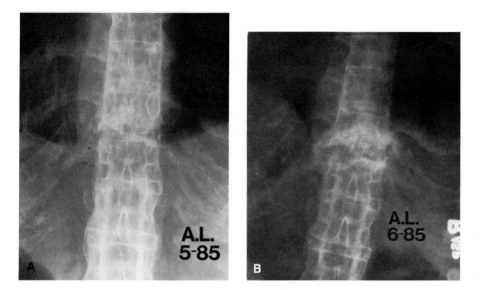

FIG. 19–20. A.L. (same patient as Fig. 19–18) also suffered a thoracolumbar fracture. Full-blown spondylodiscitis developed in only 1 month.

into a halo vest. Uncomplicated and timely healing should be anticipated, especially if the disease process is still active. Suspected delayed union at 8 to 10 weeks is best managed by posterior cervical fusion and continued protection in a halo vest for an additional 8 to 12 weeks.

An acute chin-on-chest deformity suggests an occult fracture. In some instances the deformity can be corrected by taking advantage of the fracture.[2] Gentle halo traction with gradually increased weight can achieve reduction of the flexion deformity. If a physiologic sagittal contour can be restored, the patient can be managed in a halovest. If a reduction cannot be achieved, the patient is best managed by a posterior osteotomy as previously described.

In incomplete neurologic injuries, the fracture is best managed by immediate reduction in halo traction. Generally, the severity of neurologic injury correlates with the degree of displacement or instability.[40] Internal fixation and fusion are recommended in this instance to prevent continued or further spinal cord injury. In patients with complete cord injuries, the fracture should be managed by internal fixation and fusion after reduction and a period of observation in halo traction. Internal fixation is recommended to unburden the patient from external devices and to facilitate rehabilitation.

Before any manipulation of the cervical spine, the stability of the atlantoaxial joint must be assessed. If instability is noted, Gallie fusion of the atlantoaxial joint is indicated.[8] The bone in ankylosing spondylitis is osteoporotic and fixation may be less than optimal, in which case halo-vest immobilization is still necessary.

Thoracolumbar Fractures

Fractures of the lower spine generally occur at the thoracolumbar junction as a result of the increased stresses in this region. A common consequence of ankylosing spondylitis is the progressive loss of lumbar lordosis. As the lumbar spine flattens, the posterior elements normally under compression tend to experience more tensile stresses. The apex of the normal kyphosis, T7, migrates distally to the region of the thoracolumbar junction. The thoracolumbar junction is at the fulcrum of two long lever arms created by the thoracic spine and rib cage and the lumbar spine and pelvis. The increased stresses at this region, combined with the generalized osteoporosis, contribute to the propensity to fracture. These same factors contribute to the development of spondylodiscitis or pseudarthrosis in this region.

One can be tempted to treat nondisplaced or minimally displaced fractures in this region by plaster cast or brace. Although these fractures can be treated successfully in this manner, any fracture that occurs involves all three columns because of the circumferential ankylosis of the osteoligamentous structures, and the inherent instability of these injuries is reflected by their potential to acute displacement. Trent and colleagues recognized this disposition and recommended reduction and stabilization with a Luque ring.[67]

Minimally displaced fractures with a normal sagittal contour can be stabilized posteriorly with Cotrel–Dubousset instrumentation and a posterior fusion. Compression must be achieved across the posterior elements, which cannot be obtained with the Luque method. Postoperatively, a TLSO is recommended until healing is evident because of the fragility of the bone.

A fracture with significant displacement or a concomitant kyphosis is managed by posterior and anterior spinal surgery, regardless of neurologic status. Reduction of the fracture can usually be achieved by postural methods. In some patients with severe kyphosis, the supine position must be avoided because it will extend the fracture site, possibly exacerbating neurologic compromise.

The fracture site can be used at surgery to correct the kyphotic deformity (Fig. 19-21). Posterior compression instrumentation is crucial. The surgeon should make every attempt to restore the sagittal vertical axis to its physiologic position. Moving the sagittal vertical axis in line with or dorsal to the fracture site aids stability and healing.

Simmons indicates that if the weight-bearing line can be shifted posterior to the fracture site, uncomplicated healing should be expected.[60] However, residual kyphosis in the thoracic and cervical spine usually persists. Moreover, extension of the fracture site opens the disc space in front, resulting in a significant anterior column deficit. Considering these factors and the initial three-column involvement of the fracture, anterior inlay fusion with a substantial autologous graft is recommended (Fig. 19-22). A TLSO is worn postoperatively until healing is obtained, usually 6 to 7 months.

Spondylodiscitis

The incidence of spondylodiscitis is reported to be approximately 5% of the anklosing spondylitic population.[41, 49] Simmons states that this may be underestimated, with his experience suggesting 23%.[60] Spondylodiscitis may be asymptomatic, but the majority of patients present with pain and increasing deformity.

The distribution of spondylodiscitis is the same as that for the thoracolumbar fractures. This process is regarded as a pseudarthrosis, and the basic surgical considerations are the same as for acute thoracolumbar fractures. An additional consideration in spondylodiscitis is that a localized stenosis may occur at the site of the pseudarthrosis, which should be evaluated before surgical intervention (Fig. 19-23). Compression

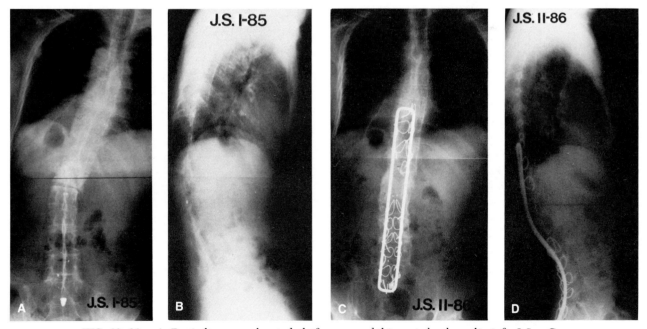

FIG. 19–21. **A, B.** A slip on an elevated platform caused this acute kyphoscoliosis for J.S. **C, D.** Frontal and sagittal contours were restored by anterior osteotomies and interbody fusion and by posterior instrumentation and fusion. Cotrel–Dubousset instrumentation is now performed.

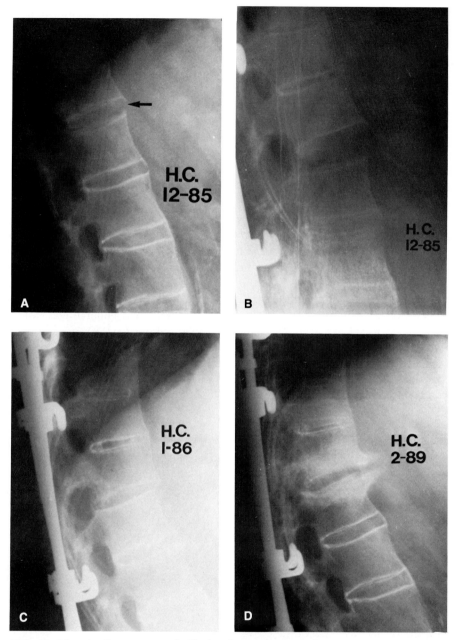

FIG. 19–22. A. Fracture revealed by break in anterior ossification. **B.** Correction of preexisting kyphosis achieved by posterior compression instrumentation across fracture level. **C.** Failed correction due to residual anterior column deficit. **D.** Resulting spondylodiscitis appearance.

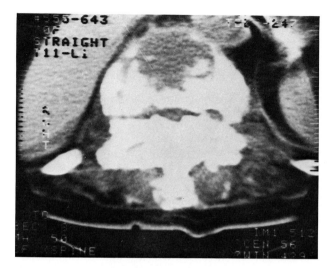

FIG. 19–23. Severe spinal stenosis at the level of the spondylodiscitis illustrated in Fig. 19–20.

of the posterior elements is important, and shifting the sagittal vertical axis dorsally is imperative. Anterior grafting is recommended as a second stage because of the residual kyphosis and the anterior column deficit.

SUMMARY

Ankylosing spondylitis is a chronic inflammatory disease that leads to pain and progressive stiffness. Its cause is still not well understood.

Medical management consists of nonsteroidal antiinflammatory medications for relief of pain. The prevention of a fixed flexion deformity of the spine is attempted through proper posture and an extension exercise program. Patient education is important in light of the proclivity toward spinal fractures with significant neurologic sequelae.

Surgical intervention is primarily indicated for patients in whom the fixed flexion deformity becomes a functional deterrent. Preoperative assessment must include an evaluation of hip motion because it is often limited. Hip arthroplasty can allow enough trunk realignment to obviate spinal osteotomy. Lumbar osteotomy is indicated for lumbar kyphosis and can often compensate for mild to moderate cervicothoracic deformity. Spinal osteotomy is a high-risk procedure, especially in the cervical spine. However, as McCaroll stated in his discussion of Smith-Peterson's 1945

paper, "there can be no objection to any procedure . . . which offers the unfortunate patient with Marie-Strümpell disease some hope of being able to look the world in the eye again."

References

1. Adams JC: Technique, dangers and safeguards in osteotomy of the spine. J Bone Joint Surg [Br] 34:226, 1952
2. Bailey RW: Surgical considerations in arthritis of the cervical spine. In Rothman R, Simeone F (eds): The Spine, pp 1002–1014. Philadelphia, WB Saunders, 1982
3. Ball J: Enthesopathy of rheumatoid and ankylosing spondylitis. Ann Rheum Dis 30:213 1971
4. Baum J, Ziff M: The variety of ankylosing spondylitis in the black race. Arthritis Rheum 14:12, 1971
5. Berens DL: Roentgen features of ankylosing spondylitis. Clin Orthop 74:20, 1971
6. Bohlman H: Acute fractures and dislocations of the cervical spine. J Bone Joint Surg [Am] 61:1119, 1979
7. Brewerton DA, Hart ED, Nicholls A, et al: Ankylosing spondylitis and HLA27. Lancet 1:904, 1973
8. Broom MJ, Raycroft JF: Complications of fractures of the cervical spine in ankylosing spondylitis. Spine 13:763, 1988
9. Bulstrode SJ, Barefoot J, Harrison RA, et al: The role of passive stretching in ankylosing spondylitis. Br J Rheumatol 26:40, 1987
10. Calin A (ed): Spondyloarthropathies. Orlando, FL, Grune and Stratton, 1984
11. Calin A: The spondyloarthropathies. In Wyngaarden J, Smith L (eds): Cecil Textbook of Medicine, 18th ed. Philadelphia, WB Saunders, 1988
12. Calin A: Seronegative spondyloarthritides. Med Clin North Am 70:323, 1986
13. Calin A: Spondyloarthropathies. In Kelly WN, Harris ED, Ruddy S, Sledge CB (eds): Textbook of Rheumatology, pp 1021–1034. Philadelphia, WB Saunders, 1989
14. Calin A: Creatine phosphokinase in ankylosing spondylitis. Ann Rheumatol 34:244, 1975
15. Calin A, Elswood J: The relationship between pelvic, spinal and hip involvement in ankylosing spondylitis—one disease process or several? Br J Rheumatol 27:393, 1988
16. Calin A, Elswood J: The natural history of juvenile-onset ankylosing spondylitis: A 24-year retrospective case-control study. Br J Rheumatol 27:91, 1988
17. Calin A, Elswood J: Ankylosing spondylitis: A review of 149 total hip replacements in 86 patients. Br J Rheumatol 26:71, 1987
18. Calin A, Fries JF: Striking prevalence of ankylosing spondylitis in "healthy" W27 positive males and females. N Engl J Med 293:835, 1975
19. Camargo FP, Cordeiro EN, Napolli MMM: Corrective osteotomy of the spine in ankylosing spondylitis. Clin Orthop 208:157, 1986

20. Carette S, Graham D, Little H, et al: The natural disease course of ankylosing spondylitis. Arthritis Rheum 26: 186, 1983
21. Chan FL, Ho EWK, Fang D, et al: Spinal pseudarthrosis in ankylosing spondylitis. Acta Radiol 28:383, 1987
22. Cruickshank B: Pathology of ankylosing spondylitis. Clin Orthop 74:43, 1971
23. Dommisse GF: The blood supply of the spinal cord. J Bone Joint Surg [Br] 56:225, 1974
24. Dommisse GF: The Arteries and Veins of the Human Spinal Cord from Birth. Edinburgh, Churchill, Livingstone and Longman, 1975
25. Ebringer RW, Cawdell DR, Oates JK, Young AC: Sequential studies in ankylosing spondylitis. Ann Rheum Dis 37:146, 1978
26. Godfrey RG, Calabrao JJ, Mills D, et al: A double-blind crossover trial of aspirin, indomethacin and phenylbutazone in ankylosing spondylitis. Arthritis Rheum 15:110, 1972
27. Gordon AL, Yudell A: Cauda equina lesion associated with rheumatoid spondylitis. Ann Intern Med 78:555, 1973
28. Graham B, van Peteghew PK: Fractures of the spine in ankylosis spondylitis, diagnosis, treatment and complications. Spine 14:803, 1989
29. Hanson CA, Shagrin JW, Duncan H: Vertebral osteoporosis in ankylosing spondylitis. Clin Orthop 74:59, 1971
30. Hehne HJ, Zielke K: Operative treatment of spinal deformities by multi-segmental osteotomies and transpedicular screws with VDS system. Orthop Trans 11:95, 1987
31. Herbert JJ: Vertebral osteotomy, technique, indications, and results. J Bone Joint Surg [Am] 30:680, 1948
32. Herbert JJ: Vertebral osteotomy for kyphosis especially in Marie-Strümpell arthritis. J Bone Joint Surg [Am] 41:291, 1959
33. Ho EKW, Chan FL, Leong JCY: Post-surgical stress fracture of the spine affected by ankylosing spondylitis. Clin Orthop 247:87, 1989
34. Hunter T, Dobo H: Spinal fractures complicating ankylosing spondylitis. Ann Intern Med 88:546, 1978
35. LaChapelle EH: Osteotomy of the lumbar spine for correction of kyphosis in a case of ankylosing spondyloarthritis. J Bone Joint Surg [Am] 28:851, 1946
36. Law WA: Lumbar spine osteotomy. J Bone Joint Surg [Br] 41:270, 1959
37. Law WA: Osteotomy of the spine. Clin Orthop 66:70, 1969
38. Lawrence JS: The prevalence of arthritis. Br J Clin Pract 17:699, 1963
39. Lichtblau PO, Wilson PD: Possible mechanism of aortic rupture in orthopedic correction of rheumatoid spondylitis. J Bone Joint Surg [Am] 38:123, 1956
40. Lipson SJ: Ankylosing spondylitis. In Kelly WN, Harris ED, Ruddy S, Sledge CB (eds): Textbook of Rheumatology, pp 2009–2012. Philadelphia, WB Saunders, 1989
41. Little H, Urowitz MB, Smythe HA, et al: Asymptomatic spondylodiscitis. An unusual feature in ankylosing spondylitis. Arthritis Rheumatol 17:487, 1974
42. Mason C, Cozen L, Adelstein L: Surgical correction of flexion deformity of the cervical spine. Calif Med 70:244, 1953
43. McMaster MJ: A technique for lumbar spinal osteotomy in ankylosing spondylitis. J Bone Joint Surg [Br] 67:204, 1985
44. McMaster PE: Osteotomy of the spine for fixed flexion deformity. J Bone Joint Surg [Am] 44:1207, 1962
45. Nashel DJ, Petrone DL, Ulmer CC, et al: C-reactive protein. A marker for disease activity in ankylosing spondylitis and Reiter's syndrome. J Rheumatol 13:364, 1986
46. Pearcy MJ, Wordsworth BP, Partek I, et al: Spinal movements in ankylosing spondylitis and the effect of treatment. Spine 10:42, 1985
47. Puschel J, Zielke K: Transpedicular vertebral instrumentation using VDS-instruments in ankylosing spondylitis. Orthop Trans 9:130, 1985
48. Romanus R, Yden S: Destructive and ossifying spondylitic changes in rheumatoid ankylosing spondylitis. Pelvo-spondylitis ossificans. Acta Orthop Scand 22:88, 1952
49. Rosen P, Graham DC: Ankylosing spondylitis (a clinical review of 128 cases). Arch Int Am Rheumatol 5:128, 1962
50. Rosenkranz W: Ankylosing spondylitis: Cauda equina syndrome with multiple spinal arachnoid cysts. Neurosurgery 34:241, 1971
51. Russel AS, Lentle BC, Percy JS: Investigation of sacroiliac disease: Comparative evaluation of radiological and radionuclide techniques. J Rheumatol 2:45,1975
52. Russel ML, Gordon DA, Ogryzlo MA, et al: The cauda equina syndrome of ankylosing spondylitis. Ann Intern Med 78:551, 1973
53. Salathé M, Jöhr M: Unsuspected cervical fractures: A common problem in ankylosing spondylitis. Anesthesiology 70:869, 1989
54. Schlosstein L, Terasaki DI, Bluestone R, Pearson CM: High association of an HLA antigen W-27 with ankylosing spondylitis. N Engl J Med 228:704, 1973
55. Scudese V, Calabro JJ: Vertebral wedge osteotomy. JAMA 186:627, 1963
56. Schwimmbeck PL, Oldstone MB: Molecular mimicry between human leukocyte antigen B27 and Klebsiella. Consequences for spondyloarthropathies. Am J Med 85:51, 1988
57. Seager K, Bashir HR, Geczy AF: Evidence for a specific B27-associated cell surface marker on lymphocytes of patients with ankylosing spondylitis. Nature 277:68, 1979
58. Sharp J, Purser DW: Spontaneous atlantoaxial dislocation in ankylosing spondylitis and rheumatoid arthritis. Ann Rheum Dis 20:47, 1961
59. Sigler JW, Bluhm GB, Ensiger DC: Clinical features of ankylosing spondylitis. Clin Orthop 74:14, 1971
60. Simmons EH: Surgery of the spine in rheumatoid arthritis and ankylosing spondylitis. In Evarts CM (ed): Surgery of the Musculoskeletal System, pp 4–85. New York, Churchill Livingstone, 1983
61. Simmons EH: The surgical correction of flexion deformity of the cervical spine in ankylosing spondylitis. Clin Orthop 86:132, 1972

62. Simmons EH: Kyphotic deformity of the spine in ankylosing spondylitis. Clin Orthop 128:65, 1977

63. Smith-Peterson MN, Larson CB, Aufranc OE: Osteotomy of the spine for correction of flexion deformity in rheumatoid arthritis. J Bone Joint Surg 27:1, 1945

64. Stretcher RM: Hereditary factors in arthritis. Med Clin North Am 39:499, 1955

65. Thomasen E: Vertebral osteotomy for correction of kyphosis in ankylosing spondylitis. Clin Orthop 194:142, 1985

66. Thompson GH, Kahn MA, Bilenker RM, et al: Spontaneous atlantoaxial subluxation as a presenting manifestation of juvenile ankylosing spondylitis. Spine 7:78, 1982

67. Trent G, Armstrong GWD, O'Neil J: Thoracolumbar fractures in ankylosing spondylitis: High risk injuries. Clin Orthop 227:61, 1988

68. Urist MU: Osteotomy of the cervical spine. J Bone Joint Surg [Am] 40:833, 1958

69. Van Rood JJ, van Leewen A, Ivany P, et al: Blind confirmation of Ceczy factor in ankylosing spondylitis. Lancet 2:943, 1985

70. Wade W, Saltzstein R, Maiman D: Spinal fractures complicating ankylosing spondylitis. Arch Phys Med Rehab 70:398, 1989

71. Weatherby C, Jaffray D, Terry A: Vascular complications associated with osteotomy in ankylosing spondylitis: A report of two cases. Spine 13:43, 1988

72. Woodruff FV, Dewing SB: Fractures of the cervical spine in patients with ankylosing spondylitis. Radiology 80:17, 1963

73. Wu PC, Fang D, Ho EKW, et al: The pathogenesis of extensive discovertebral destruction in ankylosing spondylitis. Clin Orthop 230:154, 1988

CORRECTION OF LONG, CURVED DEFORMITIES IN ANKYLOSING SPONDYLITIS

HANS-JOACHIM HEHNE

KLAUS ZIELKE

Despite intensive conservative therapy, 66% of all patients with ankylosing spondylitis develop serious kyphotic deformities.[34] The patients are no longer able to look straight ahead and are unable to perform many occupations.[28, 40] In most cases, it is impossible for these patients to drive a vehicle, and eating, drinking, and reading become increasingly difficult. The loss of visual contact results in the loss of social contact; patients become isolated and withdrawn.[10] In severe cases, the chin rests on the sternum, and the patient finds it difficult to feed himself. Owing to the stiffness of the thorax, restricted function of the lungs becomes evident.[30]

Surgical correction of the kyphotic deformity was first performed by the Smith-Petersen group and the Briggs group in the United States and by LaChapelle and Herbert in Europe.[2, 11, 16, 37] The principle was a dorsal wedge osteotomy of the vertebral arch of a lumbar segment—usually at L2 or L3—and extension of the spine. Metal implants were first reported for fixation by Lichtblau and Wilson, Dawson, and Law and Simmons.[3, 20, 22, 36] The correction was performed on the lumbar vertebrae below the kyphotic apex to achieve a large lever arm for the erection of the head.

Correction in the lumbar spine was not restricted by the ribs, and the osteotomy was below the spinal cord.

Cervical wedge osteotomies, for the high-thoracic or cervical kyphoses, were first introduced by Mason and colleagues and by Urist.[23, 39] They selected segment C7 to T1. This area is without ribs to hinder the correction, and the vertebral artery is extravertebral.

These monosegmental wedge osteotomies, with angles of up to 45°, always necessitate an annular fracture of the vertebral disc.[1–4, 6, 7, 12–15, 17–22, 24–27, 29, 35–38, 40, 41] This leads to a considerable acute extension and can cause subluxation injury to the spinal cord, nerve roots, aorta, vena cava, and abdominal vessels. Paraplegia, root lesions, paralytic ileus, occlusion of the mesenteric vessels, and aortic ruptures examined in detail by several authors were traced back to this monosegmental extension. In addition, the gastrointestinal and pulmonary problems increase the risk of the operation. It was calculated that complication rates were 50%, and the mortality rate was up to 12%. Neurologic deficits were frequent.

New techniques were developed to minimize these complications. In addition to the vertebral arch, Ziwjan, Yau, and Leong resected a wedge from the posterior wall of the vertebral body to compress the vertebra.[42, 44, 45] The pivot is moved to the center of the vertebral body, preventing a large ventral gap. Detailed statistics are not available. In 1979, to avoid the specific complications of a monosegmental correction, Püschel and Zielke began to do polysegmental osteotomies with the aim of achieving long, curved, harmonious lordosis.[9, 10, 31] At least four or, in severe kyphosis cases, six segments were osteotomized. For correction and stabilization, the compression rod system of Harrington was used initially.[8] Thirty-four patients were treated with this method.[10] Of these patients, 2 died of bronchial pneumonia and 1 after caval compression. One patient had an irreversible root lesion, and 3 developed paraplegia, which was reversed after immediate operative decompression of epidural hematomas. A wound infection resolved after removal of metal. In these cases, the mortality rate was 4%; the irreversible complications, 3%; and the reversible complications, 24%.

The results were still not acceptable. Although a correction of $40.4° ± 13.3°$ (corresponding to $10.1°$ per segment) was successful, an ideal harmonious lordosis, with equal gaps in all osteotomized segments, was accomplished in only 15 cases (44%). Nineteen patients had one or two segments constituting the correction. The dangers of monosegmental corrections were still present, and all patients experiencing complications actually had disharmonious lordosis with monosegmental or bisegmental lordosis.

Thirty-one of these patients were followed on an annual basis for 4 to 7.5 years. After 12 months, all spondyloses had completely fused. Further complications did not arise. For lordosis, there was a loss of correction in the instrumentation area of 10%, and for the overall kyphosis, 7%. Conclusions can be drawn: kyphotic deformities can be corrected through polysegmental osteotomies, and harmonious lordosis can also be achieved. However, the Harrington compression rod system did not consistently achieve an equal distribution of pressure across all osteotomized segments. Monosegmental openings were still seen. These openings lead to a disharmonious lordosis with an unsatisfactorily high complication rate. The good results obliged us to continue with the principle of polysegmental osteotomies but to exchange the metal implants for the more favorable transpedicular screws (Fig. 19-24).[9, 10, 32, 33] This principle is exactly the same as the compressive polysegmental scoliosis correction on the convex side described by Dwyer and Zielke.[5, 43] The instrumentation system developed by Zielke for the Ventral Derotation System (Universal Spinal Instrumentation System, Firma Ulrich, Ulm, West Germany) was consistently used. The diameter of the threaded rod was changed at a later stage from 3 mm to 4 mm. Since then, more than 200 patients have been operated on with this process. One hundred patients over a period of 1 year and 53 patients over a period of 2

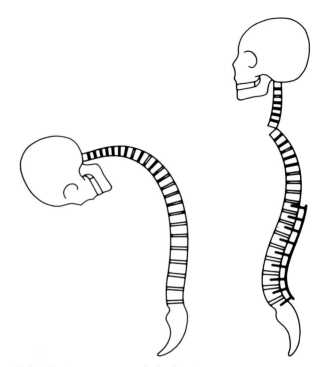

FIG. 19–24. Position of the kyphosed spine before and after polysegmental lumbar and monosegmental cervical osteotomies.

years were examined, and statistical details were recorded.

SURGICAL CONSIDERATIONS

Indications

The indications were noncompensated thoracic and thoracolumbar kyphoses greater than 70°. Total kyphoses greater than 55° and lumbar kyphosis greater than 15° in total ankylosis were also indications.

Segment Selection and Operation Technique

Usually the osteotomies are carried out on five segments. If the apical vertebra of the kyphosis is at or above L2, osteotomies are carried out between T12–L1 and L4–L5. Below L2, the osteotomies are made a segment lower, between L1–L2 and L5–S1. The number of osteotomies varies between four and seven, depending on the angle of the kyphosis. If seven osteotomies are planned, they are consistently carried out between T11–T12 and L5–S1.

To counterbalance the pressure on the screws in both the lowest and uppermost osteotomized segments, one or two segments are additionally instrumented. This means that the average instrumentation is performed from T10 to S1 (see Fig. 19-24). The operations are performed under controlled hypotensive anesthesia using nitroprusside. In 100 operations, only 1 tracheotomy was necessary. The operation is carried out with the patient in the prone position on a flexed table.

A midline longitudinal incision is made, exposing the vertebral arches from T8 to S2. Usually, the joint capsules, the interspinal ligaments, and the ligamentum flavum have ossified. The fused ligaments are resected together with the spinous process. The osteotomy is begun at the midline in the interlaminar space. The flavum is frequently ossified, and the dura is adherent. Careful dissection is needed. The osteotomy is curved laterally and cephalad in the form of a chevron through the facet joints (Fig. 19-25A). Four to 5 mm of the adjacent arches are removed, and the ventral edge is cut back to prevent possible pressure on the dura and roots during correction. The lateral oblique osteotomies have an angle of 35° to 40° to the horizontal and an approximate width of 6 to 7 mm.

If a scoliosis is present, the osteotomy is made larger on the convex side.

When all the osteotomies are complete, the instrumentation can proceed. The point of insertion of the screws at the intersection of the axis of the joint and the transverse process is marked by an awl. From here, the hole can be drilled in a slightly medial direction of about 10° through the pedicle to the front wall of the vertebral body. The pedicle wall itself should not be drilled through. The length of this hole measures between 45 and 55 mm. The transpedicular screws should be inserted immediately after drilling. The side-opening screw heads are at the end of the construct; the top-opening screws are in the middle. Occasionally, when osteoporosis is severe, the screws may not hold firmly enough. If this occurs, intrapedicular implantation of bone cement is advised. The bilateral rows of screws are connected by a threaded rod (diameter, 4 mm). Each screw requires two nuts. The nuts are screwed tightly into place. This immediately establishes a stable right angle between the screw and the rod and guarantees an independent correction of each segment.

The correction of the kyphosis is applied by tightening the peripheral nuts in the direction of the central

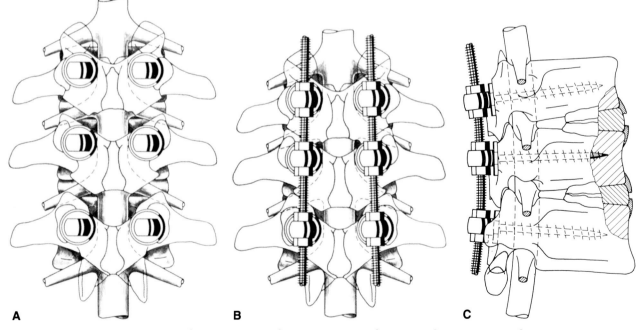

FIG. 19–25. Spinal sections. **A.** After osteotomies and screw implantation. **B.** After correction (dorsal view). **C.** After correction (lateral view).

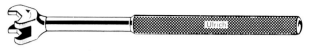

FIG. 19–26.   Double-key "Haiffa" by Zielke.

screws until the osteotomies are closed, while simultaneously straightening the table (Fig. 19-25*B*). Usually the ventral syndesmophytes yield to the correcting forces (Fig. 19-25*C*). To simultaneously tighten the nuts on either side of each screw, the double key system (Haiffa, Ulrich Co., Ulm) is used (Fig. 19-26).

Scoliosis can be corrected by exerting more compression on the convex side. After all nuts have been tightened and the remaining lengths of the rods have been trimmed, the final dorsal spondylodesis is completed with the decortication of the vertebral arches. Bone grafts obtained from the osteotomies and bone resections are placed in the wound. The average operation time of our first 100 patients was 4 hours and 15 minutes ± 55 minutes, and the intraoperative blood loss measured 1440 ± 650 ml.

Postoperative Care

Three to 4 days in intensive care with intensive breathing therapy is usually necessary. After 1 week of confinement to bed, the patient is given a torso plaster cast to be worn for 6 months and finally a Stagnara corset for another 6 months.[10] The patient is not allowed to sit down until 12 weeks after the operation.

Additional Operations

If a severe cervical kyphosis exists, it can be corrected about 2 to 4 weeks after the lumbar osteotomy (see Fig. 19-24). The Mason-Urist sitting position is used with local anesthesia. A halo cast is worn. For correction and fixation, the halo can be applied to the torso cast used for the lumbar osteotomy.

PATIENTS

One hundred patients (86 male, 14 female) had surgery in our hospital between 1983 and 1986 using this method. They were between 24 and 64 years old (average, 44 years). The diagnosis had been made an average of 14 years before. Ninety-three suffered a typical ankylosing spondylitis, and 7 had ankylosing spondylarthritis with Reiter's syndrome, psoriasis arthritis,

or ulcerative colitis. Ninety-five patients received regular conservative preoperative treatment. Owing to antirheumatic therapy, 22 patients suffered from gastritis and stomach ulcers; 22 patients experienced no vertebral pain, 17 experienced slight pain, 22 had significant pain, and 39 had severe vertebral pain. In 84 cases, the cervical spine was also affected. Forty-two had peripheral, 28 had ocular, and 12 had visceral manifestations. Thirty-two had a rheumatic coxitis or a hip prosthesis, and 22 suffered further hip flexion contracture.

The ESR measured 31 ± 19 mm, and the vital capacity was 3040 ± 830 ml. The majority of kyphotic deformities had developed gradually during the last 5 to 7 years, although 10 patients developed it only 2 years after the diagnosis. Fifty-eight kyphoses affected the complete spine (77° ± 18°), 31 affected the thoracic spine, 7 affected the cervical spine, and 4 affected the lumbar spine. There were 18 dorsal, 36 annular, and 46 ostotic (bamboo spine) types of ossification. Nineteen patients had spondylodiscitis usually localized to the lumbar spine. Forty-nine had pronounced osteoporosis, and 63 had scoliosis that measured 11° ± 5°, with a decompensation of 3.1 ± 2.5 cm.

Complications

There was no intraoperative mortality. Four elderly patients died between the second and tenth postoperative weeks. The causes of death were bronchial pneumonia, cardiac failure, and two cases of pulmonary embolism. Two root lesions were irreversible, the cause of which could not be explained. Reversible complications occurred with 20 patients, including an incomplete paraplegia (Table 19-1). This incomplete paraplegia patient was a 61-year-old woman with severe kyphosis of 131° who underwent correction of 84°. Immediate revision was performed, and a bone chip that had become embedded in the spinal canal was removed. This patient made an immediate and complete recovery; she had no problems during a follow-up period of 7 years.

There were many cases of isolated root lesions that occurred at L3; all but one healed spontaneously within the first 6 months. These lesions may be due to a temporary hematoma. In 1 female patient with a correction of 75°, the nerve deficit was reversible after removing the hematoma. One male patient required a second instrumentation because of a broken rod. Two wound infections occurred, which were controlled by

TABLE 19-1. Complications of 100 Patients After Corrective Polysegmental Osteotomies

Complications	Number of Patients
Nonreversible	
Death	4
Root lesion	2
Reversible	
Paraplegia	1*
Root lesion	11*
Wound infection	2
Broken rod	2*
Venous thrombosis	3
Pneumonia	1
Cholecystitis	1
Pancreatitis	1

* After reoperation.

debridement, closed drainage, and eventual removal of the metal implants. Four percent of the patients had fatal complications, and 22% had nonfatal complications. Of the nonfatal complications, 20% were reversible and 5% necessitated a second operation. Seventy-four percent of the patients experienced no complications, and 94% were eventually released from the hospital free of complaints.

Early Results

The lordization for all 100 patients was between 21° and 84° (mean, 45.4° ± 14.6°). The lordization for 51 patients was between 30° and 50°. The average correction for each osteotomized segment was 8.7°. Ninety-eight patients were able to achieve a horizontal visual axis from 0 to −10°, including 6 patients who had additional cervical osteotomies.

Five patients were corrected between 21° and 25° and were considered to have insufficient correction. These patients had particularly excessive syndesmophytes and severe osteoporosis. The ultimate degree of the lordosis depended on the extent of the syndesmophytic ossifications (Table 19-2). An average correction of 52° was achieved for patients with only dorsal ossifications. Those suffering ostotic syndesmophytes could only be corrected 43°.

An ideal, harmonious lordosis with equivalent gaps between all segments was achieved for 70 patients (see Table 19-2). For 23 patients, the gaps between one or two discs were more than 12°, fracture of a vertebral body occurred in 5, and dorsal compression of the vertebral body happened twice. The frequency of disharmonious lordosis correlated with the degree of the syndesmophytes. Nine of the 13 patients who had root lesions and both patients with broken rods had disharmonious lordosis.

Late Results

All patients were examined by the surgeons (Table 19-3). The results were evaluated for 53 patients followed between 24 and 48 months (mean, 34 months ± 8 months). In all cases, the spondylodeses fused completely within 12 months (Fig. 19-27). With one exception, the visual axis remained constant (Fig. 19-28). The gain in lordosis measured in the area of instrumentation was 46° ± 14°. As a result, the body height (i.e., vertical standing height) was increased by 9.5 cm ± 1.5 cm.

The loss of correction of the lordosis was 15% ± 2%;

TABLE 19-2. Lordosis and Harmonious Lordoses in 100 Corrective Polysegmental Osteotomies

Syndesmophytes	Patients	Lordosation (degrees)	Harmonious Lordoses (n)	(%)
Dorsal ossification only	18	52.0 ± 15.0	18	100
Ligamentous	36	45.2 ± 13.4	29	81
Bamboo spine	46	43.0 ± 15.4	23	50
Total (or mean)	100	45.4 ± 14.6	70	70

TABLE 19-3. Results of 53 Patients After Corrective Polysegmental Osteotomies

Examination	Body Height (cm)	Area of Instrumentation (degrees)	Total Kyphosis (degrees)	Thoracic Kyphosis Above Instrumentation (degrees)	Scoliosis (degrees)
Preoperative	160 ± 10	K 12 ± 18*	74 ± 17	42 ± 20	10 ± 5
Postoperative	170 ± 7	L 34 ± 17	44 ± 25	40 ± 19	5 ± 4
1 year control	168 ± 8	L 30 ± 16	44 ± 25	40 ± 19	5 ± 4
Final control†	168 ± 8	L 27 ± 16	46 ± 25	42 ± 20	5 ± 4
Gain of correction	10	46	30		5, 6
Loss of correction	2 (20%)	7 (15%)	3 (10%)		0, 4 (7%)

*K, kyphosis; L, lordosis.
† Follow-up ranged from 24 to 48 months (mean, 34 ± 8 months).

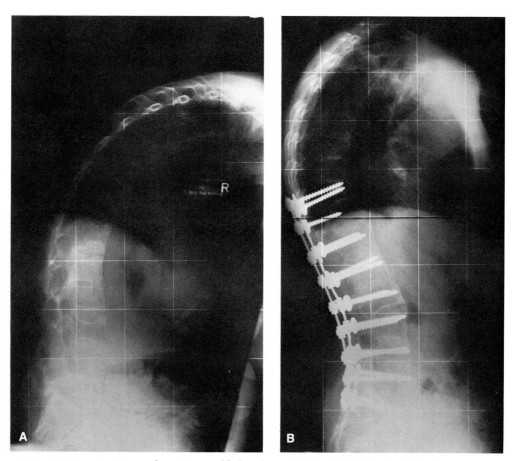

FIG. 19–27. **A.** Spine of a 62-year-old female patient with 98° kyphosis before correction. **B.** One year postoperatively; a 54° correction.

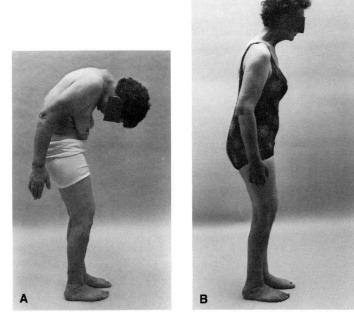

FIG. 19–28. A, B. A 61-year-old woman before and 4 years after lumbar and cervical correction with a resultant gain in body height (vertical standing height) of 34.5 cm immediately after surgery and 31.8 cm at ultimate follow-up.

for the total kyphosis, it was 10% ± 1%; and for body height, it was 20% ± 3%. The thoracic section of the kyphosis above the area of instrumentation did not change. The 41 patients with existing scoliosis were corrected by 5.6° (54%). As long as the kyphoses were identical to the length of instrumentation, a correction of 91% could be achieved. The loss of correction was 4° (7%).

A 30% or greater loss of initially increased trunk height occurred in 13 patients. In 7 patients, the loss was in the area of instrumentation; in 6, the loss was in the cervical spine or the thoracic spine above the fusions. Only 15% were free of pain preoperatively. Postoperatively, 92% were free of vertebral pain (Table 19-4). No patient claimed to have suffered severe pain. According to our score, it was concluded that 51% of the results were excellent, 30% were good, and 19% were satisfactory (Table 19-5). A self-assessment by the patients showed somewhat better results (Table 19-5).

DISCUSSION

Kyphotic deformities in ankylosing spondylitis can be straightened by a monosegmental dorsal lumbar osteotomy. However, the short curved lordosis led to numerous complications and to cosmetically unsatisfactory results. The maximal correction was restricted to

TABLE 19-4. Vertebral Pain of 53 Patients After Corrective Polysegmental Osteotomies

Examination	Vertebral Pain (%)				Total (%)
	None	*Moderate*	*Evident*	*Severe*	
Preoperative	15	17	25	43	100
Postoperative	75	23	2		100
1 year follow-up	89	9	2		100
Final follow-up*	92	4	4		100

*Follow-up ranged from 24 to 48 months (mean, 34 ± 8 months).

TABLE 19-5. Assessments of 53 Patients After Corrective Polysegmental Osteotomies

Results*	Physician Assessment		Patient Assessment	
	n	(%)	n	(%)
Excellent	27	(51)	39	(74)
Good	16	(30)	13	(24)
Satisfactory	10	(19)	1	(2)
Poor				
Total	53	(100)	53	(100)

*Follow-up ranged from 24 to 48 months (mean, 34 ± 8 months).

40 to 45°. In our hands, polysegmental osteotomies are superior to the monosegmental type. The operative lordosis desired secures 4 to 7 segments, decreasing the forces and the angle alterations per segment. Despite larger corrections being carried out, the complication rate was reduced by using Harrington compression rods. However, an even distribution of the correction to all osteotomized segments was rarely possible. In 56% of the operations, these wide, monosegmental gaps led to unacceptable complications. With the help of transpedicular screws, isolated lordosis could be performed on each segment, producing a harmonious lordosis in 70% of all cases. The average lordosis achieved per segment was 9°. For 100 operations, an average lordosis of 45° ± 15° was possible. Corrections up to 70° were also achieved, enabling the visual axis to become permanently horizontal. Cervical osteotomies were sometimes necessary.

Using these techniques, the complication rate was significantly reduced. Moreover, severe and irreversible complications seldom occurred. During the first 30 operations, 4 elderly, high-risk patients died from pulmonary and cardiac complications. Since that experience, we require candidates for surgery over 55 years old to be in excellent health except for their ankylosing spondylitis. The patients now spend 3 weeks in the hospital before the operation, during which time they are prepared medically and by physiotherapy.

Isolated cases of root lesions still present problems, although these are reversible in most cases. These occurred in 13 of the 100 operations; 10 were spontaneously reversible, 1 necessitated a second operation, and 2 remained constant. Injuries are possible through extrapedicular positioning of the screws, but the roots

will not recover if this is the case. It is assumed that in most cases root lesions are secondary to hematoma.

With the exception of one case of partial paraplegia, which was reversed by immediate reoperation, no cases of severe neural lesions, subluxations, abdominal complications, or vascular lesions occurred. Results were also good in the 7 cases in which individual ruptures or compressions of vertebral bodies occurred. In these cases of severe bamboo spine the ventral ossifications were especially strong, so the correction in these segments was carried out intracorporeally instead of extracorporeally.

For cases other than severe bamboo spine, the syndesmophytes continued to break because of the lordosating force wielded by the implants. An average lordosis correction of 43° was obtained in the bamboo spine patient, and 50° of correction was obtained in patients for whom harmonious lordosis was achieved. Preoperatively, 78% of all patients suffered vertebral pain, despite the long history. Postoperatively, 75% of the patients were immediately pain free; at the final examination 2 to 4 years after surgery, 92% were pain free.

All spondylodeses fused within 1 year. Those with wide monosegmental gaps or with the broken rods also fused. Pseudarthrosis did not occur. The fusion obviously benefits from the strong ossification tendency of the basic disease. Nevertheless, 9 patients (17%) experienced a slight return of the kyphosis inside and outside the area of fusion after 2 to 4 years. Time will tell whether the dynamic process of kyphotic deformation—the cause of which is unknown—can be halted by the operation.

References

1. Adams JC: Technique, dangers and safeguards in osteotomy of the spine. J Bone Joint Surg [Br] 34:226, 1952
2. Briggs H, Keats S, Schlesinger PT: Wedge osteotomy of spine with bilateral intervertebral foraminotomy: Correction of flexion deformity in five cases of ankylosing arthritis of the spine. J Bone Joint Surg [Br] 29:1075, 1947
3. Dawson CW: Posterior elementectomy in ankylosing arthritis of the spine. Clin Orthop 10:256, 1957
4. Donaldson JR: Osteotomy of spine for kyphosis due to Marie-Strümpell's arthritis. Indian J Surg 21:400, 1959
5. Dwyer AF: An anterior approach to scoliosis. West Pac Orthop Assoc 6:63, 1969
6. Emneus H: Wedge osteotomy of spine in ankylosing spondylitis. Acta Orthop Scand 39:321, 1968

7. Goel MK: Vertebral osteotomy for correction of fixed flexion deformity of the spine. J Bone Joint Surg [Am] 50:287, 1968

8. Harrington PR: Treatment of scoliosis. J Bone Joint Surg [Am] 44:591, 1962

9. Hehne HJ, Zielke K: Aufrichtungsosteotomien an der Wirbelsäule bei Spondylitis ankylosans—Ergebnisse und Erfahrungen nach 146 Operationen. Orthop Praxis 23:552, 1987

10. Hehne HJ, Zielke K: Die kyphotische Deformität bei Spondylitis ankylosans. Klinik, Radiologie, Therapie. Stuttgart, Hippokrates, 1990

11. Herbert JJ: Vertebral osteotomy: Technique, indications and results. J Bone Joint Surg [Am] 30:680, 1948

12. Herbert JJ: Vertebral osteotomy for kyphosis, especially in Marie-Strümpell arthritis. J Bone Joint Surg [Am] 41:291, 1959

13. Junghanns H: Aufrichtungsoperation bei Spondylitis ankylopoetica (Bechterew). Dtsch Med Wochenschr 93:1592, 1968

14. Kallio KE: Osteotomy of the spine in ankylosing spondylitis. Ann Chir Gynaecol 52:615, 1963

15. Klems H, Friedebold G: Ruptur der Aorta abdominalis nach Aufrichtungs operation bei Spondylitis ankylopoetica. Z Orthop 108:554, 1971

16. LaChapelle EH: Osteotomy of the lumbar spine for correction of kyphosis in a case of ankylosing spondylarthritis. J Bone Joint Surg 28:851, 1946

17. Law WA: Surgical treatment of the rheumatic diseases. J Bone Joint Surg [Br] 34:215, 1952

18. Law WA: Lumbar spinal osteotomy. J Bone Joint Surg [Br] 41:270, 1959

19. Law WA: Osteotomy of the cervical spine. J Bone Joint Surg 41:640, 1959

20. Law WA: Osteotomy of the spine. J Bone Joint Surg [Am] 44:1199, 1962

21. Law WA: Osteotomy of the spine. Clin Orthop 66:70, 1969

22. Lichtblau PO, Wilson D: Possible mechanism of aortic rupture in orthopaedic correction of rheumatoid spondylitis. J Bone Joint Surg [Am] 38:123, 1956

23. Mason C, Cozen L, Adelstein L: Surgical correction of flexion deformity of the cervical spine. Calif Med 79:244, 1953

24. McMaster MJ, Coventry MB: Spinal osteotomy in ankylosing spondylitis. Technique, complications, and long-term results. Mayo Clin Proc 48:476, 1973

25. McMaster MJ: A technique for lumbar spinal osteotomy in ankylosing spondylitis. J Bone Joint Surg [Br] 67:204, 1985

26. McMaster PE: Osteotomy of the spine for fixed flexion deformity. J Bone Joint Surg [Am] 44:1207, 1962

27. McMaster PE: Osteotomy of the spine for fixed flexion deformity. Prac Med Surg 73:314, 1965

28. Moll JMH: Ankylosing Spondylitis. London, Churchill Livingstone, 1980

29. Morscher E, Müller W: Operative Korrektur fixierter Kyphosen. Orthopäde 2:193, 1973

30. Ott V, Wurm H: Spondylitis Ankylopoetica. Darmstadt, Steinkopf, 1957

31. Püschel J, Zielke K: Korrekturoperation bei Bechterew-Kyphose. Indikation, Technik, Ergebnisse. Z Orthop 120:338, 1982

32. Rodegerdts U, Gisbertz D, Zielke K: Untersuchung zur dorsalen Aufrichtungsosteotomie der Kyphose. Z Orthop 123:374, 1985

33. Roy-Camille R, Demeulenaere C: Ostéosynthèse du rachis dorsal lumbaire et lambo-sacré par plaques métalliques visseès dans les pédicules vertébraux et les apophyses articulaires. Presse Med 78:1447, 1970

34. Shilling F: Spondylitis ankylopoetica. In Diethelm L et al (eds): Handbuch der Medizinischen Radiologie, vol 2. Berlin, Springer, 1974

35. Simmons EH: The surgical correction of flexion deformity of the cervical spine in ankylosing spondylitis. Clin Orthop 86:132, 1972

36. Simmons EH: Kyphotic deformity of the spine in ankylosing spondylitis. Clin Orthop 128:65, 1977

37. Smith-Petersen MN, Larson CB, Aufranc OE: Osteotomy of the spine for correction of flexion deformity in rheumatoid arthritis. J Bone Joint Surg 27:1, 1945

38. Stuart FW, Rose GK: Ankylosing spondylitis treated by osteotomy of the spine. Br Med J 1:165, 1950

39. Urist MR: Osteotomy of the cervical spine. Report of a case of ankylosing rheumatoid spondylitis. J Bone Joint Surg [Am] 40:833, 1958

40. Wiberg G: Cuneiform osteotomy of the spine in spondylarthritis ankylopoetica. Nord Med 48:1530, 1952

41. Wilson MJ, Turkell JH: Multiple spinal wedge osteotomy: Its use in a case of Marie-Strümpell spondylitis. Am J Surg 77:777, 1949

42. Yau ACMC, Leong JCY: Personal communication, 1986

43. Zielke K, Stunkat R, Beaujean F: Ventrale Derotationsspondylodese. Vorläufiger Ergebnisbericht über 26 operierte Fälle. Arch Orthop Unfallchir 85:257, 1976

44. Ziwjan JL: Lumbar correcting vertebrotomy in ankylosing spondylarthritis. Khirurgiia (Mosk) 47:47, 1971

45. Ziwjan JL: Die Behandlung der Flexionsdeformitäten der Wirbelsäule bei der Bechterewschen Erkrankung. Beitr Orthop Traumatol 29:195, 1982

CHAPTER
20

Congenital Spondylolisthesis

Perry L. Schoenecker

■

Severe anterior displacement of L5 on the sacrum and the pelvis was recognized primarily as an obstetric problem in the eighteenth and nineteenth centuries.[7, 8] Kilian introduced the term *spondylolisthesis* to describe a gradual anterior displacement of the lowest lumbar vertebra. Robert and Lambl are credited with establishing the location of a defect in the pars interarticularis as one cause of anterior lumbar slippage.[9, 18] Naugebauer examined 10 of the 17 known European specimens of "spondylolisthetic pelves." He concluded that spondylolisthesis of the lumbosacral joint occurred with and without a pars lesion of the last lumbar vertebra.[12, 13] With the advent of radiology in the early twentieth century, attention focused on identifying the defect of the pars interarticularis.[4, 11, 24]

It was not until 1932 that Capener again identified the existence of two types of spondylolisthesis—the frequently reported pars defect type and the less common type without a pars defect.[3] In 1963, Newman presented a comprehensive review of 319 cases of spondylolisthesis.[14] He distinguished between Group II (164 of 319 patients), which he described as spondylolytic spondylolisthesis and which had the pars defect, and Group I (66 of 319 patients), which he defined as congenital spondylolisthesis and which had an intact pars and true lumbosacral facet joint disassociation (Table 20-1). In Group I, the lumbosacral subluxation occurs with an intact pars with resulting deformity of both the last lumbar vertebra and the upper part of the sacrum (Fig. 20-1). The superior sacral facets are deficient, as are the sacral neural arches. The inferior lumbar facets and entire spine gradually slips forward on the sacrum as the patient assumes the upright posture. The slippage may stop as the spinous process and adjacent lamina of the lumbar spine come to rest on the posterior fibrous defect of the first sacral neural arch. If progression continues, as it often does, the pars interarticularis must elongate and attenuate but usually stays intact. In Newman's subsequent study of patients with Group I (congenital) spondylolisthesis, 34 of 66 had slippage greater than 50%.[15]

Congenital spondylolisthesis is more common in females than in males; Dandy and Shannon reported that 67% (31 of 46) of their patients were females. Heredity may be an important etiologic factor. Wynne-Davies studied 147 first-degree relatives of patients with both Group I (congenital) and Group II (spondylolytic) deformities.[26] She reported a significantly higher incidence of congenital or spondylolytic spon-

TABLE 20-1. Classification of Spondylolisthesis[14,25]

Group I	Congenital; dysplastic facets
Group II	Isthmic; spondylolytic pars defect
	A. Lytic (fatigue fracture of pars)
	B. Elongated, attenuated pars
	C. Acute pars fracture

dylolisthesis among relatives of her referenced patients, suggesting a common genetic pathway for Groups I and II.

Patients with congenital spondylolisthesis typically present for treatment earlier in life than patients with spondylolytic spondylolisthesis (Fig. 20-2). In Newman's series, 29 of the 66 patients with congenital spondylolisthesis had symptoms before the age of 19 years. Typically, patients complain of low back stiffness

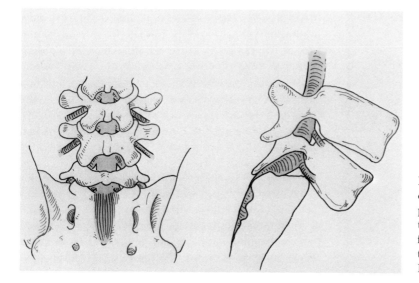

FIG. 20–1. Spondylolisthesis secondary to dysplastic L5 to S1 articulation; L5 transverse processes are diminutive and spina bifida of the sacrum is present. (Adapted and redrawn from Wiltse LL: Spondylolisthesis and its treatment. In Finneson BE (ed): Low Back Pain. Philadelphia, JB Lippincott, 1980)

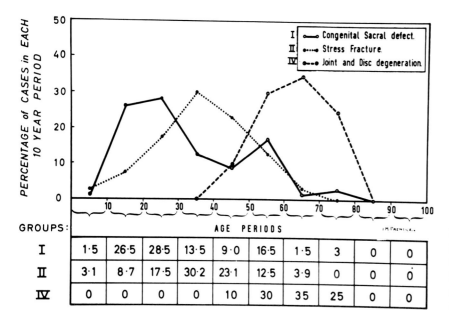

FIG. 20–2. Age of onset for congenital, spondylolytic, and degenerative spondylolisthesis. (With permission from Newman PH: The etiology of spondylolisthesis. J Bone Joint Surg [Br] 45:39, 1963)

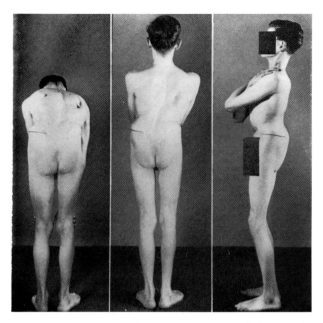

FIG. 20–3. Patient with a neurologic crisis exhibiting tight hamstrings, stiffness of the lumbar spine, and scoliosis. (With permission from Newman PH: The etiology of spondylolisthesis. J Bone Joint Surg [Br] 45:39, 1963)

and pain; often there is associated radicular pain to the buttocks or thighs. Pain radiating beyond the thighs is usually associated with a more severe deformity. In cases with slippage greater than 25%, the cauda equina may be significantly constricted.[25] This can occur anteriorly over the posterior superior dome of the sacrum or

posteriorly under the lamina of L5 or L4 (see Fig. 20-1).

Given the same degree of slippage, neurologic deficit involving the sacral nerve roots is much more likely to be seen in a patient with a Group I spondylolisthesis than in a patient with a Group II spondylolisthesis. Twenty-five of Newman's 34 cases of Group I spondylolisthesis with slippage greater than 50% had the clinical findings of cauda equina injury (Newman's syndrome).[15] Typically, patients with this neurologic crisis present with low back and leg pain, paralumbar muscle spasm, tight hamstrings, short stride length, and a waddling gait (Fig. 20-3).[16] Neurologic deficits may include diminished ankle jerks and decreased plantar flexion power of toes; more important for the patient, diminished sensation and control of the urogenic bladder and rectal sphincter can occur.

The characteristic radiographic feature of a Group I spondylolisthesis is an intact but often elongated pars and rudimentary or absent L5–S1 facet joints on the lateral radiograph. The elongation of the pars ("greyhound neck") and adjacent pedicle can best be seen on the oblique radiograph (Fig. 20-4) and compared with the typical pars defect ("Scottie dog") seen in Group II isthmic spondylolisthesis. These radiographic findings are very similar to those found in Group IIB (see Table 20-1). If the pars breaks, the radiographic finding becomes nearly indistinguishable from the pathologic findings of a patient with a Group IIA spondylolisthesis (see Table 20-1). Many high-grade isthmic spondylolistheses are spondylolytic defects superimposed

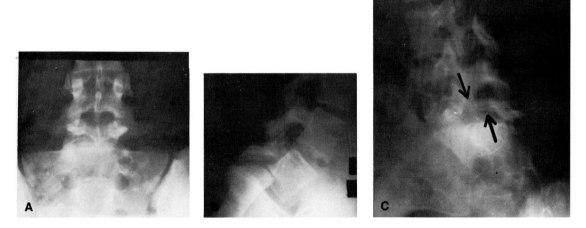

FIG. 20–4. Anterior-posterior (**A**), lateral (**B**), and oblique (**C**) radiographs of patient with dysplastic spondylolisthesis and elongation of the pars interarticularis.

on congenital slips. Thirty-four of Newman's 66 Group I patients had slippage of more than half the diameter of the vertebral body.[16] In the other cases, the slip stabilized as a result of impingement of L5 on the posterior sacral elements and on the anterior sacral buttress. Newman reported that spontaneous fusion occasionally occurs. Myelograms, computed tomography (CT), and magnetic resonance imaging (MRI) consistently show a narrowing of the spinal canal of variable severity between the posterior sacrum and the anterior border of the lowest lumbar lamina (Fig. 20-5).

The unique pathologic anatomy associated with congenital spondylolisthesis often causes encroachment of the cauda equina (see Fig. 20-1) with resultant incapacitating low back pain and leg pain. These patients have relatively little chance of obtaining significant lasting relief with nonoperative treatment. Dandy and Shannon reported that 30 of their 46 patients had a significant trial period of conservative treatment, including bedrest, traction, corset, plaster jacket, and physical therapy. Only 4 of 30 patients had lasting

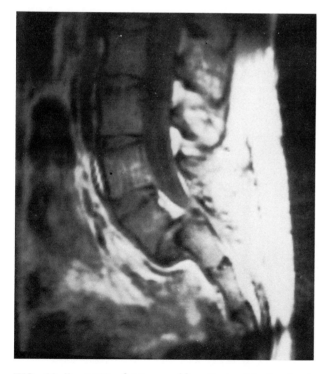

FIG. 20–5. MRI of 14-year-old patient with dysplastic spondylolisthesis showing constriction of the cauda equina over the posterior-superior dome of the sacrum.

improvement and did not require surgery. Three of these 4 were among the patients whose symptoms began in adult life. Hensinger and colleagues reported that conservative means were at least temporarily successful for 4 of 12 children with congenital spondylolisthesis.[6] Asymptomatic patients can be observed. Standing lateral radiographs taken initially and at 6-month intervals are mandatory. A low-profile thoracolumbosacral orthosis or lumbosacral corset may suffice as a temporary treatment for patients with low back pain, but one must be cautious in recommending conservative treatment for a skeletally immature patient with congenital spondylolisthesis. Further slip may lead to a significant compression of the cauda equina. Persistent symptoms of back and leg pain, lower back stiffness, and hamstring irritability are indications for proceeding with surgical treatment.

Patients with congenital spondylolisthesis are much more likely to require surgical treatment than patients with spondylolytic spondylolisthesis for slippage of the same magnitude. Forty-two of 66 patients in Newman's series with Group I spondylolisthesis eventually underwent surgical treatment.[15] In a report by Hensinger and colleagues, only 19% (14 of 78) of patients who presented had Group I pathology, but 40% (8 of 20) of the Group I patients eventually needed surgery. Similarly, in a review of 76 consecutive patients treated between 1962 and 1988 who presented for treatment of spondylolisthesis at the St. Louis Shriners Hospital, only 18 (24%) were found to have the congenital type (unpublished data). However, of the 33 patients who had surgical treatment, 14 (42%) had congenital spondylolisthesis.

Although the literature is replete with articles about the treatment of spondylolisthesis, little of it specifically addresses congenital spondylolisthesis.[6, 15] Most authors have combined groups of patients with congenital and spondylolytic spondylolisthesis in reviewing the results of surgical treatment.[1, 17, 21] Surgical treatment of congenital spondylolisthesis follows the same general guidelines as treatment of spondylolytic spondylolisthesis, except that there is greater potential for cauda equina compromise in patients with the congenital type. The majority of patients with slippage less than 25% can be satisfactorily stabilized with an in situ bilateral fusion from the sacral alae to the transverse process of L5 or L4 (Fig. 20-6). A paralumbar muscle–splitting surgical approach theoretically minimizes further instability. Pathoanatomic findings center on the

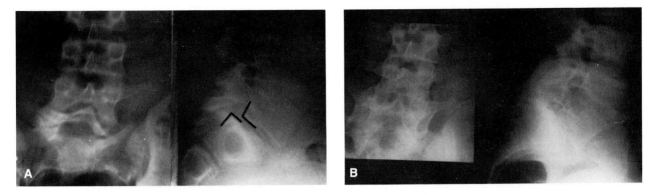

FIG. 20–6. **A.** Preoperative anterior-posterior and lateral radiographs of 13-year-old boy with 25% slip that was symptomatic. **B.** Postoperative anterior-posterior and lateral radiographs show solid fusion after in situ arthrodesis.

disassociation of the last lumbar and first sacral apophyseal joints and marked diminution of their respective facets. The posterior sacrum is typically bifid over several segments and attenuated where present. The lamina of the last lumbar vertebra rests on the fibrous defect over the midline of the sacrum. Typically, this lamina is not loose, as is seen in Group II spondylolisthesis, but is in continuity with the anteriorly displaced body and pedicles of the last lumbar vertebra. The fusion mass must extend bilaterally from the alae of the sacrum to L4 or L5. Abundant autogenous iliac bone graft can be obtained from the same incision. Postoperatively, the fusion site is usually protected with a thoracolumbosacral orthosis or lumbosacral corset to reduce the patient's activities for 4 to 6 months.

Patients with congenital spondylolisthesis presenting with greater than 25% slippage often have relative impingement of the cauda equina. A thorough preoperative neurologic examination is mandatory. Ankle jerk reflexes may be diminished. Preoperative assessment of the integrity of sacral nerve root innervation to the urinary bladder and rectal sphincter is essential. Evaluation by myelography, CT with contrast, and MRI (see Fig. 20-5) can be very helpful in assessing vertebral column deformity and the secondary distortion of the cauda equina.[2, 10] For those patients without neurologic deficit, a satisfactory outcome usually can be obtained with an in situ fusion. Because L5 is displaced far anteriorly and the posterior elements of L5 are typically diminutive, some surgeons feel the fusion should be extended to L4 to allow for an adequate

surface area and a more vertical orientation of the fusion mass.[5, 6]

Adequate decompression in conjunction with an in situ fusion may be warranted for patients with a significant neurologic deficit detected preoperatively. Decompression of the cauda equina in this uniquely abnormal anatomic setting is technically challenging. Decompression may require resection of the lamina of L5, and occasionally L4, bilateral L5 nerve root foraminotomies, and a partial superior-posterior sacroplasty and adjacent L5–S1 discectomy. With or without decompression, patients are kept recumbent postoperatively, and within 7 to 10 ten days they are placed in a double pantaloon reduction cast for 4 to 6 months (Fig. 20-7).[19] A thoracolumbosacral orthosis does nothing to immobilize the lumbosacral joint, which can only be controlled by extensions down one or both thighs. Therefore, if ambulation is permitted in the first 6 to 8 months following this extensive surgical procedure, a single pantaloon cast-brace must be utilized to further protect the lumbosacral junction. One must be aware of the potential for further slippage and the destabilizing effect of the surgical event itself. In our multicenter study, 12 cases of cauda equina syndrome occurred after an otherwise uneventful in situ fusion of severe spondylolisthesis.[20] Five of these patients had a congenital spondylolisthesis noted at the time of surgery.

Surgical reduction of a severe lumbosacral spondylolisthesis in combination with the fusion diminishes the lumbosacral kyphosis and the sagittal-plane trans-

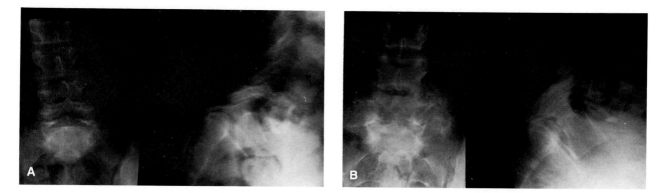

FIG. 20–7. **A.** Preoperative anterior-posterior and lateral radiographs of 15-year-old girl with severe slip. **B.** Partial reduction after L4 to S1 fusion, followed by recumbent immobilization in an extension pantaloon cast (case performed by Dr. Bridwell at St. Louis Shriners Hospital for Crippled Children). The operative reduction was attempted with Edwards instrumentation after decompression, but monitoring of sensory evoked potentials (SEPs), indicated a problem on the patient's left side, and she was unable to move her left leg and foot during a Stagnara wake-up test. She was able to move her right leg on a wake-up test and her right SEPs were normal. When L5 was allowed to fall back, the SEPs recovered, and she was able to move both legs and feet on repeat wake-up tests. Instrumentation was removed and in situ fusion was accepted. Some improvement in the sagittal angle and anterior translation between L4, L5, and the sacrum was accomplished by cast treatment, and a large solid fusion was achieved.

lation. This decreases the potential for encroachment of the cauda equina and the secondary compensatory hyperlordosis of the upper lumbar and lower thoracic spine. As with spondylolytic spondylolisthesis, surgical reduction of a high-grade congenital spondylolisthesis can probably best be obtained and maintained with posterior pedicular instrumentation.[22, 23] This reduction must be combined with decompression. This is an extremely demanding and potentially dangerous surgical technique. The indications for routine attempted instrumentation and reduction of a high-grade congenital spondylolisthesis in conjunction with fusion have not been established.

References

1. Boxall D, Bradford DS, Winter RB, Moe JH: Management of severe spondylolisthesis in children and adolescents. J Bone Joint Surg [Am] 61:479, 1979
2. Buirski G, McCall I, O'Brien J: Myelography in severe lumbosacral spondylolisthesis. Br J Radiol 57:1067, 1984
3. Capener N: Spondylolisthesis. Br J Surg 19:374, 1932
4. Chandler FA: Lesions of the isthmus (pars interarticularis) of the laminal of the lower lumbar vertebrae and their relation to spondylolisthesis. Surg Gynecol Obstet 53:273, 1931
5. Dandy DJ, Shannon MJ: Lumbosacral subluxation. J Bone Joint Surg [Br] 53:578, 1971
6. Hensinger RN, Lang JR, MacEwen GD: Surgical management of spondylolisthesis in children and adolescents. Spine 1:207, 1976
7. Herbiniaux G: Traite sur Divers Accouchments Laborieux et sur les Polypes de la Matrice. Bruxelles, J.L. DeBoubers, 1782
8. Kilian HF: Schilderungen neuer Beckenformen und ihres Verhalten im Leben. Mannheim, Verlag von Bassermann und Mathey, 1854
9. Lambl DZ: Zehn Thesen uber Spondylolisthesis. Zentralbl Gynakol Urol 9:250, 1855
10. McAfee PC, Hansen AY: Computed tomography in spondylolisthesis. Clin Orthop Rel Res 166:62, 1982
11. Meyerding HW: Spondylolisthesis. J Bone Joint Surg 13:39, 1931
12. Naugebauer F: Die Entschung der Spondylolisthesis. Centralab Gynak 5:260, 1881
13. Naugebauer FL: A New Contribution to the History & Etiology of Spondylolisthesis. New Sydenham Society Selected Monographs, vol 121, 1888
14. Newman PH: The etiology of spondylolisthesis. J Bone Joint Surg [Br] 45:39, 1963
15. Newman PH: A clinical syndrome associated with severe lumbo-sacral subluxation. J Bone Joint Surg [Br] 47:472, 1965

16. Phalen GS, Dickson JA: Spondylolisthesis and tight hamstrings. J Bone Joint Surg [Am] 43:505, 1961
17. Pizzutillo PD, Mirenda W, MacEwen GD: Posterolateral fusion for spondylolisthesis in adolescence. J Pediatr Orthop 6:311, 1986
18. Robert (uz Koblenz): Monatsschr Geburtskunde Frauenkrank 5:81, 1855
19. Scaglietti O, Frontino G, Bartolozzi P: Technique of anatomical reduction of lumbar spondylolisthesis and its surgical stabilization. Clin Orthop Rel Res 117:164, 1976
20. Schoenecker PL, Cole HO, Herring JA, et al: Cauda equina syndrome following in situ arthrodesis of severe spondylolisthesis of the lumbosacral junction. J Bone Joint Surg [Am] 72:369, 1990
21. Stanton RP, Meehan P, Lovell WW: Surgical fusion in childhood spondylolisthesis. J Pediatr Orthop 5:411, 1985
22. Steffee AD, Biscup RS, Sitkowski DJ: Segmental spine plates with pedicle screw fixation. Clin Orthop Rel Res 203:45, 1986
23. Vidal J, Fassio B, Buscayret C, Allieu Y: Surgical reduction of spondylolisthesis using a posterior approach. Clin Orthop Rel Res 154:156, 1981
24. Willis TA: The separate neural arch. J Bone Joint Surg 13:709, 1931
25. Wiltse LL, Newman PH, MacNab I: Classification of spondylolysis and spondylolisthesis. Clin Orthop Rel Res 17:23, 1976
26. Wynn-Davies R, Scott J: Inheritance and spondylolisthesis. J Bone Joint Surg [Br] 61:301, 1979

CHAPTER 21

Isthmic Spondylolisthesis

Rudolph F. Taddonio

■

Spondylolisthesis (from the Greek *spondylo*, vertebra, and *listhesis*, slide or slip) is a condition that has fascinated medical science for over 200 years. In 1782, Herbiniaux, a Belgian obstetrician, reported a patient with a difficult delivery because of the forward displacement of lumbar vertebra 5 on the first sacral segment that caused significant narrowing of the pelvic outlet.[26] As interest in the condition grew, anatomic dissection provided further elucidation. The early researchers concluded that the condition was an acute subluxation.

In 1854, Kilian coined the term *spondylolisthesis* and theorized that it was due to a gradual subluxation of the lumbosacral facet.[31] Robert in 1855, after experimentally removing the soft tissue attachments around the lumbosacral junction, concluded that displacement of the fifth vertebra on the first sacral segment could not take place if the posterior neural arch of L5 remained intact.[48] This was supported by Lambl in 1858.[34] Some controversy ensued, because many investigators had not always found spondylolysis, the neural arch defect, in association with spondylolisthesis during postmortem examinations.

Neugebauer, in 1882, attempted to resolve this clinical and experimental discrepancy by providing a description of two anatomic conditions that could produce spondylolisthesis.[43] He felt that the condition could be congenital or acquired. In the congenital form, there was failure of the L5 articular process to develop normally, unilaterally or bilaterally, with resultant elongation of the pars interarticularis and gradual slipping forward of L5 on the first sacral segment, without a break in the neural arch continuity. In the acquired type, which developed after a fracture of the pars interarticularis of L5, Neugebauer was undecided about whether the cause was primary fracture or the condition was secondary to an attenuated, weakened pars.

CLASSIFICATION OF SPONDYLOLISTHESIS

The classification most widely accepted was that proposed by Wiltse, Newman, and MacNab, based on Newman and Stone's original work studying over 300 cases.[42, 68] Five different types have been proposed: (1) dysplastic, (2) isthmic, (3) degenerative, (4) traumatic, and (5) pathologic.

This classification provides the clinician with a practical tool for diagnosis and subsequent treatment of patients with this disorder. An elegant simplification of this classification is offered by Taillard: common to all spondylolisthesis is "a failure of the bony hook" that acts as the check rein to stabilize the vertebral segment.[59] Failure of this "articular bolt," whether it is caused by congenital deficiency of ligaments in articular surfaces, fracture, or degenerative changes that produce subluxation, is the common denominator in the etiology of all spondylolistheses.

Type I: Dysplastic Spondylolisthesis. In Type I spondylolistheses, there is a congenital aplasia or hypoplasia of the L5 to S1 posterior check rein. Radiologically, hypoplasia of the L5 to S1 articulating facets and spina bifida occulta of L5 and sacrum result in loss of the bony attachments for stabilizing ligaments (Fig. 21-1). Significant slips of greater than 50% and spondyloptosis occur in this category. Dysplastic spondylolisthesis is two times more prevalent in females than males.

Although various causes have been proposed, such as a genetic defect in the ossification of the neural arch, spondylolisthesis is rarely seen before the age of 5.[7]

Type II: Isthmic Spondylolisthesis. This chapter deals primarily with isthmic spondylolisthesis and its surgical treatment in children and adults. Isthmic spondylolisthesis is classified into three subtypes:

Type IIA. Lytic spondylolisthesis, the most common type of spondylolisthesis, is rarely seen in patients younger than 5 years.[41, 50] It occurs in children more commonly at 7 or 8 years, and it stabilizes in late adolescence.[59]

Type IIB. The characteristics of this subgroup are attenuation of the pars interarticularis caused by repeated microfractures, which lead to attenuation and elongation of the pars rather than a lytic lesion (Fig. 21-2). This is probably identical to Type IIA, except that the traumatic events producing the microfracture are probably less potent and more repetitive.

Type IIC. An uncommon acute pars fracture can be the result of a severe traumatic episode, usually the result of high-velocity injury, such as a fall from a height or motor vehicle accident.

Lysis at the pars interarticularis is the common denominator in isthmic spondylolisthesis and is most prevalent at the L5 segment, followed by the L4 segment. It can be unilateral and can occur at multiple segments.[11, 46, 47] The condition has not been reported at birth or in dissected embryos, but a case of a 3-month-old infant stands as the earliest recorded.[3] Except for the rare case reports, this lesion is not usually found until after the age of 5 years.[68]

Type III: Degenerative Spondylolisthesis. Junghanns coined the term pseudospondylolisthesis in his early description of this disorder.[30] Degenerative spondylolisthesis was studied extensively by Rosenberg and found to be more common in middle-aged to elderly

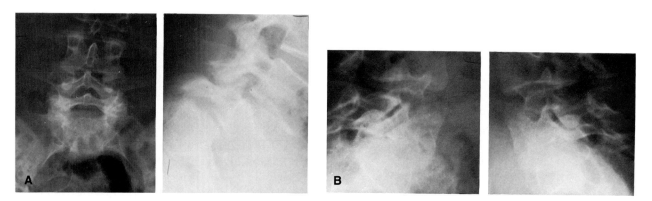

FIG. 21–1. **A.** Anterior-posterior and lateral roentgenograms of a severe Type I dysplastic spondylolisthesis, demonstrating an intact pars and subluxation of the lumbosacral facets. Owing to the severe slipping and intact pars interarticularis, this patient experienced early cauda equina compression and symptoms. **B.** Left and right oblique roentgenograms demonstrating the intact pars interarticularis.

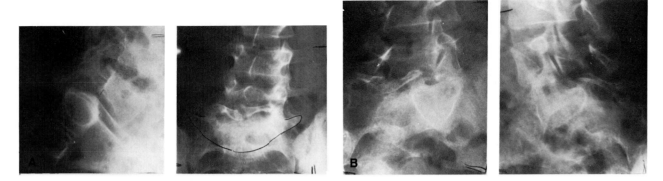

FIG. 21–2. **A.** Lateral and anterior-posterior roentgenograms of a 12-year-old boy with a severe spondylolisthesis demonstrating an elongated pars interarticularis, which had a higher degree of slippage after a stress fracture. **B.** Oblique roentgenograms demonstrating the elongated and attenuated pars interarticularis at L5 and a stress fracture of the attenuated portion.

females and to occur more frequently at the L4–L5 segment.[50] Predisposing factors are sacralization of L5 and an intercrestal line, which falls below the L4–L5 disc space. Higher stresses at the L4 to L5 articulation produce a hypermobile segment, facet joint laxity, disc degeneration, and slippage. The slippage is rarely greater than 30 to 40% and may be accompanied by pedicular kinking of the nerve root or central spinal stenosis.

Type IV: Traumatic Spondylolisthesis. Type IV spondylolisthesis is observed after a significant traumatic event that fractures a region of the posterior hook other than the pars interarticularis. Dislocations that occur with pure disruption of soft tissues secondary to severe trauma (e.g., low seatbelt injuries) should also be included in this classification. Spondylolisthesis acquisata (i.e., slipping above or below a previous fusion mass) is also included in this group and can be acutely traumatic, secondary to a pars stress fracture or degenerative in nature.[60]

Type V: Pathologic Spondylolisthesis. In Type V spondylolisthesis, there is usually a systemic bone disorder that leads to incompetence of the bony hook mechanism, allowing the slippage. Osteogenesis imperfecta, achondroplasia, Paget's disease, Albers-Schönberg disease, rheumatoid arthritis, metastatic tumors, arthrogryposis, and syphilis have all been implicated as primary conditions.[59, 68]

PREVALENCE AND PREDISPOSITION

The prevalence of spondylolisthesis is 2 to 5%.[1, 49, 61] Eisenstein studied 485 South African skeletons and found a prevalence of 3.5%, with no significant race or sex differences.[16] Stewart reported a prevalence of 50% among Alaskan natives. In Caucasian Americans studied by Wiltse, approximately 6% of the population demonstrate the lesion by the age of 18.[58, 68]

The predisposition to develop spondylolisthesis, either isthmic or dysplastic, is familial.[1, 55, 58, 68, 71] It has been shown that 15 to 50% of first-degree relatives of patients with spondylolisthesis demonstrated the lesion.[71] A third of the parents of the 400 schoolchildren studied by Baker and McHollick demonstrated the same isthmic lesion.[1] It appears that, in the general population, a combination of familial and mechanical factors predispose an individual to develop a spondylolisthesis. The pars is predisposed to stress fractures because it is the weakest component of the neural arc, and a large body of evidence supports the theory that isthmic spondylolisthesis is a fatigue fracture.[12, 13, 17, 32, 33, 54]

Rosenberg and colleagues studied 134 patients with cerebral palsy who never ambulated and found no spondylolysis or spondylolisthesis among them.[51] At the opposite extreme, Jackson studied 100 female gymnasts and reported an 11% incidence, with bilateral L5 pars defects.[27] It was his opinion that repetitive hyperextension dismounts were the reason for the increased incidence.

CLINICAL SIGNS AND SYMPTOMS

Children and Adolescents

The clinical signs and symptoms of spondylolysis or spondylolisthesis in a child or adolescent differ from those in the adult.

Children with mild to moderate slips may present with a primary complaint of low-back pain. These patients may have leg discomfort with paresthesias or may even have a painless neurologic deficit, such as a weak great toe extensor. Back pain may produce spasm and a scoliosis. The patient may present with lumbar scoliosis and low back pain, and the spondylolisthesis is discovered on a routine scoliosis x-ray evaluation.

Examination of the patient's spine usually localizes a step-off, especially if slippage is greater than 25%. This step-off is between the L4 and L5 posterior elements. In isthmic spondylolisthesis, the L5 vertebral body and the superincumbent spinal column slip forward. The L5 neural arch remains behind, creating a step-off between the L4 and the L5 segments. Range of motion of the spine may be limited by back pain and spasm and tight hamstrings. Neurologic deficits are uncommon.

In the second type of presentation, a high-grade slippage of greater than 50% occurs. These patients may present without back pain and with predominating leg pain. Occasionally, they may be totally asymptomatic and present to the physician because of an abnormal gait or spinal deformity. They usually have a hyperlordosis, a shortened trunk with an anterior abdominal crease, externally rotated hips, heart-shaped buttocks, and a waddling gait (Fig. 21-3).

Hamstring tightness is usually prevalent in the more severe slips, and the L5 nerve root can be compromised. The L5 nerve root can be compressed between the fibrocartilaginous callus of the fractured pars interarticularis, and the distorted relationship between the L5 vertebra and the cephalad edge of the S1 vertebra severely narrows the intervertebral foramina.

The sacral nerve roots of the cauda equina can be deflected and compressed in their excursion over the dome of the sacrum. This can lead to sacral nerve root symptoms that, although uncommon, can present as bowel and bladder dysfunction. Patients with even high degrees of spondylolisthesis may be totally asymptomatic and may be referred for evaluation of spinal deformity or abnormal gait.

When spondylolisthesis becomes very severe, 75 to 100%, compensating postural mechanisms develop and disrupt the normal balance between the hamstrings and spinal musculature. As L5 progressively rotates and slips forward onto S1, a true lumbosacral kyphosis develops. The sacrum becomes more vertical and the pelvis rotates into retroversion. The hip joints likewise rotate forward and the upper torso compensates to keep its sagittal vertical plumb line in balance by hyperextending. This produces hyperlordosis of the lumbar spine and a flattened kyphosis in the thoracic spine.

When the hips can no longer hyperextend enough to balance the upper torso over the sacrum, the patient's knees flex so that the trunk is thrust backward and balanced. The trunk is shortened. There may be an absence of waistline and, in severe cases, the lower ribs can come to rest upon the pelvic rim. The characteristic waddling gait associated with the heart-shaped buttocks, prominent sacrum, and tight hamstrings has been described by Phalen and Dickson.[45]

Functional or sciatic scoliosis secondary to muscle spasm, sciatic nerve root irritation, or rotatory displacement of the L5 on S1 can develop in severe slips. This type of scoliosis differs from idiopathic scoliosis, which can also be associated with this condition, in that the scoliosis has its origins in the sacrum. Associated idiopathic scoliosis may be thoracic or thoracolumbar.

In the third type of presentation, the patient is completely asymptomatic and the spondylolisthesis is only discovered on routine x-ray films, usually in evaluating scoliosis. The physical examination is generally within normal limits. If the slippage is greater than 50%, a step-off can be palpated.

Radiographic evaluation should be correlated with the risk factors described by Boxall,[5] especially in preadolescents, and follow-up should take place at regular intervals.

In general, progression usually occurs during the periods of rapid growth between the late juvenile and early adolescent periods. Progression may be slow and produce intermittent axial symptoms, with or without associated trauma, or may be quite rapid, producing severe slips with few symptoms.

In a patient who is initially discovered to have an asymptomatic spondylolisthesis, age, period of development, radiologic risk factors, recreational and sporting activities, lifestyle, future vocational capabilities, and goals must be considered.

I share the opinion of others that patients with spondylolistheses of Grades III and IV are at very high risk for progression and, even if asymptomatic, should be considered for surgical stabilization.[1, 5, 25]

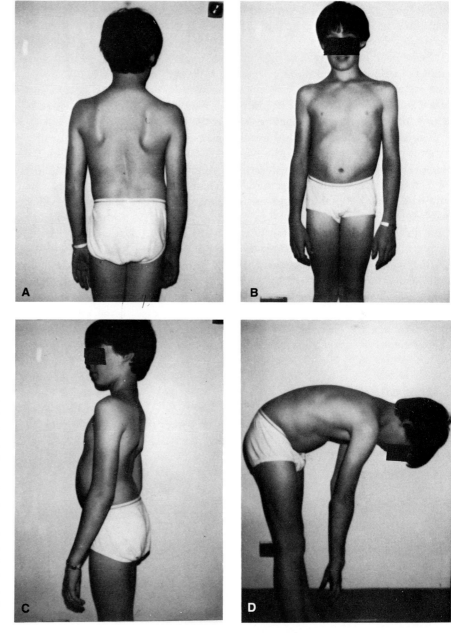

FIG. 21–3. Clinical photographs of a child with severe spondylolisthesis and spondylogenic scoliosis. **A–D.** Front, back, side, and flexion views of this deformity reveal a trunk shift and scoliosis, shortening of the patient's waistline, the compensatory flattened thoracic spine, increased lordosis, and flattened buttocks. Although there is some restriction of forward bending, it is not severe in this patient. More severe deformities increase trunk shortening, with an abdominal crease at the level of the umbilicus.

Adults

Adult patients with spondylolisthesis normally have a long history of intermittent, activity-related backache, finally reaching a point in their lives when degenerative changes produce more chronic and recurrent symptoms. The pain may be axial, with or without lower-extremity involvement.

The most commonly involved lower-extremity der-

matome is along the L5 nerve root, with associated lateral calf and great toe pain or paresthesias. Occasionally, neurologic symptoms include dorsiflexion weakness, and rarely bowel and bladder become compromised (most commonly in severe slips)).

Ruptured intervertebral discs at L5–S1 are rare; if they do occur, the affected area is usually L4–L5. Ruptured intervertebral discs may be additive in terms of nerve root compression, especially at L4–L5, where the nerve root may be compressed at the site of disc herniation and at the pars interarticularis or in the nerve root foramen.

Sciatic radiculopathy may be a presenting feature in adult patients. Some patients may present with a long history of intermittent backache accompanied by occasional sciatica, which evolves into a chronic backache with neurogenic claudication, such as that found in degenerative spinal stenosis. These are usually older patients with stable slips and severe degenerative changes occurring both at the level of the slip and the level above. The resultant degenerative changes are cumulative, and stenotic symptoms are the result of two-level involvement.

A group of adults exists who have had no recognizable symptoms in the past and who, as a result of trauma, experience low back pain with or without peripheral symptoms. Radiographic examination reveals spondylolisthesis or spondylolysis. If symptoms are new but the radiographic appearance is one of a chronic condition, the physician must establish whether the lesion is acute for medical and legal reasons.

RADIOGRAPHIC FEATURES

Radiographic confirmation of spondylolysis or spondylolisthesis secondary to an isthmic defect is essential. Standing, weight-bearing lateral and anterior-poste-rior x-ray films of the lumbar spine and pelvis should be obtained first. Even the slightest degree of forward slipping will be evident on a standing, lateral x-ray film. In most patients, a pars defect can be visualized (Fig. 21-4).

In severe slips, the anterior-posterior roentgenogram provides a curious sign termed the inverted Napoleon's hat sign. This image is produced when the L5 vertebra rolls so far forward that the anterior-posterior x-ray film is actually an axial view of the L5 vertebra (Fig. 21-5).

If the slip is barely present and the lateral x-ray film does not reveal a pars defect, oblique x-ray films outlining the "Scotty dog and its neck" may be useful. In an acute fracture, the edges of the defect are ragged, but in a long-standing situation they will be smooth and rounded. In isthmic spondylolisthesis Type IIB, in which there is an attenuation and elongation of the pars because of repeated microstress fractures that heal, a break in the neck of the Scottie dog is not seen; instead, the greyhound sign of Hensinger is a useful radiologic indicator (Fig. 21-6).[25]

Oblique tomograms of the pars interarticularis may sometimes be necessary, especially to assess healing of acute stress fractures of the pars that are undergoing conservative management.

Meyerding described an imprecise but simple method of classifying spondylolisthesis according to percentage of slippage:[40]

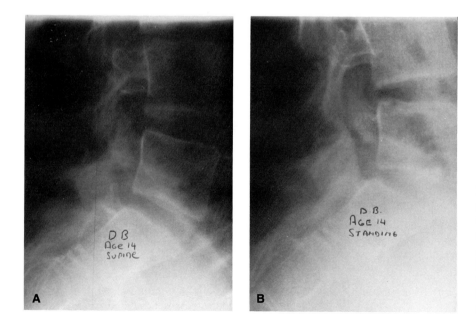

FIG. 21-4. **A.** Lateral x-ray film of a 14-year-old teenager taken in the supine position and showing a normal L4 to L5 and L5 to S1 alignment. **B.** A lateral, standing x-ray film taken of the same individual, showing a break in the pars interarticularis that is not evident in the supine position.

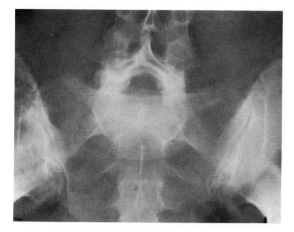

FIG. 21–5. An anterior-posterior x-ray film of a patient with a severe spondylolisthesis, demonstrating the inverted Napoleon hat sign. The L5 vertebra is rolled and slipped so far forward that the anterior-posterior film produces an axial view of this vertebra, with the transverse processes representing the rim of the hat and the body representing the dome of the hat.

Grade I—0 to 25%
Grade II—25 to 50%
Grade III—50 to 75%
Grade IV—greater than 75%

Although Grade V slippage was not originally classified by Meyerding, it has been added to indicate any slip greater than 100%; it is also called spondyloptosis.

Boxall, Bradford, Wiltse, and Winter contributed much to the understanding and standardization of the terminology and measurement of the spondylolisthesis.[5, 69] The amount of anterior displacement is measured on the standing lateral radiograph of the lumbosacral spine. It is measured as a distance between the posterior cortex of L5 and the posterior cortex of S1 and expressed as a percentage of the anterior-posterior S1 diameter (Fig. 21-7).

The sacral tilt or the angle of sacral inclination is measured on the lateral radiograph as the angle formed by a line along the posterior border of the first sacral vertebra and the vertical plane. As the spondylolisthesis progresses and the sacrum becomes more vertical, the angle of sacral inclination decreases (Fig. 21-8).

The lumbosacral kyphosis angle or the slip angle refers to the angle of sagittal rotation or sagittal roll of L5 on S1. This angle is constructed by lines drawn parallel to the anterior cortex of L5 and the posterior cortex of S1. As the L5 slip progresses and the sacrum

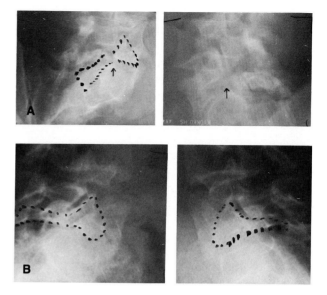

FIG. 21–6. **A.** An oblique radiograph indicating a fracture in the pars interarticularis of L5 showing the broken neck of the Scottie dog. **B.** An elongated pars interarticularis, which is intact, demonstrating the greyhound sign of Hensinger.

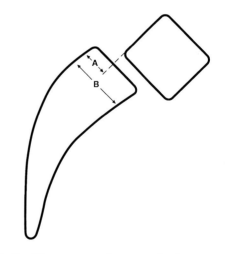

FIG. 21–7. The amount of anterior displacement or anterior slip is a percentage obtained by dividing the displacement **A,** which is the distance between the posterior cortex of the first sacral vertebra and the posterior cortex of the fifth sacral vertebra, by **B,** the maximal anterior-posterior diameter of the first sacral vertebra, and multiplying by 100.

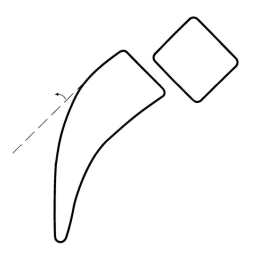

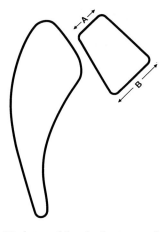

FIG. 21–10. Wedging of the olisthetic vertebra is arrived at by dividing A by B and multiplying by 100.

FIG. 21–8. Sacral inclination is arrived at by drawing a line along the posterior border of S1 (*dotted line*), intersecting it with a true vertical line, and measuring the subtended angle.

becomes more vertical, this kyphotic angle or lumbosacral kyphosis increases (Fig. 21-9).

As the body of L5 becomes more trapezoidal and becomes wedged, the posterior height decreases, and its magnitude is expressed as a percentage of the greater anterior height (Fig. 21-10).

Lumbar lordosis is measured by the Cobb method of a line drawn along the upper endplate of L1 and L5.

The sacral horizontal angle is the angle between the upper border of the sacrum and the horizontal plane. This angle decreases as the sacrum becomes more vertical and increases when the sacrum is extended and tends to become more horizontal (Fig. 21-11).

The lumbosacral joint angle is the angle between the lower border of L5 and the upper border of S1 (Fig. 21-12).

Technetium bone scanning can be particularly useful for a young patient with recent history of back pain related to trauma or excessive physical activity. In a young patient, an active pars defect that has no signifi-

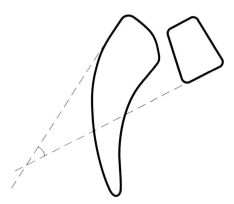

FIG. 21–9. The angle of sagittal rotation or lumbosacral kyphosis is determined by drawing a line along the anterior border of the olisthetic vertebra and measuring the angle it subtends with a line drawn along the posterior border of the first sacral segment. These two landmarks are normally unobscured on routine standing lateral x-ray films.

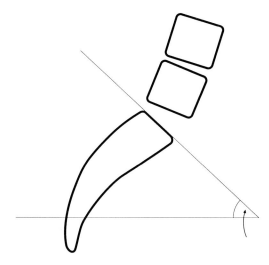

FIG. 21–11. The sacral horizontal angle is the angle subtended by a true horizontal line on a standing lateral radiograph with a line drawn parallel to the upper border of the sacrum.

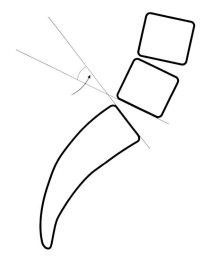

FIG. 21–12. The lumbosacral joint angle is the angle subtended by lines drawn across the upper border of the sacrum and the lower border of L5. This angle has less importance in severe slips, but it can be a useful indicator of the degree of flat back.

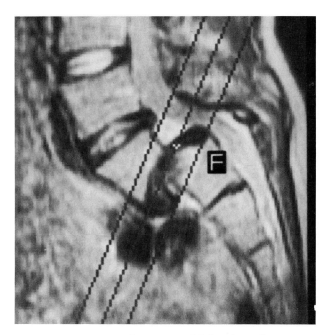

FIG. 21–13. MRI of a 22-year-old female with a severe Type II spondylolisthesis. This demonstrates the early loss of hydration of the L4–L5 disc with posterior bulging and demonstrates how the nucleus of the L5–S1 disc migrates anteriorly with the olisthetic vertebra. It is easy to visualize how the L5 nerve root could be doubly entrapped by a bulging or herniated L4–L5 disc and the fibrocartilaginous tissue of the pars interarticularis defect.

cant slippage and is positive on technetium-99 scanning could heal with immobilization. In older patients and adults, these lesions are usually inactive or minimally active, representing degenerative changes.

Magnetic resonance imaging (MRI) has become very useful in visualizing the lower lumbar nerve root structures and the degree of hydration of the L4–L5 disc. This information is very useful in planning the surgical approach because, if the L4–L5 disc is abnormal, it should be included in the levels fused (Fig. 21-13).

Computed tomography (CT) alone has not been particularly useful because it often misses the pars defect on axial cuts and tends to distort severely during the process of volume averaging for high-grade slips.

Myelographic evaluation with and without CT scanning is rarely indicated for children and adolescents because MRI is more sensitive, provides information about discs and nerve roots, and can examine the conus and spinal cord for the presence of intraspinal abnormalities. MRI is also recommended for adult patients; however, in certain instances of multilevel disease in the older adult with degenerative segments at several levels above the spondylolisthesis, myelography with sequential CT scanning can provide further diagnostic information.

RISK FACTORS FOR PROGRESSION

The most common age for spondylolisthesis to progress is between the ages of 10 and 15. Progression to any significant degree is not common in the adult, but degenerative changes that occur with age at the lumbosacral joint may increase the slip by one grade.[5, 14, 20] Progression of isthmic spondylolisthesis in the adult years is more common at L4–L5.[22]

Some patients develop a sclerotic buttress that protrudes anteriorly from the anterior body of S1, buttressing the L5 from slipping. This stabilizes the lumbosacral joint and indicates a good prognosis regarding further slippage. This is seen most commonly in adults with Grade I or II slips. The angle of slip, the lumbosacral kyphosis, and the angle of sacral inclination have been referred to by Boxall and Wiltse.[5, 69]

Risk factors in Boxall and and Bradford's study were outlined as age, sex, presence of spina bifida, low lumbar index, a high-grade S1 contour, and a congenital defect. Lordosis and a vertical sacrum were considered compensatory factors.

The most predictive single factor was the slip angle or angle of lumbosacral kyphosis. The slip angle varied directly with the lumbar index, convexity of the first sacral vertebral body, percentage of slipping, lordosis, and the sacral inclincation. Boxall thought that this one measurement could be used to represent "risk factors and associated compensatory mechanisms of severe slipping." A high slip angle was believed to have a poor prognosis for progression. Boxall recommended that patients who had slip angles of greater than 55° be considered for reduction and fusion because these patients also had a high propensity to continue slipping after fusion alone.

In lower degrees of spondylolisthesis, excessive motion during flexion-extension studies of the area in question may also portend a high risk for progression.

TREATMENT

The literature is replete with diverse methods of treating spondylolysis and spondylolisthesis, and this continues to be a controversial issue. Most patients with this disorder respond to conservative management. A small percentage require a surgical procedure, which should achieve two primary and important goals: decompression of nerve root compromise and stabilization of the spondylolisthesis with a solid bony arthrodesis.

Conservative Management

The conservative management of Grade I and II slips can include cessation of strenuous activities and bedrest. After the back pain is significantly reduced, abdominal and paraspinal muscle strengthening exercises are instituted.

Swimming, exercycle, and resistive exercises help in a spinal rehabilitation program. For patients who have persistent symptoms, immobilization in a cast or brace and nonsteroidal anti-inflammatory medication may be necessary.

Alleviation of hamstring tightness is usually an excellent clinical indicator of the success of the treatment program. Most children respond to a conservative program and remain asymptomatic in the long term.[62, 65]

Hensinger and Lang reported an excellent clinical response to conservative measures for children and teenagers with simple spondylolysis.[25] An acute pars fracture, if diagnosed early enough, may heal in a high percentage of cases with immobilization.

If a child or teenager with spondylolysis is unresponsive to conservative management, a more detailed workup is necessary to rule out the other causes of lower back pain in this age group. These include osteoid osteoma, spinal cord tumor, disc infection, juvenile herniated nucleus pulposus, neurologic disorders, and primary diseases of the nervous system (Fig. 21-14).

If objective neurologic findings are documented for a young patient with spondylolysis, a more serious disorder must be suspected. An electromyographic evaluation and MRI are the diagnostic procedures of choice. The same principles are adhered to for any child or adolescent with neurologic findings to be sure that the origin of the patient's pain is the obvious lesion on x-ray film.

A child or adolescent under the age of 10 should be followed closely during his or her growth because progression, although uncommon, may take place in an asymptomatic fashion.[65, 70]

In a child or adolescent, an asymptomatic spondylolisthesis that is discovered on a routine roentgenogram should be followed closely. Progression may occur in an asymptomatic patient; I believe that any slip greater than 50%, or progressing toward 50%, should be stabilized.[1, 5, 25]

Restricting the patient's activities is an issue that should be discussed with the parents and the patient. It seems unjustified to restrict all vigorous activities. However, restriction of vigorous contact sports and activities known to be associated with higher risk of spondylolysis, such as gymnastics, wrestling, and football, is appropriate.[27] These patients should be restricted from those vigorous activities that place them at higher risk for injury or slip progression. Advice and counseling about vocational plans and lifestyle changes are recommended for these children.

Adult patients require a different treatment protocol because low back pain and lower-extremity symptoms, rather than slip progression, are the key factors in determining whether surgical treatment is necessary. As with any adult patient who presents with back pain, with or without lower-extremity symptoms, conservative management should always be the initial treatment.

Exceptions to this rule are when the patient pre-

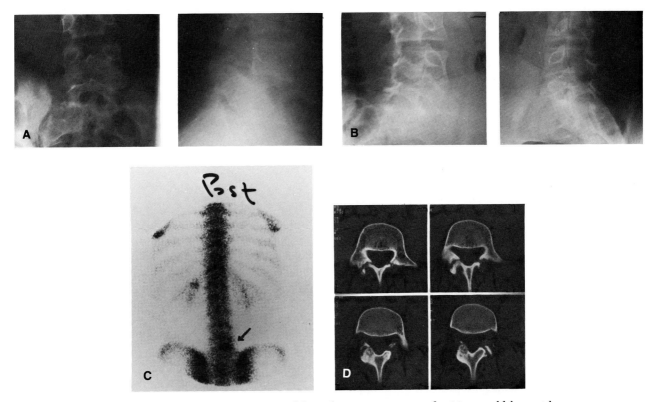

FIG. 21–14. **A.** Anterior-posterior and lateral roentgenograms of a 14-year-old boy with a vague history of trauma but with low-back pain unresponsive to appropriate conservative care. His pain became nocturnal and was relieved by aspirin during the course of his conservative care. A minimal spondylolisthesis occurs between L4 and L5, which is the last mobile segment due to the sacralization of L5 on S1. **B.** Left and right oblique roentgenograms showing the isthmic spondylolisthesis (the broken neck of the Scottie dog) at L4. **C.** The bone scan demonstrates increased uptake on the right at L4. **D.** These 2-mm CT scans demonstrate the pars interarticularis defect of L4 bilaterally and a lesion producing cortical thickening with sclerosis just proximal to the pars defect in the right lamina of L4. This is a typical osteoid osteoma with a nidus in this location.

sents with bowel and bladder symptoms and a complete workup eliminates all other causes, if the patient's axial or peripheral complaints are not relieved by conservative management and a rehabilitation program, and if the patient is not willing to accept the imposed lifestyle restrictions. Elective surgical stabilization should then be considered.

If the axial symptoms become chronic or if the lower-extremity symptoms wax and wane frequently or present as neurogenic claudication, decompression and stabilization is the treatment of choice. The adult patient with a Grade I or II slip with an insignificant previous history who develops back pain with or without peripheral symptoms should be viewed as any other patient with low back pain. Secondary gain, drug dependence, personality disorders, litigation, and other diagnoses must be taken into consideration in recommending treatment.

Grobler and colleagues distinguished between isthmic spondylolisthesis at L4–L5 and at L5–S1.[22] They noted that the average age of onset of clinical symptoms in an L4–L5 spondylolisthesis was later, that the lesion did not stabilize but continued to demonstrate features of instability, and that conservative management produced a high failure rate, often necessitating surgical stabilization. In these patients, perhaps surgical intervention should be pursued more aggressively.

Surgical Management

The goals of surgical management of spondylolysis or spondylolisthesis are to control pain unresponsive to conservative care, to correct neurologic deficits, and to correct severe spinal deformity. Although most patients, especially children, with slips less than 50% respond to conservative care, some patients with persistent symptoms, even after altering their lifestyle, require surgical intervention.

There are several indications for surgical intervention: (1) asymptomatic and symptomatic spondylolisthesis greater than 50% in a growing patient, (2) observed progression of spondylolisthesis in a growing or mature patient, (3) spinal deformity and a significantly abnormal gait that is uncorrected by conservative measures, (4) pain unresponsive to conservative treatment, and (5) neurologic involvement with lower-extremity weakness or cauda equina syndrome.

Elective surgery should always be preceded by a period of conservative care. Immobilization in a well-molded orthosis or cast may provide the clinician and patient with information about the success of spinal stabilization. If patients respond favorably to immobilization with decreased symptoms, especially axial complaints, surgical stabilization is more likely to be efficacious.

OPERATIVE TECHNIQUES

Children and Adolescents

Gill advocated removal of the loose posterior element in adult patients with spondylolisthesis and radicular symptoms, but this is never indicated in children and adolescents.[20, 21] Removal of the posterior elements without fusion is associated with a high incidence of slip progression postoperatively.[2, 4, 36, 37, 38, 62, 64, 65] Furthermore, it is associated with a higher incidence of pseudarthrosis if spinal fusion is performed.[56]

Children and adolescents do not have the stabilizing reactive bone formation from degenerative changes at the lumbosacral joint that adults do, but high success rates have been reported with intertransverse posterolateral fusion in Grades I and II slips in this young age group. Midline posterior fusion alone results in a high pseudarthrosis rate, because the loose posterior element does not provide a stable fusion bed.[37, 64]

In children and adolescents with spondylolisthesis of less than 50%, excellent surgical results may be obtained in most patients with an intertransverse fusion in situ from L5 to the sacrum. A solid fusion produces relief of back pain and relief of radicular complaints.

Hensinger and MacEwen advocated posterolateral fusion in situ in patients with severe slips of Grades III or IV. However, the results were not uniformly satisfactory, and a significant number of patients continued to have lower-extremity complaints.[25]

Buck advocated direct repair of the spondylolysis defect, but in children and adolescents, this is rarely a lesion that requires treatment; if it is unresponsive to conservative measures, other causes should be sought.[8, 9] I prefer compression arthrodesis with Cotrel–Dubousset rods, anchored to bilateral L5 pedicle screws and L5 offset lamina hooks. The pars is drilled out with a fine burr until bleeding bone is exposed, and morselized cancellous graft is impacted into the defect (see Fig. 21-13). Patients are immobilized for 6 months in an ambulatory custom-molded orthosis (Fig. 21-15).

Author's Preferred Method for Grades I and II

In a child or adolescent with Grade I or II isthmic spondylolisthesis unresponsive to conservative management, my preferred method is an intertransverse posterolateral in situ spinal fusion with autogenous iliac bone graft. An MRI is performed preoperatively to assess the state of hydration of the L4–L5 disc. Although uncommonly found in some adolescents, the L4–L5 disc may demonstrate early loss of hydration; therefore, although there is a low correlation with back pain, this level should be included in the fusion. If not, the early disc degeneration at L4–L5 may be accelerated.

Wiltse described an approach in which a cutaneous midline incision is made and the paraspinous muscles are split, providing direct access to the transverse processes and sacral alae.[66, 67] Meticulous decortication and copious bone grafting in the posterolateral gutter are performed. This is a safe approach without the potential dangers of cauda equina damage over an occult sacral spina bifida and results in a high fusion rate in children and adolescents (Fig. 21-16).

It has been my practice to place children in a bilateral pantaloon spica for 3 months and continue immobilization for another 3 months in an ambulatory, custom-molded TLSO. In adolescents past their growth spurt, a cast or custom-molded TLSO mobilization with early ambulation is adequate. The adolescent,

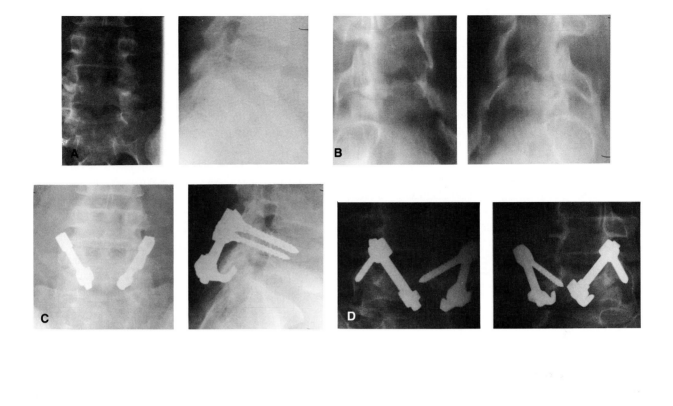

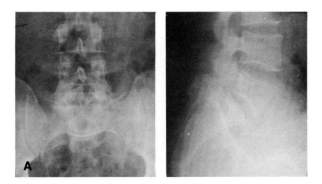

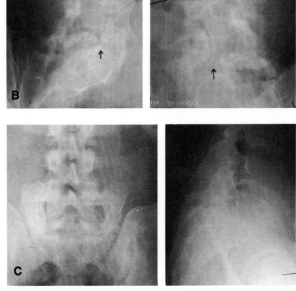

FIG. 21–16. A. Anterior-posterior and lateral roentgenograms of a mature 18-year-old patient with a Grade I isthmic spondylolisthesis of L5 on S1. Lateral view demonstrates some retrolisthesis of L4 on L5. This patient's chief complaint was lower back pain. **B.** Left and right oblique x-ray films showing the defect in the pars interarticularis at L5. **C.** Solid posterolateral arthrodesis from L4 to S1 performed through a paraspinous muscle-splitting approach.

with little growth remaining, has much less risk of progression during the healing stages of fusion than the preadolescent patient.

Grades III and IV Spondylolisthesis

Much controversy exists regarding the surgical management of high-grade slips in children and adolescents. Advocates of in situ fusion from L4 to the sacrum report good results.[25, 29, 63, 67]

Little mention is made of the correction of spinal deformity, especially the short waist and heart-shaped buttocks. Furthermore, a significant number of patients have residual radicular complaints.[25]

Capner, in 1932, was probably the first to attempt open reduction, but with little change in the degree of slippage.[10] Jenkins, in 1936, reported success in reducing the degree of slippage, but not without a high degree of risk.[28] Newman advocated skeletal traction for the reduction of spondylolisthesis, but he reported an unacceptable complication rate of bladder dysfunction.[41] Techniques employing external traction, with or without decompression, have not yielded satisfactory results and should not be employed.[28, 35]

In 1969, Harrington and Tullos reported their first cases of reduction of spondylolisthesis by employing Harrington instrumentation.[23] In 1976, Harrington and Dickson modified the technique by using a sacral bar and performing a posterior interbody fusion of the lumbosacral interspace.[24] In their reports, the instrumentation was long and reduction was not consistently maintained at follow-up. Applying vertical corrective force theoretically produced tension on the anterior longitudinal ligament, with a resultant ligamentotaxis to correct the sagittal displacement. The disadvantages of this method were the risks of bowel and bladder dysfunction after reduction and the fact that the lum-

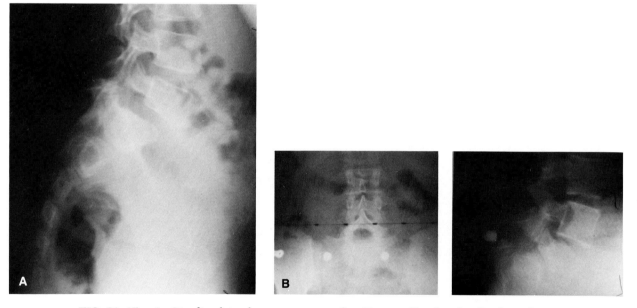

FIG. 21–17. **A.** Standing lateral roentgenogram of an 11-year-old girl with a Grade I isthmic spondylolisthesis. **B.** Anterior-posterior and lateral roentgenograms 2 years after the patient had been lost to follow-up, demonstrating progression to a severe Grade IV slip. The inverted Napoleon hat sign is evident on the anterior-posterior view, and the sacral inclination (verticalization of the sacrum) is extreme. **C.** Postoperative x-ray films demonstrating the DeWald method of posterior Harrington instrumentation from L1 through the sacrum. Bilateral sublaminar wiring of L3 and L4 and posterolateral fusion of L4 through the sacrum produced near anatomic reduction. This was followed by an anterior transperitoneal iliac strut graft interbody fusion between L5 and S1. **D.** Three years after surgery and after rod removal, demonstrating a solid anterior and posterior arthrodesis, although some loss of correction has occurred.

bosacral kyphosis with verticalization of the sacrum was not adequately addressed.

DeWald and colleagues modified the Harrington technique by instrumenting from L1 or L2 to the sacrum for reduction, performing a posterolateral spinal fusion from L4 to the sacrum, and then performing an anterior interbody fusion, adhering to the principles that severe spondylolisthesis is a lumbosacral kyphosis and that the anterior column had to be arthrodesed.[15] The long rods were removed after 6 months. In a number of patients this resulted in stiff, unfused upper lumbar spinal segments. Reduction was advocated only in children and adolescents, because the corrective forces required to effect an adequate reduction were dangerous in older patients with fixed deformities (Fig. 21-17).

Scaglietti and coworkers understood the sagittal-plane deformity of severe spondylolisthesis and the fact that it was a lumbosacral kyphosis. They advocated correction of the deformity by longitudinal traction and hyperextension by serial casting, followed by instrumentation and fusion in situ.[53] This proved to be a safe

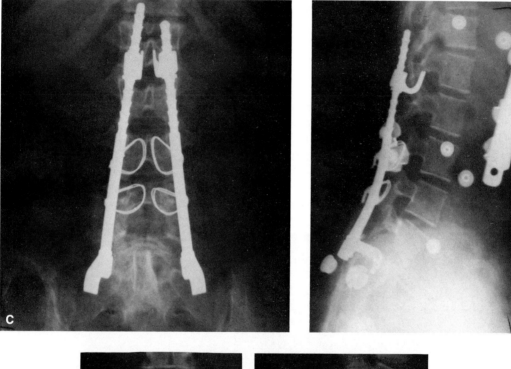

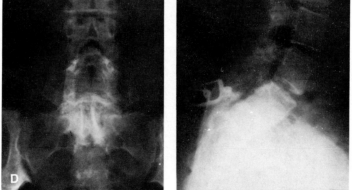

FIG. 21–17. *(continued)*

method, with resultant correction of the vertical sacrum and lumbosacral kyphosis but with incomplete reduction of L5 sagittal translation.

Sibrandij reported three cases of one-stage reduction and stabilization of severe spondylolisthesis employing axial traction with Harrington rods and screws in the L5 vertebral body to reduce the slip by pulling it backwards.[57] No complications or recurrent slipping were reported.

Author's Preferred Method for Grades III and IV

My preferred method is to employ pedicle fixation with rods or plates as a posterior first stage, combined with posterior release and partial excision of the L5–S1 intervertebral disc. Direct visualization of the neural structures is afforded by the wide L5 decompression. Pedicle screw fixation at L5 and S1 in a severe slip is exacting.

Posterior removal of the annulus and L5–S1 disc allows extension of the L5–S1 motion segment, with correction of the vertical sacrum and translation reduction of the L5–S1 ventral slip. The patient is positioned on an image table that has the capability of extending the hips during the reduction maneuver. It is imperative to obtain reduction by placing an instrument in the L5–S1 disc space and gently applying corrective force. Visualization of the L5 nerve roots is imperative and is facilitated by this approach.

Under the same anesthesia or at a second stage 10 days later, an anterior interbody fusion is performed through a Pfannenstiel incision and transperitoneal approach. This completes the circumferential fusion, providing anterior column support, which helps prevent loss of reduction postoperatively.

Meticulous attention must be paid to the dissection, and electrocautery must not be used in the prevertebral space at L5–S1 to avoid retrograde ejaculation in males, which has been reported by other authors.[15, 18, 52]

Without reduction to at least a Grade I slip, anterior interbody fusion is difficult and often inadequate. Similarly, posterior lumbar interbody fusion in high-grade slips does not afford an adequate bivertebral surface for graft coaptation and fusion (Fig. 21-18).

With appropriate surgical experience and expertise, high-grade slips in children and adolescents can be reduced safely and provide the degree of cosmetic improvement that young patients in today's society warrant.

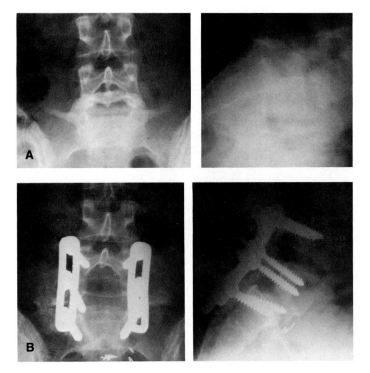

FIG. 21–18. **A.** Twenty-year-old female with a Grade IV isthmic spondylolisthesis of L5 on S1 presenting with significant axial and peripheral complaints. **B.** Anterior-posterior and lateral roentgenograms 4 months after surgery demonstrating reduction of the spondylolisthesis to Grade I with Steffee plates and pedicle screws accompanied by posterolateral fusion and anterior interbody fusion between L5 and S1.

Adults with Isthmic Spondylolisthesis

Most adults requiring a surgical approach have low back pain and leg pain as their presenting problems. Both problems should be addressed at surgery. Unless the patient has significant degenerative changes at the lumbosacral joint and presents with a neurogenic claudication syndrome secondary to spinal stenosis, a decompressive procedure should always be followed by stabilization.

If the L5–S1 disc is removed, even in the more degenerated spine, further slipping can occur, producing recurrent leg symptoms and new axial complaints.

The many reports of surgery to reduce and stabilize high-grade spondylolisthesis are replete with neurologic compromise of the bowel, bladder, and nerve root structures. The extent of successful fusion depends on the patient's age, weight, smoking habits, and intercurrent illness.

My preferred technique is in situ pedicle screw fixation from L4 to the sacrum, combined with adequate decompression of all nerve root structures in Grade I or II slips. The addition of a copious posterolateral spinal fusion with autologous bone graft should result in a high rate of fusion. All patients should be immobilized in a low-profile orthosis for at least 6 months.

With Grade III or IV spondylolisthesis, an L5 posterior element and nerve root decompression is usually adequate, but occasionally a more aggressive proximal decompression must be carried out and the fusion extended to L3. If the dome of the sacrum produces cauda equina compromise, it can be osteotomized to make more room for the descending dural sac.

Pedicular fixation with rod or plate contouring is necessary, as is a meticulous posterolateral spinal fusion. These patients have been managed in a low-profile orthosis with a unilateral pantaloon attachment to further immobilize the lumbosacral joint for 3 months. It is then converted to a simple lumbosacral orthosis with removal of the pantaloon extension for another 3 months.

The passage of sublaminar wires under the S1 lamina is dangerous and does not afford adequate fixation. It can lead to cauda equina damage, with resultant bowel and bladder compromise. Despite good results, I abandoned this method completely (Fig. 21-19).

In severe spondylolisthesis (Grade IV or V), some authors have suggested totally resecting the body of L5

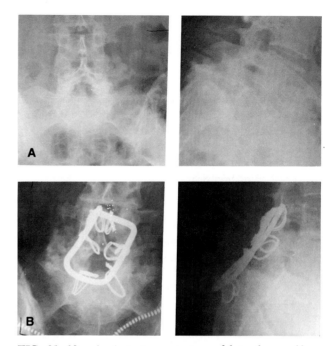

FIG. 21–19. **A.** Anterior-posterior and lateral x-ray films of a 30-year-old female with severe isthmic spondylolisthesis of L5 on S1. **B.** Anterior-posterior and lateral roentgenograms showing in situ fusion from L3 through the sacrum with sublaminar wires around L3, L4, and the first sacral lamina. Posterolateral fusion relieved the symptoms.

and replacing L4 on S1 in combination with posterior instrumentation and arthrodesis.[19] This procedure must be done both anteriorly and posteriorly in the same sitting to gain control and maintain correction of the deformity. It requires visualization of the L4 and L5 nerve roots anteriorly and posteriorly to be sure that they are completely free and remain free of impingement after resection is completed. This is a demanding exercise with significant potential for neurologic compromise.

SUMMARY

Spondylolisthesis is a fascinating, fairly common disorder. The enormous body of literature generated over the years on this topic is proof that there is still much to be learned. The treatment of severe degrees of slippage, especially in the adult population, is still undefined.

Most young patients respond to conservative care

with modification of vigorous activity. When the patient does require surgery, the simplest and safest approach for providing stabilization of the lumbosacral spine and relief of nerve root compromise should be used.

Reduction of severe slips, especially in children and adolescents, has the theoretical advantage of normalizing sagittal alignment and improving cosmesis. In adults, however, reduction is still not widely accepted because of its attendant risks.

References

1. Baker DR, McHollick W: Spondyloschisis and spondylolisthesis in children. J Bone Joint Surg [Am] 38:933, 1956
2. Barash HL, Galante JO, Lambert CN, Ray RD: Spondylolisthesis and tight hamstrings. J Bone Joint Surg [Am] 52:1319, 1970
3. Borkow SE, Kleiger B: Spondylolisthesis in newborn. A case report. Clin Orthop 81:73, 1971
4. Bosworth DM, Fielding JW, Demarest L, Bonaquist M: Spondylolisthesis: A critical review of a consecutive series of cases treated by arthrodesis. J Bone Joint Surg [Am] 37:767, 1955
5. Boxall D, Bradford DS, Winter RB, Moe JH: Management of severe spondylolisthesis in children and adolescents. J Bone Joint Surg [Am] 61:479, 1979
6. Bradford DS: Treatment of severe spondylolisthesis. A combined approach for reduction and stabilization. Spine 4:423, 1979
7. Brailsford JF: Spondylolisthesis. Br J Radiol 6:666, 1933
8. Buck JE: Direct repair of the defect in spondylolisthesis. J Bone Joint Surg [Br] 52:432, 1970
9. Buck JE: Further thoughts on direct repair of the defect in spondylolysis. J Bone Joint Surg [Br] 61:123, 1979
10. Capner N: Spondylolisthesis. Br J Surg 19:347, 1932
11. Colonna PC: Spondylolisthesis. Analysis of two hundred and one cases. JAMA 154:398, 1954
12. Cyron BM, Hutton WC: Variations in the amount and distribution of cortical bone across the partes interarticulares of L5. A predisposing factor in spondylolysis? Spine 4:163, 1979
13. Cyron BM, Hutton WC, Troup JDG: Spondylolytic fractures. J Bone Joint Surg [Br] 58:462, 1976
14. Dandy DJ, Shannon MJ: Lumbosacral subluxation (Group I spondylolisthesis). J Bone Joint Surg [Br] 53:578, 1971
15. DeWald RL, Faut MM, Taddonio RF, et al: Severe lumbosacral spondylolisthesis in adolescents and children. Reduction and staged circumferential fusion. J Bone Joint Surg [Am] 63:619, 1981
16. Eisenstein S: Spondylolysis. A skeletal investigation of two population groups. J Bone Joint Surg [Br] 60:488, 1978
17. Farfan HF, Osteria V, Lamy C: The mechanical etiology of spondylolysis and spondylolisthesis. Clin Orthop 117:40, 1976
18. Flynn JC, Hoque MA: Anterior fusion of the lumbar spine. J Bone Joint Surg [Am] 61:1143, 1979
19. Gaines RW, Nichols WK: Treatment of spondyloptosis by two-stage L5 vertebrectomy and reduction of L4 onto S1. Spine 10:680, 1985
20. Gill GG, Manning JG, White HL: Surgical treatment of spondylolisthesis without spine fusion. J Bone Joint Surg [Am] 37:493, 1955
21. Gill GG, White HL: Surgical treatment of spondylolisthesis without spine fusion. Acta Orthop Scand 85 (suppl), 1965
22. Grobler L, Haugh L, Wiltse L, Frymoyer J: L4–5 isthmic spondylolisthesis: Clinical and radiologic review in 52 cases. Presented at the Fifth Annual Meeting of the Federation of Spine Associates, New Orleans, LA, February 11, 1990
23. Harrington PR, Tullos HS: Spondylolisthesis in children. Observations and surgical treatment. Clin Orthop 79:75, 1971
24. Harrington PR, Dickson JH: Spinal instrumentation in the treatment of severe progressive spondylolisthesis. Clin Orthop 117:157, 1976
25. Hensinger RN, Lang JR, MacEwen GD: Surgical management of spondylolisthesis in children and adolescents. Spine 1:207, 1976
26. Herbiniaux, G: Traite sur Divers Accouchments Laborieux et sur les Polypes de la Matrice. Bruxelles, J.L. DeBoubers, 1782
27. Jackson DW, Wiltse LL, Cirincione RJ: Spondylolysis in the female gymnast. Clin Orthop 117:68, 1976
28. Jenkins JA: Spondylolisthesis. Br J Surg 24:80, 1936
29. Johnson JR, Kirwan EO: The long-term results of fusion in situ for severe spondylolisthesis. J Bone Joint Surg [Br] 65:43, 1983
30. Junghanns H: Spondylolisthesis ohne Spalt im Zeischengdenk-Stuck. Arch Orthop Unfallchir 29:118, 1931
31. Kilian HF: Schilderungen neuer Beckenformen und ihres Verhaltens in Leven. Mannheim, Verlag von Basserman & Mathy, 1854
32. Krenz J, Troup JDG: The structure of the pars interarticularis of the lower lumbar vertebrae and its relation to the etiology of spondylolysis. J Bone Joint Surg [Br] 55:735, 1973
33. Lafferty JF, Winter WG, Gambaro SA: Fatigue characteristics of posterior elements of vertebrae. J Bone Joint Surg [Am] 59:154, 1977
34. Lambl W: Beitrage zur Geburtskunde und Gynackologie. Von F.W. v. Scanzoni, 1858
35. Lance EM: Treatment of severe spondylolisthesis with neural involvement. A report of two cases. J Bone Joint Surg [Am] 48:883, 1966
36. Laurent LE: Spondylolisthesis in children and adolescents: A study of 173 cases. Acta Orthop Belgica 35:717, 1969
37. Laurent LE, Osterman K: Operative treatment of spondylolisthesis in young patients. Clin Orthop 117:85, 1976
38. Marmor L, Bechtol CO: Spondylolisthesis: Complete slip following the Gill procedure. A case report. J Bone Joint Surg [Am] 43:1068, 1961

39. McPhee IB, O'Brien JP: Reduction of severe spondylolisthesis. Spine 4:430, 1979
40. Meyerding HW: Spondylolisthesis. Surg Gynecol Obstet 54:371, 1932
41. Newman PH: A clinical syndrome associated with severe lumbosacral subluxation. J Bone Joint Surg [Br] 47:472, 1965
42. Newman PH, Stone KH: The etiology of spondylolisthesis, with special investigation. J Bone Joint Surg [Br] 45:39, 1963
43. Neugebauer FL: Aetiologie der sogenannten Spondylolisthesis. Arch Gynak Munchen 35:375, 1882
44. Osterman K, Lindholm TS, Laurent LE: Late results of removal of the loose posterior element (Gill's operation) in the treatment of lytic lumbar spondylolisthesis. Clin Orthop 117:121, 1976
45. Phalen GS, Dickson JA: Spondylolisthesis and tight hamstrings. J Bone Joint Surg [Am] 43:505, 1961
46. Porter RW, Park W: Unilateral spondylosis. J Bone Joint Surg [Br] 64:345, 1982
47. Ravichandran G: Multiple lumbar spondylolyses. Spine 5:552, 1980
48. Robert HLF: Eine eigenthumliche angeborene Lordose wahrscheinlich bedingt durch eine Verschiebung des Korpers des letzten Lendenwirbels aud die vordere Flache des ersten Kreuzbeinwirbels (Spondylolisthesis Kilian), nebst Bemerkungen uber die Mechanik dieser Beckenformation. Monatschr Geburtsk Frauen Berl 5:81, 1855
49. Roche MD, Rowe GG: The incidence of separate neural arch and coincident bone variations. J Bone Joint Surg [Am] 34:491, 1952
50. Rosenberg NJ: Degenerative spondylolisthesis, predisposing factors. J Bone Joint Surg [Am] 57:467, 1975
51. Rosenberg NJ, Bargar WL, Friedman B: The incidence of spondylolysis and spondylolisthesis in nonambulatory patients. Spine 6:35, 1981
52. Sacks S: Anterior interbody fusion of the lumbar spine. J Bone Joint Surg [Br] 47:211, 1965
53. Scaglietti O, Frontino C, Bartolozzi P: Technique of anatomic reduction of lumbar spondylolisthesis and its surgical stabilization. Clin Orthop 117:164, 1976
54. Shah JS, Hampson WGJ, Jayson MIV: The distribution of surface strain in the cadaveric lumbar spine. J Bone Joint Surg [Br] 60:246,1978
55. Shahriaree H, Sajadi K, Rooholamini SA: A family with spondylolisthesis. J Bone Joint Surg [Am] 61:1256, 1979
56. Sherman FC, Rosenthal RK, Hall JC: Spine fusion for spondylolysis and spondylolisthesis in children. Spine 4:59, 1979
57. Sibrandij S: Reduction and stabilization of severe spondylolisthesis. J Bone Joint Surg [Br] 65:40, 1983
58. Stewart TD: The age incidence of neural arch defects in Alaskan natives, considered from the standpoint of etiology. J Bone Joint Surg [Am] 35:937, 1953
59. Taillard WF: Etiology of spondylolisthesis. Clin Orthop 117:30, 1976
60. Tietjen R, Morgenstern JM: Spondylolisthesis following surgical fusion for scoliosis. Clin Orthop 117:176, 1976
61. Torgerson WR, Dotter WE: Comparative roentgenographic study of the asymptomatic and symptomatic lumbar spine. J Bone Joint Surg [Am] 58:850, 1976
62. Turner RH, Bianco AJ Jr: Spondylolysis and spondylolisthesis in children and teenagers. J Bone Joint Surg [Am] 53:1298, 1971
63. Velikas EP, Blackburn JS: Surgical treatment of spondylolisthesis in children and adolescents. J Bone Joint Surg [Br] 63:67, 1981
64. Wiltse LL: Etiology of spondylolisthesis. Clin Orthop 10:48, 1957
65. Wiltse LL: Spondylolisthesis in children. Clin Orthop 21:156, 1961
66. Wiltse LL: Spondylolisthesis: Classification and etiology. In American Academy of Orthopaedic Surgeons Symposium on the Spine, pp 143–168. St. Louis, CV Mosby, 1969
67. Wiltse LL, Jackson DW: Treatment of spondylolisthesis and spondylolysis in children. Clin Orthop 117:92, 1976
68. Wiltse LL, Newman PH, Macnab I: Classification of spondylolysis and spondylolisthesis. Clin Orthop 117:23, 1976
69. Wiltse LL, Winter RB: Terminology and measurement of spondylolisthesis. J Bone Joint Surg [Am] 65:768, 1983
70. Wiltse LL, Widell EH, Jackson DW: Fatigue fracture: The basic lesion in isthmic spondylolisthesis. J Bone Joint Surg [Am] 57:17, 1975
71. Wynne-Davis R, Scott JHS: Inheritance and spondylolisthesis. A radiographic family survey. J Bone Joint Surg [Br] 61:301, 1979

CHAPTER
22

Surgical Treatment of Spondylolisthesis: The Harms Technique

Jurgen Harms
Heinrich Boehm
Klaus Zielke

■

The treatment of spondylolisthesis remains controversial, as is evidenced by a published debate between Nachemson and Wiltse in 1976.[35] The methods of treatment range from posterior fusion in situ of even the most severe slips to instrumentation, reduction, and circumferential fusion of lesser slips. The divergent opinions about treating spondylolisthesis are partially due to the variable natural history of the deformity and the lack of correlation between the patient's impairment and the radiographic measurements (Fig. 22-1). The inability to accurately define and describe spinal instability adds to the confusion regarding the appropriate treatment of spondylolisthesis of all grades.

CLASSIFICATION

Although the classification system of Wiltse has merit, it does not distinguish among the underlying causes of the spondylolisthesis.[36] Regardless of the influence of genetics or growth on the appearance of a defect in the "articular bolt" (pars interarticularis), the mechanical conditions determine the mode of its evolution.[1, 13, 14, 18, 19, 24, 27, 31, 32, 37]

A retrospective analysis of 200 of our spondylolisthesis cases demonstrated three main groups: isthmic defect, isthmic dysplasia, and degenerative spondylolisthesis. Each group is composed of patients with fairly uniform presentations, etiologies, and natural histories. Acute traumatic spondylolisthesis and pathologic spondylolisthesis (e.g., tumor or infection) represent exceptional and unusual types.

Isthmic Defect

The isthmic defect type of spondylolisthesis is generally diagnosed in the 30- to 40-year-old individual who is engaged in physically demanding work. Recently, this condition has been noticed in younger patients who are engaged in high-level athletics. The lytic defect occurs through a pars interarticularis of normal size and shape. The slippage occurs as the involved disc begins to degenerate, allowing laxity in the annulus and the longitudinal ligaments (Fig. 22-2).

The defect may occur at any lumbar level, but it is most common at the lumbosacral joint. The slippage rarely exceeds 50% and never progresses to ptosis unless decompression (without concomitant successful fusion) is performed. The sacral inclination is normal or increased. This deformity does not produce lum-

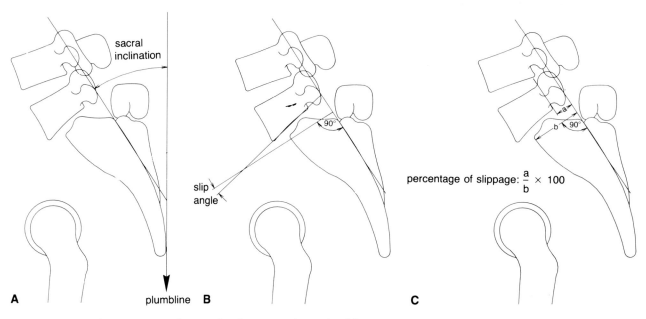

FIG. 22–1.   **A.** The sacral inclination is the angle of the posterior sacrum to vertical. Normal is 40 to 60° of lordosis.   **B.** The slip angle is measured according to the method described by Boxall.[3] Normal is 0 to 5°.   **C.** The normal percentage of slipping is zero.

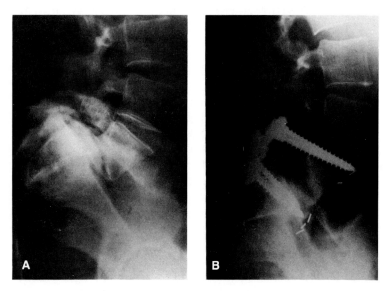

FIG. 22–2.   **A.** Isthmic defect type of spondylolisthesis with posterior elements of normal size. Sacral inclination is normal at 40° and slippage is 59%.   **B.** Solid fusion 5 months after dorsoventral reduction and stabilization.

bosacral kyphosis and does not markedly affect posture.

Isthmic Dysplasia

The isthmic dysplasia group is largely composed of juveniles and adolescents. Progression of the slippage and neurologic symptoms, including spondylolisthetic crisis, are relatively common. Radiographically, the pars interarticularis is attenuated and elongated. A lytic defect may or may not be present, but there is usually a congenital anomaly of the lumbosacral joint, such as spina bifida occulta (Fig. 22-3). The deformity occurs exclusively at the lumbosacral joint and is the only type in our series to progress to spondyloptosis. In contrast to the isthmic defect type, the slip angle increases and the sacral inclination diminishes, producing lumbosacral kyphosis and postural derangement secondary to verticalization of the sacrum.

Degenerative Spondylolisthesis

The group of patients with degenerative spondylolisthesis typically consists of 50- to 70-year-old women who present with complaints of neurogenic claudication. The cause is usually degeneration of the three-joint complex or rheumatoid arthritis.[28] The deformity is the result of forward slipping of a vertebra, usually of L4 or L5, with intact posterior elements (Fig. 22-4). The slippage rarely exceeds 20 to 30%, but

owing to the intact posterior elements and concomitant degenerative arthropathy, a mild slippage can produce substantial spinal stenosis.

TREATMENT

Theoretically, the most elegant treatment of spondylolysis would be direct repair of the lytic isthmic defect. However, repair of the pars defect remains a questionable undertaking with a high failure rate.[5]

Decompression

In the low-grade isthmic defect and the isthmic dysplasia types of spondylolisthesis, neurologic deficit is rare. Decompression procedures, such as those proposed by Gill or Crock, add to the instability.[7, 10] The results of decompression are rated only fair or better in approximately 75% of the cases in a 5-year follow-up.[1, 2, 8, 16, 17, 20] Progression of the slippage in 25% of the patients and a reoperation rate of 12% are not acceptable results in our opinion.[25]

Wiltse has denied the need for decompression and advocates fusion in situ for improving neurologic symptoms and signs.[33, 34] Numerous reports have supported the excellent results achieved by his method. However, those results must be interpreted in terms of the techniques available at the time and the expectations of the patient and the surgeon.

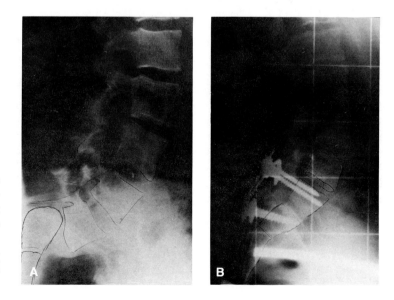

FIG. 22–3. **A.** High-grade, isthmic dysplasia type of spondylolisthesis. The pars interarticularis is attenuated and elongated without lysis. Sacral inclination approaches zero due to compensatory verticalization of the pelvis. **B.** Instrumentation with anterior and posterior fusion yielded remarkable reduction of lumbosacral kyphosis.

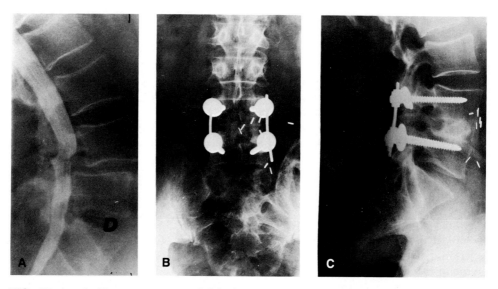

FIG. 22–4. **A.** Degenerative spondylolisthesis produces significant stenosis despite only moderate slippage because of the intact posterior elements. Sacral inclination and slip angle are slightly increased, but this does not represent a lumbosacral kyphosis. **B, C.** Solid monosegmental fusion 4 years after surgery. Neighboring motion segments are untouched.

Posterior Stabilization

Posterior fusion, even with instrumentation, has a high risk of failure and likelihood of additional iatrogenic destruction. The contact area for fusion and the strength of the transverse processes are limited, producing a high pseudarthrosis rate.[16] Often, at least one healthy neighboring motion segment is altered or included in the fusion. This may be secondary to the purposeful inclusion of the next proximal segment in the fusion or a result of impingement of pedicle instrumentation on the zygapophyseal joints of the next open segment.

Despite a solid posterior arthrodesis, pain may persist owing to residual anterior motion through the intervertebral disc space.[21] If the indication for surgery is painful instability, it seems illogical to perform a posterior fusion alone. Moreover, because the spondylolisthetic deformity in most cases is a kyphosis of the lumbosacral joint, permanent monosegmental correction can only be maintained by a solid anterior column.

Anterior Stabilization

Anterior interbody fusion alone is not the solution for the stabilization of spondylolisthesis. This technique has had a high rate of pseudarthrosis, and we aban-

doned it 10 years ago.[23] Another shortcoming is the inability to achieve reduction in more severe grades of slippage.[22] Direct decompression of the neural elements is not possible from the anterior approach, and iatrogenic neurologic impairment may result from nerve root compression by the displaced fibrocartilaginous tissue in the isthmic defect after vertebral manipulation.

Circumferential Stabilization

One-stage combined approaches are currently much more realistic owing to advances in anesthesia and surgical technique.[6] The combined approach permits safe and direct control of both spinal columns, which is essential in radical treatments.

In our opinion, if painful instability is accepted as a surgical indication, the monosegmental lesion of the anterior and posterior column necessitates a monosegmental reconstruction of both columns.

OPERATIVE TECHNIQUE

The aim of surgical treatment of spondylolisthesis is to restore the patient's occupational and recreational function. This goal is achieved by stabilization of the monosegmental instability, reversal of neurologic compromise, normalization of lumbosacral geometry, and maintenance of the above by solid bony fusion.

In 1983, Harms developed his method of reduction and monosegmental transpedicular stabilization of spondylolisthesis. Initially, Zielke instrumentation was employed, but the instrumentation was subsequently modified to provide greater application for posterior insertion.

Posterior Instrumentation

The patient is prone on a frame. General anesthesia and induced hypotension are routinely used. The spine is exposed through a midline incision with subperiosteal stripping.

If root compression exists or is anticipated after reduction due to the fibrocartilaginous tissue in the isthmic defect, the posterior elements are removed. Nerve root decompression may be performed at this point or after the next step, which is screw insertion. The screws are inserted into the pedicles of the two corresponding levels. In dysplastic spondylolisthesis, the superior joint is often frontally oriented. To avoid irritation of the joint and to increase rotational stability of the construct, the screws are inserted as laterally as possible and directed medially in a convergent fashion (Fig. 22-5). Partial excision of the inferior facet of the next upper segment is unacceptable.

The site for insertion in the lumbar spine is the intersection of a horizontal line bisecting the transverse process and a vertical line 2 mm medial to the lateral aspect of the superior facet. Because this oblique insertion is difficult to control, it is crucial to perforate the corticalis centrally above (posterior to) the pedicle. Drilling at low speed, intermittently using the 3.2-mm drill like a probe to ascertain bony contact, allows proper placement even in an attenuated dysplastic pedicle. The site of sacral insertion is the inferolateral aspect of the sacral facet. We feel that if the implant adapts to the spine, rather than vice versa, one screw in the sacrum should be sufficient, even in osteopenia. The use of methylmethacrylate to augment screw fixation, as recommended by some authors, is not advisable.[21, 30]

Reduction of the spondylolisthesis is achieved in three steps. The first is the application of longitudinal corrective force by the means of unilateral or, in severe cases, bilateral Harrington rods from L3 to the sacral ala.[11] Second, during gradual axial correction, an assistant pulls the spinous process of the superior vertebra dorsally. A threaded 4-mm rod is engaged in the screw-

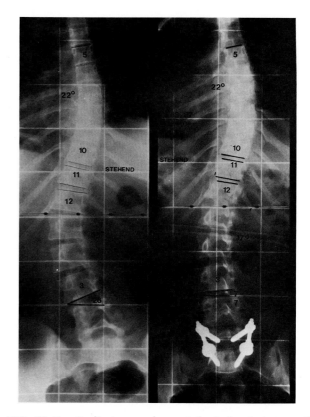

FIG. 22–5. Scoliosis secondary to isthmic dysplasia type of spondylolisthesis. Notice lateral insertion and medial direction of pedicle screws. The convergent construct adds to rotational stability.

heads.[12] The third step is the tightening of the nuts on the threaded rod with the Harrington rods still in place. According to the principles of kyphosis surgery, the mechanism of correction is the shortening of the posterior column by compression. Monosegmental transpedicular correction is continued until a normal lumbosacral profile is achieved. The Harrington rods are then removed, and the transpedicular implant remains for definitive stabilization (Fig. 22-6).

In severe grades of spondylolisthesis, the spine may not demonstrate sufficient mobility to achieve full reduction or the L5 nerve roots may become entrapped between the L5 pedicle and the dome of the sacrum. In these instances, the definitive stabilization is delayed until the anterior surgery is accomplished. The insertion of large corticocancellous interbody grafts mobilizes the spine and restores the height of the lumbosacral disc space, opening the stenotic L5 foraminae. The grafts also provide a fulcrum for further posterior compression and reduction.

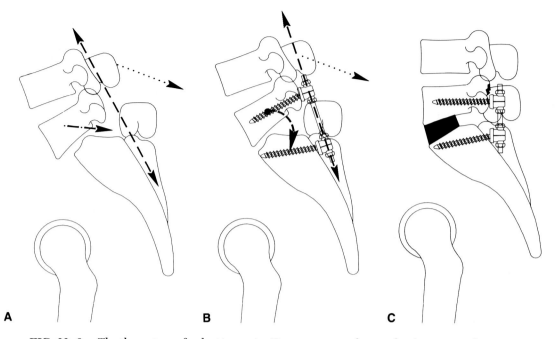

FIG. 22–6. The three steps of reduction. **A.** First, temporary longitudinal corrective force is applied between L3 and sacrum (*dashed arrow*). Second, manual posterior traction is applied using the spinous process of the next upper vertebra (*dotted arrow*). **B.** Third, transpedicular monosegmental compression reverses the slipping moment (*dash-dot arrow*). **C.** Anterior interbody spondylodesis.

After the definitive stabilization, a final inspection of the involved nerve roots is mandatory. If the "rattle fragment" (loose posterior element) is intact, it may be replanted by transarticular screws on either side. This is not done in degenerative or dysplastic spondylolisthesis. In those cases the dura is routinely covered by a free fat graft. For interbody fusion, three corticocancellous bone blocks from the posterior iliac crest may be taken from the same incision or from a separate one directly over the posterior iliac crest. No posterior fusion is attempted. The wound is then closed.

Anterior Fusion

In 94% of our cases, the anterior fusion was performed under the same anesthesia. The patient is supine, with the table hyperextended at the waist. The lumbosacral disc is approached by a midline, transperitoneal exposure.[9] The L4–L5 disc is approached by a left lumbar, retroperitoneal exposure.[15] The anterior and anterolateral aspect of the disc is exposed by blunt dissection. The median sacral, ascending lumbar, and seg-

mental vessels are identified, ligated, and transected. The anterior longitudinal ligament is incised in a "saloon-door" fashion and retracted laterally to provide protection to the superior hypogastric plexus and the iliac vessels. The disc is removed, the endplates are decorticated, and two or three bone blocks are inserted. Readaptation of the anterior ligament wings avoids bleeding from decorticated endplate surfaces; wound closure is routine.

Results

From 1983 to 1989, 230 patients with spondylolysis, spondylolisthesis, and spondyloptosis were treated by the Harms technique. The isthmic defect type constituted 45% of this series, isthmic dysplasia type accounted for 26%, and degenerative spondylolisthesis constituted 27%. The remaining 2% consisted of acute traumatic spondylolisthesis. The levels of involvement included L3–L4 (5%), L4–L5 (31%), L5–S1 (63%), and one case of a lumbarized S1 on S2. Degenerative spondylolisthesis was noted exclusively at the L4–L5

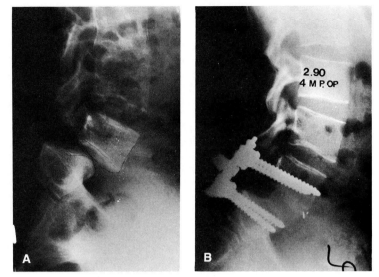

FIG. 22–7. **A.** Isthmic dysplasia type of spondylolisthesis with sacral inclination of only 20°. **B.** Solid fusion at 4 months with restoration of normal sacral inclination to 40°. Notice advanced instrumentation, including adjustable screw heads and a transverse stabilizing device.

level, and dysplastic spondylolisthesis occurred only at the last mobile segment. Isthmic dysplasia was the only one to progress to ptosis.

There were no mortalities. Of the 180 patients followed for more than 1 year, two patients developed a pseudarthrosis. Initially, when the 3.2-mm rod was employed, 6 cases of rod breakage were reported. Both pseudarthrosis patients had broken rods. No breakage of the 4-mm rod or pedicle screws was observed. One wound infection required surgical drainage, but the implant was not removed. Five patients developed deep vein thrombosis. No additional neurologic injury—in particular, no case of retrograde ejaculation[29]—was noted.

SUMMARY

The Harms technique of dorsoventral reduction and stabilization of spondylolisthesis is effective and safe. The aim of surgery should be to restore normal sagittal profile, not to stabilize the spine in a deformed position. Although normal sagittal contour can vary widely, the value of 30° of sacral inclination is 10° too low in our opinion.[4, 26] The growing interest in the sagittal profile should provide more substantial data about the normal range of lumbosacral kyphosis.

The normal lumbosacral sagittal angle found in the isthmic defect and the degenerative type must not be altered by surgical intervention. Conversely, the ratio-

nal treatment of the isthmic dysplasia type must be directed at correction of the pathologic hyperkyphosis (Fig. 22-7). The goals of surgical intervention should be to approximate normal anatomic conditions by creating either a surgical sacralization or a block of two vertebrae without sacrifice of additional motion segments.

References

1. Amuso SJ, Mankin HJ: Hereditary spondylolisthesis and spina bifida. A report of a family in which the lesion is transmitted as an autosomal dominant. J Bone Joint Surg [Am] 49:507, 1967
2. Amuso SJ, Neff RS, Coulson DB, Laing PG: The surgical treatment of spondylolisthesis by posterior element resection. A long-term follow-up study. J Bone Joint Surg [Am] 52:529, 1970
3. Boxall D, Bradford DS, Winter RB, Moe JH: Management of severe spondylolisthesis in children and adolescents. J Bone Joint Surg [Am] 61:479, 1979
4. Bradford DS: Spondylolysis and spondylolisthesis. In Bradford DS, Lonstein J, Ogilvie J, Winter R (eds): Moe's Textbook on Scoliosis and Other Deformities. Philadelphia, WB Saunders, 1987
5. Buck JE: Direct repair of the defect in spondylolisthesis. Preliminary report. J Bone Joint Surg [Br] 52:432, 1970
6. Cloward RB: Posterior lumbar interbody fusion updated. Clin Orthop 193:16, 1985
7. Crock HV: Normal and pathological anatomy of the lumbar spinal nerve root canals. J Bone Joint Surg [Br] 63:487, 1981
8. Davis IS, Bailey RW: Spondylolisthesis long-term follow-up study of treatment with total laminectomy. Clin Orthop 88:46 1972

9. Freebody D, Bendall R, Taylor RD: Anterior trans-peritoneal lumbar fusion. J Bone Joint Surg [Br] 53:617, 1971

10. Gill GG, Manning JG, White HL: Surgical treatment of spondylolisthesis without spine fusion. Excision of the loose lamina with decompression of the nerve root. J Bone Joint Surg [Am] 37:493, 1955

11. Harms J, Rolinger H: Die operative Behandlung der Spondylolisthese durch dorsale Aufrichtung und ventrale Verblockung. Z Orthop 120:343, 1982

12. Harms J, Stoltze D: Die operative Behandlung der BWS- und LWS-Frakturen mit dem USI-System. In Stuhler TH (ed): Fixateur Externe—Fixateur Interne. Berlin, Springer-Verlag, 1989

13. Harrington PR, Tullos HS: Spondylolisthesis in children. Observations and surgical treatment. Clin Orthop 79:76, 1971

14. Harris RI, Wiley JJ: Acquired spondylolysis as a sequel to spine fusion. J Bone Joint Surg [Am] 45:1159, 1969

15. Hodgson AR, Wongs K: A description of a technic and evaluation of results in anterior spinal fusion for deranged intervertebral disk and spondylolisthesis. Clin Orthop 56:133, 1968

16. Johnson JR, Kirwan EOG: The long-term results of fusion in situ for severe spondylolisthesis. J Bone Joint Surg [Br] 65:43, 1983

17. Johnsson K-E, Willner S, Johnsson K: Postoperative instability after decompression for lumbar stenosis. Spine 11:107, 1986

18. Kettelkamp DB, Wright DG: Spondylolysis in the Alaskan Eskimo. J Bone Joint Surg [Am] 53:563, 1971

19. Laurent LE, Östermann K: Operative treatment of spondylolisthesis in young patients. Clin Orthop 117:85, 1976

20. Lee CK: Lumbar spinal instability (olisthesis) after extensive posterior spinal decompression. Spine 8:429, 1983

21. Lee CK, Langrana NA: Lumbosacral spinal fusion. Spine 9:574, 1984

22. Louis R, Maresca C: Stabilisation chirurgicale avec réduction des spondylolyses et des spondylolisthésis. Int Orthop 1:215, 1977

23. Magerl F, Wörsdorfer O: 10-Jahres-Resultate von lumbalen interkorporellen Spondylodesen. Orthopäde 8:192, 1979

24. Newman PH: The etiology of spondylolisthesis. With a special investigation by Stone KH. J Bone Joint Surg [Br] 45:39, 1963

25. Östermann K, Lindholm TS, Laurent LE: Late results of removal of the loose posterior element (Gill's operation) in the treatment of lytic lumbar spondylolisthesis. Clin Orthop 117:121, 1976

26. Pasquet A: Etude des Paramètres Descriptifs de la Colone Vertébrale Humaine vue de Profil. Lyon, Thèse Ingénier, 1980

27. Pfeil E: Spondylolysis and Spondylolisthesis bei Kindern. Z Orthop 109:17, 1969

28. Rosenberg N:Degenerative spondylolisthesis. Surgical treatment. Clin Orthop 117:112, 1976

29. Sacks S: Anterior interbody fusion of the lumbar spine. J Bone Joint Surg [Br] 47:211, 1965

30. Steffee AD, Sitkowski DJ: Reduction and stabilization of Grade IV spondylolisthesis. Clin Orthop 227:82, 1988

31. Stewart TD: The age incidence of neural arch defects in Alaskan natives, considered from the standpoint of ethiology. J Bone Joint Surg [Am] 35:937, 1953

32. Taillard W: L'ethiologie du spondylolisthésis. Rev Chir Orthop 7:90, 1971

33. Wiltse LL, Bateman G, Hutchinson RH, Nelson WE: The paraspinal sacrospinal-splitting approach to the lumbar spine. J Bone Joint Surg [Am] 50:919, 1968

34. Wiltse LL, Jackson DW: Treatment of spondylolisthesis and spondylolysis in children. Clin Orthop 117:92, 1976

35. Wiltse LL, Nachemson A: Spondylolisthesis [editorial]. Clin Orthop 117:23, 1976

36. Wiltse LL, Newman PH, Macnab I: Classification of spondylolysis and spondylolisthesis. Clin Orthop 117:23, 1976

37. Wiltse LL, Widell EH, Jackson DW: Fatigue fracture: The basic lesion in isthmic spondylolisthesis. J Bone Joint Surg [Am] 57:17, 1975

CHAPTER
23

Treatment of Lumbosacral Spondyloptosis by Spondylectomy and Reduction

Robert W. Gaines, Jr.
W. Kirt Nichols

Debate about the optimal treatment for patients with spondyloptosis continues. The three most serious issues clouding rational decisions about treatment are the relative rarity of high-grade lesions, lack of a commonly accepted definition for spondyloptosis, and inclusion of patients with spondyloptosis in reports of patients with less severe (third- and fourth-degree) slips.

For this discussion, spondyloptosis is defined as the most severe form of L5 spondylolisthesis, one that permits vertical descent of the entire vertebral body of L5 below the end plate of S1 (Fig. 23-1).

Suggestions for treatment taken from the literature range from Wiltse's claim of successful functional results from fusion in situ in 8 cases, to Bradford's high complication rate from attempted two-stage reduction of L5 onto the sacrum, to DeWald's partially successful reduction with distractive force rods.[1, 2, 7]

Although Wiltse was able to achieve union with no neurologic complications in his 8 patients, other experienced surgeons using a so-called conservative surgical approach (i.e., fusion in situ or cast reduction) reported neurologic complications after treating high-grade spondylolisthesis.[7] Schoenecker reported L5 root problems and, much more importantly, permanent motor and sensory bowel and bladder dysfunction from cauda equina damage.[8] Bradford and DeWald reported a worrisome incidence of bowel and bladder loss after attempted restoration of L5 onto S1.[1, 2] Edwards successfully used his device to reduce moderate slips, but he did not suggest it for spondyloptosis.[3]

Other authors have reported techniques for reduction of L5 onto S1, but they did not distinguish spondyloptosis from less severe forms of spondylolisthesis. All of these reports included motor and sensory deficits in the L5 root in a small but significant number of patients when L5 was reduced onto S1. These reports also included bowel and bladder deficits.[6, 9]

Transfeldt and Steffee (personal communication) reported severe upper lumbar root (L2, L3, L4) deficits from lumbar plexus stretch when attempting to reduce L5 onto S1 for patients with spondyloptosis.[10]

The two-stage procedure shown in Figures 23-2 to 23-4 was developed because of dissatisfaction with previous techniques. The object was to restore sagittal plane balance and avoid nerve root damage from spinal and nerve root stretching during reduction. The procedure was designed to neither shorten nor lengthen the spine and to provide the experienced surgeon with

(text continues on page 596)

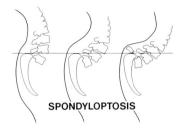
SPONDYLOPTOSIS

FIG. 23–1.   Spondyloptosis exists if the entire vertebral body of L5 exists on a vertical plane below the top of S1. The tilt angle varies considerably.

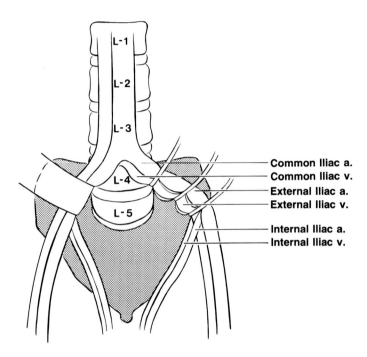

Common Iliac a.
Common Iliac v.
External Iliac a.
External Iliac v.

Internal Iliac a.
Internal Iliac v.

FIG. 23–2.   Anterior approach for resection of the L4–L5 disc, the vertebral body of L5, and the L5–S1 disc is done through an incision extended transversely across both rectus abdominus muscles. The great vessels are mobilized laterally after they are carefully identified, and the structures to be resected are visualized between the bifurcation of the vena cava and aorta.

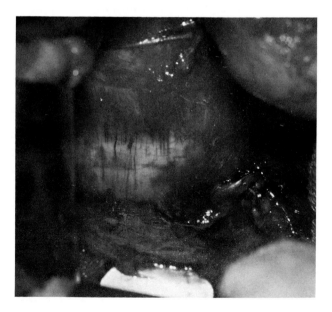

FIG. 23–3.   Here the L4 vertebral body, the L4–L5 disc, and the L5 vertebral body are identified. A malleable retractor is directly caudal to the inferior aspect of L5. The L5–S1 disc cannot be visualized at this point in the procedure because it lies directly underneath the vertebral body of L5, between L5 and the anterior-superior surface of the sacrum. The L4–L5 disc is excised first. Next, the L5 body is excised back to the base of the pedicles. Then the L5–S1 disc is excised. Bleeding is controlled with gelfoam and bipolar cautery, and a bolus of gelfoam is left in the resection gap.

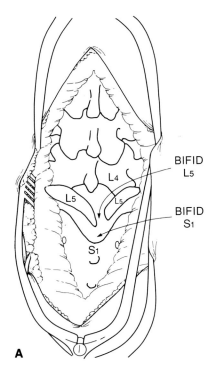

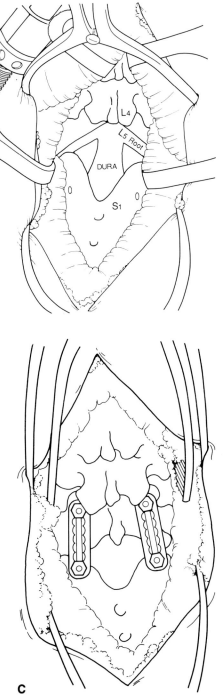

FIG. 23–4. A. Second-stage procedure begins with exposure of L2 to S3. All patients have bifid S1 segment, and most have bifid L5 segment. **B.** Harrington hooks and outriggers are applied between L2 and sacral ala to gently distract the interval between L4 and S1. All L5 posterior elements, including the pedicle, superior articular process, and transverse process, are resected with great care, protecting the dura, L5 roots, and cauda equina. The S1 endplate is decorticated. **C.** After the resection is completed, the outriggers are gently loosened, the L4–S1 interval is gently approximated, and the internal fixation devices are applied. The realignment of L4 and S1 requires minimal effort. Bone from the L5 body resection, kept frozen between stages, is added in the intertransverse area of L4–S1 as a graft. No extra iliac graft is used. The L5 and S1 roots are clearly identified and protected as the L4–S1 interval is approximated.

excellent exposure of the nerve roots and cauda equina so that they could be protected. Moreover, all of the structural barriers to reduction were to be surgically excised so that restoration of spinal alignment could be achieved with minimal effort.

MATERIALS AND METHODS

All four patients shown in Figures 23-5 through 23-23 show severe distortion of their sagittal contour with marked forward displacement of the trunk, posterior prominence of the posterior iliac crest, a more vertical orientation of the sacrum, and marked extension of the lumbar lordotic curve into the thoracic area in an attempt to rebalance the trunk in the sagittal plane.

All of the patients in this series were severely functionally disabled and virtually housebound by back and leg pain. Weinstein and colleagues reported patients who were not severely functionally disabled by relatively high-grade spondylolisthesis.[5] None of the patients in this series complained primarily of their postural distortion, although on questioning all noticed the uniqueness of posture that they had accepted as normal for them.

The first two cases were reported in 1985.[4] Table 23-1 lists the 5 patients operated on with this procedure at the University of Missouri—Columbia Hospital. Three other patients operated on by the author at other hospitals are not included here because follow-up on these patients is not adequate.

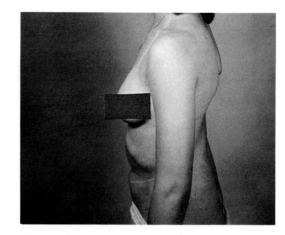

FIG. 23–6. Postoperative photograph of J.P. Trunk length is essentially the same as preoperative length. Forward tilting of the pelvis is obvious, as is improvement in sagittal contour.

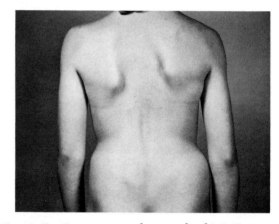

FIG. 23–7. Preoperative photograph of J.P. Paraspinous spasm is obvious, as is trunk foreshortening.

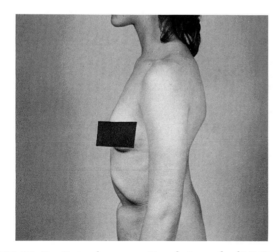

FIG. 23–5. Lateral preoperative photograph of J.P. Crease across her abdomen is obvious, as is the posterior rotation of the iliac crest.

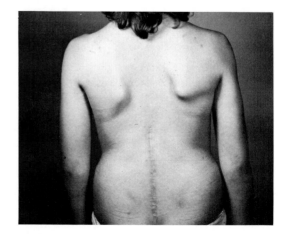

FIG. 23–8. Postoperative photograph of J.P. Absence of muscle spasm is seen, as is maintenance of trunk height.

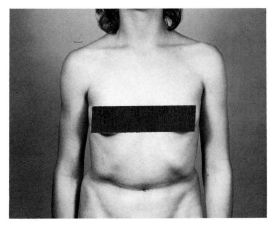

FIG. 23–9. Preoperative photograph of J.P. Trunk foreshortening is obvious, with the crease across the abdomen.

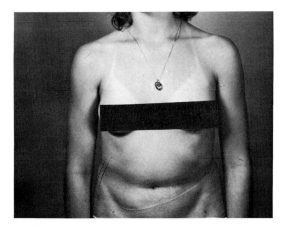

FIG. 23–10. Postoperative photograph of J.P. Same trunk length is visualized.

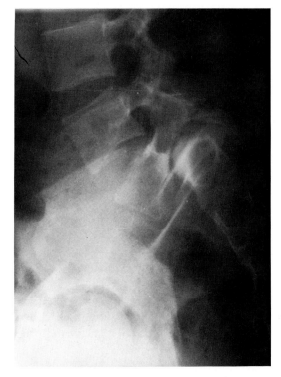

FIG. 23–11. Preoperative lateral x-ray film of patient E.K. (1980).

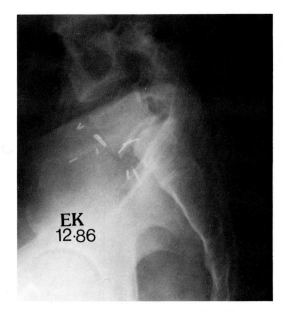

FIG. 23–12. Postoperative lateral x-ray film of patient E.K. showing reduction of L4 onto S1.

Each patient had virtually the same procedure as the one I previously reported.[4] The only departure was that R.P. and N.D. (see Table 23-1) had internal fixation of their osteotomies with the Steffee plating system. This dramatic improvement in the internal fixation of the osteotomy has permitted only 6 weeks of bedrest for the last 2 patients and the reexploration of a solid fusion mass and plate and screw removal at 4 months after the second stage.

As indicated in Table 23-1, each of these patients has been carefully and closely followed from the time of surgery until the reconstruction was solidly healed and the implants were removed. Subsequently, the patients have been seen every other or every third year.

(text continues on page 602)

TABLE 23-1. Clinical Information for All Patients

Initials	Age	Symptoms	Past Medical History	Deformity	Preoperative Neurologic Examination	Slip Angle	Surgery Date	Length of Follow-up	Fusion Solid	Postoperative Neurologic Status (Permanent)	Postoperative Pain	Postoperative Occupation	Postoperative Bowel/Bladder Fx	Estimated Blood Loss 1st stage/2nd stage (ml)
B.B.	24	B/L*	Down's syndrome	Severe	Restricted SLR	80°	1980	10 yrs	Yes	No	No	Independent at home	Normal	1980/1850
E.K.	17	B/L	—	Severe	Restricted SLR	45°	1980	9 yrs	Yes	No	No	State Highway Department worker	Normal	3260/4800
J.P.	17	B/L	—	Severe	Restricted SLR	35°	1982	7 yrs	Yes	No	No	Student	Normal	1100/1500
R.S.	16	B/L	—	Severe	Restricted SLR	50°	1985	4 yrs	Yes	No	No	Fast food restaurant/ student	Normal	2340/850
N.D.	20	B/L	—	Severe	Restricted SLR	45°	1988	18 mos	Yes	No	No	Student	Normal	2100/1800

*B/L, back and leg pain.

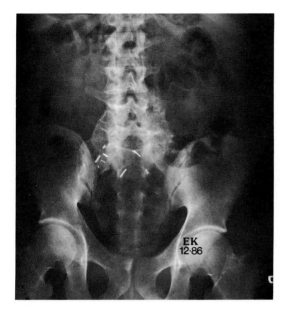

FIG. 23–13. Postoperative anterior-posterior x-ray film of patient E.K. (7-year follow-up).

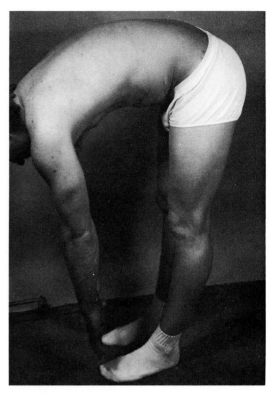

FIG. 23–15. Eight-year follow-up of patient E.K. Lateral bending photograph showing excellent lumbar motion.

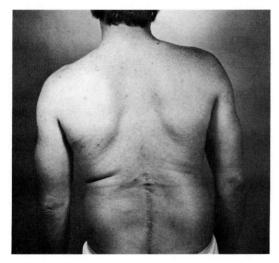

FIG. 23–14. Eight-year postoperative follow-up of patient E.K.

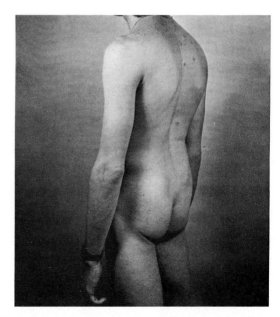

FIG. 23–16. Preoperative lateral photograph of R.S. showing posterior pelvic prominence and extension of lumbar lordosis into the midthoracic area.

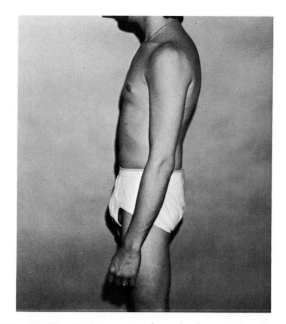

FIG. 23–17. Postoperative lateral photograph of R.S. showing improvement of sagittal contour. Characteristically, the anterior displacement of L4 relative to the sacrum is almost completely corrected.

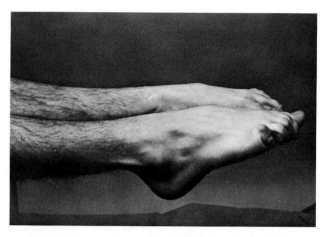

FIG. 23–19. Postoperative foot plantar flexion of R.S.

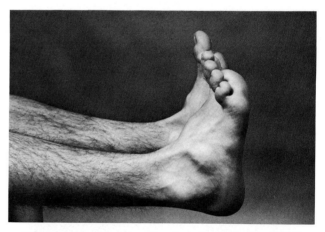

FIG. 23–20. Postoperative foot dorsal flexion of R.S.

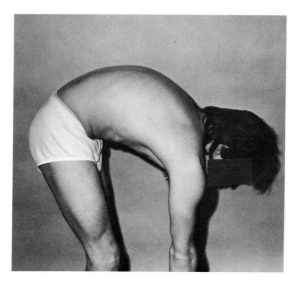

FIG. 23–18. Postoperative lateral bending photograph of R.S. showing excellent lumbar motion.

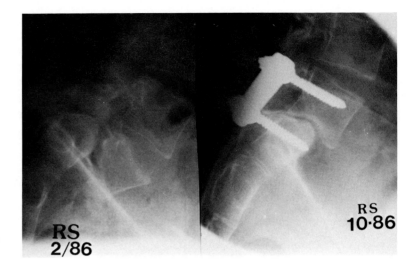

FIG. 23–21. Preoperative and postoperative lateral x-ray films of R.S.

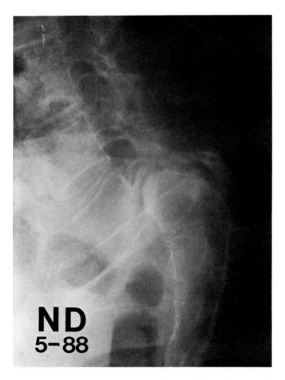

FIG. 23–22. Preoperative lateral x-ray film of N.D. showing spondyloptosis with high tilt angle.

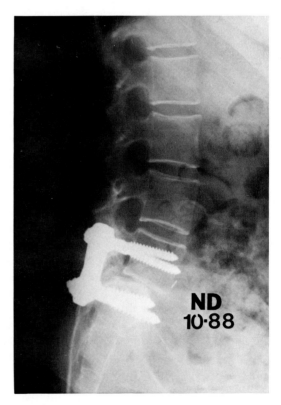

FIG. 23–23. Postoperative lateral film showing L4 reduced onto S1. In this case, there is some improvement in the sagittal Cobb angle between L4 and S1 and significant correction of the anterior translational deformity.

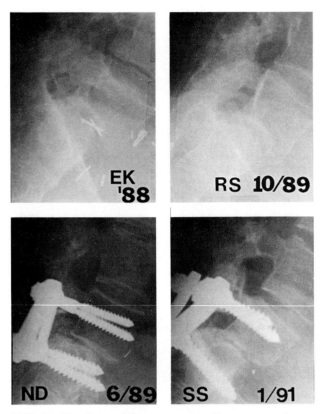

FIG. 23–24. Latest follow-up x-rays of four patients demonstrate interbody union at long-term follow-up. (Patient S.S., not included in this series because of short follow-up, underwent the surgical procedure 7 months earlier.)

RESULTS

Each patient was relieved of his or her preoperative symptoms. All patients noticed an improvement in spinal alignment. All of the patients are engaging in lifestyles compatible with their family background and educational potential, with only a relatively minor influence on their activities from a solid spinal reconstruction. They try to avoid repeated heavy bending and lifting, particularly from a twisted position.

None of the patients has leg pain. Three (J.P., R.S., N.D.) of the 5 patients had mild sensory deficits in the L5 dermatome after the second-stage procedure. These deficits cleared within 6 months after the surgery.

Two of the 5 patients had mild motor weakness (4/5 strength) in the toe and foot dorsiflexors after the first stage (J.P.) or second stage (R.S.). This weakness abated within 2 months after surgery and was com-

pletely gone in both patients after 6 months. None of the patients has shown the upper lumbar deficit in the L2, L3, or L4 roots reported by Transfeldt.[10]

Although these patients have been carefully checked for signs and symptoms of bowel or bladder deficit during all phases of treatment, none has had any suggestion of bowel or bladder difficulty. No patient complains of thoracolumbar pain.

SUMMARY

Although reports exist of patients having minimal symptoms with spondyloptosis, all of my patients have been severely functionally disabled by back pain or leg pain or both. The severe deformity at the base of the spine has produced severe thoracolumbar dysfunction due to sagittal plane imbalance, even in patients with solid lumbosacral fusions in situ.

The procedure described, although elaborate, has produced very satisfactory restoration of the sagittal contour in all of the patients operated, relief of the patients' preoperative back and leg pain, and freedom from nerve root tension.

Although minor dysfunction of the L5 nerve root has been a frequent part of the postoperative recovery, no patient has pain or permanent deficit in the L5 root. Most importantly, no patient has had bowel, bladder, sexual, motor, or sensory dysfunction.

The short-level fusion benefits these young patients, and the short period of bedrest necessary when firm internal fixation (the VSP plates and screws) has been used has made this procedure the primary reconstructive option for patients with spondyloptosis.

No posterior interbody fusions have been done in this series. However, all patients have gone on to have spontaneous interbody fusion. This was accomplished by removing the cartilaginous endplate from the inferior aspect of L4 and the superior aspect of S1 and gaining apposition of these two bony surfaces during the reduction of the deformity (Fig. 23-24).

References

1. Bradford DS: Treatment of severe spondylolisthesis. A combined approach for reduction and stabilization. Spine 4:423, 1979
2. DeWald RL, Faut MM, Taddonio RF, Neuwirth MG: Severe lumbosacral spondylolisthesis in adolescents and

children. Reduction and staged circumferential fusion. J Bone Joint Surg [Am] 63:619, 1981

3. Edwards C: Prospective evaluation of a new method for complete reduction of L5–S1 spondylolisthesis using corrective forces alone. Presented at the American Academy of Orthopaedic Surgeons, New Orleans, Louisiana, 1990

4. Gaines RW, Nichols WK: Treatment of spondyloptosis by two-stage L5 vertebrectomy and reduction of L4 onto S1. Spine 10:680, 1985

5. Harris IE, Weinstein SL: Long-term follow-up of patients with Grade III and IV spondylolisthesis. Treatment with and without posterior fusion. J Bone Joint Surg [Am] 69:960, 1987

6. McPhee IB, O'Brien JP: Reduction of severe spondylolisthesis. A preliminary report. Spine 4:430, 1979

7. Peek RD, Wiltse LL, Reynolds JB, et al: In situ arthrodesis without decompression for Grade III or IV isthmic spondylolisthesis in adults who have severe sciatica. J Bone Joint Surg [Am] 71:62, 1989

8. Schoenecker PL, Cole HO, Herring JA, et al: Cauda equina syndrome after in situ arthrodesis for severe spondylolisthesis at the lumbosacral junction. J Bone Joint Surg [Am] 72:369, 1990

9. Sijbrandij S: Reduction and stabilisation of severe spondylolisthesis. A report of three cases. J Bone Joint Surg [Br] 65:40, 1983

10. Transfeldt EE, Dendrinos GK, Bradford DS: Briefly noted: Paresis of proximal lumbar roots after reduction of L5–S1 spondylolisthesis. Spine 14:884, 1989

CHAPTER
24

Reduction of Spondylolisthesis

Charles C. Edwards

■

The history of orthopedics is dominated by a quest for the straight (*ortho*) child (*paedia*). Over the years, investigators and clinicians have sought to wrench deformity and the pathomechanics that accompany it from one disease after another. As the 20th century comes to a close, both surgeons and patients expect surgical treatments to yield anatomic length and alignment for the extremities. In contrast, fusion in situ remains the standard treatment for the spondylolisthesis deformity.

Is there a role for reduction in the treatment of spondylolisthesis? To answer this question, one must consider the degree to which the current standard—in situ fusion—meets our expectations, the added advantages of reduction, and any offsetting risk or morbidity associated with the reduction alternative.

PATHOMECHANICS OF SPONDYLOLISTHESIS

The body's center of gravity lies anterior to the lumbosacral joint. As a result, the lumbar spine tends to slip forward and rotate anteriorly into flexion about the sacral dome. In the normal spine, the inferior facets of L5 buttress against the superior facets of S1 to block slippage and rotation. The pars defect or elongation that characterizes spondylolisthesis functionally cleaves the inferior facets from L5, allowing the lumbar spine to slip forward. Resulting anterior shear forces in the lumbosacral disc cause progressive disc degeneration, loss of anterior column height, and lumbrosacral kyphosis. Depending on the patient's age when this scenario begins, the L5 and sacral architecture, the degree of sacral lordosis, and the amount of ligamentous laxity, the deformity progresses or remains stable.

When the slip progresses in childhood or adolescence, the posterior portion of the fifth lumbar vertebra comes to rest on the anterior portion of S1 (Fig. 24-1). Concentration of axial loads over such a small area erodes or remodels the postero-inferior corner of L5 and the anterosuperior corner of the sacrum. The result is a trapezoidal or wedge-shaped L5 body and a rounded sacral dome. Once this geometry occurs, the rate of anterior lumbar tilt accelerates, and the lumbar spine proceeds to rotate around the dome with progressive lumbosacral kyphosis.

To stand erect, the patient must compensate for every degree of lumbosacral kyphosis. This compensation is accomplished in several ways. First, the patient

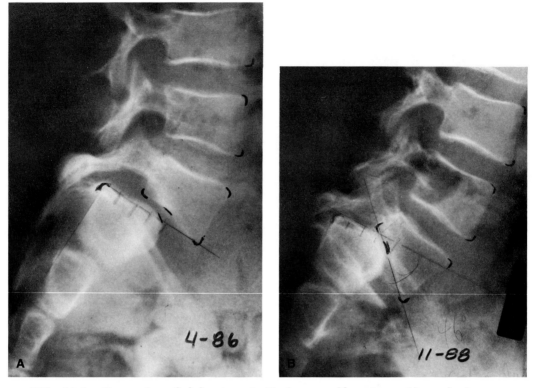

FIG. 24–1. Progression of deformity. **A.** Twelve-year-old patient with grade 3 spondylolisthesis. **B.** Nineteen months later, there is complete loss of the disc space, erosion and remodeling of the posteroinferior corner of L5, rounding of the anterior sacral dome, and rotation of the lumbar spine about the sacral dome into lumbosacral kyphosis.

arches the lumbar spine into maximum lordosis. Second, the hamstrings and iliopsoas muscles contract to rotate the pelvis into a more vertical position. If these measures are not sufficient, the patient must flex the hips and knees to restore an erect posture and sagittal balance. The lumbosacral kyphosis (slip angle) and compensatory thoracolumbar hyperlordosis are reflected clinically by the anteriorly protruding inferior rib cage and the flattened buttocks that characterize the spondylolisthesis deformity.

The advanced deformity is always associated with foreshortening of the trunk. This is caused by the accordion effect of lumbosacral kyphosis with compensatory thoracolumbar lordosis combined with the slippage of L5 from the top of the sacrum into the pelvis. Loss of trunk height is responsible for such clinical signs as waist line absence and flank creases. It is also most likely responsible for 12–40% reduced abdominal and

erector spinae muscle strength in spondylolisthesis patients,[28, 39] since these muscles become shorter than their optimal length on the Blix curve. In high-grade spondylolisthesis and spondyloptosis, the rib cage often abuts against the iliac crest, adding another source of discomfort. Substantial loss of trunk height is responsible for a disproportionate body; this condition, combined with the absence of a waist and redundant belly and flank tissues, is often cosmetically offensive to the young women most frequently afflicted with high-grade spondylolisthesis.

Radicular pain and varying degrees of nerve root dysfunction are present in roughly half of spondylolisthesis patients requiring surgery.[11, 24, 46] Anterior translation of L5 on the sacrum stretches the sacral roots over the posterosuperior corner of the sacral endplate. If rapid slippage occurs, a cauda equina syndrome with bowel and bladder dysfunction may follow. More commonly, the fifth lumbar roots are compressed as they approach the L5 foramina. Typically, they are trapped under the fibrocartilage that fills the pars defect or its adjacent osteophyte.

SHORTCOMINGS OF IN SITU FUSION

Some authors consider the results of in situ fusion to be highly satisfactory for all grades of adolescent spondylolisthesis without significant further slippage or nonunion.[30, 50] However, most spine surgeons encounter a rate of pseudarthrosis, progression, and other problems higher than that considered acceptable for other spine reconstructive procedures.

Pseudarthrosis

It is noteworthy that large lumbosacral fusion studies that report union rates according to diagnosis cite a lower union rate for spondylolisthesis fusions (72%) than other primary conditions (83% average).[9, 22, 64] If series with more than 50 cases are considered, the average union rate for in situ iliac fusions is 76%.[2, 9, 29, 37, 52, 71] Series that use posterolateral iliac fusion report a higher union rate (81%)[3, 51, 52, 68] than those that use only posterior fusion (75%).[2, 9, 29, 37, 52] The average union rate for grade 3 + slips in adolescents[3, 37, 71] is about the same as for grade 1 slips in adults.[2, 52] This information is particularly sobering in view of Bradford's observation that, of 10 symptomatic patients thought to have solid in situ fusion by radiography, 7 actually had a pseudarthrosis at the time of surgical exploration.[7] Hence, the true union rate for primary posterolateral in situ fusion for spondylolisthesis is probably in the range of 60–70%. Most of the nonunions eventually cause mild to moderate pain.[2, 19]

Loss of Motion Segments

The vast majority of in situ fusions for spondylolisthesis are from L4 to the sacrum, with extension to L2 or L3 for high-grade slips. Fusion across normal joints above the slip is sometimes recommended to improve union rates by placing the fusion mass in a more vertical orientation and providing more graft contact area. However, proximal extension of the fusion reduces lumbar motion segments and concentrates more load than necessary at the first open joint.

Further Slippage

Even when solid fusion is achieved for the unreduced spondylolisthesis deformity, it often fails to arrest slip progression, because the same anterior bending and shear forces that dissuade union in the first place persist even after successful fusion. Tension forces that work against the graft can bend and elongate the immature fusion. They also may cause successive fatigue failure and repair of the mature fusion, with further progression of lumbosacral kyphosis.

Most English-language studies of in situ fusion for spondylolisthesis acknowledge progression of deformity despite apparently solid arthrodesis.[2, 10, 28, 34, 37, 44, 48, 72] The reported incidences of slip progression include 11%,[37] 14%,[28] 20%,[2] 26%,[3] 37%,[44] 57%,[48] and 72%,[10] for an average reported incidence of 33%. The slip angle (lumbosacral kyphosis) tends to progress to a greater extent than L5–S1 displacement. Average slip angle progression is reported at 15–20°.[2, 3, 51] Both Gill laminectomy[2, 51] and lack of postoperative immobilization[10, 51] encourage slip progression. Nevertheless, slip progression can occur even when patients are kept supine for several months[2, 37] or when the L5 arch is left in place.[3, 10, 28, 37, 48, 51, 72] A high preoperative slip angle also increases the chance of late progression. Boxall noted that 40% of patients with a slip angle of more than 55° progressed in the presence of solid arthrodesis.[3] Dandy found that the majority of progression occurs during the 6 months following surgery, after the patient begins to ambulate.[10] However, on the average, approximately 2% additional translation and 1–2° angulation occur per year for at least several years.[3, 10]

Neurologic Deficit

In situ fusion in adolescent patients with slips that exceed 50% carries the risk of neurologic injury. Dandy reported minor motor or sensory deficits in 12% of patients after posterolateral in situ fusion.[10] Despite using a bilateral paraspinous muscle–splitting approach, Maurice published three case reports with permanent cauda equina syndrome, reduced perineal sensation, and bowel or bladder dysfunction.[41] This serious complication occurs more frequently than once thought. In 1989, Schoenecker and colleagues identified 12 cases of cauda equina syndrome with loss of bowel and bladder control that developed after in situ fusion for adolescent patients with grade 3 or 4 spondylolisthesis. Posterolateral fusion was performed through a bilateral paraspinous muscle—splitting incision in four patients and through the midline in eight patients without known dural injury. The procedures were performed by six experienced spinal surgeons, who report a combined incidence of 6% (12 in 189 cases) for cauda equina syndrome complications after in situ fusion. Schoenecker postulated that muscle relaxation after general anesthesia and surgical dissection led to additional slippage, which stretched sacral roots over the posterosuperior corner of the sacrum. Patients most at risk were those with an initial slip angle of more than 45°.[58]

Residual Deformity

Fusing a high-grade spondylolisthesis deformity in place leaves the patient with abnormal spinal mechanics and often a tarnished self-image. Patients with more than 30° of lumbosacral kyphosis must hold their thoracolumbar spine in maximal hyperextension to maintain sagittal balance. This causes muscle fatigue and can lead to facet changes and disc degeneration. Retrolisthesis is reported above the in situ fusion in 24% of cases.[28] Late degenerative changes secondary to abnormal spine mechanics may account for much of the mild but continuous low back and thigh pain experienced by 30% of patients after "successful" in situ fusion.[52, 56]

Patients with higher degrees of lumbosacral kyphosis develop an abnormal waddling gait secondary to the vertical pelvis, hip, and knee flexion that are required for sagittal balance. The combination of protruding ribs from anterior translation and thoracolumbar hyperlordosis, loss of trunk height, flattened buttocks, and crouched stance is unsightly. Unfortunately, most high-grade spondylolistheses occur in adolescent girls who often find their own appearance distressing. Osterman recently observed that, despite solid union, 8 of 10 girls in his series of in situ fusion for spondyloptosis considered their own result cosmetically poor.[48]

POTENTIAL ADVANTAGES OF REDUCTION AND FIXATION

Since reduction, fixation, and fusion involve more extensive surgery than in situ fusion alone, it must offer clear advantages to be worthy of consideration. Most current reduction techniques include segmental pedicle screw fixation, thus the advantages of reduction and secure fixation are considered together.

Stops Progression of Deformity. Fixation, preferably in a reduced position, eliminates the approximately one-third chance of progression seen despite successful in situ fusion. Reduction increases the likelihood that fixation will remain secure by reducing the anterior bending forces that work against the instrumentation.

Lessens Postoperative Pain. Effective fixation blocks anterior shear at the unstable lumbosacral joint to greatly reduce the back pain associated with ambulation during the first weeks after spinal fusion. In my experience, secure internal fixation reduces total analgesic consumption by more than 50% of that required by patients without fixation.

Permits Full Nerve Decompression. Since removal of the fifth arch is thought to make the spine more unstable, some authors advise against root decompression even in the face of mild radiculopathy; they explain that pain will subside and function will improve after future remodeling.[2, 28, 51, 67] However, the majority of investigators favor root decompression for prompt pain relief and optimum nerve recovery.[3, 10, 11, 24, 29, 37, 40, 43, 45, 49, 53, 60, 63] Root pain or deficit is present in as many as 70% of surgical candidates.[11, 24, 46] The clinical signs, symptoms, and surgical exploration show that most radiculopathy is due to compression of the fifth lumbar root by the pars fibrocartilage.[3] Decompression requires removal of the fibrocartilage attached to the loose arch of L5, a treatment first described by Gill.[24] Internal fixation makes it possible to fully decompress all symptomatic L5 roots without fear of residual instability or progressive slippage.

Sacral radiculopathy is caused by the stretching of the sacral roots over the posterosuperior corner of the sacrum. Loss of the Achilles reflex and other signs of compression of the first two sacral roots are reported in as many as 29% of patients who require surgery for high-grade spondylolisthesis.[37] Root compression of S2–S4, with bowel and bladder dysfunction, generally occurs only in patients with rapidly progressing high-grade slips. Spondylolisthesis reduction is the ideal treatment for sacral radiculopathy. Restoring the lumbar spine to its proper position over the sacrum relieves anterior pressure from the sacral roots, shortens their course, and, hence, relaxes the cauda equina.

Promotes Union. Arthrodesis can be difficult to achieve in spondylolisthesis for three reasons: (1) rotation of the lumbar spine around the sacrum shifts the body's central axis anterior to the lumbosacral graft; the resulting flexion moment subjects the graft to considerable tensile forces; (2) the slip itself (anterior displacement) first decreases and then eliminates axial loading across the lumbosacral interspace; and (3) without the buttressing effect of the L5 facets posteriorly or the sacral endplate inferiorly, the lumbosacral graft is subjected to considerable anteroinferior shear forces. Reduction addresses each of these biomechanic irregularities to increase the chance of successful union. Correction of the slip angle restores the body's central axis over the sacrum to greatly reduce the bending moment and tensile stress that works against the lumbosacral graft. Correcting the slip itself restores axial loading across the lumbosacral interspace. Pedicular fixation of the aligned spine then eliminates shear.

Limits Fusion Length. Fusion across normal joints above the slip has been recommended as a way to partially compensate for the abnormal biomechanics and achieve a reasonable rate of union. When normal biomechanics are restored via correction of the deformity, it is possible to restrict instrumentation and fusion to the affected lumbosacral joint in most cases. Even for the most severe cases of spondyloptosis with L4–L5 joint pathology or associated scoliosis, it is possible to limit the proximal extent of fusion to L4.

Restores Body Posture and Mechanics. Full correction of the spondylolisthesis deformity (lumbosacral kyphosis, loss of height, and anterior translation) restores normal spine mechanics and body posture. Correction of lumbosacral kyphosis eliminates the *need* for patients to maintain maximum lumbar lordosis, pelvic tilt, or hip flexion for sagittal balance. Thus there is spontaneous correction of compensatory lumbar and thoracolumbar lordosis, reduction in muscle fatigue,[6] and a more efficient gait. Restoration of trunk height improves the length-tension relationship of paraspinous and abdominal muscles for more efficient spinal function.[23]

Improves Appearance and Self-Image. In agreement with DeWald[13] and Bradford,[6] we find that most adolescents with high-grade spondylolisthesis deformities are disturbed about their abnormal posture, proportions, body contours, and gait. This concern results in a poor self-image and, frequently, personality disorders. Full reduction of the deformity can dramatically improve the patient's self-image (Fig. 24-2). Correction of lumbosacral kyphosis eliminates the crouched posture, waddling gait, and protruding rib cage and improves buttock contour. Restoration of trunk height eliminates abdominal folds and restores normal waist contours and body proportions. Patients with major preoperative deformity emerge several inches taller and far more attractive. Adolescent females, in particular, become happier, more outgoing, and generally have more positive family and peer relationships.

The theoretical advantages of spondylolisthesis reduction-fixation are substantial. However, two questions remain: (1) Can full reduction be accomplished for most patients? (2) If so, can it be achieved without excessive risk and morbidity relative to in situ fusion?

DEVELOPMENT OF A REDUCTION CAPABILITY

Traction-Cast Reduction

The first attempts to correct the deformity of spondylolisthesis with closed-reduction techniques used traction, posture manipulations under anesthesia, and extension casts followed by anterior or posterior fusion and months of bed rest. The fascinating history of spondylolisthesis reduction began with Scherb, a German surgeon. In 1921, he reported successful reduction of spondylolisthesis in a remarkably flexible 14-year-old girl, which was maintained with a panlumbar tibial graft at 1 year follow-up.[57]

Jenkins from New Zealand was the first to actually describe a reduction technique. In 1936, he reported the case of a 16-year-old boy with a rapidly progressing slip, which he reduced with longitudinal traction and a pelvic sling. He placed a tibial dowel from the anterior aspect of L5 into the sacrum, which maintained reduction for more than a year;[33] unfortunately, the graft eventually resorbed and the deformity recurred.[39]

In 1951, Harris renewed interest in spondylolisthesis reduction with a preoperative traction technique that combined longitudinal femoral pin traction with anterior traction through anterior iliac crest tongs to flex and translate the sacrum. After posterolateral fusion, he resumed traction and then incorporated the tongs in a pantaloon cast for 3 months.[27] Lance first used Steinmann pins rather than tongs for improved iliac fixation.[36]

Some authors found that partial reduction could be

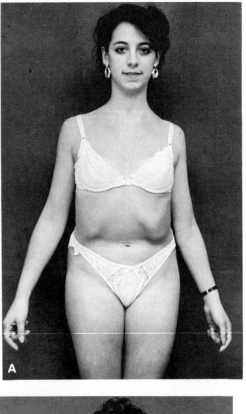

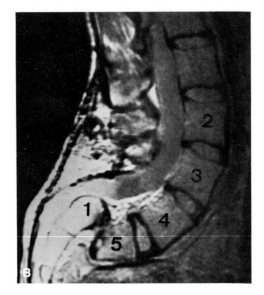

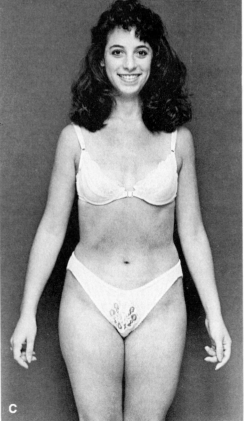

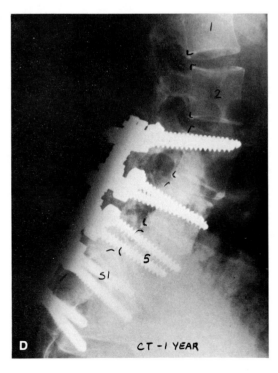

FIG. 24–2.

610

obtained in children with this method if postoperative traction and casting was employed.[36, 44, 66] On the other hand, Newman found traction-reduction "while possible in a few instances was never maintained during graft consolidation" and cited four cases of major neurologic deficit that complicated traction reduction.[44]

Two reports in 1976 reactivated interest in closed-reduction techniques for spondylolisthesis. Scaglietti emphasized the importance of longitudinal traction with hips in maximal extension so as to flex the pelvis and, thus, counteract lumbosacral kyphosis. He applied an extension double pantaloon Minerva cast with patients in traction on a fracture table. Despite 4 months of preoperative traction-casting and 10 months of postoperative cast protection, Scaglietti only achieved about 50% correction; thus, he abandoned the technique in favor of internal fixation.[56] In the same year Snijder[62] and, later, others[3, 39] reported that preoperative traction was unnecessary. Snijder also reported the successful use of posterior traction wires from the lumbar lamina to an outrigger worn on the patient's back to help maintain reduction during graft consolidation.[62] Ohki and associates combined intraoperative halo-femoral traction with Snijder's spinous process wiring technique.[47]

Despite these advances, the great majority of reports on traction-cast reduction of spondylolisthesis remained negative. It never enjoyed widespread use because of concerns about neurologic deficit and unpredictable reduction results. Several authors reported motor deficits in one-third or more patients while in traction before or after posterior surgery.[5, 7, 39] Most investigators concluded that traction-cast reductions are unpredictable since they rely on the flexibility of the deformity[40] and generally fail to achieve satisfactory correction.[3, 21, 40, 44, 56, 60, 66]

Bradford and coworkers have achieved the most favorable results with closed reduction by limiting the technique to young patients with intermediate deformity and by synthesizing the most effective elements of prior techniques (Fig. 24-3).[5] Details of their technique and results are discussed later under "Current Options for Spondylolisthesis Reduction."

Posterior Distraction Instrumentation

In 1967, Paul Harrington first used *internal* traction for reduction of spondylolisthesis. He placed distraction rods between the lamina of L1 and a transiliac "sacral" bar in a 13-year-old girl. By distracting the spine, he was able to correct much of the slippage via ligamentotaxis. Following a Gill laminectomy and lateral iliac fusion, the patient was treated in a bilateral spica cast.[25] The use of distraction instrumentation was rapidly embraced by Vidal, Scaglietti, DeWald, and others.[13, 56, 73] Scaglietti improved the surgical construct with alar hooks rather than a transiliac rod for distal fixation.[56] Unfortunately, the rods tended to rotate into flexion around their single-point of distal hook fixation on the sacrum or iliac rod. Resulting progressive loss of reduction was noted by Harrington and other early investigators.[3, 26, 56] In an effort to prevent forward rotation and slippage, Harrington[26] and Vidal[73] bolstered the anterior column with an interbody fusion from the posterior approach, and Scaglietti performed a second stage interbody fusion from the anterior approach.[56]

Reduction results from distraction instrumentation were generally unsatisfactory. Final correction of 50–60% of the slip was possible, but no improvement was seen in the slip angle or in the correction of abnormal vertical sacral inclination.[7, 26, 56] Most of these panlumbar distraction rod fusions caused considerable flattening of the lumbar lordosis. This was of great concern

◀ **FIG. 24–2.** Correction of clinical deformity. **A.** Clinical photo of patient with spondyloptosis demonstrates typical stigmata of anterior rib cage protrusion, loss of trunk height and waist, flank skin folds, and hip flexion contractures. **B.** Preoperative sagittal magnetic resonance imaging demonstrating spondyloptosis with marked lumbar compensatory hyperlordosis. **C.** Appearance after instrumented reduction of spondyloptosis. Trunk height is restored with the appearance of a waistline and loss of abdominal folds. Sagittal spine alignment is corrected with elimination of rib cage prominence. **D.** Postoperative radiograph. Reduction was accomplished with the application of corrective forces only; there was no need to cross the abdomen or enter the disc space. Disruption of L3–L4 facets from a prior failed in situ fusion attempt made it necessary to extend instrumentation proximally to L3.

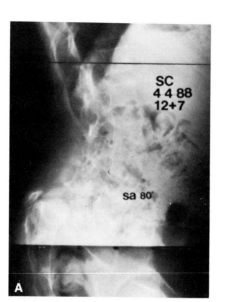

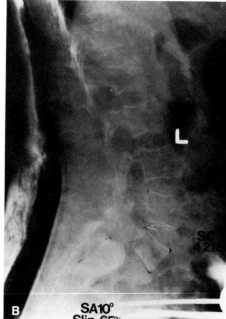

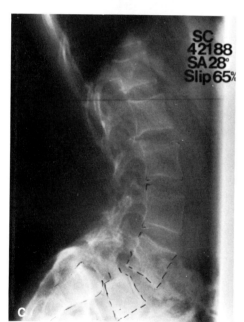

FIG. 24–3. Extension cast reduction of spondylolisthesis. **A.** Preoperative lateral radiograph of spondyloptosis in child of 12 years with progressive and flexible deformity. **B.** Lateral radiograph after posterior fusion and traction-cast reduction. Iliac wing pins-in-plaster are used to flex the sacrum and reduce lumbosacral kyphosis. **C.** Post-treatment radiograph after removal of the extension-cast. Slip angle has improved from 80° before the operation to 28°. (Case courtesy of David Bradford, M.D.)

to patients with spondylolisthesis, since lumbar hyperlordosis is required to compensate for lumbosacral kyphosis and to maintain sagittal balance.

During the late 1970s, efforts were made to shorten the length of the distraction instrumentation or at least the number of fused vertebrae. Minneapolis surgeons began rodding long, from T12 to the sacrum, but fusing only L4–S1 with subsequent rod removal.[3] Vidal[73] and Kaneda[35] used much shorter rods that extended from L3 or L4 to the sacrum. Alignment results were still unsatisfactory. In the largest current distraction rod series, Kaneda presented 39 cases. Slippage was slightly inproved from 26% only to 21%, but with a 7° *worsening* of the slip angle.[35]

Anterior-Posterior Resection Reductions

With the limitations of closed-reduction techniques and the liabilities of posterior distraction rods, surgeons turned to more extensive operations in the quest for a more effective reduction capability. Combined anterior and posterior surgery for spondylolisthesis reduction was first described in 1956 by Denecke in a German publication.[12] He performed anterior resection of the inferior L5 body, followed by posterior resection of the sacral dome to shorten the spine. From the posterior approach, he then inserted a reduction instrument between L5 and S1 to lever L5 back in place on the sacrum. Axial Steinmann's pins were used to fix the reduction.

In 1973, DeWald undertook staged anterior and posterior surgery for adolescents with grade 3 and 4 slips. He began with posterior laminectomy with or without sacral dome resection, posterolateral grafting, and reduction of the deformity by distracting with Harrington rods while manually extending the pelvis during surgery. The second stage consisted of anterior discectomy with further reduction, using large iliac wedge grafts for anterior strut support. Patients had 3 months of bed rest in the pantaloon cast and a third operation to remove their L1 to S1 Harrington rods. Thirteen of his 14 patients achieved reductions that averaged 86% slip correction and moderate correction of lumbosacral kyphosis.[13]

In 1979, both McPhee and O'Brien[39] and Bradford[4] reported multistage surgery for correction of grade 3 and 4 slips without the use of distraction instrumentation. They began with posterior laminectomy and fu-

sion, followed by 2 to 3 weeks of halo-femoral traction in extension. Bradford then obtained additional correction anteriorly by using a lever between L5 and S1 and placement of a dowel graft,[4] while McPhee and O'Brien obtained fixation with an anterior axial screw.[39] Patients were treated in a bilateral spica extension cast for 4 months in bed. In a subsequent report, Bradford added a third-stage procedure to place posterior Harrington compression or Luque rods for fixation.[7] In 1988, Dick described a four-stage surgical sequence for reduction of grade 3 and 4 spondylolisthesis.[15] He began with percutaneous placement of external fixation pins in the pedicles of L4 and S1 for preliminary distraction. This procedure was followed by anterior discectomy and grafting, then posterior placement of an internal fixator, with manual reduction of the deformity by pulling back then angulating the L4 screws to reverse lumbosacral kyphosis. Patients could be ambulated shortly after surgery in a brace. The fourth stage consisted of fixator removal at 1 year.

Six major studies have reported the results of using the anterior and posterior techniques outlined above.[4, 7, 15, 39, 46, 55] All were essentially confined to adolescents with grade 3 or 4 slips. Correction of translation (slip) averaged approximately 45% in two series,[7, 15] and as high as 73% for the others.[4, 39, 46, 55] For patients with severe slips, correction of lumbosacral kyphosis ranged from a 20° improvement in slip angle[15, 55] to a 63° improvement in Bradford's most recent series.[7] With all aspects of the spondylolisthesis deformity considered (slip, kyphosis, height shortening), it appears that DeWald's open-reduction technique, which combined anterior resection, posterior distraction rods, and extension cast recumbency, yielded the best initial correction.[13]

Unfortunately, the complication rate for multistage anterior and posterior reduction methods is high. Series reporting detailed information on complications cited an approximate 30% incidence of neurologic deficit and a 10–20% incidence of dislodgment with or without complete loss of reduction.[4, 7, 13, 15] In the treatment of high-grade slips, additional surgery was often needed to regraft delayed unions or nonunions.[7] In summary, these series documented that adolescents with grade 3 and 4 slips could consistently obtain substantial reduction of their deformity. However, their clinical indications remained quite limited owing to the magnitude and number of procedures required, the high rate of complication, and length of recumbency.

Vertebrectomy

In an effort to improve spinal alignment for patients with true spondyloptosis, a few surgeons have advanced the concept of spine shortening to include resection of the entire fifth vertebra. This process relaxes surrounding soft tissues and the cauda equina to facilitate reduction and minimize deficit from lumbar root stretching. Gaines provided the first description of this procedure in the English literature.[23] He began with anterior resection of the fifth vertebral body. He then removed the posterior elements of L5 and reduced the slip with the aid of Harrington distraction instrumentation between L2 and the ala. He performed a lateral L4-to-sacral fusion and stabilized the reduction with Harrington compression rods attached from over the lamina of L4 to the first sacral foramina. His patients were placed on bed rest in a spica cast for 5 months. Other surgeons have reported five additional cases using this procedure.[7, 8, 32]

Results published to date suggest that L5 vertebrectomy achieves full correction of spine alignment and the slip angle with moderate correction of the slip from spondyloptosis to a grade 1 or 2 listhesis.[7, 8, 32] On the other hand, complications are substantial. Two of seven cases developed residual weakness of L5 innervated muscles, and two required additional surgery to repair delayed unions or nonunions.[7, 16, 23] Because of its risk and magnitude, vertebrectomy is typically reserved for selected spondyloptosis patients with fixed deformities for whom less extensive procedures offer little chance of success.[6]

Pedicle Fixation

The advent of pedicle screw fixation addressed many shortcomings of prior techniques. At first, pedicle screws were tried in conjunction with distraction rod techniques to help limit postoperative loss of correction. In 1967, Harrington wired L5 pedicle screws to distraction rods at the completion of reduction.[25] This practice was followed by Vidal[73] and later by Zielke,[76] who connected L5 screws to distraction rods by means of a cross plate. However, Harrington was quick to note that the screws provided little advantage and discontinued their use after a few cases.[26] Years later, it was shown that with only one level of sacral fixation, the rods rotate around this axis of distal fixation into flexion with loss of translational correction.[17]

Next, several surgeons added pedicle fixation to the multistage anterior-posterior reduction resection methods for better maintenance of correction and for sufficient fixation to permit early ambulation. In 1973, Louis began using plate fixation after spondylolisthesis reduction.[38] First, he resected the anterior disc and reduced the deformity by traction, extension, and L5–S1 leverage; he used fibular struts to hold open the disc space supplemented with either an axial fibular dowel or screw across the bodies of L5 and S1. His second stage of surgery consisted of a posterior fusion fixed with cancellous screws and a plate. The plate served as a tension band, working in conjunction with the anterior graft, to permit patient ambulation in a plaster cast. He reported 189 grade 1 to 3 slips, with excellent correction of both the slip and kyphosis, a moderate improvement in trunk height, and permanent neurologic deficit in only 6% of his cases.

Dick also used pedicle fixation as part of a multistage reduction method.[14] He began with preliminary traction via percutaneous pins, followed by anterior discectomy and grafting, then posterior reduction using Schanz pedicle screws as handles, which were subsequently held in place with an internal fixator. The final stage consisted of fixator removal. Dick treated somewhat higher grade 3 and 4 slips. He obtained approximately 60% correction of the slip and kyphosis but had a 20% incidence of residual neurologic deficit.[15]

A third group of surgeons began to use pedicle screws to apply active posterior translation for low- to moderate-grade slips. This procedure was made possible by a screw bolt described by Matthiass and Heine in 1973.[40] The screw bolt was threaded into L5. A slotted plate was placed over the bolt portion. By tightening a nut over the plate, it was possible to pull L5 posteriorly on the sacrum. Roy-Camille and coworkers also used plates with screw bolts for partial spondylolisthesis reduction and fixation in a single-stage posterior procedure.[54] After posterior release, they used fracture table traction, pelvic extension, distraction forceps, and a plate with L4 and L5 threaded bolts to obtain approximately 55% slip correction in 11 of 12 patients with primarily grade 3 slips; their permanent L5 deficit rate was 9%.

Sijbrandij combined both instrumented distraction and posterior translation for reduction followed by tension band screw fixation in a one-stage posterior procedure.[60] First, he resected the L5–S1 disc and endplates, with further sacral dome resection when necessary, to minimize lumbar root tension during reduction. He obtained partial reduction by distracting with L1–S1 Harrington rods and then posteriorly translating L5 with screw bolts attached to the rods with temporary hooks. He then performed an interbody L5–S1 fusion from the same posterior approach. He removed the distraction rods and stabilized the spine with a one-level tension band by directly connecting the L5 screw bolts to Zielke "sacral" bars placed into both iliac wings.[76] He reported only 3 cases using this technique but achieved more than 80% correction of both slip and slip angle.

Posterior Levered Reduction

Since moderate slips are always associated with varying degrees of forward tilt (kyphosis) and loss of height, it became clear that posterior translation from plates and screws alone was generally unable to correct most spondylolisthesis deformities. To gain the necessary height and lordosis, some used traction and fracture table positioning during surgery,[42, 54] others used temporary distraction rods,[60] while another group of surgeons used manual leverage to gain height and lordosis. Brown and associates described a novel "crowbar" reduction method with laminar wires attached to an outrigger. After discectomy, a lever on the outrigger reduced the slip, which was then fixed with pins passed from each iliac wing across the sacrum and into the body of L5.[8]

In 1973, Schollner[59] developed and Matthiass[40] published the more direct posterior leverage method, employed by many of the surgeons today who use Steffee plates. Posterior levered reduction is a single-stage procedure for spondylolisthesis but is not well suited for spondyloptosis. It consists of five surgical steps: (1) removal of the L5 arch and disc with sacral dome resection when necessary for shortening;[62] (2) application of distraction by manually raising L5 with a lever placed in the L5–S1 disc space; (3) posterior translation by shortening a screw bolt on a slotted plate; (4) posterior interbody fusion (PLIF) for anterior support (as recommended by Harrington in 1971) combined with a posterolateral iliac fusion[26]; and (5) pedicle screw fixation to allow early patient ambulation. The slotted plate employed by Schollner[59] and Matthiass[40] preceded use of pedicle screws. The plate was affixed to the sacrum by distal flanges, which fit into the dorsal foramina of S2. They used a Cobb elevator in the disc space to raise L5 and recommended monitoring nerve conduction during reduction. Matthiass reported 48 adolescents with lumbosacral spondylolisthesis treated with posterior levered reduction. He obtained good correction of deformity in 47, but one-third experi-

enced postoperative neurologic deficits, most of which resolved.[40]

Steffee recently reported results of 14 patients with grade 3 and 4 slips treated with the Schollner-Matthiass technique. To gain height, he levered a "persuader" within the L5–S1 disc space. For posterior translation, he used screw bolts in conjunction with his VSP slotted plate. Reduction was done while monitoring sensory-evoked potentials. Steffee stressed the importance of using a PLIF for anterior support. Good reduction was maintained in 11 patients with both interbody and lateral fusions; however, the 3 patients without interbody fusion lost reduction (Fig. 24-4).[65]

Gradual Instrumented Reduction

The concept of gradual instrumented reduction for spondylolisthesis was developed during the mid-1980s by Edwards and other members of the Spinal Fixation Study Group, a select group of spinal surgeons trained and monitored in these techniques. Our goal was to achieve *full* correction of the spondylolisthesis deformity with less surgery and morbidity than alternative methods. To accomplish this goal, we combined four concepts: (1) the simultaneous application of three corrective forces, (2) two-point sacral fixation, (3) viscoelastic stress relaxation, and (4) restoration of full anatomic alignment to obviate the need for interbody grafting (PLIF). To simultaneously apply the three corrective forces, it is necessary to use instrumentation with three-dimensional adjustability. Accordingly, we employed the Modular Spinal System, which included finely ratcheted rods for initial distraction and adjustable connectors between the rods and pedicle screws to effect posterior translation of the lumbar spine and flexion of the sacrum.

Three Corrective Forces

Since the spondylolisthesis deformity results from anterior slippage, loss of height, and lumbosacral kyphosis, we postulated that full reduction might be possible by simultaneously applying the opposite forces of distraction, posterior translation of the lumbar spine, and sacral flexion (lordosis).[17] In the same year as our initial report (1985), Balderston and Bradford described a traction-cast technique with halo-femoral traction, pelvic fixation pins to flex the sacrum, and laminar wires attached to an outrigger for posterior translation.[1, 5] Prior instrumentation techniques had not allowed a gradated application of distraction, posterior translation, and lumbosacral lordosis. As a result,

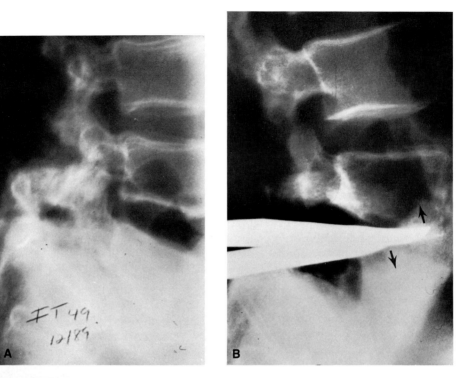

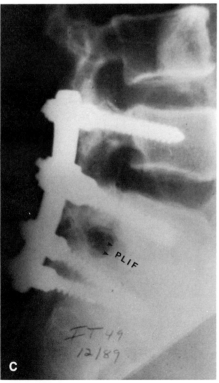

FIG. 24–4. Levered plate reduction of spondylolisthesis. **A.** Preoperative lateral radiograph of symptomatic grade 3 spondylolisthesis. **B.** Intraoperative radiograph of levered reduction maneuver. After discectomy, the "persuader" is placed between L5 and the sacrum to restore height before correction of the translational deformity with screw-bolts and plates. **C.** Radiograph after correction of slip (PLIF) with posterior interbody fusion (*arrows*) and plates to maintain reduction. (Case courtesy of Dr. Arthur Steffee)

earlier instrumented reductions were usually incomplete.[42, 54, 74]

Two-Point Sacral Fixation

To provide lumbosacral lordosis, the lumbar spine must be extended and the sacrum flexed. To maximize the necessary rotational force (extension moment) to accomplish these goals, two-point fixation on the sacrum is required. Accordingly, we found considerably better maintenance of spondylolisthesis reduction with screw fixation at both S1 and S2 rather than just S1.[17]

Stress Relaxation

To lessen the magnitude of surgery and risk of neurovascular injury, we employed viscoelastic stress relaxation and avoided manual manipulations. As symbolized by the crooked tree of Andre, the use of corrective forces over time to reduce deformity is a longstanding principle of orthopedics. The earliest traction-cast techniques for reducing spondylolisthesis made use of tissue creep. DeWald and others have recognized the advisability of gradually correcting the spondylolisthesis deformity at surgery.[13, 28, 40, 56, 60] However, it was not known to what *extent* stress relaxation could be employed at surgery until we learned that even spondyloptosis could be fully corrected in adolescents or adults by applying the three corrective forces over several hours.[20] Hence, by continuously replenishing the forces of distraction, posterior translation, and sacral flexion, contracted anterior structures gradually lengthen until they return to their original dimensions, resulting in *full* correction of most spondylolisthesis deformities (Fig. 24-5).

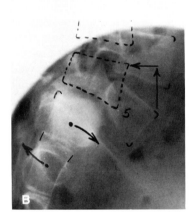
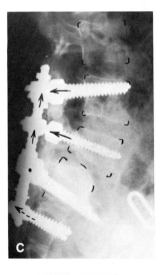
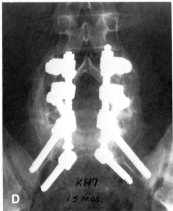

FIG. 24–5. The biomechanics of instrumented reduction. **A.** Edwards' hypothesis. **B.** Lateral coned-down radiograph of grade 4 spondylolisthesis shows characteristic loss of height, anterior translation, and lumbosacral kyphosis. *Arrows* demonstrate the opposite corrective force needed for reduction: (1) distraction, (2) posterior translation, and (3) sacral flexion (lumbosacral lordosis). **C.** Postoperative radiograph demonstrates full correction from the application of the three corrective forces alone. The patient proceeded to painless fusion without radiculopathy or other complications. **D.** AP radiograph of the same case at 15 months with consolidation of the lateral fusion masses.

Anatomic Alignment

Restoration of normal alignment eliminates the need for anterior grafting. With anatomic alignment, excess anterior bending forces at the lumbosacral junction are eliminated, and posterior grafts are no longer subjected to excessive tensile stress. As a result, lateral fusions can be expected to unite and strengthen with time. Hence, it should no longer be necessary to routinely resect the disc and place interbody grafts anterior to the dura.

To test this reduction hypothesis, we conducted a prospective study of 25 consecutive patients. All were treated with a single-stage posterior procedure using corrective forces alone without discectomy or even discotomy, followed by early ambulation in a brace. The procedure maintained 91% slip correction and 88% correction of lumbosacral kyphosis in addition to restoration of normal trunk height. Two patients with spondyloptosis had transient root deficits, but patients with grade 2–4 slips remained completely free of neurologic complications.[18] Successful use of this method has also been reported by Bradford[6] and West.[75] The detailed results of 180 cases documented by members of the Spinal Fixation Study Group are discussed later in this chapter.

INDICATIONS FOR REDUCTION-FIXATION

Until recently, the magnitude and morbidity of the multistage operations required for reduction of most spondylolisthesis deformities inspired restrictive indications for reduction. However, with the increased advantages associated with *anatomic* alignment and the reduced risk associated with gradual instrumented reduction, the indications for spondylolisthesis reduction-fixation are beginning to broaden. Indeed, from my recent experience and current data from the Spinal Fixation Study Group, the likelihood of complications from reduction and fixation of grade 1–4 spondylolisthesis is no more than that reported in comparable series from in situ fusion. It should be noted, however, that the difficulty and complication rate for correcting high-grade spondyloptosis is considerably greater. Accordingly, the discussion of indications focuses on spondylolisthesis and borderline spondyloptosis. The reduction of true spondyloptosis is still considered an investigational procedure.

Prerequisites

Safe and effective correction of spondylolisthesis is greatly facilitated by lumbosacral mobility and adequate bone stock and is complicated by L5–S1 autofusion or surgical arthrodesis. Hence, if preoperative flexion-extension or standing-supine films show no L5–S1 motion and tomograms or computed tomography (CT) scans suggest arthrodesis, we are reticent to advise attempted reduction without anterior release.

Adequate bone stock is necessary for instrumented reduction. Since these procedures rely on pedicle screw fixation, the patient's vertebrae must be large enough to accommodate available screw sizes. A preoperative CT scan can help make this determination. Below the age of 10, vertebrae are often too small for pedicle screw reduction-fixation. Likewise, good screw purchase requires adequate bone quality. Accordingly, old patients or those with severe osteoporosis are not candidates for reduction techniques.

Indications

Reduction is indicated when the advantages of reduction are greater and the risk of failure less than in situ fusion with or without root decompression. If the surgeon is well trained in current reduction methods, available data support the following indications.

Cauda Equina Syndrome. Sacral root stretch that causes loss of normal bowel and bladder control or plantar flexion weakness in the lower extremities is best treated with reduction. Since the sacral roots are tented over the posterior corner of the sacral endplate, restoring canal alignment relaxes the cauda equina and relieves anterior pressure from the sacral roots.

Progressive Slip That Surpasses 40–50%. Laurent correlated age with degree of slip and concluded that a slip of more than 30° in a young person tends to progress.[37] It is well known that the majority of progressions occur in late childhood and early adolescence.[3, 10, 30, 35] Hence, when documented progression surpasses 40% in the child, reduction-fixation-fusion is recommended. As the slip progress to 50%, the surface contact between the lumbar spine and sacrum is only 38% of normal and then rapidly diminishes with further slip progression.[61] More than 50% slip in the adult suggests unusual instability and a greater likelihood for nonunion, progression, or even cauda equina syndrome after in situ fusion. In these cases, the risk of deficit may well be greater after in situ fusion than after reduction-fixation with current methods.[18]

Major Deformity That Causes Decompensation or Distress. We agree with Bradford that the clinical consequences of major deformity are great enough to warrant the higher than usual rate of complications encountered when reducing high-grade spondylolisthesis.[6] Specifically, our clinical experience suggests that the advantages of reduction well outweigh the risks for majority deformities with either loss of sagittal compensation or major negative psychological impact. Restoration of anatomic alignment for these patients can dramatically improve their spinal mechanics, appearance, and self-image.

Major Pain or Deficit Plus Two or More Risk Factors. The likelihood that surgical failure or complications will arise from in situ fusion appears to be increased by the eight factors listed below. Conversely, several of these factors simplify reduction and decrease its risks. Therefore, it seems reasonable to afford surgical candidates the advantages of reduction when two or more of the risk factors listed below are present.

In Situ Risk Factors. Factors known to increase the tendency for pseudarthrosis, slip progression, neurologic deficit, or late symptoms from abnormal spine mechanics after in situ fusion include:

1. *Lumbosacral kyphosis or slip angle of 25° or more.* Lumbosacral kyphosis is measured from the perpendicular of the lines that describe the posterior cortex of the proximal sacral bodies and the superior endplate of L5. In the normal spine, 5° or more of lordosis is present at the lumbosacral junction; hence, 25° of kyphosis represents a 30° deformity. The slip angle is measured from the undersurface of L5. It therefore indicates both lumbosacral kyphosis and the wedge deformity of L5.

2. *Trapezoidal L5.* Trapezoidal deformity (wedging) of the fifth vertebral body may be considered an independent risk factor when the posterior vertebral body height is less than 75% of anterior vertebral body height. Bosworth found that slip progression was proportional to the amount of L5 wedging.[2] During his study, patients with minor wedging slipped 9.5%; those

with a 25% difference in anterior versus posterior body height slipped 21%.

3. *Rounded sacral endplate.* Patients with obliteration or rounding of the anterior aspect of the first sacral endplate tend to have progressive slipping.[3, 37, 61, 66] They probably progress because the rounded sacral dome provides little support for the anterior column of the lumbar spine.

4. *Hyperlordosis that exceeds 50° L2–S1.* Lumbar hyperlordosis increases the vertical inclination of the lumbosacral joint. Increased vertical shear results, which most likely delays arthrodesis and promotes further slippage with possible neurologic sequelae.[3]

5. *L5 radiculopathy that requires decompression.* Several investigators have observed an increased rate of pseudarthrosis or nonunion after L5 laminectomy and root decompression.[2, 6, 68] Nevertheless, many spondylolisthesis patients who come to surgery have L5 pain or weakness. Full decompression at the time of surgery is highly desirable since it can fully relieve their radicular pain and speed root recovery.[3, 10, 11, 24, 29, 37, 40, 43, 45, 49, 53, 60, 63]

6. *Female adolescents.* Young females are most likely to slip further and attach more importance to the cosmetic advantages of reduction than other patient groups. The spondylolisthesis deformity tends to progress further in females than in males. During Bosworth's study, females slipped 25% and males only 14%.[2] Osterman studied 87 adolescents with severe slips; he noted that the 10 most severe deformities in his series occurred in females.[48] Most progression of deformity occurs during adolescence;[3, 10, 37] slip progression has also been observed in several patients after pregnancy.

7. *Excess lumbosacral mobility.* Significant slippage usually follows disc space narrowing and stiffening. Thus, more than 3 mm of translation or 10° of angulation between flexion-extension or standing-supine radiographs probably represent unusual mobility. These numbers are only approximate guidelines, since specific correlative studies have not been completed. Nevertheless, it is important to assess L5–S1 motion, since excess lumbosacral mobility tends to shift the risk-benefit ratio balance toward reduc-

tion-fixation. The mobile spine is more difficult to fuse in situ without progression or nonunion but easier and less risky to reduce than more fixed deformities.

8. *Signs of sacral root stretch.* Schoenecker and associates felt that sacral root signs may be a precursor to the most serious complication of in situ fusion, the cauda equina syndrome.[58] They recently documented that two thirds of their 12 cases of cauda equina syndrome that complicated in situ fusion had at least subtle signs of sacral root dysfunction before surgery. The following findings may indicate early sacral root stretch: (1) a strongly positive Lasègue's sign,[37] (2) decreased Achilles reflex, or (3) early bowel and bladder dysfunction.

CURRENT OPTIONS FOR SPONDYLOLISTHESIS REDUCTION

When reduction, fixation, and fusion are indicated, the method that offers the greatest potential advantage with the least morbidity must be selected for each case. After surveying results from the numerous methods reported for reduction of spondylolisthesis, I have identified three techniques that appear to best address the needs of each patient category. These include (1) posterior release followed by extension casting for children with highly flexible deformities, (2) posterior instrumentation for patients in whom reduction-fixation-fusion is indicated, and (3) anterior resection with posterior pedicle fixation for adults with very fixed or high-grade spondyloptosis.

Posterior Grafting with Extension Casting

Indications

This approach has evolved from the traction-cast techniques of the past. It is most effective in reducing the kyphotic aspect of the spondylolisthesis deformity but has little effect on translation. Since the amount of corrective force that can be applied by cast is somewhat limited, this technique is best reserved for young patients with primarily kyphotic and very flexible deformities. It is a good choice for children; their small bones do not pose a problem since no instrumentation is required. Moreover, children are better able to toler-

ate months of recumbency in a hyperextension cast than adolescents or adults.

Technique

The largest recent series and best results are reported by Bradford.[5] He treated 22 children and adolescents with an average slip of 50% and slip angle of 33°. One week after standard L4–S1 posterolateral fusion, he places patients in longitudinal traction on a Risser frame. To reduce lumbosacral kyphosis, he extends the legs and applies pressure directly over the back of the sacrum with the patient awake. A localizer cast that includes one leg is applied to maintain extension. Some patients can be ambulated, but most are kept supine in the cast for 3 months.

For patients with higher grade slips and less malleable deformities, Bradford often adds three techniques to improve correction: (1) removal of the posterior arch of L5 to facilitate reduction, (2) insertion of Hoffman half pins into each ilium with incorporation of these into an extension cast to maintain pelvic flexion and lumbosacral extension, and (3) attachment of percutaneous wires from the L2–L4 lamina to an outrigger on the cast to maintain the posterior position of the lumbar spine relative to the sacrum.[1,5]

Results

Long-term results demonstrated a two-thirds reduction of the slip angle (33–12°) but little change in trunk height or the amount of slip (50% preoperative to 40% slip at fusion). Slight improvement in both parameters was seen with time owing to differential growth of the unfused anterior column and to sacral dome remodeling after correction of sagittal alignment. Surgical complications were limited to transient L5 weakness in two patients who were placed in halo-femoral traction and nonunion in one patient with complete loss of correction. Partial loss of reduction tended to occur in patients with more than 70% slip, Gill laminectomy, or when residual deformity left the L4 body anterior to the axial plane of the proximal sacrum, the so-called *stable zone.*[5,6]

Posterior Instrumented Reduction

Indications

Posterior instrumented reduction provides the most gain with the least amount of surgery and risk for patients older than age 10 with unfused spondylolisthesis or borderline spondyloptosis. It may be combined with posterior sacral dome resection for patients with spondyloptosis to prevent excess stretching of the lumbar roots.

Technique

Gradual Instrumented Reduction.   The deformity is reduced in a single-stage posterior operation (Fig. 24-6). First, the L5 roots are fully decompressed to expose the L5 pedicles. Screws are inserted at L5 and across the ala at S1 and S2. There is no need to cross the canal or disturb the disc. Height is gradually restored with ratcheted Universal rods attached to the screws. Posterior translation of the lumbar spine and flexion of the sacrum is effected by gradually shortening adjustable connectors between the L5 screws and Universal rods. When radiographs document full reduction, the instrumentation is locked and iliac fusion performed. For high-grade slips (grade 4 and 5) fixation is extended to L4, and sensory evoked potentials (SEP) and wake-up test nerve monitoring are employed.

Posterior Levered Reduction.   When fully adjustable instrumentation is not available, some surgeons use the posterior levered reduction technique described by Matthiass[40] and advocated by Steffee[65] for grade 2–4 slips. This technique requires mobilizing the dura, performing a L5–S1 discectomy, and placing a lever within the disc space to regain height. Translation is effected by screw bolts attached to the VSP plates. The plates are then contoured for lordosis and reapplied, and a lateral fusion is performed. As an alternative to the use of a lever in the L5–S1 disc space, I suggest a temporary distraction rod placed between L1 or L2 and the sacral ala to gain height before posterior translation. Results of the levered reduction technique have not been published in detail; however, some surgeons who use both techniques have found the less-invasive gradual instrumented reduction advantageous.[6]

Results

Results of 25 patients were recently presented by Edwards.[18] Eighteen had grade 2 to 4 spondylolisthesis and seven spondyloptosis. Patients ranged from age 12 to 59, with an average age of 25. Slip correction averaged 91% at 2 year follow-up. The 33° preoperative slip angle was 90% reduced to 4° (average) kyphosis. In addition, 35 mm (average) trunk height (L1–S1) was restored, with 43 mm restoration in patients with spondyloptosis. Patients were ambulated at discharge in a total contact orthosis with one-thigh extension. Complications for patients with spondylolisthesis were remarkably few. One patient with borderline spondyloptosis developed unilateral dorsiflexion weakness. There were zero dislodgments, one donor site infection, and one patient who required repair of nonunion.

Similar results were obtained for 180 spondylolisthesis patients treated by members of the Spinal Fixation Study Group. Complication rates from the series include 3% transient radiculopathy, 1% neurologic deficit, 1% infection, and 2% S2 screw pull-out for grade 1 to 4 spondylolisthesis. Solid fusion was achieved in 88% of patients with 1-year follow-up. Although instrumented reduction is a technically challenging operation, results to date suggest that it is highly effective in the treatment of spondylolisthesis

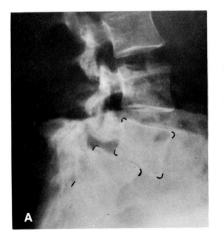
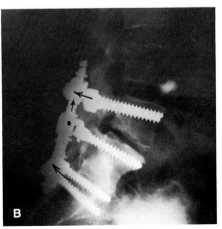

FIG. 24–6. Instrumented reduction of a low-grade slip. **A.** Lateral radiograph of symptomatic 45% slip. **B.** Postoperative radiograph demonstrates full correction of deformity from the gradual application of distraction, posterior translation, and sacral flexion without the need for discectomy. Edwards instrumentation crosses only one disc space. (Case courtesy of Neil Kahanovitz, M.D.)

with complication rates that do not exceed those for in situ fusion.

In contrast, results from the treatment of true spondyloptosis with a single-stage instrumented reduction without sacral dome resection have been less satisfactory. Although anatomic alignment can usually be accomplished,[6, 18, 75] the incidence of complications has been similar to reports for anterior-posterior resection-reduction methods. Accordingly, one-stage instrumented reduction without discectomy is now reserved for patients with spondylolisthesis. For patients with spondyloptosis, sacral dome resection and staged posterior reduction techniques are added to lower the risks of reduction.

Anterior-Posterior Resection Reduction

Indications

Combined anterior and posterior methods require more extensive surgery and present greater risk and morbidity than other current options. Hence, they are best reserved for deformities beyond the scope of extension cast or posterior instrumented reductions. The anterior-posterior resection operation sacrifices the anterior endplates, thus eliminating the slight autoreduction that occurs when a posterior fusion tethers posterior growth while anterior elongation and remodeling continue. For this reason, spine resection reduction is most appropriate for skeletally mature patients. Combined anterior and posterior surgery is indicated when high-grade spondylolisthesis is complicated by anterior fusion and for chronic high-grade spondyloptosis.

Autofusion between the inferior endplate of L5 and the anterior aspect of the sacrum is suggested when no motion is seen on either standing-supine or flexion-extension motion studies. It is confirmed with tomograms or CT scans. Initial open anterior osteotomy is safer than attempted blind posterior osteotomy.

High-grade spondyloptosis is defined by flexion tilt and loss of height that have progressed to the point where the entire fifth vertebral body lies at or below the dome of the sacrum on standing films. Chronicity of the deformity is suggested by lack of perceptible motion on standing-supine or flexion-extension radiographs. The amount of lengthening that can be tolerated by the lumbar roots during reduction is inversely proportional to the duration of the deformity. Hence, shortening the length of the anterior spinal column helps protect against radiculopathy during reduction of

chronic high-grade spondyloptosis. If only discectomy and sacral dome resection are required, they are best carried out from the posterior approach; however, if additional shortening is required, the inferior portion of L5 or even the entire vertebral body can be resected. For most surgeons, this procedure is best accomplished through an anterior approach.

Technique

Before surgery for reduction of high-grade spondyloptosis, it is important to carefully plan anterior and posterior osteotomies from preoperative radiographs. A standing radiograph and maximum flexion radiograph are selected. Spine cutouts can be used, or the radiographs can be superimposed. The flexion radiograph is used to represent the postoperative position of the lumbar spine after reduction eliminates the need for compensatory hyperlordosis. The fifth lumbar vertebra on the flexion film is placed in a reduced position, with T12 or L1 residing directly over the sacrum. The ideal location for the sacral dome and L5 osteotomies is marked on the standing film. To determine the correct amount of resection (shortening), L4 is positioned so that its distance from S1 is increased by no more than 3–4 cm postoperatively.

The anterior stage of surgery begins with the patient positioned supine and the table extended. The lumbar spine is approached through the midline, and the peritoneum is opened along the course of the right iliac artery. Care is taken to dissect and protect the presacral plexus, which controls sexual function. It is displaced to the left, and the middle sacral artery is ligated. A 2-mm drill bit is inserted into the body of L5 and radiographed to adjust the level and inclination of the osteotomy to match the preoperative plan. In most cases, the L5–S1 disc cannot be seen. To facilitate subsequent union, bone removed from the L5 body can be used for L4–L5 interbody grafting or morselized and replaced under the osteotomized surface of L5. Use of morselized graft has been found effective by Dick.[14]

The second stage is scheduled 1 to 2 weeks later. It is best to avoid halo-femoral traction during this interval since most reported root complications associated with combined anterior and posterior spondylolisthesis reductions have occurred during periods of unmonitored traction. To further minimize the risk of root injury, we advise removal of the posterior L5 arch (Gill) with complete dissection and decompression of the L5 and S1 roots. The dura can now be safely mobilized.

Before the sacral dome osteotomy, we drill a 2-mm bit across the dome and adjust its position with the aid of intraoperative radiography until it matches the preoperative plan. Sacral dome osteotomy and posterior discectomy are then performed. Reduction is accomplished over several hours according to the gradual instrumented reduction method described later in this chapter.

Results of Anterior-Posterior Resection Reduction

I and others have performed a number of resection reductions using the technique described above, though no series has yet been published. Nevertheless, by combining our results with the results of similar procedures reported by Bradford[7] and DeWald,[13] we estimate that an experienced spinal surgeon can now expect 80 to 90% correction of lumbosacral kyphosis with good axial alignment. Reduction of translation (slip) to a residual 10 to 30% is usually accomplished and is limited only by the degree of root stretch that can be tolerated with preservation of normal function. Some degree of fixed thoracolumbar lordosis often remains in patients with longstanding and severe spondyloptosis.

Complications are frequent but rarely catastrophic if the recommended procedures are carefully followed. Approximately 30% of patients will develop root deficits. About half of these will eventually resolve. The most common deficit is unilateral foot drop. The nonunion rate is 10 to 15%, with occasional loss of midsacral fixation. In addition, less frequent general complications include infection (after posterior surgery) and ileus, pulmonary problems, bowel obstruction, iliac thrombosis, and sexual dysfunction in males (after anterior surgery).

AUTHOR'S PREFERRED METHOD: GRADUAL INSTRUMENTED REDUCTION

The gradual posterior reduction method combines simultaneous and gradated distraction, posterior translation of the proximal spine, and flexion of the sacrum to reduce all aspects of the spondylolisthesis deformity. After reduction, the instrumentation counteracts anterior shear forces at L5–S1 and permits axial loading across the graft to promote union.

Instrumentation

To generate the three corrective forces, we use four components of the Edwards' Modular Spinal System (Scientific Spinal, Ltd):

1. *Spinal (sacral) screws.* These are blunt-tip, self-tapping, self-guiding screws that are inserted only after palpating all sides of a 3.5-mm pilot hole. Screws are available in 5-mm-length increments. The midsacral screws articulate directly with the rods, whereas proximal screws have a linkage between the screw and rod. Edwards screws have the same outer diameter but a greater thread cross-sectional area than other spinal screws to maximize pull-out strength and eliminate the need for using cement supplementation at L4 or L5 in the treatment of spondylolisthesis.[65]

2. *Anatomic hooks.* The L-shaped hooks serve as a linkage between the rods and screws at S1. Anatomic hooks are available in three heights. These heights make it possible to set the rods at the correct sagittal inclination so that contouring is unnecessary.

3. *Universal rods.* The rods permit bidirectional ratcheting in 1/16 in. gradations for gradual distraction during reduction and compression after reduction.

4. *Adjustable connectors.* These are positioned between the spinal screws in L5 and the Universal rods. Shortening the connectors translates the lumbar spine posteriorly while flexing the sacrum.

The instrumentation is designed for optimum biocompatibility so that additional surgery to remove it is rarely necessary. For example, the system is articulated by movable linkages so that screws can be inserted from any position, to avoid adjacent unfused facet joints. Its composite modulus (overall stiffness) is similar to bone so as not to stress-shield the underlying vertebrae. Construct profile is relatively low so as not to irritate overlying tissues.

Reduction of Spondylolisthesis

Preoperative Planning

Preoperative studies should include a standing lateral radiograph of the entire lumbar spine to assess sagittal alignment, an anteroposterior (AP) projection to assess pedicle size and possible scoliosis, and bending films to determine the degree of lumbosacral mobility and the amount of fixed thoracic lordosis. In young patients whose adequate pedicle size (7 mm cortical diameter) cannot be documented on the AP radiograph, a CT scan is helpful. Likewise, we have found CT scanning to be the most useful test in delineating the presence and location of autofusion when no motion can be seen on bending or standing-supine films. Scoliosis is found in approximately 30% of patients who require surgery for spondylolisthesis (range 23–48%).[2, 21, 31, 37, 39, 69] The scoliosis may be due to spasm and corrects with fixation and fusion of the spondylolisthesis,[21, 39] or it may be torsional with a structural component.[21] The structural variety tends to have asymmetric slippage at the lumbosacral joint, which acts as the apex of the curve with rotational scoliosis extending proximally to the upper lumbar vertebrae. When torsional-structural scoliosis is significant, we recommend extending instrumentation to L4, leaving the concave connectors in distraction, while compressing the convex side of the scoliosis after reduction of the spondylolisthesis.

Before surgery, either cutouts or superimposed radiographs are used to select the final position for the reduced lumbar spine. The proximal cutout or radiograph is held in the desired position on the sacrum to simulate normal spine alignment. The corrected position of the posterior elements of L4 and L5 is marked on the standing preoperative lateral view. A straight line is drawn from the midsacrum to a point 0.5 inch posterior to the desired position for the posterior elements of L4. This line represents the optimal sagittal inclination of the Universal rod at surgery. The distance between this line and the posterior sacrum at its superior end indicates the correct hook linkage (low or medium) between the S1 screws and Universal rods.

Surgical Dissection and Screw Placement

After a generous midline incision, the L5 lamina is removed by first dividing the distal ligamentum flavum, grasping the spinous process with a towel clip to gradually rotate the lamina cephalad while peeling dural fat and veins from its undersurface, and then dividing the proximal ligamentum flavum from inside out. The L5 lamina is then avulsed from the fibrocartilaginous tissue that fills the pass defect, one side at a time.

Next, the L5 roots are fully decompressed. The roots are covered by the medial edge of the superior facet of L5. To locate the root, first osteotomize the medial-inferior tip of the L4 inferior facet. This exposes the articular cartilage of the L5 superior facet. Place a small angled Kerrison punch into the canal at this point and begin resecting the osteophytic margin of the L5 superior facet in a cephalo-caudad direction. The medial edge of the facet is contiguous with an osteophyte that forms at the junction of the pedicle and pars nonunion (Fig. 24-7). This osteophyte must also be removed to decompress the root and identify the medial and inferior cortex of the pedicle. Decompression should be continued laterally with the Kerrison to remove ligaments between the transverse process and sacral ala. The L5 root should be left completely free from the spinal canal to the anterior surface of the sacral ala. In addition to decompressing the root, this dissection releases the contracted iliolumbar ligaments to facilitate reduction.[13]

Before the L5 screws are placed, it is helpful to curette off the cartilage and debris that overlie the pedicle stump just lateral and superior to the L5 root. Next, the medial and inferior walls of the pedicle are palpated to select an entry point on the L5 pedicle stump 4 mm from the medial and inferior cortices. If L5 is the most proximal level for instrumentation, the entry point should be more lateral, so screw placement does not disrupt the L4–L5 facet capsule. A depression is made with a burr at the point of entry. A lateral

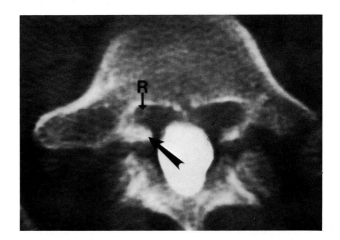

FIG. 24–7. Osteophytes over L5 roots. Computed tomographic scan at the level of L5 pedicles shows the characteristic osteophytes at the base of the pars nonunion. The osteophyte (*arrow*) covers the 5th lumbar root (R). This osteophyte must be removed to decompress the 5th lumbar root and visualize the medial cortex of the pedicle before screw insertion.

radiograph or image taken with the patient on the operating table should then be consulted to orient the screw parallel to the superior endplate of L5. A straight 3-0 curette is used as a probe and twisted in an inferior and medial direction to parallel the ridge at the infero-medial border of the pedicle, through the pedicle, and across the L5 vertebral body; 2-mm bits are then placed into the L5 pedicle probe holes for subsequent radiographic confirmation of position.

Fixation of L4 is recommended for grade 4 slips and some grade 3 slips with substantial lumbosacral kyphosis or scoliosis. In high grade slips, the L4–L5 facet directly overlies the L5 pedicle. In addition, it is prone to L4–L5 disc retrolisthesis, instability,[37] and early degenerative changes[15] from forced hyperextension. The entry site for L4 screws should be approximately 4 mm distal and lateral to the center of the pedicle to avoid injuring the L3–L4 facet capsule. The screws are then directed medially and superiorly, aiming toward the anterosuperior corner of the L4 vertebral body.

Sacral screws are placed across the ala at S1 and S2. The entry site for S1 screws is 3–4 mm lateral to the small dimple found at the base of the superior facet of S1. The 2-mm drill bits are inserted perpendicular to the long axis of the proximal sacrum in the sagittal plane and inclined 30° laterally in the transverse plane to the anterior cortex of the lateral ala.

Screw placement for S2 requires the most care since midsacral screws are more prone to failure than other screws in the spondylolisthesis construct. The entry point is two thirds of the way from the inferior wall of the first dorsal foramen to the superior wall of the second dorsal foramen of the sacrum on the vertical (y) axis, and two thirds the distance from the midline to the foramina on the horizontal (x) axis. The posterior cortex is opened with a burr just lateral to the lateral cortex of the spinal canal. The drill bits for S2 should be directed 35° laterally in the transverse plane and converge toward it about 5°–10° toward the S1 bits in the sagittal plane. The bits should be adjusted until a depth of at least 40 mm is achieved.

Drill bit positions are then checked and adjusted as needed with the aid of AP and lateral images or radiographs. The orientation of each bit is then replicated with a 3.5-mm bit to enlarge the holes in preparation for screw placement. The L5, S1, and S2 screws are all carefully drilled just across the anterior cortex for maximum holding power. After the seating reamer is used, the depth of each screw hole is checked, and the appropriate length screws are selected and screwed into place with a hex screwdriver. Screw lengths are double-checked again with a lateral image.

Spondylolisthesis Construct Assembly and Reduction

To assemble the spondylolisthesis construct, Universal rods are placed through the holes in the distal screws and affixed with narrow washers at the distal end of the rods. The appropriate anatomic hook (low or medium) is selected as the S1 linkage to place the rod at the desired vertical inclination. The hook is oriented distally and held in place with a proximal washer. When instrumentation extends only to L5, ring connectors are passed over the proximal end of the rods with their stems lateral to the rods and articulated with the L5 screws. When fixation extends to L4, ring connectors are used at L4 and snap connectors at L5. The snap connectors angulate more to better accommodate lumbosacral kyphosis. Before reduction is initiated, an 18-gauge wire is tightened between the distal end of the rods to negate some of the lateral pull-out load on the S2 screws during reduction.

To reduce the deformity, first shorten the connectors until resistance is felt, then gradually distract the connectors to restore disc space height. Sequentially shorten (tighten) and distract (ratchet) the connectors to two-finger tightness every 10 minutes (Fig. 24-8). Follow the reduction on the image to determine the relative amount of distraction vs. translation required at approximately 30-minute intervals. Allow 30

Spondylolisthesis

REDUCTION SEQUENCE

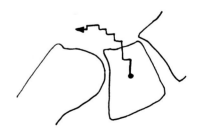

FIG. 24–8. Instrumented reduction sequence. When reducing the spondylo deformity with corrective forces alone, distraction forces are used initially to regain height, followed by equal steps of posterior translation and distraction, then by posterior translation only, and finally release of all distraction to permit axial loading through the anterior column.

to 60 minutes per grade for stress relaxation and reduction of the deformity. In the final stages of reduction, progressively release all distraction and further shorten the connectors until normal alignment is achieved. Ideally, the proximal connectors "bottom out," locking these otherwise mobile linkages. At the conclusion of reduction, all distraction forces should be removed and gentle compression applied to facilitate axial loading of the graft. Stop washers are then placed on the cephalad side of the connectors. The connector positions are locked and their stems cut off (Fig. 24-9).

Grafting and Bracing

Iliac bone graft is harvested through the midline incision. The sacral ala, transverse processes, and lateral aspect of the superior facets, and possibly L4 lamina, are decorticated if this was not done earlier in the procedure. The posterolateral graft is packed into place. A fat graft is placed over the exposed dura and roots, and the incision is closed. Several days after surgery, the patient is placed on a Risser frame to construct a plaster mold for a polypropylene total-contact orthosis. The clam shell orthosis extends from below the nipples to the pubic bone with an extension around one thigh. The patient begins to ambulate in this leg-in orthosis approximately 7 to 10 days after surgery and is then discharged home. After about 3 months, the thigh extension is removed; the remaining lumbosacral brace is worn for an additional 1 to 2 months, depending on the age of the patient.

Reduction of Spondyloptosis

Both the advantages and risks of reduction are greatest for patients with true spondyloptosis. Correction of deformity increases the distance through which lumbar roots must travel and stretches contracted anterior ligamentous structures. Hence, spinal instrumentation is subjected to much greater stresses than during reduction of spondylolisthesis. Accordingly, the likelihood of lumbar root deficit, fixation failure, and nonunion is greater after reduction of spondyloptosis.

Careful planning and incorporation of several new techniques can substantially reduce the incidence of these complications. Preoperative planning is required to determine the amount of spinal shortening (if any) needed to keep lumbar root stretch within tolerable limits, to arrange for neurologic monitoring during reduction, and to provide for second-stage surgery (if necessary) to safely complete the reduction. To de-

crease the rate of reduction and the stresses that act against both contracted tissues and spinal instrumentation, we employ auxiliary internal distraction rods and overhead posterior traction and often delay ambulation for several weeks.

Neural Limits of Single-Stage Reduction

In spondyloptosis, the lumbar spine slips anteriorly, shortens, and rotates into flexion to shorten the course of the lumbar roots. The distance between the lumbar neural foramina and either the exit of the femoral nerve from the pelvis under the ilioinguinal ligament or the exit of the sciatic nerve at the sciatic notch is shortened by several inches. With time, these nerves contract, eventually limiting the amount of correction that can be obtained without shortening the spine itself.

Since the nerves course anterior and inferior to the spine, correction of the lumbosacral kyphosis by extending the spine causes the greatest stretch on the mid lumbar roots, whereas restoring height and posterior translation causes proportionally more lengthening of the low lumbar roots. The risk to midlumbar roots is greatest in patients with fixed compensatory hyperlordosis of the thoracolumbar spine, since structural changes do not permit relaxation of the lordosis on correction of the lumbosacral kyphosis. Differential stretching of midlumbar roots with transient postoperative deficits has been observed by the author in two cases and by Transfeldt and colleagues in one.[70]

From my ongoing analysis, it appears that the risk of neural deficit increases with the degree of kyphotic deformity (slip angle), rigidity of the lumbar lordosis, duration of the deformity, age of the patient, speed of reduction, and amount of cord length restoration. For example, we find that the spine of a late adolescent patient with a grade 4 to 5 slip and a 50° slip angle tolerates up to about 3 cm of lengthening between L4 and the sacrum in one surgical session. More axial lengthening is possible when the slip has progressed rapidly, in especially flexible deformities, in younger patients, and when the slip angle is low (Fig. 24-10). Less single-stage lengthening is tolerated for those with high slip angles, longstanding deformities, older age groups, or previously fused or rigid deformities.

If preoperative planning with radiographs shows that more axial lengthening is required than lumbar roots can tolerate, then, according to these guidelines, two courses of action can be followed: (1) shorten the spine to permit single-stage lengthening within tolerable limits, and/or (2) stage the reduction to give lum-

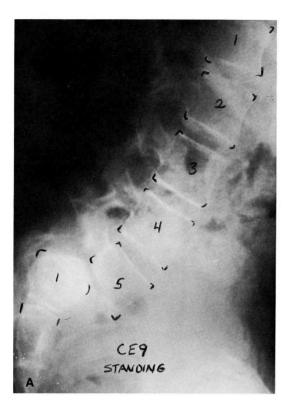

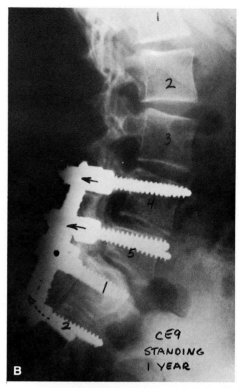

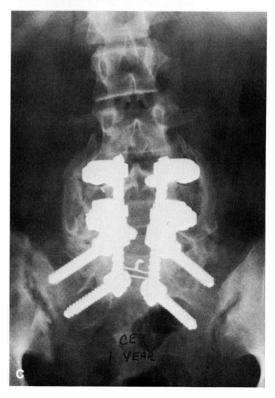

FIG. 24–9. Instrumented reduction of grade 4 spondylolisthesis.
A. Lateral radiograph of 12-year-old girl with grade 4 spondylolisthesis. **B.** Postoperative radiograph shows full restoration of normal
spine alignment using corrective forces alone. The patient proceeded
to painless fusion without radiculopathy or other complications.
C. AP radiograph 1 year after surgical reduction shows consolidated
lateral fusion.

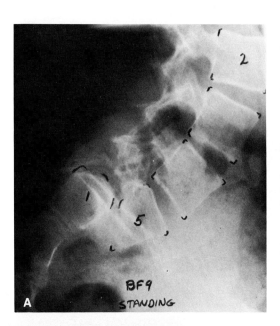

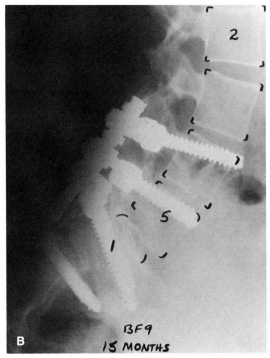

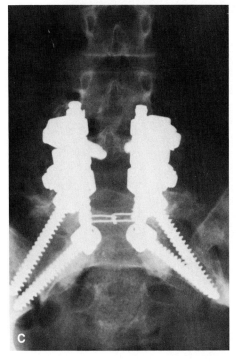

FIG. 24–10. Instrumented reduction of low-grade spondyloptosis. **A.** Preoperative radiograph of 13-year-old girl with 100% slip and early rotation of L5 about the rounded sacral dome into the pelvis. This deformity represents the most that should be attempted without either staged reduction or spine shortening. **B.** Lateral radiograph 15 months after surgery demonstrates full correction of deformity using corrective forces alone without discectomy, traction, or anterior surgery. The patient proceeded to painless fusion without radiculopathy or other complications. **C.** AP radiograph demonstrates methacrylate supplementation to reinforce midsacral screw fixation.

bar roots more time for stress relaxation. If only 1 cm of shortening is needed, this amount can be safely achieved with a sacral dome osteotomy from the posterior approach. If additional shortening is required, the AP resection procedures are necessary.

Nerve Function Monitoring

The use of sensory evoked potential monitoring of the peroneal and posterior tibial nerves during reduction of high-grade spondylolisthesis was described by Gaines in 1985 and has since come into general use.[23] It is probably not necessary when treating grade 1 to 3 slips with the gradual instrumented reduction method, since neither we nor members of the Spinal Fixation Study Group have experienced lasting radiculopathy after reduction of spondylolisthesis with slip angles of less than 45°. For greater slip angles, or in all cases with borderline or true spondyloptosis, neurologic monitoring *should* be performed during reduction.

We recommend wake-up testing as well for *all* cases with spondyloptosis, since we have had patients with completely normal SEP tracings throughout reduction but with weakness of ankle dorsiflexion on wake-up testing, which persisted after surgery. The baseline wake-up test should be performed at the beginning stage of reduction, again at two-thirds reduction, and finally after full reduction. In addition, wake-up tests should be performed after any sustained lessening in SEP amplitude or increase in latency. A 30 to 50% drop in amplitude is considered significant. The critical action of the wake-up test is active ankle dorsiflexion. For patients who require considerable reduction of kyphosis, knee extension should be checked as well.

Supplemental Traction

We recommend two forms of supplemental traction during reduction of spondyloptosis—alar rods and posterior traction. They extend the time for stress relaxation without extending the length of surgery. They also protect the bone-screw interface from overload during reduction.

Alar rods are placed soon after opening the wound. High anatomic hooks are inserted under the lamina of L1 and into holes burred into the superior aspect of both sacral ala. The ratcheted Universal rods are contoured so that they lie parallel to the spine proximally, then bend laterally out of the way of the L5 root dissection, and turn again to parallel the spine until inserting distally into the alar hooks. The alar rods are sequentially distracted to two-finger tightness. This raises the

L5 pedicles from the pelvis to facilitate L5 root dissection and screw placement. The alar rods are removed when the spondylolisthesis construct is assembled. Temporary alar rods are safer than halo-femoral traction in that they do not lengthen the entire spinal column.

After L4 screws are inserted, we assemble overhead traction for posterior translation. This traction removes much of the pull-out load from the S2 screws during reduction, which greatly decreases the chance of bone-screw interface failure. To assemble the overhead traction, we attach sterile 18-gauge wire from the L4 screws to traction rope. Each rope passes through two pulleys that hang from a bridge constructed of traction frame bars that passes transversely over the operating table. Ten to 30 lbs of weight are added to the end of each rope, depending on the relative amount of posterior translation needed at various stages to gradually steer the L5 vertebra around the sacral dome.

Optional Sacral Dome Resection

If the preoperative planning radiographs suggest that more distraction is required for reduction than is likely to be tolerated by the lumbar roots for a particular case, posterior osteotomy of the sacral dome is performed. First, the L5 and S1 roots, together with the dural sac, must be fully mobilized. A 2-mm bit is then drilled into the sacral dome and adjusted until it corresponds with the position and inclination planned for the osteotomy on the preoperative radiograph. Usually, as much as 1 cm can be safely resected. The posterior annulus is then sharply divided from its L5 origin. The resected sacral dome is removed together with the lumbosacral disc. If an unduly prominent ridge projects posteriorly from the inferior edge of L5, it can be resected at the same time.

Staged Reduction

The alar rods and overhead traction usually accomplish the first one third of reduction before assembly of the spondylolisthesis construct. Alar rods are then removed, but the L4 overhead traction is attached to the proximal end of the Universal rods. Reduction is completed in small increments using the spondylolisthesis construct as described under "Reduction of Spondylolisthesis."

Staging the reduction makes it possible to correct most cases of spondyloptosis without resorting to the more extensive AP resection procedures. Reduction is continued until significant amplitude drop on SEP or reduced function on the wake-up test is seen. In the correction of spondyloptosis, this drop typically occurs with about a grade 2 slip and 30° of slip angle remaining. The instrumentation is then locked in place and the wound is closed. Patients are log rolled and kept at bed rest for 1 to 2 weeks until they return to the operating room to complete the reduction (Fig. 24-11). If reduction cannot be completed at the second stage, the rods are contoured into slight kyphosis. If fatigue failure of the bone about an S2 screw is seen, the screw is replaced by directing it more cephalad and lateral into the anterolateral corner of the ala and, perhaps, by supplementing fixation with methacrylate placed in the doughy state. During gradual reduction, iliac grafting is performed between L4 and the sacrum.

After surgery, most spondyloptosis patients follow the same regimen as described earlier for spondylolisthesis. However, if there is significant osteoporosis, question about the quality of fixation, or restoration of less than anatomic spine alignment, patients may remain recumbent in their brace for 4 to 6 weeks. If anatomic alignment is not achieved for any reason, then secondary anterior grafting should be performed and the patient left recumbent for the traditional 3 to 4 months.[7]

Current Expectations for Spondyloptosis Reduction

I have been using these techniques for the treatment of low- to intermediate-grade spondyloptosis for the past 2 years. The techniques have permitted more correction of deformity with less surgery and fewer complications than previously obtained. From our experience to date, gradual posterior reduction supplemented by the techniques outlined above can successfully address all but the most severe grades of spondyloptosis. With careful preoperative planning and adherence to the details of gradual posterior reduction, one can expect reduction to nearly anatomic spinal alignment, a 10 to 30% slip and 5 to 20° residual kyphosis. Complications vary according to the initial severity and duration of deformity, amount of prior surgery, and age of the patient. Average expectations are for 15% transient deficit and, perhaps, a 10% incidence of lasting radiculopathy, typically unilateral weakness of ankle dorsiflexion. We have not seen any case of cauda equina syndrome or weakness in plantar flexion. Failure of fixation at S2 with loosening and partial pull-out after final reduction can be predicted in approximately 8% of cases. With restoration of anatomic alignment and axial loading, we expect union rates slightly below the 88% documented for cases of spondylolisthesis treated by the Spinal Fixation Study Group with these methods. Despite our favorable early experience, gradual instrumented reduction for spondyloptosis remains investigational and long-term follow-up is not yet available.

FUTURE ROLE OF SPONDYLOLISTHESIS REDUCTION

The concept of reducing spondylolisthesis has been controversial. Prior methods rarely achieved full correction of the deformity and were associated with con-

FIG. 24–11. Two-stage instrumented reduction with spine shortening for severe spondyloptosis. **A.** Standing lateral radiograph of 28-year-old female demonstrates severe spondyloptosis with both L4 and L5 completely below the dome of the sacrum. **B.** Lateral radiograph at conclusion of first stage. The anterior spinal column has been shortened by resecting the sacral dome and anterior beak of L5 from the posterior approach. The severe deformity has been partially reduced with the very gradual but progressive application of distraction, posterior translation, and sacral flexion until SEP and wake-up test monitoring suggested borderline changes in root function. **C.** Standing final lateral radiograph. One to two weeks after the initial osteotomy and reduction, gradual reduction is completed and all distractive forces released to permit axial loading through the anterior column. **D.** Preoperative clinical photo with anterior rib cage protrusion, loss of trunk height and waistline, flank creases, thoracic hyperlordosis, fixed hip, and knee flexion contractures. **E.** Photograph 2 months after surgery with correction of both sagittal alignment and trunk height. Clinical changes include loss of flank creases, restoration of waistline, and reduction in acute thoracolumbar lordosis with near-complete correction of hip and knee flexion contractures.

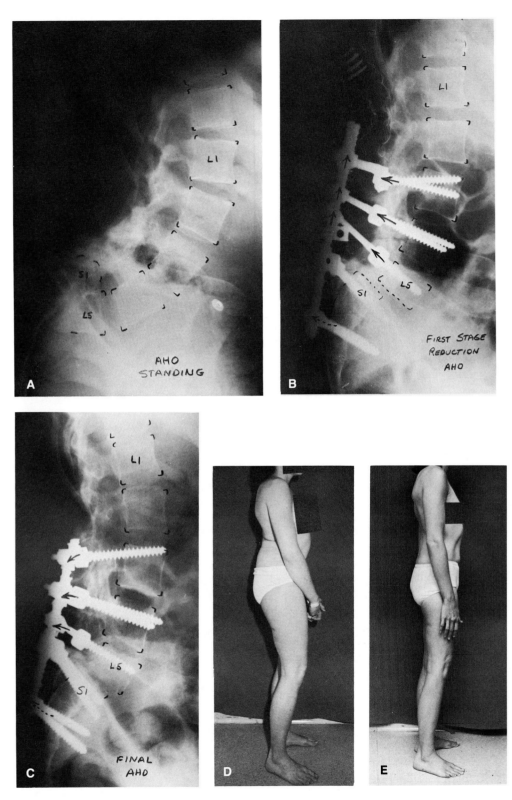

FIG. 24–11.

siderably more complications than in situ fusion. However, with recent surgical advances, patients can now obtain the many advantages of reduction without excessive risk and, in some cases, with fewer complications than attempted fusion without reduction.

The longstanding acceptance of residual deformity has eventually yielded to a new standard of anatomic reduction many times before in orthopedics, but the process is lengthy. If significant clinical improvement is possible in the face of residual deformity, it would be unwise to consciously accept a far greater risk of complications just to add physiologic and psychological advantages well beyond present expectations. However, when methods are developed that make it possible to realize these new expectations without a significant increase in complication or morbidity, it becomes time to reevaluate our standards for "clinical success."

Not so long ago, most displaced femoral shaft fractures were treated with prolonged skeletal traction followed by a spica cast or cast brace. Moderate shortening and angulation were considered acceptable if painless union was achieved. Initial attempts at open reduction with plate or nail fixation were seen by many as overly complex and prone to complication. Eventually, closed nailing techniques and image intensification were perfected, and full restoration of length and alignment with early mobilization were possible without increased complications. Yet, more than 2 decades lapsed between the early reports of excellent success with this method and its acceptance as the standard of care for femoral fractures.

The idea of correcting deformity and restoring normal body mechanics has great appeal for any reconstructive surgeon. Reports that document the effectiveness and relative safety of new methods for reduction-fixation of spondylolisthesis are beginning to appear, and the benefits of spondyloptosis reduction are seen to outweigh the liabilities. Yet it is with good reason that incorporation of these new procedures occurs gradually. All spondylolisthesis reduction or even fixation procedures are technically difficult operations. Full correction of major spondylolisthesis deformity is a truly demanding operation for even the most experienced spinal surgeon. It requires hands-on training, case feedback, and a long learning curve to master the planning and reduction techniques necessary for excellent results. As these techniques are gradually mastered, however, reduction of spondylolisthesis will set a new standard for surgeons and improve the quality of life for patients with symptomatic spondylolisthesis.

References

1. Balderston RA, Bradford DS: Technique for achievement and maintenance of reduction for severe spondylolisthesis using spinous process traction wiring and external fixation of the pelvis. Spine 10:376, 1985
2. Bosworth DM, Fielding JW, Demarest L, Bonaquist M: Spondylolisthesis: A critical review of a consecutive series of cases treated by arthrodesis. J Bone Joint Surg 37A:767, 1955
3. Boxall D, Bradford DS, Winter RB, Moe JH: Management of severe spondylolisthesis in children and adolescents. J Bone Joint Surg 61A:479, 1979
4. Bradford DS: Treatment of severe spondylolisthesis: A combined approach for reduction and stabilization. Spine 4:423, 1979
5. Bradford DS: Closed reduction of spondylolisthesis: An experience in 22 patients. Spine 13:580, 1988
6. Bradford DS, Boachie-Adjei O: Reduction of spondylolisthesis. In Evarts CM (ed): Surgery of the Musculoskeletal System, 2nd ed, pp 2129–2142. New York, Churchill Livingstone, 1990
7. Bradford DS, Gotfried Y: Staged salvage reconstruction of grade IV and V spondylolisthesis. J Bone Joint Surg 69A:191, 1987
8. Brown CW, Heinig CF, Odom JA, et al: A new method of reduction and fusion of symptomatic spondylolisthesis: The "crowbar" procedure. Orthop Trans 8:403, 1984
9. Cleveland M, Bosworth DM, Thompson FR: Pseudarthrosis in the lumbosacral spine. J Bone Joint Surg 30A:302, 1948
10. Dandy DJ, Shannon MJ: Lumbo-sacral subluxation. J Bone Joint Surg 53B:578, 1971
11. Davis IS, Bailey RW: Spondylolisthesis: Long-term follow-up study of treatment with total laminectomy. Clin Orthop 88:46, 1972
12. Denecke H: Reposition der luxierten wirbelsaule bei spondylolisthese. Verh Deutsch Orthop Ges 44:404, 1956
13. DeWald RL, Faut MM, Taddonio RF, Neuwirth MG: Severe lumbosacral spondylolisthesis in adolescents and children. J Bone Joint Surg 63A:619, 1981
14. Dick W: The "Fixateur Interne" as a versatile implant for spine surgery. Spine 12:882, 1987
15. Dick WT, Schnebel B: Severe spondylolisthesis: Reduction and internal fixation. Clin Orthop 232:70, 1988
16. Dimar JR, Hoffman G: Grade 4 spondylolisthesis: Two-stage therapeutic approach of anterior vertebrectomy and anterior-posterior fusion. Orthop Rev 15:49, 1986
17. Edwards CC: Reduction of spondylolisthesis: Biomechanics and fixation. Orthop Trans 10:543, 1986
18. Edwards CC: Prospective evaluation of a new method for complete reduction of L5–S1 spondylolisthesis using corrective forces alone. Orthop Trans 14:549, 1990
19. Edwards CC, Weigel MC: Treatment of 56 lumbosacral nonunions with compression instrumentation. Orthop Trans 14: 1990 (in press)

20. Edwards CC, White JB, Levine AM: One-stage reduction of spondyloptosis using corrective forces alone: A new surgical option. Orthop Trans 12:136, 1988
21. Fisk JR, Moe JH, Winter RB: Scoliosis, spondylolysis, and spondylolisthesis: Their relationship as reviewed in 539 patients. Spine 3:14, 1978
22. Flatley TJ, Derderian H: Closed loop instrumentation of the lumbar spine. Clin Orthop 196:273, 1985
23. Gaines RW, Nichols WK: Treatment of spondyloptosis by two stage L5 vertebrectomy and reduction of L4 onto S1. Spine 10:680, 1985
24. Gill GC, Manning JG, White HL: Surgical treatment of spondylolisthesis without spine fusion. J Bone Joint Surg 37A:493, 1955
25. Harrington PR, Tullos HS: Reduction of severe spondylolisthesis in children. South Med J 62:1, 1969
26. Harrington PR, Tullos HS: Spondylolisthesis in children. Clin Orthop 79:75, 1971
27. Harris RI: Spondylolisthesis. Ann R Coll Surg Engl 8:259, 1951
28. Harris IE, Weinstein SL: Long-term follow-up of patients with grade III and IV spondylolisthesis. J Bone Joint Surg 69A:960, 1987
29. Henderson ED: Results of the surgical treatment of spondylolisthesis. J Bone Joint Surg 48A:619, 1966
30. Hensinger RN, Lang JR, MacEwen GD: Surgical management of spondylolisthesis in children and adolescents. Spine 1:207, 1976
31. Hodgson AR, Wong SK: A description of a technic and evaluation of results in anterior spinal fusion for deranged intervertebral disk and spondylolisthesis. Clin Orthop 56:133, 1968
32. Huizenga BA: Reduction of spondyloptosis with 2-stage vertebrectomy. Orthop Trans 7:21, 1983
33. Jenkins JA: Spondylolisthesis. Br J Surg 24:80, 1936
34. Johnson JR, Kirwan EO: The long-term results of fusion in situ for severe spondylolisthesis. J Bone Joint Surg 65B:43, 1983
35. Kaneda K, Satoh S, Nohara Y, Oguma T: Distraction rod instrumentation with posterolateral fusion in isthmic spondylolisthesis. Spine 10:383, 1985
36. Lance EM: Treatment of severe spondylolisthesis with neural involvement. J Bone Joint Surg 48A:883, 1966
37. Laurent LE, Osterman K: Operative treatment of spondylolisthesis in young patients. Clin Orthop 117:85, 1976
38. Louis R: Fusion of the lumbar and sacral spine by internal fixation with screw plates. Clin Orthop 203:18, 1986
39. McPhee IB, O'Brien JP: Reduction of severe spondylolisthesis. Spine 4:430, 1979
40. Matthiass HH, Heine J: The surgical reduction of spondylolisthesis. Clin Orthop 203:34, 1986
41. Maurice HD, Morley TR: Cauda equina lesions following fusion in situ and decompressive laminectomy for severe spondylolisthesis. Spine 14:214, 1989
42. Mazel C, Roy-Camille R, Saillant G, Bouchet T: Spondylolisthesis: Treatment and results. Orthop Trans 11:500, 1987
43. Monticelli G, Ascani E: Spondylolysis and spondylolisthesis. Acta Orthop Scand 46:498, 1975

44. Newman PH: A clinical syndrome associated with severe lumbo-sacral subluxation. J Bone Joint Surg 47B:472, 1965
45. Newman PH: Stenosis of the lumbar spine in spondylolisthesis. Clin Orthop 115:116, 1976
46. O'Brien JP, Mehdian H, Jaffray D: Reduction of severe lumbosacral spondylolisthesis. Orthop Trans 12:620, 1988
47. Ohki I, Inoue S, Murta T, et al: Reduction and fusion of severe spondylolisthesis using halo-pelvic traction with wire reduction device. Int Orthop 4:107, 1980
48. Osterman K, Seitsalo S: Fusion in situ in severe spondylolisthesis. Orthop Trans 12:605, 1988
49. Phalen GS, Dickson JA: Spondylolisthesis and tight hamstrings. J Bone Joint Surg 43A:505, 1961
50. Reynolds JB, Wiltse LL: The treatment of severe spondylolisthesis in the young. Orthop Trans 13:27, 1989
51. Riley P, Gillespie MB: Severe spondylolisthesis: Results of posterolateral fusion. Orthop Trans 9:119, 1985
52. Rombold C: Treatment of spondylolisthesis by posterolateral fusion, resection of the pars interarticularis, and prompt mobilization of the patient. J Bone Joint Surg 48A:1282, 1966
53. Rosenberg NJ: Degenerative spondylolisthesis: Surgical treatment. Clin Orthop 117:112, 1976
54. Roy-Camille R, Saillant G, Mazel C: Internal fixation of the lumbar spine with pedicle screw plating. Clin Orthop 203:7, 1986
55. Savini R: Surgical treatment of severe spondylolisthesis. Orthop Trans 10:11, 1986
56. Scaglietti O, Frontino G, Bartolozzi P: Technique of anatomical reduction of lumbar spondylolisthesis and its surgical stabilization. Clin Orthop 117:164, 1976
57. Scherb R: Zur indikation und technik der Albee-de Quervainschen operation. Schweiz Med Wochenschr 2:763, 1921
58. Schoenecker PL, Cole HO, Herring JA, et al: Cauda equina syndrome after in situ arthrodesis for severe spondylolisthesis at the lumbosacral junction. J Bone Joint Surg 72A:369, 1990
59. Schollner D: Ein neues verfahren zur reposition und fixation bei spondylolisthesis. Orthop Praxis 4:270, 1975
60. Sijbrandij S: A new technique for reduction and stabilization of severe spondylolisthesis. J Bone Joint Surg 63B:266, 1981
61. Sijbrandij S: A new technique for the reduction and stabilization of severe spondylolisthesis. Int Orthop 9:247, 1985
62. Snijder JGN, Seroo JM, Snijder CJ, Schijvens AWM: Therapy of spondylolisthesis by repositioning and fixation of the olisthetic vertebra. Clin Orthop 117:149, 1976
63. Stanton RP, Meehan P, Lovell WW: Surgical fusion in childhood spondylolisthesis. J Pediatr Orthop 5:411, 1985
64. Stauffer RN, Coventry MB: Posterolateral lumbar spine fusion. J Bone Joint Surg 54A:1195, 1972
65. Steffee AD, Sitkowski DJ: Reduction and stabilization of grade IV spondylolisthesis. Clin Orthop 227:82, 1988
66. Taillard W: Le spondylolisthesis chez l'enfant et l'adolescent. Acta Orthop Scand 24:115, 1954–1955

67. Takeda M: A newly devised "three-one" method for the surgical treatment of spondylolysis and spondylolisthesis. Clin Orthop 147:228, 1980

68. Ternes JP, Alexander AH, Burkus JK: Treatment of spondylolisthesis with posterolateral fusion. Orthop Trans 13:166, 1989

69. Tojner H: Olisthetic scoliosis. Acta Orthop Scand 33:291, 1963

70. Transfeldt EE, Dendrinos GK, Bradford DS: Paresis of proximal lumbar roots after reduction of L5–S1 spondylolisthesis. Spine 14:884, 1989

71. Turner RH, Bianco AJ: Spondylolysis and spondylolisthesis in children and teenagers. J Bone Joint Surg 53A:1298, 1971

72. Vercanteren M, et al: Reduction of spondylolisthesis with severe slipping. Acta Orthop Belg 47:502, 1981

73. Vidal J, Fassio B, Buscayret C, Allieu Y: Surgical reduction of spondylolisthesis using a posterior approach. Clin Orthop 154:156, 1981

74. Waters PM, Emans JB, Hall JE: Technique for maintenance of reduction of severe spondylolisthesis using L4–S4 posterior segmental hyperextension fixation. Orthop Trans 11:499, 1987

75. West JL, Bradford DS: Grade IV spondylolisthesis. Orthop Consult 9:1, 1988

76. Zielke K, Strempel AV: Posterior lateral distraction spondylodesis using the twofold sacral bar. Clin Orthop 203:151, 1986

Index

NOTE: A *t* following a page number indicates tabular material, an *f* following a page number indicates an illustration, and a *c* following a page number indicates a case study. Drugs are listed under their generic names. When a trade name is listed, the reader is referred to the generic name.

A

ABCs. *See* Aneurysmal bone cysts
Abdomen, patient positioning to avoid pressure on, 24
Abdominal assessment, nursing, 10–11
Abdominal signs, in metastatic disease, 1198
ABGs (arterial blood gases)
    and evaluation of pulmonary risk, 20*t*
    preoperative assessment of
        in Duchenne's muscular dystrophy, 318
        in neuromuscular scoliosis, 286–287
Achondroplasia, spinal problems in, 467*t*
    craniovertebral junction disorders, 1126
    spinal stenosis, 474–476
    thoracolumbar kyphosis, 469
Acid phosphatase, serum, in metastatic disease, 1202
Actinomyces, infection after discography caused by, 704
Activities of daily living, postoperative difficulty in performing, nursing care plan for, 6*t*
Activity modification, in cervical spondylosis, 787
Adenocarcinoma of lung, as primary in metastatic disease, 1229
ADI. *See* Atlanto-dental interval
Adjacent segment disease, in failed back syndrome, 727
Adult scoliosis, 249–277. *See also* Scoliosis
    cosmesis in, 265
    Cotrel-Dubousset instrumentation in, 261–265

current problems in, 249–252
definition of, 249
degenerative, 273–276
and extension of fusions in lumbar spine, 270–272
nonsurgical care in, 254
pain assessment in, 252–253, 256–257
patient evaluation in, 252–253
in patients over age of fifty, 267–269
postoperative care and, 256
restoration of iatrogenic lumbar lordosis and, 272–273, 274*f*
roentgenologic findings in, 253–254
sacral fusions and, 269–270
severe rib deformities in, treatment of, 265–273
structural disabilities in, 266–267
surgical indications in, 254–256
surgical techniques in, 257–265
Zielke instrumentation in, 257–261
Aerobics, low-impact, in adult scoliosis, 254
AIBF (anterior interbody fusion). *See* Anterior fusion, interbody
Alar ligaments, 1109
Alar staples, for pelvic fixation, 354
Alkaline phosphatase, in metastatic disease, 1202
ALL. *See* Anterior longitudinal ligament
Allograft
    freeze-dried, sources of, 762*t*
    fresh frozen, sources of, 762*t*
    irradiation, sources of, 762*t*
Alpha-fetoprotein determinations, in myelomeningocele, 418

Ambulation, cast or brace breakdown causing difficulty with, 7*t*
Amplifiers, differential, for recording system in evoked potential monitoring, 35
Analgesia
    in adult scoliosis, 254
    in cervical disc herniation, 753
    in cervical spondylosis, 787
    epidural corticosteroid, in sciatica due to disc herniation, 677
    in postoperative pain management, 26–27
        epidural opioid, 27
        intrapleural, 27
        patient-controlled, 27
Anemia, in metastatic disease, 1202
Anesthesia, 19–29
    cardiac evaluation and, 19–20
    double-lumen tubes for, 23
    epidural
        in sciatica due to disc herniation, 677
        steroid injection and, 27–28
    evaluation and risk assessment for, 19–20
    fiberoptic intubation for, 22–23
    hypotensive, 25–26
        in posterior spinal fusion, 98
        in spinal stenosis surgery, 644
        in Zielke instrumentation in adults, 259–260
    intubation for, 22–23
    local, in cervical spondylosis, 787
    for microlumbar discectomy, 680
    monitoring of, 21–22

1

for congenital kyphosis in myelomeningocele, 337
for scoliosis in myelomeningocele,
334–335
for radiation-induced scoliosis and kyphoscoliosis, 488
for Scheuermann's kyphosis, 508–509
for scoliosis
in dwarfs, 469–471
skeletal maturity and, 98
for senile kyphosis, 518
for spinal muscular atrophy, 310–311
for spinal stenosis, 640
wheelchair seating, in neuromuscular
scoliosis, 284, 285f
Os odontoideum, 1035–1036, 1125–1126
Osteitis, radiation, 1208
Osteoblastoma, 1144t, 1145, 1170–1171c,
1173c
scoliosis and, 142, 145–146c
Osteochondroma, 1144t, 1145, 1157–1159c
Osteochondrosis, intervertebral. *See also*
Disc degeneration
in metastatic disease, 1191
Osteoclast activating factor, and predisposition to metastatic seeding, 1190
Osteogenesis imperfecta, spinal deformities in, 491–498
incidence of, 491–493
natural history of, 493
surgery for, 494–495f, 496–498
assessment before, 496
complications of, 498
indications for, 496
postoperative care and, 498
technique for, 496–498
treatment of, 493–496
Osteoid osteoma, 1144t, 1145, 1169c
scoliosis and, 142
Osteoporosis
in ankylosing spondylitis, 528
kyphosis and, 518, 519–520
and progression of deformity in postmenopausal women, 254
and Zielke instrumentation in adults,
257
Osteosarcoma, 1148t, 1149, 1166–1167c
Osteosynthesis, compression, of traumatic
spondylosis of C2, according to
Judet, 1084–1088
Osteotomy
in ankylosing spondylitis
cervical
for fixed flexion deformity, 535–539
for long/curved deformities, 547
dorsal wedge, for long/curved deformities, 547
for fixed flexion deformity, 530–535
complications of, 539–540

indications for, 530
preoperative assessment for, 530–
531
for long/curved deformities
additional operations and, 550
complications of, 550–551
early results of, 551
indications for, 548
late results of, 551–553
postoperative care and, 550
segment selection for, 548–550
technique for, 548–550
lumbar, for fixed flexion deformity,
531–534
monosegmental, for long/curved deformities, 547
polysegmental, 547–548, 548–550
complications of, 550–551
early results of, 551
late results of, 551–553
thoracic, for fixed flexion deformity,
534–535
vertebral, through enlarged posterior
approach, 1245–1249, 1250f
Z-shaped, 806
Otitis media, serous, after transoral or
transmandibular procedures, 74

P
Paget's osteosarcoma, 1166–1167c
Pain
in adult scoliosis, 250–252
evaluation of, 252–253, 256–257
as surgical indication, 254–256
in ankylosing spondylitis, 527
from cauda equina injury, 864t
centralization of within spinal cord, in
failed back syndrome, 729–730
in cervical spondylosis, 776–777
after chemonucleolysis, 709
from conus medullaris injury, 864t
deafferentation, in failed back syndrome,
730
in herniated cervical disc, 751
in idiopathic scoliosis, associated conditions and, 142
in lumbar disc disease, 675–677
in metastatic spinal disease, 1197–1198
radiation affecting, 1206
persistence of after surgery. *See* Failed
back syndrome
postoperative
management of, 26–27
nursing care and, 5t, 11
after spinal fusion, 100
in spinal stenosis, 638–639
in spondylolisthesis, 568, 569
degenerative, 657–658
in tethered spinal cord, 422

from thoracolumbar cord injury, 864t
Palatal flaps, 71
Pancoast tumor, differentiation of from cervical disc herniation, 751–752
Pancytopenia, in advanced metastatic spinal disease, 1202
Pantaloon cast, postoperative, in congenital
kyphosis in myelomeningocele,
337
Paracondylar area, 1108
Paralysis, iatrogenic, after scoliosis surgery,
157
Paralytic kyphosis, and myelomeningocele,
335–337, 338–339f
Paralytic spinal deformity (paralytic
scoliosis), 279–322. *See also specific disorder* and Pelvic obliquity
in adults, 266–267
arthrogryposis and, 311–314
cerebral palsy and, 296–301
Charcot-Marie-Tooth disease and, 304
Cotrel-Dubousset instrumentation for,
347–364
complications of, 364
etiologic considerations and, 347
local strategy for, 348
overall strategies for, 347–348
postoperative care and results of,
363–364
Duchenne's muscular dystrophy and,
315–318
Friedreich's ataxia and, 301–304
in myelomeningocele, 327
neuromuscular, 280–295
Cotrel-Dubousset instrumentation for,
347–364
spinal cord injury and, 306–307
spinal muscle atrophy and, 307–311,
312f
syringomyelia and, 304–306
and uncontrolled deformities in child,
295–296
VDS for, 168, 169f
Paramedian retroperitoneal approach, to
anterior lumbar spine, 85–93
Paraparesis, primary tumors of spine presenting with, 1146t
Paraplegia, secondary to neurofibromatosis, 447
Paravertebral ossification, in ankylosing
spondylitis, 529
Paresthesias, in metastatic spinal disease,
1197
Pars interarticularis, 1109
in congenital spondylolisthesis, 557,
559
Pathologic burst fractures, thoracic and
lumbar, 924–926, 927f
Pathologic spondylolisthesis (type V), 567

Spondyloepiphyseal dysplasia (*continued*)
  odontoid hypoplasia in, 468
  spinal problems in, 467t
Spondylolisthesis
  anterior fusion in treatment of, 590
  anterior-posterior resection reduction
      for, 613, 622–623
  anterior stabilization in treatment of,
      588
  circumferential stabilization in treatment
      of, 588
  classification of, 558t, 565–567, 570–
      571, 585–587
  congenital, 557–563
    age of onset for, 558f
    classification of, 558t
    incidence of, 557–558
    neurologic deficits in, 559
    pathology of, 560
    radiographic features of, 559–560
    surgical treatment of, 560–562
    symptoms of, 558–559
  Cotrel-Dubousset instrumentation for,
      363
  decompression procedures in treatment
      of, 587
  degenerative (type III), 566–567, 587,
      657–674
    age of onset for, 558f
    anterior interbody fusion for,
        667–668
    clinical presentation of, 657–658
    decompression for, 661
    differential diagnosis of, 658
    fusion for, 661–668
    internal fixation for, 668–671
    intertransverse process fusions for,
        665–667
    nonoperative treatment of, 659
    pathogenesis of, 658–659
    pedicle screw fixation for, 668–671
    posterior lumbar interbody fusions for,
        666–667f, 667
    surgery for, 660–661, 662–663f
      and anterior retroperitoneal ap-
          proach to lumbar spine, 671,
          672–673f
      authors' recommendations for, 661
      complications of, 671–673
      indications for, 659
      postoperative care and, 673
      preoperative evaluation and, 659–
          660
      techniques for, 661–671
    in dwarfs, 467t, 476
    dysplastic (type I), 566. *See also* Spon-
        dylolisthesis, congenital
    gradual instrumented reduction for,
        615–618, 621, 623–626
      anatomic alignment and, 618

grafting and bracing for, 626
  instrumentation techniques in, 623
  preoperative planning for, 623–624
  reduction techniques in, 623–626
  and spondylolisthesis construct assem-
      bly and reduction, 625–626
  stress relaxation and, 617
  surgical dissection and screw place-
      ment for, 624–625
  three corrective forces and, 615–617
  two-point sacral fixation and, 617
Harms technique for surgical treatment
    of, 585–592
high-grade. *See* Spondyloptosis
in situ fusion in treatment of, shortcom-
    ings of, 607–608
isthmic (type II), 565–583, 585–587
  in adults, 585–587
    clinical signs and symptoms of,
        569–570
    operative techniques for, 581
  in children and adolescents, 587
    clinical signs and symptoms of, 568,
        569f
    operative techniques for, 576–580
  classification of, 566
    according to slippage, 570–571
  clinical signs and symptoms of, 568–
      570
  conservative management of, 574–575
  definition of, 566
  operative techniques for, 576–581
  predisposition to, 567
  prevalence of, 567
  radiographic features of, 570–573
  risk factors for progression of, 573–
      574
  surgical management of, 576
  treatment of, 574–576
in Marfan's syndrome, 459–466
  treatment of, 462–463
motion segment loss complicating fusion
    for, 607
in neurofibromatosis, 457
neurologic deficit complicating fusion for,
    607–608
operative technique for, 589–591
  results of, 590
pathologic (type V), 567
pathomechanics of, 605–607
pedicle fixation for, 614–615
postdecompression, 647–649
posterior distraction instrumentation for,
    611–613
posterior grafting with extension casting
    for, 620
posterior instrumentation in treatment
    of, 589–590
posterior instrumented reduction for,
    620–622

posterior levered reduction for, 615,
    616f, 621
posterior stabilization in treatment of,
    588
pseudoarthrosis complicating fusion for,
    607
reduction of, 605–634
  advantages of, 608–609, 610f
  authors' preferred method for, 623–
      626
  current options for, 620–623
  development of techniques for, 609–
      618
  future role of, 630–632
  indications for, 618–620
  prerequisites for, 618
residual deformity complicating fusion
    for, 608
slip progression complicating fusion for,
    607
spondylolytic, age of onset for, 558f
surgery for, 589–591. *See also specific
    type*
  in congenital disease, 560–562
  Harms technique for, 585–592
  in isthmic disease, 576–581
    in adults, 581
    in children and adolescents, 576–
        580
  results of, 590
traction-cast reduction for, 609–611, 612f
traumatic (type IV), 567
  of C2 (hangman's fracture), 1037–
      1039, 1122
    surgical versus nonsurgical manage-
        ment of, 1040t
  treatment of, 574–576, 587–588. *See
      also* Spondylolisthesis, surgery for
  in Marfan's syndrome, 462–463
vertebrectomy for, 614
Spondylolisthesis construct, assembly of,
    625–626
Spondylolysis
  acquisita, and failed back syndrome, 727
  age of onset for, 558f
  in children and adolescents, clinical
      signs and symptoms of, 568
  in dwarfs, 467t, 476
  radiographic features of, 570–573
  traumatic of C2, compression osteo-
      synthesis for, 1084–1088
  treatment of, 574–576
Spondylometaphyseal dysplasia, spinal
    problems in, 467t
Spondyloptosis. *See also* Spondylolisthesis
  reduction of, 626–630, 631f
    anterior-posterior resection, 622–623
    current expectations for, 630
    and nerve function monitoring, 629
    and sacral dome resection, 629

ISBN 0-397-51236-8

90000